Handbook of Cancer Chemotherapy

Seventh Edition

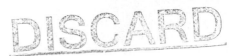

Handbook of Cancer Chemotherapy

Seventh Edition

Editor

Roland T. Skeel, MD
Professor of Medicine
College of Medicine
University of Toledo
and
Division of Hematology and Oncology
University of Toledo Medical Center
Toledo, Ohio

Lippincott Williams & Wilkins
a Wolters Kluwer business
Philadelphia · Baltimore · New York · London
Buenos Aires · Hong Kong · Sydney · Tokyo

Acquisitions Editor: Jonathan W. Pine, Jr.
Managing Editor: Anne E. Jacobs
Project Manager: Alicia Jackson
Senior Manufacturing Manager: Benjamin Rivera
Associate Director of Marketing: Adam Glazer
Design Coordinator: Holly McLaughlin
Cover Designer: Becky Baxendell
Production Service: Laserwords Private Limited, Chennai, India
Printer: RR Donnelley-Crawfordsville

© 2007 by **LIPPINCOTT WILLIAMS & WILKINS, a Wolters Kluwer business**
530 Walnut Street
Philadelphia, PA 19106 USA
LWW.com

First Edition, 1982   Fourth Edition, 1995
Second Edition, 1987   Fifth Edition, 1999
Third Edition, 1991   Sixth Edition, 2003

Library of Congress Cataloging-in-Publication Data
Handbook of cancer chemotherapy / editor, Roland T. Skeel.—7th ed.
    p. ; cm.
    Includes bibliographical references and index.
    ISBN 978-0-7817-6531-2
    1. Cancer—Chemotherapy—Handbooks, manuals, etc. I. Skeel, Roland T.
    [DNLM: 1. Neoplasms—drug therapy—Handbooks. 2. Antineoplastic
Agents—administration & dosage—Handbooks. QZ 39 H2355 2007]
    RC271.C5H36 2007
    616.99′4061—dc22

              2007007798

Contents

IV. Selected Aspects of Supportive Care of Patients with Cancer

Appendices

Contributing Authors

Haitham S. Abu-Lebdeh, MD   *Consultant, Department of Internal Medicine, Mayo Clinic; Assistant Professor, Department of Medicine, Mayo Clinic College of Medicine, Rochester, Minnesota*

Stephen Andrews, MD   *Associate Professor, Department of Gynecologic Oncology, University of Toledo Medical Center; Chief, Division of Gynecologic Oncology, University of Toledo Medical Center, Toledo, Ohio*

Rachid Baz, MD   *Fellow, Department of Special Hematology / Medical Oncology, Cleveland Clinic Foundation, Cleveland, Ohio*

Tracy T. Batchelor, MD   *Associate Professor, Department of Neurology, Harvard Medical School; Executive Director, Stephen E. and Catherine Pappas Center for Neuro-Oncology; Associate Neurologist, Department of Neurology, Massachusetts General Hospital, Boston, Massachusetts*

Robert S. Benjamin, MD   *Department of Sarcoma Medical Oncology, Division of Cancer Medicine, University of Texas, M.D. Anderson Cancer Center, Houston, Texas*

Al B. Benson, III, MD, FACP   *Professor, Department of Medicine, Associate Director for Clinical Investigations, Northwestern University, Feinberg School of Medicine, Robert H. Lurie Comprehensive Cancer Center; Faculty, Department of Medicine, Northwestern Memorial Hospital, Chicago, Illinois*

Joseph S. Chan, MD   *Fellow, Department of Hematology and Medical Oncology, Oregon Health and Science University, Oregon Health Science Cancer Institute, Portland, Oregon,*

Rekha T. Chaudhary, MD   *Assistant Professor, Department of Medicine, Division of Hematology / Oncology, University of Toledo Medical Center, Toledo, Ohio*

Mary E. Cianfrocca, MD   *Assistant Professor, Department of Medicine, Northwestern University, Feinberg School of Medicine, Chicago, Illinois*

Charles S. Cleeland, MD, PhD   *Chairman, Department of Symptom Research, University of Texas, M.D. Anderson Cancer Center, Houston, Texas*

Joan M. Duggan, MD   *Associate Professor, Department of Internal Medicine, Physiology and Molecular Medicine, University of Toledo; Division of Infectious Diseases, University of Toledo Medical Center, Toledo, Ohio*

April F. Eichler, MD *Instructor, Department of Neurology, Harvard Medical School; Assistant in Neurology, Department of Neurology, Stephen E. & Catherine Pappas Center for Neuro-Oncology, Massachusetts General Hospital, Boston, Massachusetts*

Michael J. Fisch, MD, MPH, FACP *Associate Professor, Department of General Oncology; Medical Director, Community Clinical Oncology Program Research Base, University of Texas, M.D. Anderson Cancer Center, Houston, Texas*

Kathleen S. N. Franco-Bronson, MD *Adjunct Professor, Department of Psychiatry, University of Toledo Medical Center, Toledo, Ohio; Associate Dean of Admissions and Student Affairs, Department of Education and Neuroscience, Cleveland Clinic Lerner College of Medicine / Cleveland Clinic Foundation, Cleveland, Ohio*

Olga Frankfurt, MD, MS *Instructor, Department of Medicine, Division of Hematology and Oncology, Northwestern University, Feinberg School of Medicine, Robert H. Lurie Comprehensive Cancer Center; Staff Physician, Department of Medicine, Division of Hematology and Oncology, Northwestern Memorial Hospital, Feinberg School of Medicine, Robert H. Lurie Comprehensive Cancer Center, Chicago, Illinois*

John P. Greer, MD *Professor, Department of Medicine, Vanderbilt University School of Medicine, Nashville, Tennessee*

Mohamad A. Hussein, MD *Professor of Oncology and Medicine, Department of Interdisciplinary Oncology; Leader Multiple Myeloma Clinical Research, Clinical Director, Department of Interdisciplinary Oncology, Division of Malignant Hematology, University of South Florida College of Medicine & The H. Lee Moffitt Cancer and Research Institute, Tampa, Florida*

Chatchada Karanes, MD *Director, Cord Blood Transplant Program, Department of Hematology and Hematopoietic Cell Transplant, City of Hope Cancer Center, Duarte, California*

Samir N. Khleif, MD *Chief, Cancer Vaccine Section, Center for Cancer Research, National Cancer Institute, Bethesda, Maryland*

James M. Leonardo, MD, PhD *Clinical Associate Professor, Department of Medicine, New York, New York; Associate Director, Bassett Regional Cancer Program, May Imogene Bassett Hospital, Cooperstown, New York*

Karen S. Milligan, MD *Senior Hematology / Oncology Fellow, Leo Jenkins Cancer Center, East Carolina University, Brody School of Medicine, Greenville, North Carolina*

Iman Mohamed, MD, FACP, MRCP(UK), MPH   *Associate Professor, Department of Medicine, University of Toledo; Division Chief of Hematology & Oncology, Medical Director of the Breast Center, Department of Medicine, University of Toledo Medical Center, Toledo, Ohio*

David S. Morgan, MD   *Associate Professor, Department of Medicine, Vanderbilt University School of Medicine; Division of Hematology and Oncology, Vanderbilt University Medical Center Nashville, Tennessee*

Craig R. Nichols, MD   *Professor, Department of Medicine, Hematology, and Medical Oncology, Oregon Health and Science University, Oregon Health Science Cancer Institute, Portland, Oregon*

Harlan A. Pinto, MD   *Associate Professor, Department of Medicine, Stanford University School of Medicine; Chief of Medical Oncology Section, Veterans Affairs Palo Alto Health Care System, Palo Alto, California*

Walter D. Y. Quan, Jr., MD   *Director of Cancer Immunotherapy, Leo Jenkins Cancer Center; Associate Professor, Department of Medicine, East Carolina University, Brody School of Medicine; Medical Director, 3 West Oncology, Pitt County Memorial Hospital, Greenville, North Carolina*

NurJehan Quraishy, MD   *Clinical Assistant Professor, Department of Pathology, Health Science Campus, University of Toledo; Medical Director, American Red Cross Blood Services, Toledo, Ohio*

Roberto Rodriguez, MD   *Staff Physician, Division of Hematology and Hematopoietic Cell Transplantation, City of Hope Cancer Center, Duarte, California; Staff Physician, Department of Hematology / Oncology, Southern California Permanente Medical Group, Los Angeles, California*

Scott B. Saxman, MD   *Director, Office of Medical Services, Peace Corps, Washington, DC*

Joan H. Schiller, MD   *Professor, Department of Hematology / Oncology, University of Texas, Southwestern Medical School; Chief, Department of Hematology / Oncology, University of Texas Southwestern Medical Center, Dallas, Texas*

Roland T. Skeel, MD   *Professor, Department of Medicine, College of Medicine, University of Toledo and Division of Hematology and Oncology, University of Toledo Medical Center, Toledo, Ohio*

Mary R. Smith, MD   *Professor, Department of Medicine and Pathology, University of Toledo; Division of Hematology and Oncology, University of Toledo Medical Center Toledo, Ohio*

Richard S. Stein, MD   *Professor, Department of Medicine, Vanderbilt University School of Medicine, Nashville, Tennessee*

Sophie Sun, MD   *Assistant Instructor, Department of Hematology / Oncology, University of Texas Southwestern Medical Center, Dallas, Texas*

Martin S. Tallman, MD   *Professor, Department of Medicine, Division of Hematology and Oncology, Northwestern University, Feinberg School of Medicine; Attending Physician, Department of Medicine, Northwestern Memorial Hospital, Chicago, Illinois*

Janelle M. Tipton, MSN, RN, AOCN   *Oncology Clinical Nurse Specialist and Adjunct Instructor of Nursing University of Toledo, University of Toledo Cancer Center, Toledo, Ohio*

Mikhail Vinogradov, MD   *Fellow, Department of Hematology / Oncology, East Carolina University, Brody School of Medicine, Greenville, North Carolina*

Paul R. Walker, MD, FACP   *Clinical Associate Professor, Department of Internal Medicine, Division of Hematology / Oncology, East Carolina University, Brody School of Medicine; Attending in Medical Oncology, Pitt County Memorial Hospital, Greenville, North Carolina*

Peter White, MD   *Emeritus Professor, Department of Medicine, College of Medicine University of Toledo, Toledo, Ohio*

Kristi S. Williams, MD   *Associate Professor, Department of Psychiatry, University of Toledo, Toledo, Ohio*

Preface

Advances in the treatment of cancer have continued at an intense pace over the 25 years since the *Handbook of Cancer Chemotherapy* was first published in 1982. This is reflected in the expansion of the list of clinically useful antineoplastic drugs from 43 to over 115 and the growth of the *Handbook* from 280 pages to over 750 pages with the current edition. While the number and benefit of cytotoxic agents has continued to grow over this time, the greatest change has been the development and demonstrated efficacy of a new class of systemic treatments called molecular targeted therapy, which has resulted from the wealth of biologic discoveries and insights into the etiology and behavior of cancer that have taken place over the last quarter century. Although the ultimate role that these new agents will play in the control of cancer remains to be seen, they have clearly changed the face of cancer treatment and will undoubtedly become more dominant in cancer treatment over the next decade. For this reason, we have expanded the coverage of these agents in the discussion of the biologic and pharmacologic basis for chemotherapy, in the description of characteristics and use of chemotherapeutic and biologic agents, and in the chapters on the treatment of individual cancers.

As with previous editions of this book, primary indications, usual dosage and schedule, special precautions, and expected toxicities have been added for new drugs and biologic agents that oncologists have begun to use in the past 5 years, and new data have been added to the information for many of the older agents. Each of the chapters dealing with specific cancer sites has been revised to reflect current best medical practice and to point the way toward future advances. The section on supportive care has been updated to highlight those issues and pharmacologic agents that are most essential to the daily care of patients with cancer. Because cancer screening is so important to reducing the number of cancer deaths, current American Cancer Society screening guidelines have been continued in the appendix, along with an updated list of helpful Internet addresses for cancer information.

The *Handbook* continues to be a practical pocket or desk reference, with a wide range of information for oncology specialists, nononcology physicians, house officers, oncology nurses, pharmacists, and medical students. It can even be read and understood by many patients and their families who want to be able to find practical information about their cancer and its treatment. Unlike many other books, the *Handbook* combines in one place the most current rationale and the specific details necessary to safely administer chemotherapy for most adult cancers.

The realization of a more specific, less toxic, and more effective medical treatment for cancer—which has been stimulated by the tremendous recent increase in information on the molecular basis of cancer—is still in its early days, but patients have already reaped the benefits of these developments. Growing from the first agents rituximab, trastuzumab, and imatinib (which 10 years ago were just entering the clinical practice arena), there are now a host of other molecular targeted therapies. Prominent among the new agents now in clinical use are those that target signal transduction pathways crucial for delivering messages from the outside environment into the nucleus to enable it to carry on the crucial processes of survival of the cell, including cell proliferation and differentiation. Other new agents target the cancer cell milieu through inhibition of angiogenesis, selectively impede degradation of proteins involved in cell proliferation and survival, or modulate other intracellular pathways critical to maintenance of the cancer phenotype.

Cure of cancer with less toxic systemic treatment has been a long-term aspiration for many people: those engaged in cancer research, physicians who daily are faced with anxious patients who have cancer, and others in the health professions. It has also been a fervent hope of patients and their families. Although cure is possible for some common tumors, particularly when there is only micrometastasis, and for some more advanced tumors such as lymphomas, for most patients chemotherapy remains palliative, at best. When curing and minimizing the cancer can no longer be achieved, then expert, compassionate supportive care becomes the essential and appropriate focus of the oncology team.

Progress is always slower than patients, physicians, and basic scientists would like. Current research that joins the expertise and discoveries of the basic scientist, systematic investigation through clinical trials by the clinician, and their interaction in "translational" research continues to offer a realistic expectation of accelerated progress in the control of cancer in the decades ahead.

Roland T. Skeel, MD

Basic Principles and Considerations of Rational Chemotherapy

CHAPTER 1

Biologic and Pharmacologic Basis of Cancer Chemotherapy and Biotherapy

Roland T. Skeel and Samir N. Khleif

I. **General mechanisms by which chemotherapeutic agents control cancer.** The purpose of treating cancer with chemotherapeutic agents is to prevent cancer cells from multiplying, invading, metastasizing, and ultimately killing the host (patient). Most traditional chemotherapeutic agents currently in use appear to exert their effect primarily on cell proliferation. Because cell multiplication is a characteristic of many normal cells as well as cancer cells, most cancer chemotherapeutic agents also have toxic effects on normal cells, particularly those with a rapid rate of turnover, such as bone marrow and mucous membrane cells. The goal in selecting an effective drug, therefore, is to find an agent that has a marked growth-inhibitory or controlling effect on the cancer cell and a minimal toxic effect on the host. In the most effective chemotherapeutic regimens, the drugs are capable not only of inhibiting but also of completely eradicating all neoplastic cells while sufficiently preserving normal marrow and other target organs to permit the patient to return to normal, or at least satisfactory, function and quality of life.

Ideally, the cell biologist, pharmacologist, and medicinal chemist would like to look at the cancer cell, discover how it differs from the normal host cell, and then design a chemotherapeutic agent to capitalize on that difference. Until recently less rational means were used for most of the chemotherapeutic agents that are now in use. The effectiveness of agents was discovered by treating either animal or human neoplasms, after which the pharmacologist attempted to discover why the agent worked as well as it did. With few exceptions, the reasons why chemotherapeutic agents are more effective against cancer cells

1

than against normal cells have been poorly understood. With the rapid expansion of information about cell biology and the factors within the neoplastic cell that control cell growth, the strictly empiric method of discovering effective new agents has changed. For example, antibodies against the protein product of the overexpressed *HER2/neu* oncogene have been demonstrated to be effective in controlling metastatic breast cancer and reducing recurrences after primary therapy in patients whose tumors overexpress this gene. Discovery of the constitutively activated Bcr-Abl tyrosine kinase created as a consequence of the chromosomal translocation in chronic myelogenous leukemia (CML) has led to an exciting new era of orally administered small molecular inhibitors of critical molecular changes in cancer cells and their environment. These sentinel events have presaged the development of a host of new therapeutic agents that are directed at known specific targets within and around the cancer cell. These targets have been selected, because they are altered in the cancer cell and are critical for cancer cell growth, invasion, and metastasis. This increased understanding of cancer cell biology has already provided more specific and selective ways of controlling cancer cell growth in several human cancers and will continue to dominate drug development for systemic therapy in the decade to come.

Inhibition of cell multiplication and tumor growth can take place at several levels within the cell and its environment:

- Macromolecular synthesis and function
- Cytoplasmic organization and signal transduction
- Cell membrane and associated cell surface receptor synthesis, expression, and function
- Environment of cancer cell growth

A. Classic chemotherapy agents. Most agents currently in use, with the exception of immunotherapeutic agents and other biologic response modifiers, appear to have their primary effect on either macromolecular synthesis or function. This effect means that they interfere with the synthesis of deoxyribonucleic acid (DNA), ribonucleic acid (RNA), or proteins or with the appropriate functioning of the preformed molecule. When interference in macromolecular synthesis or function in the neoplastic cell population is sufficiently great, a proportion of the cells die. Some cells die because of the direct effect of the chemotherapeutic agent. In other instances, the chemotherapy may trigger differentiation, senescence, or apoptosis, the cell's own mechanism of programmed death.

Cell death may or may not take place at the time of exposure to the drug. Often, a cell must undergo several divisions before the lethal event that took place earlier finally results in the death of the cell. Because only a proportion of the cells die as a result of a given treatment, repeated doses of chemotherapy must be used to continue to reduce the cell number (Fig. 1.1). In an ideal system, each time the dose is repeated, the same proportion of cells—not the same absolute number—is killed. In the example shown in Fig. 1.1, 99.9% (3 logs) of the cancer cells are killed with each treatment, and there is a 10-fold (1-log) growth between treatments, for a net reduction of 2 logs with each treatment. Starting at 10^{10} cells (approximately

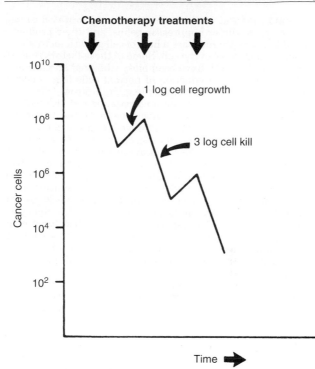

Figure 1.1. **The effect of chemotherapy on cancer cell numbers. In an ideal system, chemotherapy kills a constant proportion of the remaining cancer cells with each dose. Between doses, cell regrowth occurs. When therapy is successful, cell killing is greater than cell growth.**

10 g or 10 cm^3 leukemia cells), it would take five treatments to reach fewer than 10^0, or 1, cell. Such a model makes certain assumptions that rarely are strictly true in clinical practice:

- All cells in a tumor population are equally sensitive to a drug.
- Drug accessibility and cell sensitivity are independent of the location of the cells within the host and of local host factors such as blood supply and surrounding fibrosis.
- Cell sensitivity does not change during the course of therapy.

The lack of curability of most initially sensitive tumors is probably a reflection of the degree to which these assumptions do not hold true.

B. Biologic response modifiers and molecular targeted therapy (MTT). Within individual cells and cell populations are intricate interrelated mechanisms that promote or suppress cell proliferation, facilitate invasion or metastasis when the cell is malignant, lead to cell differentiation, promote (relative) cell immortality, or set the cell on the path to inevitable death (apoptosis). These activities are controlled in large part by normal genes and, in the case of cancer, by mutated cancer promoter genes, tumor suppressor genes, and their products. Included in these products are a host of cell growth factors that control the machinery of the cell. Some of these factors that affect normal cell growth have been biosynthesized and are now used to enhance the production of normal cells (e.g., epoetin and filgrastim) and to treat cancer (e.g., interferon [IFN]).

The recent expansion of our understanding of the biologic control of normal cells and tumor growth at the molecular level has only begun to offer improved therapy for cancer, although it has helped explain differences in response among populations of patients. New discoveries in cancer cell biology have provided insights into apoptosis, cell cycling control, angiogenesis, metastasis, cell signal transduction, cell surface receptors, differentiation, and growth factor modulation. New drugs in clinical trials have been designed to block growth factor receptors, prevent oncogene activity, block the cell cycle, restore apoptosis, inhibit angiogenesis, restore lost function of tumor suppressor genes, and selectively kill tumors containing abnormal genes. Further understanding of each of these holds a great potential for providing powerful and more selective means to control neoplastic cell growth and may lead to effective cancer treatments in the next decade.

II. Tumor cell kinetics and chemotherapy. Cancer cells, unlike other body cells, are characterized by a growth process whereby their sensitivity to normal controlling factors has been partially or completely lost. As a result of this uncontrolled growth, it was once thought that cancer cells grew or multiplied faster than normal cells and that this growth rate was responsible for the sensitivity of cancer cells to chemotherapy. Now it is known that most cancer cells grow less rapidly than the more active normal cells as in the bone marrow. Therefore, although the growth rate of many cancers is faster than that of normal surrounding tissues, growth rate alone cannot explain the greater sensitivity of cancer cells to chemotherapy.

A. Tumor growth. The growth of a tumor depends on several interrelated factors.

1. Cell cycle time, or the average time for a cell that has just completed mitosis to grow, redivide, and again pass through mitosis, determines the maximum growth rate of a tumor but probably does not determine drug sensitivity. The relative proportion of cell cycle time taken up by the DNA synthesis phase may relate to the drug sensitivity of some types (S phase specific) of chemotherapeutic agents.

2. Growth fraction, or the fraction of cells undergoing cell division, contains the portion of cells that are sensitive to drugs whose major effect is exerted on cells that are dividing actively. If the growth fraction approaches 1 and the cell death rate is low, the tumor-doubling time approximates the cell cycle time.

3. Total number of cells in the population (determined at some arbitrary time at which the growth measurement is started) is clinically important because it is an index of how advanced the cancer is; it frequently correlates with normal organ dysfunction. As the total number of cells increases, so does the number of resistant cells, which in turn leads to decreased curability. Large tumors may also have greater compromise of blood supply and oxygenation, which can impair drug delivery to the tumor cells as well as the sensitivity to both chemotherapy and radiotherapy.

4. Intrinsic cell death rate of tumors is difficult to measure in patients but probably makes a major and positive contribution by slowing the growth rate of many solid tumors.

B. Cell cycle. The cell cycle of cancer cells is qualitatively the same as that of normal cells (Fig. 1.2). Each cell begins its growth during a *postmitotic period*, a phase called G_1, during which enzymes necessary for DNA production, other proteins, and RNA are produced. G_1 is followed by a period of DNA *synthesis* (S), in which essentially all DNA synthesis for a given cycle takes place. When DNA synthesis is complete, the cell enters a *premitotic period* (G_2), during which further protein and RNA synthesis occurs. This gap is followed immediately by *mitosis* (M), at the end of which actual physical division takes place, two daughter cells are formed, and each cell again enters G_1. G_1 phase is in equilibrium with a *resting state* called G_0. Cells in G_0 are relatively inactive with respect to macromolecular synthesis and are consequently insensitive to many chemotherapeutic agents, particularly those that affect macromolecular synthesis.

C. Phase and cell cycle specificity Most classic chemotherapeutic agents can be grouped according to whether they depend on cells being in cycle (i.e., not in G_0) and, if they depend on the cell being in cycle, whether their activity is greater when the cell is in a specific phase of the cycle. Most agents cannot be assigned to one category exclusively. Nonetheless, these classifications can be helpful in understanding drug activity.

1. Phase-specific drugs. Agents that are most active against cells in a specific phase of the cell cycle are called *cell cycle phase–specific drugs*. A partial list of these drugs is shown in Table 1.1.

a. Implications of phase-specific drugs. Phase specificity has important implications for cancer chemotherapy.

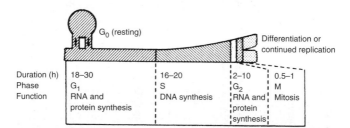

Figure 1.2. Cell cycle time for human tissues has a wide range (16 to 260 hours), with marked differences among normal and tumor tissues. Normal marrow and gastrointestinal lining cells have cell cycle times of 24 to 48 hours. Representative durations and the kinetic or synthetic activity are indicated for each phase. RNA, ribonucleic acid; DNA, deoxyribonucleic acid.

Table 1.1. Cell cycle phase–specific chemotherapeutic agents

Phase of Greatest Activity	Class	Type	Characteristic Agents
Gap 1 (G_1)	Natural product	Enzyme	Asparaginase
	Hormone	Corticosteroid	Prednisone
G_1/S junction	Antimetabolite	Purine analog	Cladribine
DNA synthesis (S)	Antimetabolite	Pyrimidine analog	Cytarabine, fluorouracil, gemcitabine
	Antimetabolite	Folic acid analog	Methotrexate
	Antimetabolite	Purine analog	Thioguanine, fludarabine
	Natural product	Topoisomerase I inhibitor	Topotecan
	Miscellaneous	Substituted urea	Hydroxyurea
Gap 2 (G_2)	Natural product	Antibiotic	Bleomycin
	Natural product	Topoisomerase II inhibitor	Etoposide
	Natural product	Microtubule polymerization and stabilization	Paclitaxel
Mitosis (M)	Natural product	Mitotic inhibitor	Vinblastine, vincristine, vindesine, vinorelbine

DNA, deoxyribonucleic acid.

(1) Limitation to single-exposure cell kill. With a phase-specific agent, there is a limit to the number of cells that can be killed with a single instantaneous (or very short) drug exposure because only those cells in the sensitive phase are killed. A higher dose does not kill more cells.

(2) Increasing cell kill by prolonged exposure. To kill more cells requires either prolonged exposure to, or repeated doses of, the drug to allow more cells to enter the sensitive phase of the cycle. Theoretically, all cells could be killed if the blood level or, more importantly, the intracellular concentration of the drug remained sufficiently high while all cells in the target population passed through one complete cell cycle. This theory assumes that the drug does not prevent the passage of cells from one (insensitive) phase to another (sensitive) phase.

(3) Recruitment. A higher number of cells could be killed by a phase-specific drug if the proportion of cells in the sensitive phase could be increased (recruited).

b. Cytarabine. One of the best examples of a phase-specific agent is cytarabine (ara-C), which is an inhibitor of DNA synthesis and is therefore active only in the S phase (at standard doses). When used in doses of 100 to 200 mg/m^2 daily (i.e., not "high-dose ara-C"), ara-C is rapidly deaminated *in vivo* to an inactive compound, ara-U, and rapid injections result in very short effective levels of ara-C. As a result, single doses of ara-C are nontoxic to the normal hematopoietic system and are generally ineffective for treating leukemia. If the drug is given as a daily rapid injection, some patients with leukemia respond well but not nearly as well as when ara-C is given every 12 hours. The apparent reason for the greater effectiveness of the 12-hour schedule is that the S phase (DNA synthesis) of human acute nonlymphocytic leukemia cells lasts for approximately 18 to 20 hours. If the drug is given every 24 hours, some cells that have not entered the S phase when the drug is first administered will not be sensitive to its effect. Therefore, these cells can pass all the way through the S phase before the next dose is administered and will completely escape any cytotoxic effect. However, when the drug is given every 12 hours, no cell that is "in cycle" will be able to escape exposure to ara-C because none will be able to get through one complete S phase without the drug being present.

If all cells were in active cycle, that is, if none were resting in a prolonged G_1 or G_0 phase, it would be theoretically possible to kill any cells in a population by a continuous or scheduled exposure equivalent to one complete cell cycle. Experiments with patients who have acute leukemia have shown that if tritiated thymidine is used to label cells as they enter DNA synthesis, it may be 7 to 10 days before the maximum number of leukemia cells have passed through the S phase. This means that, barring permutations caused by itself or other drugs, for ara-C to have a maximum effect on the leukemia, the repeated exposure must be continued for a 7- to 10-day period. Clinically, continuous infusion or administration of ara-C every 12 hours for 5 days or longer appears to be most effective for treating patients with newly diagnosed acute nonlymphocytic leukemia. However, even with such prolonged exposure, it appears that a few of the cells do not pass through the S phase.

2. Cell cycle–specific drugs. Agents that are effective while cells are actively in cycle but are not dependent on the cell being in a particular phase are called *cell cycle–specific* (or *phase-nonspecific*) *drugs*. This group includes most of the alkylating agents, the antitumor antibiotics, and some miscellaneous agents, examples of which are shown in Table 1.2. Some agents in this group are not totally phase-nonspecific; they may have greater activity in one phase than in another, but not to the degree of the phase-specific agents. Many agents also appear to have some activity in cells that are not in cycle, although not as much as when the cells are rapidly dividing.

3. Cell cycle–nonspecific drugs. A third group of drugs appears to be effective whether cancer cells are in cycle or are resting. In this respect, these agents are similar to photon irradiation; that is, both types of therapy are effective, irrespective of whether or not the cancer cell is in cycle. Drugs in this category are called *cell cycle–nonspecific drugs* and include mechlorethamine (nitrogen mustard) and the nitrosoureas (see Table 1.2).

D. Changes in tumor cell kinetics and therapy implications. As cancer cells grow from a few cells to a lethal tumor

Table 1.2.   Cell cycle–specific and cell cycle–nonspecific chemotherapeutic agents

Class	Type	Characteristic Agents
Cell cycle–specific		
Alkylating agent	Nitrogen mustard	Chlorambucil, cyclophosphamide, melphalan
	Alkyl sulfonate	Busulfan
	Triazene	Dacarbazine
	Metal salt	Cisplatin, carboplatin
Natural product	Antibiotic	Dactinomycin, daunorubicin, doxorubicin, idarubicin
Cell cycle–nonspecific		
Alkylating agent	Nitrogen mustard	Mechlorethamine
	Nitrosourea	Carmustine, lomustine

burden, certain changes occur in the growth rate of the population and affect the strategies of chemotherapy. These changes have been determined by observing the characteristics of experimental tumors in animals and neoplastic cells growing in tissue culture. Such model systems readily permit accurate cell number determinations to be made and growth rates to be determined. (Because tumor cells cannot be injected or implanted into humans and permitted to grow, studies of growth rates of intact tumors in humans must be limited largely to observing the growth rate of macroscopic tumors.)

   1. Stages of tumor growth. Immediately after inoculation of a tissue culture or an experimental animal with tumor cells, there is a *lag phase*, during which there is little tumor growth; presumably, the cells in this phase are becoming accustomed to the new environment and are preparing to enter into cycle. The lag phase is followed by a period of rapid growth called the *log phase*, during which there are repeated doublings of the cell number. In populations in which the growth fraction approaches 100% and the cell death rate is low, the population doubles within a period approximating the cell cycle time. As the cell number or tumor size becomes macroscopic, the doubling time of the tumor cell population becomes prolonged and levels off (*plateau phase*). Most clinically measurable human cancers are probably in the plateau phase, which may account, in part, for the slow doubling time observed in many human cancers (30 to 300 days). Because the rate of change in the slope of the growth curve during the premeasurable period is unknown for most human cancers, extrapolation from two points when the mass is measurable to estimate the onset of the growth of the malignancy is subject to considerable error. The prolongation in tumor-doubling time in the plateau phase may be due to a smaller growth fraction, a change in the cell cycle time, an increased intrinsic death rate (predominantly apoptosis, which is a programmed and highly orchestrated cell death that occurs both naturally and under the influence of many types of chemotherapy), or a combination of these factors. Factors responsible for these changes include decreased nutrients or growth promotion factors, increased inhibitory metabolites or inhibitory growth factors, and inhibition of growth by other cell–cell interactions. In the intact host, new blood vessel formation is a critical determinant of these factors.

   2. Growth rate and effectiveness of chemotherapy. Chemotherapeutic agents are most effective during the period of logarithmic growth. As might be expected, this result is particularly true for the antimetabolites, which are largely S phase specific. As a result, when human tumors become macroscopic, the effectiveness of many chemotherapeutic agents is reduced because only part of the cell population is dividing actively. Theoretically, if the cell population could be reduced sufficiently by other means such as surgery or radiotherapy, chemotherapy would be more effective because a higher fraction of the remaining cells would be in logarithmic growth. The validity of this theoretical premise is supported by the varying degrees of success of surgery plus chemotherapy or radiotherapy plus chemotherapy in the treatment of breast cancer, colon cancer, Wilms' tumor, ovarian cancer, small cell anaplastic cell carcinoma of the lung, non–small cell carcinoma of the lung, head and neck cancers, and osteosarcomas.

III. Combination chemotherapy. Combinations of drugs are frequently more effective in producing responses and prolonging life than are the same drugs used sequentially. Combinations are likely to be more effective than single agents for several reasons.

  A. Reasons for effectiveness of combinations

    1. Prevention of resistant clones. If 1 in 10^5 cells is resistant to drug A and 1 in 10^5 cells is resistant to drug B, it is likely that treating a macroscopic tumor (which generally would have more than 10^9 cells) with either agent alone would result in several clones of cells that are resistant to that drug. If, after treatment with drug A, a resistant clone has grown to macroscopic size (if the same mutant frequency persists for drug B), resistance to agent B will also emerge. If both drugs are used at the outset of therapy or in close sequence, however, the likelihood of a cell being resistant to both drugs (excluding, for a moment, the situation of pleiotropic drug resistance) is only 1 in 10^{10}. Therefore, the combination confers considerable advantage against the emergence of resistant clones. Compounding the problem of pre-existing resistant clones is the resistance that develops through spontaneous mutation in the absence of drug exposure. The use of multiple drugs with independent mechanisms of action or alternating non–cross-resistant combinations (as well as the use of surgery or radiotherapy to eliminate macroscopic tumor) theoretically minimizes the chances for outgrowth of resistant clones and increases the likelihood of remission or cure.

    2. Cytotoxicity to resting and dividing cells. The combination of a drug that is cell cycle specific (phase nonspecific) or cell cycle nonspecific with a drug that is cell cycle phase specific can kill cells that are dividing slowly as well as those that are dividing actively. The use of cell cycle–nonspecific drugs can also help recruit cells into a more actively dividing state, which results in their being more sensitive to the cell cycle phase–specific agents.

    3. Biochemical enhancement of effect

      a. Combinations of individually effective drugs that affect different biochemical pathways or steps in a single pathway can enhance each other. This may apply to some newer agents whereby blocking more than one molecular target in the interacting signal transduction pathways may magnify the interference of cell proliferation compared with that seen with either agent alone.

      b. Combinations of an active agent with an inactive agent can potentially result in beneficial effects by several mechanisms, but has limited clinical utility.

        (1) An intracellular increase in the drug or its active metabolites, by either increasing influx or decreasing efflux (e.g., calcium channel inhibitors with multiple agents affected by multidrug resistance [MDR] due to P-glycoprotein overexpression)

(2) Reduced metabolic inactivation of the drug (e.g., inhibition of cytidine deaminase inactivation of ara-C with tetrahydrouridine)

(3) Cooperative inhibition of a single enzyme or reaction (e.g., leucovorin enhancement of fluorouracil inhibition of thymidylate synthetase)

(4) Enhancement of drug action by inhibition of competing metabolites (e.g., N-phosphonoacetyl-L-aspartic acid inhibition of *de novo* pyrimidine synthesis with resultant increased incorporation of 5-fluorouridine triphosphate into RNA)

4. Sanctuary access. Combinations can be used to provide access to sanctuary sites for reasons such as drug solubility or affinity of specific tissues for a particular drug type.

5. Rescue. Combinations can be used in which one agent rescues the host from the toxic effects of another drug (e.g., leucovorin administration after high-dose methotrexate).

B. Principles of agent selection. When selecting appropriate agents for use in a combination, the following principles should be observed:

1. Choose individually active drugs. Do not use a combination in which one agent is inactive when used alone unless there is a clear, specific biochemical or pharmacologic reason to do so, for example, high-dose methotrexate followed by leucovorin rescue or leucovorin followed by fluorouracil. *This principle may not be applicable to the combined use of chemotherapeutic agents with biologic response modifiers or molecular targeted agents* because the cooperativity of chemotherapy and these drugs may not depend on the independent cytotoxic effects of these nonclassic agents.

2. When possible, choose drugs in which the dose-limiting toxicities differ qualitatively or in time of occurrence. Often, however, two or more agents that have marrow toxicity must be used, and the selection of a safe dose of each is critical. As a starting point, two cytotoxic drugs in combination can usually be given at two-thirds of the dose used when the drugs are given alone. Whenever a new drug combination is tried, a careful evaluation of both expected and unanticipated toxicities must be carried out. Unexpected results such as the increased cardiotoxicity of the combination of trastuzumab with doxorubicin may occur, and this latter case has precluded the use of these agents together.

3. Select agents for a combination for which there is a biochemical or pharmacologic rationale. Preferably, this rationale has been tested in an animal tumor system and in the appropriate model system, and the combination has been found to be better than either agent alone.

4. Be cautious when attempting to improve on a successful two-drug combination by adding a third, fourth, or fifth drug simultaneously. Although this approach may be beneficial, two undesirable results may be seen:

    a. An intolerable level of toxicity that leads to excessive morbidity and mortality

    b. Unchanged or reduced antitumor effect because of the necessity to reduce the dose of the most effective drugs to a level below which antitumor responses are not seen, despite the theoretical advantages of the combination. Therefore, the addition of each new agent to a combination must be considered carefully, the principles of combination therapy closely followed, and controlled clinical trials carried out to compare the efficacy and toxicity of any new regimen with a more established (standard) treatment program.

  C. Clinical effectiveness of combinations. Combinations of drugs have been clearly demonstrated to be better than single agents for treating many, but not all, human cancers. The survival benefit of combinations of drugs compared with that of the same drugs used sequentially has been marked in diseases such as acute lymphocytic and acute nonlymphocytic leukemia, Hodgkin's lymphoma, non–Hodgkin's lymphomas with more aggressive behavior (intermediate and high grade), breast carcinoma, anaplastic small cell carcinoma of the lung, colorectal carcinomas, ovarian carcinoma, and testicular carcinoma. The benefit is less notable in cancers such as non–small cell carcinoma of the lung, non–Hodgkin's lymphomas with favorable prognoses, head and neck carcinomas, carcinoma of the pancreas, and melanoma, although reports exist for each of these tumors in which combinations are better in one respect or another than single agents.

IV. Resistance to antineoplastic agents. Resistance to antineoplastic chemotherapy is a combined characteristic of a specific drug, a specific tumor, and a specific host, whereby the drug is ineffective in controlling the tumor without excessive toxicity. Resistance of a tumor to a drug is the reciprocal of selectivity of that drug for that tumor. The problem for the medical oncologist or pharmacologist is not simply to find an agent that is cytotoxic but to find one that selectively kills neoplastic cells while preserving the essential host cells and their function. Were it not for the problem of resistance of human cancer to antineoplastic agents or, conversely, the lack of selectivity of those agents, cancer chemotherapy would be similar to antibacterial chemotherapy in which complete eradication of infection is regularly observed. Such a utopian state of cancer chemotherapy has not yet been achieved for most human cancers. The problem of resistance and ways to overcome or even exploit it remain an area of major interest for the oncologist, pharmacologist, and cell biologist. This reductionist description glosses over the fact that each of these factors is a consequence of the complex genetic characteristics and changes of the cancer cell as it evolves.

    Resistance to antineoplastic chemotherapeutic agents may be either natural or acquired. *Natural resistance* refers to the initial unresponsiveness of a tumor to a given drug, and *acquired resistance* refers to the unresponsiveness that emerges after initially successful treatment. There are three basic categories of resistance to chemotherapy: kinetic, biochemical, and pharmacologic.

  A. Cell kinetics and resistance. Resistance based on cell population kinetics relates to cycle and phase specificity, growth fractions and the implications of these factors for responsiveness to specific agents, and schedules of drug administration. A particular problem with many human tumors is that they are in a plateau growth phase with a small growth fraction. This factor renders many of the cells insensitive to the antimetabolites and relatively unresponsive to many of the other chemotherapeutic agents. Strategies to overcome resistance due to cell kinetics include the following:

1. Reducing tumor bulk with surgery or radiotherapy
2. Using combinations to include drugs that affect resting populations (with many G_0 cells)
3. Scheduling of drugs to prevent phase escape or to synchronize cell populations and increase cell kill

B. Biochemical causes of resistance. Resistance can occur for biochemical reasons including the inability of a tumor to convert a drug to its active form, the ability of a tumor to inactivate a drug, or the location of a tumor at a site where substrates are present that bypass an otherwise lethal blockade. How cells become resistant is only partially understood. There can be decreased drug uptake, increased efflux, changes in the levels or structure of the intracellular target, reduced intracellular activation or increased inactivation of the drug, or increased rate of repair of damaged DNA. In one pre–B-cell leukemia cell line, *bcl-2* overexpression or decreased expression of the homolog *bax* renders cells resistant to several chemotherapeutic agents. Because bcl-2 blocks apoptosis, it has been proposed that its overexpression blocks chemotherapy-induced apoptosis. The interrelationship between mutations of *p53, HER2,* and a host of other oncogenes and tumor suppressor genes and resistance to the cytotoxic effects of radiotherapy, chemotherapeutic, hormonal, and biologic agents, when better understood, may further our understanding of resistance and provide new therapeutic strategies.

Multidrug resistance (MDR), also called *pleiotropic drug resistance*, is a phenomenon whereby treatment with one agent confers resistance not only to that drug and others of its class but also to several other unrelated agents. MDR is commonly mediated by an enhanced energy-dependent drug efflux mechanism that results in lower intracellular drug concentrations. With this type of MDR, overexpression of a membrane transport protein called *P-glycoprotein* (P meaning pleiotropic or permeability) is observed commonly. Other MDR proteins are those found in human lung cancer lines and the lung resistance protein. These proteins appear to have differing expression in different sets of neoplasms. Drugs that are effective in reversing resistance to P-glycoprotein do not reverse other MDR proteins. Combination chemotherapy can overcome biochemical resistance by increasing the amount of active drug intracellularly as a result of biochemical interactions or effects on drug transport across the cell membrane. Calcium channel blockers, antiarrhythmics, cyclosporin A analogs (e.g., PSC-833, a nonimmunosuppressive derivative of cyclosporin D), and other agents have been found to modulate the MDR effect *in vitro*, but limited beneficial effects have been observed clinically.

The use of a second agent to rescue normal cells may also permit the use of high doses of the first agent, which can overcome the resistance caused by a low rate of conversion to the active metabolite or a high rate of inactivation. Another way to overcome resistance is to follow marrow-lethal doses of chemotherapy by post-therapy infusion of stem cells obtained from the peripheral blood or bone marrow. This technique is effective for the treatment of lymphomas, chronic granulocytic leukemia, multiple myeloma, and a few other cancers. A more widely applicable technique may be to combine high-dose chemotherapy with blood cell growth factors, for example, granulocyte colony-stimulating factor (G-CSF) and granulocyte–macrophage colony-stimulating factor (GM-CSF) or oprelvekin (interleukin [IL]-11) to stimulate platelets. These and other marrow-protective and marrow-stimulating agents are being used increasingly and may enhance the effectiveness of chemotherapy in the treatment of several types of cancer. High-dose therapy is discussed more extensively in Chapter 5.

C. Pharmacologic causes of resistance. Apparent resistance to cancer chemotherapy can result from poor tumor blood supply, poor or erratic absorption, increased excretion or catabolism, and drug interactions, all leading to inadequate blood levels of the drug. Strictly speaking, this result is not true resistance; but to the degree that the insufficient blood levels are not appreciated by the clinician, resistance appears to be present. The variation from patient to patient at the highest tolerated dose has led to dose modification schemes that permit dose escalation when the toxicities of the chemotherapeutic regimen are minimal or nonexistent as well as dose reduction when toxicities are great. This regulation is particularly important for some chemotherapeutic agents for which the dose–response curve is steep or for patients who have genetically altered drug metabolism, such as can occur with irinotecan. Selection of the appropriate dose on the basis of predicted pharmacologic behavior is essential for some agents, not only to avoid serious toxicity but also to optimize effectiveness. This has been applied successfully to dose selection of carboplatin by predicting the time × concentration product (area under the curve) based on the individual patient's creatinine clearance.

True pharmacologic resistance is caused by the poor transport of agents into certain body tissues and tumor cells. For example, the central nervous system (CNS) is a site that many drugs do not reach well. Several drug characteristics favor transport into the CNS, including high lipid solubility and low molecular weight. For tumors that originate in the CNS or metastasize there, the drugs of choice should be those that achieve effective antitumor concentration in the brain tissue and that are also effective against the tumor cell type being treated.

D. Nonselectivity and resistance. Nonselectivity is not a mechanism for resistance but rather an acknowledgment that for most cancers and most drugs, the reasons for resistance and selectivity are only partially understood. Given a limited understanding of the biochemical differences between normal and malignant cells prior to the last 10 years, it is gratifying that chemotherapy has been as successful as frequently as it has. With the burgeoning of knowledge about the cancer cell, there is reason to hope that in 20 years, we will view current chemotherapeutic regimens as a fledgling—if not crude—beginning and will have found many more tumor molecular target–directed agents that have a high potential for curing the human cancers that now resist effective treatment.

V.   Molecular targeted therapy (MTT)—introduction. MTT is a new approach to cancer treatment, which resulted from the plethora of molecular and biologic discoveries into the etiology of cancer that took place over the last quarter of a century. Many agents are currently being tested in clinical trials, a few have already been approved by the U.S. Food and Drug Administration (FDA) for clinical use, and their wide integration into the mainstream of therapy for cancer is expected to increase at an accelerated pace during the next 10 years.

Agents in this type of therapy are vastly different from the traditional chemotherapeutic agents that constitute most therapy described throughout the chapters of this book, in that they are designed with the intention to specifically target molecules that are uniquely or abnormally expressed within cancer cells, thereby sparing normal cells. This is possible because agents that qualify as molecularly targeted therapeutics take advantage of the special molecular characteristics of cancer cells to exert their mechanism of action. Within the remainder of this section, we will discuss drugs that are already available for clinical use, provide a brief description of the mechanism of action of these agents and the pathways they target, and address promising agents that may be coming soon to the clinic.

A. Characteristics and classification for MTT
   1. An ideal molecule for targeted therapy should have the following characteristics:

- The molecule is uniquely expressed in cancer cells; hence the therapeutic agent will specifically target the cancer and not the normal cells.
- The molecule is important for the maintenance of the malignant phenotype; therefore, once the target has been effectively hit, the cancer cell will not be able to develop resistance against the therapeutic agent by suppressing the function of or expelling the molecule from the cell.

   The degree to which target molecules do not embody these characteristics coupled with nonspecificity of the therapeutic agent determines in part the limitations of current targets and agents.

   2. Classification and type of MTT. The classification of MTT is a moving target. These therapies can be classified on the basis of the type of treatment, whether it is antibody based, small molecules, gene therapy etc., or based on the molecular target strategy of these agents. In this chapter, we will be using a combination of both approaches to classify these therapies.

B. Strategies for MTT development
   1. Function-directed therapy. This is a strategy that is intended to restore the normal function or abrogate the

abnormal function of the defective molecule or a pathway in the tumor cell. This is accomplished by reconstituting the normal molecule, inhibiting the production of a defective molecule, or aborting, altering, or reversing a newly acquired function. Some of the agents that will be discussed here under this category would target specific cellular pathways, for example, signal transduction pathway; angiogenesis, protein degradation, and immune modulators.

2. Phenotype-directed therapy. This is a therapeutic strategy that is intended to target the unique phenotype of the cancer cell where killing is more dependent on nonspecific mechanism rather than targeting a specific pathway as outlined in Section V.B.1. in the preceding text. Such agents include monoclonal antibodies (MoAbs), immunotoxins, immunoconjugates, and vaccine therapy.

In this chapter we will classify the agents based on the pathway that they target, if the molecular outcome of the mechanism of action is known; otherwise, the agent will be classified on the basis of the type of therapy.

VI. MTT—molecular and functional mechanisms

A. Cell signaling–targeted therapy. Targeting signal transduction is an important approach for therapy against cancer because the signal transduction pathways are crucial for delivering messages from the outside environment into the nucleus to enable it to carry on the crucial processes of survival of the cell including cell proliferation and differentiation. Many pathways are involved in signal transduction in the cell. These signals are initiated from the cell surface by the interaction of molecules (ligands) such as hormones, cytokines, and growth factors with cell receptors. These cell receptors, in turn, transfer the signal through a network of molecules to the nucleus that will lead to the transcription of new molecules responsible for engineering the desired outcome.

In cancer cells, these pathways are found to be altered through the mutation of some of their components. This leads to the dysregulation of the function of the pathways leading to uncontrolled proliferation and inhibition of apoptosis. Accordingly, targeting the components of these pathways is a prime goal for the development of MTT. The components of these pathways include the following:

- The ligand
- The receptors for these ligands—most of which are kinase receptors
- The cascade of proteins that form these pathways, which are mainly protein kinases; other proteins are also present

Two of these pathways—the phosphoinositide 3-OH kinase (PI3K) and the RAS-Raf-MAP kinase pathways—are the most critical for the malignant transformation and most therapeutic interventions are being developed to target these pathways as will be discussed in the subsequent text.

Strategies that are followed to target signal transduction pathways include the following:

- Blocking of the ligand–receptor binding: this leads to the inhibition of the initiation of the signal. This can be done by either blocking circulating ligands or blocking ligand binding to the extracellular domain of the receptor. Many antibodies have been developed for this purpose and will be discussed in the subsequent text

- Inhibition of receptor protein kinases. This leads to the prevention of phosphorylation of the intracellular kinase domain of the receptor, hence aborting the cascade of protein reaction in the cell signaling pathways. This can be accomplished by blocking adenosine triphosphate (ATP) binding to the receptor
- Inhibition of intracellular signaling proteins

1. Blocking of the ligand–receptor binding. Blocking receptors and ligand-receptor interaction is currently achieved by utilizing specific MoAbs. MoAbs are biologic agents that are designed with the intention to specifically target membrane proteins that carry an extracellular domain. The MoAbs can exert their antitumor effect through multiple potential mechanisms including blocking the targeted receptor and preventing its function in transmitting proliferative signals to the nucleus, activating antibody-dependent cellular cytotoxicity, or helping in internalizing the receptor and hence delivering toxic agents into the cells. The MoAb technology has been very much improved, in the last decade, by humanizing these biologic agents to form chimeric antibodies or, in some cases, fully humanized antibodies. Substitution with the human Fc portion of the molecule for the murine equivalent leads to significant decrease in the ability to generate human antimouse antibody (HAMA), although human antichimera antibodies (HACAs) may still occur for those MoAbs that are not fully humanized. This has made these biologic agents more usable in the treatment of cancer, particularly when repetitive dosing is needed. Here, this section will discuss MoAbs that are generated for specific signal transduction receptors. In Section VI.E., we will discuss those MoAbs that are generated against membrane nonreceptor antigens.

a. Epidermal growth factor receptor (EGFR) family. The EGFR is a family of proteins that includes at least four receptors: EGFR1, Her-2-*neu* (erbB2), Her3 (erbB3), Her4 (erbB4). These receptors are glycoproteins that consist of three domains: an extracellular ligand-binding domain, a transmembrane domain, and an intracellular domain that contains tyrosine kinase activity. Binding of the ligands to the receptor leads to the activation of the intracellular tyrosine kinase and phosphorylation of the receptor, which, in turn, lead to downstream signal transduction pathway activation. The activation of this pathway leads to biologic effects that promote cell activation and proliferation and enhance survival. Agents have been developed against the first two receptors, EGFR and Her-2-*neu*, to treat cancer through the inhibition of this pathway. Some of these agents are antibodies that bind the external binding domain and inhibit the receptors, and others are small molecules that inhibit the tyrosine kinase activity of the internal domain.

(1) EGFR1-targeted therapy. EGFR1 is the first member of the EGFR family. It is activated by binding to epidermal growth factor (EGF) and to transforming growth factor alpha (TGF-α). EGFR1 is found to be overexpressed in many cancers including 50% to 70% of colon, lung, and breast cancer. Several antibodies are currently being developed to target EGFR; two have already been approved by the FDA for clinical use in patients with cancer:

- **Cetuximab** is a humanized IgG1 chimeric MoAb that binds to the external ligand-binding domain of EGFR1. It binds to the EGFR with a much higher affinity than does either EGF or TGF-α. It has been found that cetuximab can enhance the effect of both chemotherapy and radiation therapy. It has been found that the combination of cetuximab and irinotecan to treat patients with advanced colorectal carcinoma who express EGFR in their tumors and failed irinotecan therapy can improve disease response from 10.8% to 22.9% and the disease-free survival from 1.5 to 4.1 months over the use of cetuximab alone. Accordingly, cetuximab was initially approved by FDA in combination with irinotecan to treat patients with advanced colon cancer who failed irinotecan or as a single agent in patients who cannot tolerate irinotecan. Many clinical trials are currently being conducted to test cetuximab in first-line therapy in combination with other chemotherapeutic regimens including FOL-FOX4 (see Chapter 8). Clinical trials are also being conducted to test the efficacy of cetuximab in other diseases, the most advanced of which is in head and neck cancers for which cetuximab has also received FDA approval. Significant survival advantage has been demonstrated in one phase III trial adding cetuximab to high-dose radiation therapy in patients with locally advanced disease. Median survival was found to be 54 months in the combination arm versus 28 months in the radiation therapy alone arm. Other trials are currently being conducted, evaluating the addition of cetuximab to cisplatin in the metastatic setting.

- **Panitumumab** is the only fully humanized MoAb that has been developed against EGFR. This gives it the advantage of being less likely to stimulate the development of anti-antibodies. Panitumumab was found to bind to EGFR with higher affinity than cetuximab. Serious toxicity has been reported only rarely, and as a consequence it does not require premedication for human use. Phase III trials of panitumumab have shown efficacy when given alone or in combination with chemotherapy in colorectal cancer with significant improvement in disease-free survival (DFS). Other diseases in which there are some promising results with this agent include non−small cell lung and renal cancers.

- **EMD27000** is another antibody that is currently being developed against EGFR. It is a humanized IgG1 MoAb that has been found to have some activities seen in colon cancer in clinical trials.

(2) Her-2-*neu* (HER2, erbB2)-targeted therapy. HER2 is the second member of the EGFR family. It is a 185-kd protein with 632 amino acids. It has the same basic structure as the other family members. However, no conjugate ligand has been identified for HER2. There have been no mutations identified in the *HER2* gene in human cancers; however, it is overexpressed in many epithelial cancers including colon, pancreas, genitourinary, and 30% of breast cancers. HER2 works through the PI3K/Akt and MAPK pathway and its overexpression leads to inhibition of apoptosis and increase in cell proliferation.

- **Trastuzumab** was one of the first MTTs to be introduced in clinical use. It is a humanized (chimeric) MoAb that binds the HER2 receptor. The FDA approved it in 1998 for the use in patients with metastatic breast cancer with tumors that overexpress the HER2 protein. In a large, multicenter phase III study in patients with metastatic breast cancer that overexpressed HER2, it was demonstrated that trastuzumab, when used as first-line therapy in combination with chemotherapy (with either the combination of anthracyclines and cyclophosphamide or paclitaxel as a single agent), can significantly increase both the duration of response and the overall survival. Trastuzumab is used in patients with breast cancer in two settings: as a single agent for second-line therapy or in combination with paclitaxel as first-line therapy. Furthermore, it has been found that trastuzumab is effective in the adjuvant setting for patients whose tumors overexpress HER2 protein. The optimal duration of treatment, however, is still undefined.

  Whereas the mechanism of action of trastuzumab is not entirely clear, it is believed to act through one or more of the following mechanisms: binding to the receptor, thereby inhibiting the tyrosine kinase signaling pathway; activating antibody-dependent cellular cytotoxicity; induction of apoptosis; inducing G1 arrest by modulating the cyclin-dependent kinases; inhibition of angiogenesis; and enhancing chemotherapy-induced antibody dependent cell-mediated cytotoxicity (ADCC).

b. Vascular endothelial growth factor (VEGF). The VEGF family of proteins is one of the specific positive regulators of angiogenesis. It is composed of at least six different growth factors. Of these, the VEGF-A is the one member that exerts the most influence on the angiogenesis process. The VEGF proteins bind to three tyrosine-kinase receptors, VEGFR1 (vascular endothelial growth factor receptor1/Flt-1), VEGFR2 (KDR/Fetal liver kinase1, Flk-1) and VEGFR3 (Flt-4). Neuropilin-1 is a fourth receptor that can bind specifically to one of the VEGF isoforms, namely, VEGF165, which enhances its binding to VEGFR1. VEGFR2, through its interaction with VEGF, is thought to be the main mediator in tumor associated angiogenesis and metastatic processes whereas VEGFR1 plays a role in hematopoiesis. VEGF is expressed or overexpressed in many tumors including lung, breast, gastrointestinal stromal tumors (GISTs), ovarian, and in particular renal cancers, where the expression has been found to be high. Accordingly, targeting these molecules to abrogate their ability to stimulate tumor-associated angiogenesis constitutes a logical therapeutic strategy to control cancer. Both antibodies and small molecules have been developed as targeted therapies utilizing this pathway. Here we will discuss the antibodies. The small molecules will be discussed in the following section.

- **Bevacizumab** is a humanized murine anti-VEGF MoAb. Its mechanism of action is by binding VEGF and blocking the binding to the VEGF receptors, and hence, inhibiting the tumor-induced angiogenesis process. Clinical trials have demonstrated that the addition of bevacizumab to standard chemotherapy can improve the outcome in advanced disease. In colon cancer, it has been shown that the addition of bevacizumab to fluorouracil and leucovorin improved time to progression from 5.2 to 9 months with an increase in response rate from 17% to 40%. Adding bevacizumab to irinotecan, fluorouracil and leucovorin (IFL) improved median survival from 15.6 to 20 months. The addition of bevacizumab to FOLFOX4 (see Chapter 8) also resulted in higher median survival using the combination. Bevacizumab as a single agent showed inferior results compared with standard chemotherapy. Currently the drug is approved by the FDA for use as first-line treatment for advanced colon cancer in combination with fluorouracil-based chemotherapy. The drug has also been shown to be effective in other tumors including non–small cell lung cancer (NSCLC) where the addition of bevacizumab to the combination of paclitaxel and carboplatin showed higher response rate, longer disease-free survival, and median survival. Similar data was seen in advanced renal cell cancer. Trials are under way to test the effect of bevacizumab in many other tumors in both the advanced and the adjuvant setting. The use of bevacizumab has been shown to almost double the incidence of arterial thrombosis and to increase the incidence of hemorrhage and hypertension in certain cases. Hemoptysis seems to be a particular risk in squamous cell lung cancer.

2. Inhibition of receptor tyrosine kinases (RTKs). Kinases are enzymes that have the capability of attaching a phosphate moiety to another protein. This occurs on a side chain of a serine, threonine, or tyrosine moiety, by which these kinases are classified. The phosphorylation of proteins then regulates the behavior of these proteins whether with binding activity, enzymatic activity, or trafficking within the cell, or with their degradation. As a consequence, the phosphorylation process is a crucial biochemical reaction in controlling the behavior of a cell. Their critical role in cancer is shown by the observation that mutations in these kinases may lead to drastic outcomes including, in some instances, uncontrolled proliferation. Receptor serine/threonine kinases will be discussed in another section; here we will discuss the RTKs.

RTKs are a combination of families of receptors that share several structural and functional features. These kinases are glycoprotein receptors with extracellular, transmembrane, and intracellular domains. Whereas the transmembrane domain acts as an anchor for the receptor within the membrane of the cell, the extracellular domain contains a binding site for a specific multipeptide ligand, which, when it binds, initiates signaling events that are specific to the receptor. The cytoplasmic domain contains a catalytic protein tyrosine kinase region and a regulatory region, which are integral to the transmission of the signal downstream to the nucleus. The autophosphorylation of the receptor's kinase region initiates a cascade of signal transduction that leads to cell proliferation, survival/apoptosis, migration, adhesion, and promotion of angiogenesis. Some of the subfamilies in this group of receptors include the platelet-derived growth factor receptor (PDGFR), EGFR, VEGFR, fibroblast growth factor receptor (FGFR), and others. These RTKs are overexpressed or mutated in many human cancers. Therefore, the ability to target RTK activity is an attractive strategy for cancer therapy. A few small molecules have already been introduced into clinical practice and many others are currently in clinical trials. Here we will discuss some of these molecules:

- **Erlotinib** is an orally available small molecule with the chemical structure of N-(-3-ethynylphenyl)-6,7-bis (2-methoxyethoxy)-4-quinazolinamine. This compound is a reversible inhibitor of EGFR and it exhibits its function through the inhibition of the intracellular phosphorylation of tyrosine kinase by competing with ATP in binding the intracellular domain of the tyrosine kinase region. Accordingly, it blocks signal transduction of the EGFR, leading to the inhibition of the downstream effect of the pathway including the inhibition of cell propagation and survival, and angiogenesis. Erlotinib is a highly selective inhibitor for EGFR tyrosine kinase region; concentrations that reach more than 1,000-fold higher are required for the inhibition of other tyrosine kinases. Erlotinib has been shown to be effective in few tumors. In phase III placebo-controlled clinical trials in patients with locally advanced or metastatic NSCLC, erlotinib resulted in a median survival of 6.7 months versus 4.7 months when used as a second-line therapy. In pancreatic cancer, the addition of erlotinib to gemcitabine was found to improve median survival by 13.8 days over gemcitabine alone with increase in 1-year survival from 17% to 24%. Accordingly, erlotinib has been approved by the FDA in November 2005 for the treatment of patients with locally advanced or metastatic NSCLC as a second- or third-line therapy. It was also approved as a first-line therapy in combination with gemcitabine for locally advanced or metastatic pancreatic carcinoma. The most common toxicities included skin rash (12%) and diarrhea (5%). Erlotinib showed no major benefit when used as a first-line therapy in combination with platinum-based chemotherapy in advanced NSCLC. Clinical trials are currently being conducted in testing erlotinib in combination with other agents as first-line therapy for advanced NSCLC.

- **Gefitinib** is another small molecule that is designed to effectively inhibit the tyrosine kinase domain of the EGFR. This compound initially showed an effect in randomized phase II trials with symptomatic improvement in advanced NSCLC. On the basis of these results, the drug was approved as a third-line therapy for this disease by the FDA in 2003. However, further placebo-controlled phase III studies as frontline showed no survival benefit. Accordingly, the drug is being re-evaluated by regulatory agencies. The drug had a new label approved by the FDA that states that the medicine can be used in patients with cancer who have already taken the medicine and whose doctor believes it is helping them.

- **Sunitinib** is an ATP competitive inhibitor that leads to the inhibition of the phosphorylation of the kinase and further signal transduction in multiple RTKs. It functions as an inhibitor to a closely related family of RTK including PDGFR-α and -β, VEGFR, stem cell factor receptor KIT, Fms-like tyrosine kinase-3 receptor (FLT-3), and the RET oncoprotein. Accordingly, the antitumor effect of sunitinib is multifactorial. It inhibits cell proliferation and has an antiangiogenesis effect. The antiangiogenesis effect of sunitinib comes from the inhibition of both the VEGFR and PDGFR that is important for the recruitment of pericytes. Because of the inhibition of both these RTKs, this agent has a stronger inhibiting effect than those that target VEGF alone. Furthermore, KIT and PDGFR play an important role in the development of the stromal gastrointestinal tumors. Therefore, sunitinib will be expected to play a role in the inhibition of such tumors. Because angiogenesis is the hallmark of renal cell carcinoma that has been shown to have overexpression of VEGF and platelet-derived growth factor (PDGF), sunitinib would be expected to play a therapeutic role in this disease. A recent multinational phase III clinical trial comparing sunitinib to IFN-α as a first-line treatment in advanced renal cell carcinoma showed a major advantage in overall survival of 11 months as compared with 5 months for the IFN. Sunitinib has been approved by the FDA as first-line therapy for advanced renal cell cancers. Furthermore, more than 85% of GISTs possess activating mutations of the KIT kinase and another 5% are associated with mutation in the PDGFR. On the basis of its mechanism of action, sunitinib forms a natural candidate for the treatment of GIST. Clinical trials demonstrated efficacy in GIST patients who failed imatinib. An open-label multicenter phase I/II trial showed an overall survival of 19.8 months in patients who failed imatinib. It has been approved for GIST patients whose disease has progressed or who are unable to tolerate treatment with imatinib. Trials are being conducted to test sunitinib in breast and neuroendocrine tumors.

3. Inhibition of intracellular signaling proteins and protein kinases. This mechanism is directed at a group of proteins that function in a network of communicating cascades to transfer the signal from the receptors into the nucleus to produce an intended biologic effect including, cell proliferation, apoptosis, angiogenesis, etc. When mutated, these proteins produce dysregulated pathways that cause the development of a transformation status of the cell. Most of these proteins are kinases—nonreceptor tyrosine kinases or serine/threonine kinases. The non-receptor tyrosine kinases are cytoplasmic kinases, many of which are attached to and closely linked to membrane receptors, and they are usually activated by the binding of ligand to their associated receptors; some of these kinases include src, abl, and JAK. The serine/threonine tyrosine kinases are intracellular kinases, some of which play a crucial role in carcinogenesis. They include raf, Akt, and MEK. On the basis of this mechanism, small molecules designed to block or reverse the effect of these pathways have been developed, some of which are already in clinical use. In general, these targeted therapies that inhibit the intracellular signal proteins and protein kinases can act on multiple targets, some of which include receptor kinases; therefore, they can also be classified as receptor kinase inhibitors. For the sake of simplicity, this chapter will deal with those that primarily inhibit intracellular protein in this section and will allude to their other roles within the description of the drug.

- **Imatinib mesylate** is one of the first targeted therapy small molecules to be used in clinical practice. It is primarily a protein kinase inhibitor that is designed to inhibit Bcr-Abl tyrosine kinase. The Bcr-Abl fusion protein is the product of the translocation between the *Bcr* and *Abl 1* genes. The *Abl 1* gene encodes a nonreceptor tyrosine kinase whereas the Bcr produces a serine/threonine kinase. The product of the translocation produces a phosphorylated protein that activates many pathways including the RAS, PI3K, and STAT, which leads to malignant transformation.

Through the inhibition of the Bcr-Abl tyrosine kinase, imatinib mesylate induces apoptosis in Bcr-Abl-positive cells. Imatinib mesylate binds Abl 1 and leads to inhibition of the active tyrosine kinase of the fusion protein. It has been found to be active against Bcr-Abl-positive CML and Bcr-Abl-positive acute lymphocytic leukemia (ALL). In early studies, it was found to produce superior results over the combination of IFN-α and cytarabine in CML, and subsequent experience has shown that it produces both hematologic and cytogenetic remissions that are often long term and sustainable. Imatinib has also been found to inhibit the receptor kinases PDGF, stem cell factor, and cKIT. As noted in the preceding text, cKIT is mutated in 85% of GIST tumors. Imatinib was tested in and found effective in GIST. The current FDA-approved indications for imatinib include CML that is Philadelphia chromosome−positive, whether newly diagnosed, in chronic phase, in accelerated phase or blast crisis, or after failure of IFN-α therapy, or recurrence after stem cell transplant. It is also indicated in malignant cKIT-positive GIST that is unresectable or metastatic. Studies are currently under way to evaluate the role of imatinib in the adjuvant setting in GIST patients; in addition, indications in other diseases are currently under testing. Clinically significant resistance to imatinib is being increasingly noted and has been found to occur in patients who develop mutations within the kinase domain in the Bcr-Abl proteins. Therefore, the need to develop alternatives is very important. Some of the alternative kinase inhibitors are discussed in the subsequent text.

- **Dasatinib** is an oral inhibitor of multiple tyrosine kinases including Bcr-Abl. Other families of kinases that it inhibits include cKIT and PDGFR. Clinical data with dasatinib showed that 31% to 38% of imatinib-resistant and 75% of imatinib-intolerant patients with chronic phase CML reached major cytogenetic response. In addition, 30% to 59% of patients with advanced CML and Ph+ ALL showed major hematologic response. No clinical data are available yet to show increase in survival. It is indicated for patients with chronic, accelerated, and myeloid or lymphoid blast phase of CML who are intolerant or resistant to prior therapy with imatinib. It is also indicated in patients with Ph+ ALL.
- **Nilotinib** is another Abl kinase inhibitor. Similar to imatinib, it acts by competing with the ATP-binding site of Bcr-Abl. Nilotinib differs from imatinib by having a higher binding activity to Abl kinase with higher inhibitory activity in imatinib-sensitive cell lines. In recently published studies, nilotinib was found to induce both hematologic and cytologic responses in Ph+ CML patients who are resistant to imatinib.
- **Sorafenib** is a drug used for the treatment of advanced renal cell cancer. It is a small molecular inhibitor of C-Raf kinase that leads to the inhibition of the Raf/MEK/ERK signaling pathway. The Raf protein is a serine/threonine kinase, it is part of the Ras pathway, and it gets activated

when Ras, in response to the activation of an RTK, recruits and phosphorylates Raf kinase at the membrane site. Raf, in turn, phosphorylates the MEK that activates and phosphorylates ERK. ERK then enters the nucleus where it activates many other transcription factors leading to cellular proliferation. Aberration in this pathway leads to deregulation of proliferation, resulting in transformation of the cell. Raf has been found to be mutated in many tumors. Therefore, inhibition of this kinase is a reasonable target in cancer treatment. Sorafenib has also been found to be a strong inhibitor of both VEGFR-2 and PDGF kinase. In a large, phase III study, interim results showed that Sorafenib can reduce the risk of death by 23% compared with placebo in advanced renal cell carcinoma.

B. Angiogenesis-targeted therapy. Angiogenesis is a biologic process that is crucial for the development of tumors. Tumors have exploited this physiologic process to provide the milieu to permit the growth of both primary and metastatic cancers. Although the antineoplastic effect of antiangiogenesis therapy is mediated through its effect on the environment for the cancer cell growth, the initial mechanism of current therapies is based on molecular targeting, which is described in Sections VI.A.1.b and VI.A.2.

C. Protein degradation–targeted therapy. Protein degradation is one of the mechanisms by which cell function is regulated. The ubiquitin–proteosome pathway plays a very important role in this regard. The proteosome is a large complex of proteins that degrades other proteins after being tagged with a ubiquitin chain. It exerts its degradation capability through coordinated catalytic activities of its three proteolytic sites that lead to chymotryptic, tryptic, and post–glutamyl peptide hydrolytic-like activities. Many key proteins in cell cycle, apoptosis, and angiogenesis pathways are regulated by degradation, including the p53, p21, p27 (important cell cycle) proteins; NF-κB, a key transcription factor that is activated by the proteosomes, translocates to the nucleus and leads to the transcription of many crucial proteins including cytokines; and ICAM-1, VCAM, and E selectin (cell adhesion molecules).

- **Bortezomib** is a dipeptidyl boronic acid derivative that inhibits the 26S proteosome, the principal regulator of the intracellular protein degradation. It is the first of its class to be approved for clinical use. Bortezomib can selectively inhibit the chymotryptic site of the proteosome. This leads to a selective inhibition of the degradation of proteins involved in cell proliferation and survival regulation, and, as a consequence, apoptosis is induced. Bortezomib has been found to be effective, particularly in myeloma. A phase III trial that randomized patients with myeloma, who failed one to three previous therapies, to bortezomib versus high-dose dexamethasone has found that bortezomib resulted in a superior outcome with respect to response frequency, time to progression, and overall survival. Currently bortezomib is approved by the FDA for the treatment of patients with multiple myeloma who have received at least one prior therapy.

Active research to identify other active proteosome inhibiting agents is ongoing.

D. Immune modulation–targeted therapy. Immune modulators (IMiDs) are a new family of medications that are derivatives of thalidomide and known to be immunomodulatory drugs. These compounds are generated by minor structural modifications on thalidomide that leads to enhancement of its efficacy and improvement in the side effect profile including the neurologic toxicity and prothrombotic effects of thalidomide. The mechanism of action of this group of compounds is not clearly defined. Many pathways have been shown to be triggered by these medications including caspase-8, proteosome, NFκB, and the antiangiogenesis pathways.

- **Lenolidomide** is one of the new-generation immunomodulators. It has been found to be active in refractory multiple myeloma. In one phase II clinical trial, the response rate reached 24% with more than 50% reduction in monoclonal protein in patients with relapsed or refractory disease. When combined with dexamethasone in newly diagnosed multiple myeloma patients, 91% of patients achieved an objective response including 11% with complete response. Compared with thalidomide, it showed no significant somnolence, constipation, or neuropathy. It is approved for the use of patients with multiple myeloma in combination with dexamethasone in patients who received at least one prior therapy, and in patients with myelodysplastic syndrome with 5q deletion who are transfusion dependent.

E. Phenotype-directed targeted therapy

   1. Non–receptor protein-directed MoAbs. These are a group of antibodies that are developed to recognize specific antigens on the surface of cancer cells, not for the purpose of blocking a specific pathway or receptor proteins, but rather to induce direct cytotoxic effect. These MoAbs may be used alone or as a delivery system for cellular toxins, radionuclides, or chemotherapy.

   a. Unconjugated antibodies

   - **Rituximab** is an IgG1-κ murine–human chimeric MoAb that is generated against the CD20 antigen. CD20 is expressed on the cell surface of the B cells and hence on the surface of B-cell lymphoma. Rituximab is indicated for the treatment of relapsed or refractory B-cell non–Hodgkin's lymphoma and chronic lymphocytic leukemia that expresses CD20 marker. Rituximab is also being increasingly used in combination with chemotherapy (e.g., cyclophosphamide, vincristine, doxorubicin, and prednisone), particularly in the more aggressive non–Hodgkin's lymphomas.

   - **Alemtuzumab** is a humanized IgG1-κ murine–human chimeric MoAb that is directed against CD52 cell surface glycoprotein. CD52 is expressed on the surface of normal and malignant B and T cells, natural killer cells, monocytes, and macrophages. Alemtuzumab is indicated for the treatment of B-cell chronic lymphocytic leukemia in patients who have failed fludarabine. Patients who have recently been treated with this MoAb should not receive any live viral vaccines because of the immune suppression effect of the medication.

b. Cellular toxin conjugated antibodies

- **Gemtuzumab ozogamicin** is a humanized IgG4-κ antibody against the CD33 antigen conjugated with calicheamicin. Calicheamicin is a cytotoxic agent that is isolated from fermentation of the bacterium *Micromonospora echinospora* ssp *calichensis*. The CD33 antigen is a sialic acid–dependent adhesion protein that is expressed on the surface of immature cells of the myelomonocytic lineage and the surface of leukemic blast cells but not on the normal pluripotent hematopoietic stem cells. When this fusion antibody binds to the CD33 receptors, it gets internalized into the cell, after which the calicheamicin is cleaved and released. The calicheamicin in turn binds to the minor grooves of the DNA, leading to DNA breaks and apoptosis.

    Gemtuzumab is indicated for the treatment of the first relapse of myeloid leukemia that expresses CD33 in older patients (more than 60 years old) who are not candidates for chemotherapy. Clinical trials have shown that, when given as single agent, gemtuzumab may lead to 16% complete response and 30% overall response with a median time to remission of 60 days.

c. Radioimmunoconjugate antibodies

- **Ibritumomab tiuxetan (Zevalin, IDEC-Y2B8)** is a murine monoclonal anti-CD20 antibody conjugated to tiuxetan that chelates to the pure β-emitting yttrium 90 (^{90}Y). The mechanism of action includes antibody-mediated cytotoxicity and cellularly targeted radiotherapy (radioimmunotherapy [RIT]). It is indicated for use in non–Hodgkin's lymphoma that is follicular, B-cell CD20 positive, and rituximab refractory. Experimentally it is used in non–Hodgkin's lymphoma that has relapsed or is refractory to other agents, but not refractory to rituximab. It should be used with caution in patients with 25% or more marrow involvement with lymphoma, prior external beam radiotherapy to 25% or more of the bone marrow, or a history of HAMAs or HACAs. Because the drug does not emit γ radiation, hospitalization is not required. Neutropenia and thrombocytopenia are common and are related to the radionuclide dose. At the higher end of the dosing, 25% of patients will develop nadir neutrophil counts of less than 500/μL. Low-grade nausea and vomiting are common. Infusion-related fever, chills, dizziness, asthenia, headache, back pain, arthralgia, and hypotension are occasional.

- **Iodine 131 (^{131}I)-Tositumomab (Bexxar).** ^{131}I-Tositumomab is a murine IgG2a monoclonal anti-CD20 antibody radiolabeled with ^{131}I, an emitter of both β and γ radiation. The mechanism of action includes antibody-mediated cytotoxicity and cellularly targeted

RIT. It is indicated in non–Hodgkin's lymphoma, which is chemotherapy refractory, CD20 positive, low grade, or transformed low grade. Before dosimetric and therapeutic doses, patients are premedicated with acetaminophen 650 mg and diphenhydramine 50 mg. A saturated solution of potassium iodide, two to three drops orally three times daily, is given beginning 24 hours before the dosimetric dose and continuing for 14 days after the therapeutic dose to prevent uptake of ^{131}I by the thyroid. It must be used cautiously in patients with 25% marrow involvement with lymphoma, prior external beam radiotherapy to 25% of the bone marrow, or a history of HAMAs or HACAs.

2. **Immunotoxins**

- **Denileukin diftitox (Ontak).** Denileukin diftitox is a recombinant construct that includes a fragment of the IL-2 protein (Ala$_1$- Thr$_{133}$) linked to a fragment of the diphtheria toxin fragment A and B (Met$_1$-Thr$_{387}$). This construct is designed to bind to the CD25 component of the IL-2 receptor (IL-2R) on the surface of the targeted cells that express the receptor; in turn, the complex becomes internalized into the cytoplasm and releases the toxin to exhibit its damaging effect. The high-affinity IL-2R is normally present on the activated T and B lymphocytes and activated macrophages. However, cutaneous T-cell lymphoma (CTCL) also expresses high-affinity IL-2R, which forms an appropriate target.

In two different clinical studies, investigators have shown that 30% of patients with CTCL demonstrate clinical response, including approximately 10% complete response. Therefore, the indications for this agent include persistent or recurrent CTCL that expresses the IL-2R CD25.

VII. **Other biologic therapies**
  A. **Bone marrow–supportive agents**
   1. **Erythrocyte growth factors**
      a. **Epoetin** is a recombinant growth factor, identical to endogenous human erythropoietin, which promotes the proliferation and differentiation of committed erythroid precursors. It is indicated to be used in patients with nonhematologic malignancies who have chemotherapy-induced anemia to minimize transfusion requirements during therapy. It is not indicated in these patients when they have anemia due to other causes such as iron deficiency, bleeding, or hemolysis. Erythropoietin takes time to work, and a decision on the effectiveness should not be made before 4 to 8 weeks. If transfusion requirement does not change after 8 weeks, the dose may be increased. The dose should be withheld if the hematocrit increases to more than 40% and resumed with 25% reduction when the hematocrit is reduced to 36%. If the patient fails to show improvement after increasing the dose to 60,000 U (900 U/kg)/week, it is unlikely that the patient will respond and other causes of the anemia should be looked for carefully. Rarely it may

induce pure red cell aplasia with associated neutralizing antierythropoietin antibodies.

b. Darbepoetin is an erythropoiesis-stimulating protein closely related to erythropoietin that has a threefold longer terminal half-life than epoetin. Its indications are similar to epoetin.

2. **Myeloid–monocytic growth factors**

a. G-CSF (filgrastim). G-CSF is a 175–amino acid growth factor with proliferative activity for bone marrow progenitors committed to the neutrophil line. As discussed elsewhere in this volume, G-CSF is widely used in the setting of cytotoxic chemotherapy for solid tumors and leukemia to accelerate recovery of neutrophils and lessen the risk of bacterial infection. Filgrastim is indicated under the following conditions:

- The likelihood of first-cycle febrile neutropenia is 20% or higher. It should be considered when the risk is 10% to 20%, depending on patient and cancer-related factors.
- Further cycles of chemotherapy are needed after an occurrence of febrile neutropenia, and maintenance of dose intensity rather than dose reduction is appropriate.
- High-dose chemotherapy followed by peripheral blood stem cell or autologous bone marrow support has been used.
- The patient has established febrile neutropenia, **and** when the infection is life threatening or is expected to require prolonged antibiotic or antifungal therapy.

b. Granulocyte–macrophage colony-stimulating factor (sargramostim). GM-CSF is a 127–amino acid growth factor that exhibits its predominant proliferative effects on multipotent stem cells, inhibits neutrophil migration, potentiates the functions of neutrophils and macrophages, and results in production of a spectrum of cytokines from these activated cells. GM-CSF is used mainly for the following indications: to shorten neutrophil recovery time after induction therapy in acute myelogenous leukemia and accelerate myeloid recovery after bone marrow transplantation.

3. **Megakaryocyte growth factor; IL-11 (oprelvekin).** IL-11 is a 177–amino acid growth factor that is a member of the same family of growth factors as G-CSF. IL-11 is a thrombopoietic growth factor that stimulates the proliferation of megakaryocyte progenitor cells and induces megakaryocyte maturation, leading to increase in platelets. Therefore, it is indicated in the acceleration of the recovery of platelets after cytotoxic chemotherapy and has been approved for clinical use for that purpose.

B. **Other biologic therapy**

1. **IL-2 (Proleukin).** IL-2 is a cytokine that is secreted by activated T cells. IL-2 binds to a specific cell surface receptor on activated T lymphocytes and leads to T-cell proliferation. In addition, IL-2 can also activate natural killer cells. Through these mechanisms and perhaps

others, IL-2 has been found to exhibit antitumor properties. In clinical trials, it has been found that IL-2 has
antitumor activity when used alone in high doses in patients with renal cell carcinoma and malignant melanoma.
High-dose IV therapy with IL-2 given as a single agent has
received FDA approval for the treatment of patients with
metastatic renal cell carcinoma and metastatic melanoma.
Careful selection of patients for such an intensive therapy
is mandatory, especially for the cardiopulmonary status.
This therapy is associated with significant toxicity and
should be administered only by physicians experienced in
its use.

2. IFN-α (IFN-α 2a, IFN-α 2b). The IFNs are a family
of small molecular weight proteins and glycoproteins that
are secreted by activated T cells and other cells secondary
to viral infection. There are three major types of IFNs:
α, β, and γ. IFN-α is produced by T cells, B cells, and
macrophages when exposed to the appropriate antigens,
IFN-β is produced by fibroblasts when exposed to viral
infection, and IFN-γ is produced by T cells after stimulation
with IL-2 or specific or nonspecific antigens. IFN-α is the
only one of the IFNs that is approved by the FDA for
human cancer therapy. Approved indications include hairy
cell leukemia, melanoma with high risk of recurrence after
resection, follicular lymphoma as initial treatment for the
aggressive types, in combination with anthracyclines, and
acquired immune deficiency syndrome–related Kaposi's
sarcoma.

SUGGESTED READINGS

Adjei AA, Hidalgo M. Intracellular signal transduction pathway
proteins as targets for cancer therapy. *J Clin Oncol* 2005;23:
5386–5403.

Baguley BC, Holdaway KM, Fray LM. Design of DNA intercalators to
overcome topoisomerase II-mediated multi-drug resistance. *J Natl
Cancer Inst* 1990;82:398–402.

Baserga R. The cell cycle. *N Engl J Med* 1981;304:453–459.

Chen YL, Law PY, Loh HH, et al. Inhibition of PI3K/Akt signaling: an
emerging paradigm for targeted cancer therapy. *Curr Med Chem
Anticancer Agents* 2005;5:575–589.

Clarkson B, Fried J, Strife A, et al. Studies of cellular proliferation
in human leukemia. 3. Behavior of leukemic cells in three adults
with acute leukemia given continuous infusions of 3H-thymidine
for 8 or 10 days. *Cancer* 1970;25:1237–1260.

Cohen SJ, Cohen RB, Meropol NJ, et al. Targeting signal transduction pathways in colorectal cancer–more than skin deep. *J Clin
Oncol* 2005;23:5374–5385.

Endicott JA, Ling U. The biochemistry of P-glycoprotein-mediated
multidrug resistance. *Annu Rev Biochem* 1989;58:137–171.

Ferrara N, Hillan KJ, Novotny W, et al. Bevacizumab (Avastin), a
humanized anti-VEGF monoclonal antibody for cancer therapy.
Biochem Biophys Res Commun 2005;333:328–335.

Friedland ML. Combination chemotherapy. In: Perry MC, ed. *The
chemotherapy source book*. Baltimore: Williams & Wilkins, 1996:
63–78.

Giaccone G. HER1/EGFR-targeted agents: predicting the future for patients with unpredictable outcomes to therapy. *Ann Oncol* 2005;16:538–548.

Goldie JH. Drug resistance. In: Perry MC, ed. *The chemotherapy source book*. Baltimore: Williams & Wilkins, 1992:54–66.

Goldie JH, Coldman AJ. A mathematical model for relating drug sensitivity of tumors to their spontaneous mutation rate. *Cancer Treat Rep* 1979;63:1727–1733.

Kinzler KW, Vogelstein B. Cancer therapy meets p53. *N Engl J Med* 1994;331:49–50.

Motzer RJ, Hoosen S, Bello CL, et al. Sunitinib malate for the treatment of solid tumours: a review of current clinical data. *Expert Opin Investing Drugs* 2006;15:553–561.

Normanno N, De Luca A, Bianco C, et al. Epidermal growth factor receptor (EGFR) signaling in cancer. *Gene* 2006;366:2–16.

Quintas-Cardama A, Cortes JE. Chronic myeloid leukemia: diagnosis and treatment. *Mayo Clin Proc* 2006;81:973–988.

Schabel FM Jr. The use of tumor growth kinetics in planning "curative" chemotherapy of advanced solid tumors. *Cancer Res* 1969;29: 2384–2398.

Schlessinger J. Cell signaling by receptor tyrosine kinases. *Cell* 2000;103:211–225.

Sharkey RM, Goldenberg DM. Targeted therapy of cancer: new prospects for antibodies and immunoconjugates. *CA Cancer J Clin* 2006;56:226–243.

Sikic BI. Modulation of multidrug resistance: at the threshold. *J Clin Oncol* 1993;11:1629–1635.

Simon MA. Receptor tyrosine kinases: specific outcomes from general signals. *Cell* 2000;103:13–15.

Slingerland JM, Tannock IF. Cell proliferation and cell death. In: Tannock IF, Hill RP, eds. *The basic science of oncology*. New York: McGraw-Hill, 1998:134–165.

Smith J. Erlotinib: small-molecule targeted therapy in the treatment of non-small-cell lung cancer. *Clin Ther* 2005;27:1513–1534.

Smith RA, Dumas J, Adnane L, et al. Recent advances in the research and development of RAF kinase inhibitors. *Curr Top Med Chem* 2006;6:1071–1089.

Tokunaga E, Oki E, Nishida K, et al. Trastuzumab and breast cancer: developments and current status. *Int J Clin Oncol* 2006;11: 199–208.

Tucker GC. Integrins: molecular targets in cancer therapy. *Curr Oncol Rep* 2006;8:96–103.

Vignot S, Faivre S, Aguirre D, et al. mTOR-targeted therapy of cancer with rapamycin derivatives. *Ann Oncol* 2005;16:525–537.

Yarbro JW. The scientific basis of cancer chemotherapy. In: Perry MC, ed. *The chemotherapy source book*. Baltimore: Williams & Wilkins, 1996:3–18.

Table 4.1. Useful chemotherapeutic agents

Class and Type	Agents
Alkylating agents	
Alkyl sulfonate	Busulfan
Ethylenimine derivative	Thiotepa (triethylenethiophosphoramide)
Metal salt	Carboplatin, cisplatin, oxaliplatin
Nitrogen mustard	Chlorambucil, cyclophosphamide, estramustine, ifosfamide, mechlorethamine, melphalan
Nitrosourea	Carmustine, lomustine, streptozocin
Triazene	Dacarbazine, temozolamide
Antimetabolites	
Antifolates	Methotrexate, pemetrexed, raltitrexed, trimetrexate
Purine analogs	Cladribine, clofarabine, fludarabine, mercaptopurine, nelarabine, pentostatin, thioguanine
Pyrimidine analogs	Azacitidine, capecitabine, cytarabine, decitabine, floxuridine, fluorouracil, gemcitabine
Natural products	
Antibiotics	Bleomycin, dactinomycin, daunorubicin, doxorubicin, epirubicin, idarubicin, mitomycin, mitoxantrone, valrubicin
Enzyme	Asparaginase
Microtubule polymer stabilizer	Docetaxel, paclitaxel
Mitotic inhibitor	Vinblastine, vincristine, vindesine, vinorelbine
Topoisomerase I inhibitors	Irinotecan, topotecan
Topoisomerase II inhibitors	Etoposide, teniposide
Hormones and hormone antagonists	
Androgen	Fluoxymesterone and others
Androgen antagonist	Bicalutamide, flutamide, nilutamide
Aromatase inhibitor	Aminoglutethimide, anastrozole, letrozole, exemestane
Corticosteroid	Dexamethasone, prednisone
Estrogen	Diethylstilbestrol
Estrogen antagonist (selective estrogen receptor modulator)	Fulvestrant, raloxifene, tamoxifen, toremifene

Systemic Assessment of the Patient with Cancer and Long-Term Consequences of Treatment

Roland T. Skeel

I. **Establishing the diagnosis**

A. **Pathologic diagnosis is critical.** Although it might seem obvious that the diagnosis of cancer must be firmly established before chemotherapy or any other treatment is administered, the critical nature of an accurate diagnosis warrants a reminder. As a rule, there must be cytologic or histologic evidence of neoplastic cells, together with a clinical picture consistent with the diagnosis of the cancer under consideration. Commonly, patients present to their physician with a complaint such as a cough, bleeding, pain, or a lump; through a logical sequence of evaluation, the presence of cancer is revealed on a cytologic or histologic specimen. Less frequently, lesions are discovered fortuitously during routine examination, evaluation of an unrelated disorder, or systematic screening for cancer. With some types of cancer, pathologists can establish the diagnosis on the basis of small amounts of material obtained from needle biopsies, aspirations, or tissue scrapings. Other cancers require larger pieces of tissue for special staining, immunohistologic evaluation, flow cytometry, examination by electron microscopy, or more sophisticated studies such as evaluation for gene rearrangement or genetic profiles.

It is often helpful to confer with the pathologist before obtaining a specimen to determine what kind and size of specimen is adequate to establish the complete diagnosis. When a tissue diagnosis of cancer is made by the pathologist, it is incumbent on the clinician to review the material with the pathologist. This practice is good medicine (and good learning); it also allows the clinician to tell the patient that he or she has actually seen the cancer. In addition, it prevents the physician from administering chemotherapy without a firm pathologic diagnosis. The pathologist often gives a better consultation—not just a tissue diagnosis—when the clinician shows a personal interest.

B. **Pathologic and clinical diagnosis must be consistent.** Once the tissue diagnosis is established, the clinician must be certain that the pathologic diagnosis is consistent with the clinical findings. If the two are not consistent, a search must be made for additional information, clinical or pathologic, that allows the clinician to make a unified diagnosis. A pathologic diagnosis, like a clinical diagnosis, is also an opinion with varying levels of certainty. The first part of the pathologic diagnosis—and usually the easier part—is an opinion about whether the tissue examined is neoplastic. Because most pathologists rarely render a diagnosis of cancer unless the degree of certainty is high, a positive diagnosis of cancer is generally reliable. The clinician must be more cautious if the diagnosis rendered states that the tissue is "highly suggestive of" or "consistent with the diagnosis of." Absence of definitively diagnosed cancer in a specimen does not, however, mean that cancer is not present; it means only that it could not be diagnosed on the tissue obtained, and clinical circumstances must establish if additional tissue sampling is necessary. A second part of the pathologist's diagnosis is an opinion about the type of cancer and the tissue of origin. This determination is not necessary in all circumstances but is usually helpful in selecting the most appropriate therapy and making a determination of prognosis.

C. Treatment without a pathologic diagnosis. There are rare circumstances in which treatment is undertaken before a pathologic diagnosis is established. Such circumstances are clearly exceptions, however, and involve less than 1% of all patients with cancer. Therapy is begun without a pathologic diagnosis only when the following conditions are met:

1. Withholding prompt treatment or carrying out the procedures required to establish the diagnosis would greatly increase a patient's morbidity or risk of mortality.
2. The likelihood of a benign diagnosis is remote.

Two examples of such circumstances are a primary tumor of the midbrain and superior vena cava syndrome with no accessible supraclavicular nodes and no endobronchial disease found on bronchoscopy in a patient in whom the risk of bleeding from mediastinoscopy is deemed greater than the risk of administering radiotherapy for a disease of uncertain nature.

II.   Staging. Once the diagnosis of cancer is firmly established, it is important to determine the anatomic extent or stage of the disease. The steps taken for staging vary considerably among cancers because of the differing natural histories of the tumors.

A. Staging system criteria. For most cancers, a system of staging has been established on the basis of the following factors:

1. Natural history and mode of spread of the cancer
2. Prognostic import for the staging parameters used
3. Value of the criteria used for decisions about therapy.

B. Staging and therapy decisions. In the past, surgery and radiotherapy were used to treat patients with cancer in early stages, and chemotherapy was used when surgery and radiotherapy were no longer effective or when the disease was in an advanced stage at presentation. In such circumstances, chemotherapy was only palliative (except for gestational choriocarcinoma), and in the absence of exquisitely sensitive tumors or strikingly potent drugs, the likelihood of increasing the survival was low. As knowledge has increased about the genetic determinants of cancer growth, tumor cell kinetics, and the development of resistance, the value of early intervention with chemotherapy has been transposed from animal models to human cancers. To plan this intervention and evaluate its effectiveness, careful staging has become increasingly important. Only when the exact extent of disease has been established can the most rational plan of treatment for the individual patient be devised, whether it is surgery, radiotherapy, chemotherapy, or biologic therapy—alone or in combination.

Although no single staging system is universally used for all cancers, the system developed jointly by the American Joint Committee on Cancer (AJCC) and the TNM Committee of the International Union Against Cancer (IUCC) is most widely used for staging solid tumors. It is based on the status of the primary tumor (T), regional lymph nodes (N), and distant metastasis (M). For some cancers, tumor grade (G) is also taken into account. The stage of the tumor is based on a condensation of the total possible TNM and G categories to create stage groupings, usually stages 0, I, II, III, and IV, which are relatively homogeneous with respect to prognosis. When relevant to the specific cancers whose chemotherapy is discussed in Section III of this handbook, the staging system or systems most commonly used for that cancer are discussed.

III. Performance status. The performance status refers to the level of activity of which a patient is capable. It is an independent measure (independent of the anatomic extent or histologic characteristics of the cancer) of how much the cancer or comorbid conditions have affected the patient and a prognostic indicator of how well the patient is likely to respond to treatment.

A. Types of performance status scales. Two performance status scales are in wide use:

1. The Karnofsky performance status scale (Table 2.1) has ten levels of activity. It has the advantage of allowing discrimination over a wide scale but the disadvantages of being difficult to remember easily and perhaps of making discriminations that are not clinically useful.

2. The Eastern Cooperative Oncology Group (ECOG) Performance Status Scale (Table 2.2) has the advantages of being easy to remember and making discriminations that are clinically useful.

3. According to the criteria of each scale, patients who are fully active or have mild symptoms respond more frequently to treatment and survive longer than patients who are less active or have severe symptoms. A clear designation of the performance status distribution of patients in therapeutic clinical trials is therefore critical in determining the comparability and generalizability of trials and the effectiveness of the treatments used.

B. Use of performance status for choosing treatment. In the individualization of therapy, the performance status is often a useful parameter to help the clinician decide whether the patient will benefit from treatment or will be made worse. For example, unless there is some reason to expect a dramatic response of a cancer to chemotherapy, treatment is often withheld in patients with an ECOG Performance Status Scale score of 4 because responses to therapy are infrequent and toxic effects of the treatment are likely to be good.

C. Quality of life (QOL). A related but partially independent measure of performance status can be determined based on patients' own perceptions of their QOL. QOL evaluations have been shown to be independent predictors of tumor response and

Table 2.1. Karnofsky performance status scale

Functional Capability	Level of Activity
Able to carry on normal activity; no special care needed	100%—Normal; no complaints, no evidence of disease 90%—Able to carry on normal activity; minor signs or symptoms of disease 80%—Normal activity with effort; some signs or symptoms of disease
Unable to work; able to live at home; cares for most personal needs; needs varying amount of assistance	70%—Cares for self; unable to carry on normal activity or to do active work 60%—Requires occasional assistance but is able to care for most of own needs 50%—Requires considerable assistance and frequent medical care
Unable to care for self; requires equivalent of institutional or hospital care	40%—Disabled; requires special medical care and assistance 30%—Severely disabled; hospitalization indicated, although death not imminent 20%—Very sick; hospitalization necessary; active supportive treatment necessary 10%—Moribund; fatal processes progressing rapidly 0%—Dead

survival in some cancers, and they are important components in a comprehensive assessment of response to therapy. For some cancers, improvement in QOL measures early in the course of treatment is the most reliable indicator of survival.

IV. Response to therapy. Response to therapy may be measured by survival, disease-free survival, objective change in tumor size or in tumor product (e.g., immunoglobulin in myeloma), and subjective change.

    A. Survival. One goal of cancer therapy is to allow patients to live as long and with the same QOL as they would have if they did not have the cancer. If this goal is achieved, it can be said that the patient is cured of the cancer (although biologically the cancer may still be present). From a practical standpoint, we do not wait to see if patients live a normal life span before saying that a given treatment is capable of achieving a cure, but we follow up on a cohort of patients to see if their survival within a given time span is different from that in a comparable cohort without the cancer. For the evaluation

Table 2.2. Eastern Cooperative Oncology Group (ECOG) Performance Status Scale

Grade	Level of Activity
0	Fully active; able to carry on all predisease performance without restriction (Karnofsky 90%–100%)
1	Restricted in physically strenuous activity but ambulatory and able to carry out work of a light or sedentary nature, e.g., light housework, office work (Karnofsky 70%–80%)
2	Ambulatory and capable of all self-care but unable to carry out any work activities; up and about >50% of waking hours (Karnofsky 50%–60%)
3	Capable of only limited self-care; confined to bed or chair >50% of waking hours (Karnofsky 30%–40%)
4	Completely disabled; cannot carry on any self-care; totally confined to bed or chair (Karnofsky 10%–20%)

of response to *adjuvant therapy* (additional treatment after surgery or radiotherapy that is given to treat potential non-measurable, micrometastatic disease) or *neoadjuvant therapy* (chemotherapy or biologic therapy given as initial treatment before surgery or radiotherapy), survival analysis (rather than tumor response) must be used as the definitive objective measure of antineoplastic effect. With neoadjuvant therapy, tumor response and resectability are also partial determinants of effectiveness. Disease-free survival is often a useful comparator in clinical studies of adjuvant therapy, as return of disease most often represents loss of curability.

It is, of course, possible that a patient may be cured of the cancer, that is, the cancer that was treated, but die early owing to complications associated with the treatment, including second cancers. Even with complications (unless they are acute ones such as bleeding or infection), survival of patients who have been cured of the cancer is likely to be longer than if the treatment had not been given, although shorter than if the patient had never had the cancer.

If cure is not possible, the reduced goal is to allow the patient to live longer than if the therapy under consideration were not given. It is important for physicians to know if, and with what likelihood, any given treatment will result in a longer life. Such information helps physicians to choose whether to recommend treatment and the patient to decide whether to undertake the recommended treatment program.

It is usually helpful to learn from the patient what his or her goals of therapy are and to have a frank discussion about whether those goals are realistic. This can avoid unnecessary surprises and anger at some later time, which can occur when the patient has set a goal that is not realistic and the physician has not discussed what may or may not reasonably be expected as a consequence of therapy.

B. Objective response. Although survival is important to the individual patient, it is determined not only by the treatment undertaken but also by biologic determinants of the patient's individual cancer and subsequent treatment; therefore, survival does not give an early measurement of treatment effectiveness. Tumor regression, on the other hand, frequently occurs early in the course of effective treatment and is therefore a readily used measurement of treatment benefit. Tumor regression can be determined by a decrease in size of a tumor or the reduction of tumor products.

1. Tumor size. When tumor size is measured, responses are usually classified by the new Response Evaluation Criteria in Solid Tumors (RECIST) methodology published in the *Journal of the National Cancer Institute* in 2000 (Therasse et al. 2000), and available at *http://ctep.cancer.gov/guidelines/recist.html*.

a. Baseline lesions are characterized as "measurable" (20 mm or more in longest diameter with conventional techniques, 10 mm or more in longest diameter with spiral computed tomography scan) or "nonmeasurable" (smaller lesions and truly nonmeasurable lesions). To assess response, all measurable lesions up to a maximum of five per organ and ten in total are designated as "target" lesions and measured at baseline. Only the longest diameter of each lesion is measured. The sum of the longest diameters of all target lesions is designated the *baseline sum longest diameter*. There are a variety of lesions in cancer that cannot be measured. These include many metastatic lesions to the bone, effusions, lymphangitic disease of the lung or skin, and lesions that have necrotic or cystic centers.

b. Response categories are based on measurement of target lesions:

(1) Complete response is the disappearance of all target lesions.

(2) Partial response is a decrease of at least 30% in the sum of the longest diameters of target lesions, using as reference the baseline sum longest diameter.

(3) Progressive disease is an increase of 20% or more in sum of the longest diameters of target lesions, taking as reference the smallest sum longest diameter recorded since the treatment started, or the appearance of one or more new lesions.

(4) Stable disease is when there is neither sufficient shrinkage to qualify for partial response nor sufficient increase to qualify for progressive disease.

c. Time to progression is an additional indicator that is often used. It takes into account the fact that from the patient's perspective, complete response, partial response, and stable disease may be meaningless distinctions so long as the tumor is not causing symptoms or impairment of function. It also takes into account that some agents result in disease stability for a substantial period, despite failure to produce measurable disease shrinkage. This is particularly true of the use of biologic targeted agents where it has been shown that time to progression for some cancers is substantially prolonged, despite no measurable reduction in tumor size.

Time to progression can also be used as an indicator of disease status when there was no measurable disease at the outset of treatment or when the therapeutic modalities were not comparable. For example, if one wanted to compare the results of surgery alone with those of chemotherapy alone, time to progression from the onset of treatment would allow a valid comparison of the effectiveness of the treatments, whereas the traditional tumor response criteria would not. Time to progression therefore places each of the agents or modalities on an even basis.

d. If survival curves of patient populations having different categories of response are compared, patients with a complete response frequently survive longer than those with a lesser response. If a sizable number of complete responses occur with a treatment regimen, the survival rate of patients treated with that regimen is likely to be significantly greater than that of patients who are untreated. When the number of complete responders in a population rises to approximately 50%, the possibility of cure for a small number of patients begins to appear. With increasing percentages of complete responders, the frequency of cures is likely to increase correspondingly.

Although patients who have partial response to a treatment usually survive longer than those who have stable disease or progression, it is often not easy to demonstrate that the overall survival of the treated population is better than that of a comparable untreated group. In part, this difficulty may be due to a phenomenon of small numbers. If only 15% to 20% of a population responds to therapy, the median survival rate may not change at all, and the numbers may not be high enough to demonstrate a significant difference in survival duration of the longest surviving 5% to 10% of patients (the "tail" of the curves) for treated and untreated populations. It is also possible that the patients who achieve a partial response to therapy are those who have less aggressive disease at the outset of treatment and therefore will survive longer than the nonresponders regardless of therapy. These caveats notwithstanding, most clinicians and patients welcome even a partial response as a sign that offers hope for longer survival and improved QOL.

2. Tumor products. For many cancers, objective tumor size changes are difficult or impossible to document. For some of these neoplasms, tumor products (hormones, antigens, antibodies) may be measurable and may provide a good, objective way to evaluate tumor response. Two examples of such markers that closely reflect tumor cell mass are the abnormal immunoglobulins (M proteins) produced in multiple myeloma and the beta human chorionic gonadotropin (β-hCG) produced in choriocarcinoma and testicular cancer. Other markers such as prostate-specific antigen (PSA) or carcinoembryonic antigen (CEA) are not quite as reliable but are, nonetheless, helpful measures of response of tumor to therapy.

3. Evaluable disease. Other objective changes may occur but are not easily quantifiable. When these changes are not easily measurable, they may be termed *evaluable*. For example, neurologic changes secondary to primary brain tumors cannot be measured with a caliper, but they can be evaluated using neurologic testing. An arbitrary system of grading the degree of severity of the neurologic deficit can be devised to permit surrogate evaluation of tumor response. Evaluable disease is not a category of the RECIST criteria.

4. Performance status changes may also be used as a measure of objective change, although in many respects, the performance status is more representative of the subjective than the objective status of the disease.

C. Subjective change and quality-of-life considerations. A subjective change is one that is perceived by the patient but not necessarily by the physician or others around the patient. Subjective improvement and an acceptable QOL are often of far greater importance to the patient than objective improvement: if the cancer shrinks, but the patient feels worse than before treatment, he or she is not likely to believe that the treatment was worthwhile. It is not valid to look at subjective change in isolation, however, because temporary worsening in the perceived state of well-being may be necessary to achieve subsequent long-term improvement.

This point is particularly well illustrated by the combined-modality treatment in which chemotherapy is used to treat micrometastases after surgical removal of the macroscopic tumor. In such a circumstance, the patient is likely to feel entirely well after the primary surgical procedure, but the side effects of chemotherapy increase the symptoms and make the patient feel subjectively worse for the period of treatment. The winner's stakes are valuable, however, because if the chemotherapy treatment of the micrometastases is successful, the patient will be cured of the cancer and can be expected to have a normal or near-normal life expectancy rather than dying from recurrent disease. Most patients agree that the temporary subjective worsening is not only tolerable but also well worth the price if cure of the cancer is a distinct possibility. This judgment depends on the severity and duration of symptoms, functional impairment, and perceptions of illness during the acute phase of the treatment; the benefit (increased likelihood of survival) anticipated as a result of the treatment; and the potential long-term adverse consequences of the treatment.

When chemotherapy is given with a palliative intent, patients (and less often physicians) may be unwilling to tolerate significant side effects or subjective worsening. Fortunately, subjective improvement often accompanies objective improvement, so patients in whom there is measurable improvement of the cancer also feel better. The degree of subjective worsening that each patient is willing to tolerate varies, and the patient and physician together must discuss and evaluate whether the chemotherapy treatment program is worth continuing. Such discussions should include a clear presentation of the scientific facts that include objective survival and tumor response data together with whatever QOL information has been documented for the treatment proposed. Moreover, the expressed desires and the social, economic, psychological, and spiritual situations of the patient and his or her family must be sensitively considered.

A word of caution about discussions of response and survival is important. Patients can understand the notion of response rates more easily than survival probabilities. For example, a 50:50 chance of the cancer shrinking helps them to understand the goals and expectations of therapy and does not lead to undue anxiety over time. On the other hand, providing median or expected survival estimates is more problematic intellectually and, more particularly, emotionally. It is, therefore, usually best to give the patient a range of expected survival rather than a number. For example, the physician can say, "Some patients may have progression of their disease and possibly die within 6 months, but others may go on feeling fairly well and functioning well for 2 or more years." This helps the patient and family not to focus on a single number ("They said I only had 13 months to live") and to avoid some of the feeling of impending doom.

V. Toxicity

A. Factors affecting toxicity. One of the characteristics that distinguishes cancer chemotherapeutic agents from most other drugs is the frequency and severity of anticipated side effects at usual therapeutic doses. Because of the severity of the side effects, it is critical to monitor the patient carefully for adverse reactions so that therapy can be modified before the toxicity becomes life threatening. Most toxicity varies according to the following factors:

1. Specific agent
2. Dose
3. Schedule of administration
4. Route of administration
5. Predisposing factors in the patient, including genetic variants (e.g., homozygosity for the UGT1A1*28 allele, a variation of a uridine diphosphate glucuronosyltransferase gene and its corresponding enzyme (UGT1A1), which is responsible for glucuronidation of bilirubin and involved in deactivation of irinotecan's toxic active metabolite SN-38), which may be known and be predictive for toxicity or be unknown and resulting in unexpected toxic effects.

B. Clinical testing of new drugs for toxicity. Before the introduction of any agent into wide clinical use, the agent must undergo testing in carefully controlled clinical trials. The first set of clinical trials are called *phase I trials*. They are carried out with the express purpose of determining toxicity in humans and establishing the maximum tolerated dose, although with antineoplastic agents, they are done only in patients who might benefit from the drug. Such trials are undertaken only after extensive tests in animals have been completed. Much human toxicity is predicted by animal studies, but because of significant species differences, initial doses used in human studies are several times lower than doses at which toxicity is first seen in animals. Phase I trials are carried out using several schedules, and the dose is escalated in successive groups of patients once the toxicity of the prior dose has been established.

At the completion of phase I trials, there is usually a great deal of information about the spectrum and anticipated severity of acute drug effects (toxicity). However, because patients in phase I trials often do not live long enough to undergo many months of treatment, chronic or cumulative effects may not be discovered. Discovery of these toxicities may occur only after widespread use of the drug in phase II trials (to establish the spectrum of effectiveness of the drug), in phase III trials (to compare the new drug or combination with standard therapy), or from post marketing reports (when even larger numbers and less rigorously selected patients are treated).

C. Common acute toxicities. Some toxicities are relatively common among cancer chemotherapeutic agents. Common acute toxicities include the following:

1. Myelosuppression with leukopenia, thrombocytopenia, and anemia
2. Nausea, vomiting, and other gastrointestinal effects
3. Mucous membrane ulceration
4. Alopecia.

Aside from nausea and vomiting and acute cholinergic gastrointestinal effects, most of these toxicities occur because of the cytotoxic effects of chemotherapy on rapidly dividing normal cells of the bone marrow and epithelium (e.g., mucous membranes, skin, and hair follicles).

D. Selective toxicities. Other toxicities are less common and are specific to individual drugs or classes of drugs. Examples of drugs and their related toxicities include the following:

1. Anthracyclines and anthracenediones: cardiomyopathy
2. Asparaginase: anaphylaxis (allergic reaction), pancreatitis
3. Bleomycin: pulmonary fibrosis
4. Cisplatin: renal toxicity, neurotoxicity
5. Epidermal growth factor receptor (EGFR) inhibitors: acneiform rash
6. Fludarabine, cladribine, pentostatin: prolonged suppression of cellular immunity with heightened risk for opportunistic infection
7. Ifosfamide and cyclophosphamide: hemorrhagic cystitis
8. Ifosfamide: central nervous system toxicity
9. Mitomycin: hemolytic–uremic syndrome (HUS) and other endothelial cell injury phenomena
10. Monoclonal antibodies (e.g., rituximab, trastuzumab): hypersensitivity reactions
11. Paclitaxel: neurotoxicity, acute hypersensitivity reactions
12. Procarbazine: food and drug interactions
13. Vascular endothelial growth factor (VEGF) inhibitors: gastrointestinal perforation, impaired wound healing
14. Vinca alkaloids: neurotoxicity.

E. Recognition and evaluation of toxicity. Anyone who administers chemotherapeutic agents *must* be familiar with the expected and unusual toxicities of the agent the patient is receiving, be prepared to avert severe toxicity when possible, and be able to manage toxic complications when they cannot be avoided. The specific toxicities of commonly used individual chemotherapeutic agents are detailed in Chapter 4.

For the purpose of reporting toxicity in a uniform manner, *criteria* are often established to grade the severity of the toxicity. For many years, a simplified set of criteria was used by several National Cancer Institute (NCI)-supported clinical trial groups for the most common toxic manifestations. Although this document was helpful, it was, in many respects, incomplete. To address this issue, a new set of more comprehensive toxicity criteria was developed in 1999. An updated version of these criteria, Common Terminology Criteria for Adverse Events v3.0 (CTCAE) was published in 2003 and is now available on the Internet at *http://ctep.cancer.gov/reporting/ctc .html*. A host of other helpful information can be obtained on the Internet at *http://ctep.cancer.gov/*. All new clinical trials approved by the NCI Cancer Therapy Evaluation Program (CTEP) use these new toxicity criteria. Such standardization is important in the evaluation of the toxicity of cancer treatment.

F. Acute toxicity management. Prevention and treatment of bone marrow suppression can be partially achieved using filgrastim, sargramostim, epoetin, and oprelvekin. Treatment of its infectious, bleeding, and anemia consequences is discussed in Chapters 28 and 29. Management of nausea and vomiting, mucositis, and alopecia as well as diarrhea, nutrition problems, and drug extravasation are discussed in Chapter 27. Other acute toxicities are discussed with the individual drugs in Chapter 4. Long-term medical problems are a special issue and are highlighted in the subsequent section.

VI. **Late physical effects of cancer treatment**

A. **Late organ toxicities.** Late organ toxicities may be minimized by limiting doses when thresholds are known. In most instances, however, individual patient effects cannot be predicted. Treatment is primarily symptomatic.

1. **Cardiac toxicity** (e.g., congestive cardiomyopathy) is most commonly associated with high total doses of the anthracyclines (doxorubicin, daunorubicin, epirubicin), but also with other agents, including high-dose cyclophosphamide, trastuzumab and imatinib. When mediastinal irradiation is combined with these chemotherapeutic agents, cardiac toxicity may occur at lower doses. Although evaluation of ventricular ejection fraction with echocardiography or nuclear radiography studies has been useful for closely monitoring the effects of the anthracyclines on the cardiac ejection fraction, studies have reported late onset of congestive heart failure during pregnancy or after the initiation of vigorous exercise programs in adults who were previously treated for cancer as children or young adults. The cardiac reserve in these previously treated patients with cancer may be marginal. It is probable that there are some changes that take place even at low doses, and it is only because of the great reserve in cardiac function that effects are not measurable until higher doses have been used. Mediastinal

irradiation also may accelerate atherogenesis and lead to premature symptomatic coronary artery disease.

Because of the large number of women with breast cancer who are treated with doxorubicin as part of an adjuvant chemotherapeutic regimen, this group is of special concern and warrants ongoing clinical follow-up.

2. Pulmonary toxicity has been classically associated with high doses of bleomycin (>400 U). However, a number of other agents have been associated with pulmonary fibrosis (e.g., alkylating agents, methotrexate, nitrosoureas). Premature respiratory insufficiency, especially with exertion, may become evident with aging.

3. Nephrotoxicity is a potential toxicity of several agents (e.g., cisplatin, methotrexate, nitrosoureas). These agents can be associated with both acute and chronic toxicities. Other nephrotoxic agents such as amphotericin or aminoglycosides may exacerbate the problem. Even usually benign agents such as the bisphosphonates may be a problem. Rarely, some patients may require hemodialysis as a result of chronic toxicity.

4. Neurotoxicity has been particularly associated with the vinca alkaloids, cisplatin, oxaliplatin, epipodophyllotoxins, and taxanes. Peripheral neuropathy can cause considerable sensory and motor disability. Autonomic dysfunction may produce debilitating postural hypotension. Whole-brain irradiation, with or without chemotherapy, can be a cause of progressive dementia and dysfunction in some long-term survivors. This is particularly a problem for patients with primary brain tumors and for some patients with small cell lung cancer who have received prophylactic therapy. Survivors of childhood leukemia have developed a variety of neuropsychological abnormalities related to central nervous system prophylaxis that included whole-brain irradiation.

It has become evident over the years that some patients (up to one in five) who have received adjuvant chemotherapy for carcinoma of the breast also have measurable cognitive deficits such as difficulties with memory or concentration. This appears to be greater for women who have received high-dose chemotherapy than for those women who have received standard-dose chemotherapy, and in both groups, the incidence is higher than in control women. It is not uncommon for patients to refer to the effects of chemotherapy with complaints about memory being worse than it was, not being able to calculate numbers in their head, or just having "chemo-brain."

5. Hematologic and immunologic impairment is usually acute and temporally related to the cancer treatment (e.g., chemotherapy or radiation therapy). In some instances, however, there can be persistent cytopenias, as with alkylating agents. Immunologic impairment is a long-term problem for patients with Hodgkin's disease, which may be due to the underlying disease as well as to the treatments that are used. Fludarabine, cladribine, and pentostatin cause profound suppression of CD4 and CD8 lymphocytes and render patients treated susceptible to opportunistic infections. Patients who have undergone splenectomy are also at risk of overwhelming bacterial infections. Complete immunologic reconstitution may take 2 years after marrow-ablative therapy requiring stem cell reconstitution.

B. Second malignancies

1. Acute myelogenous leukemia may occur secondary to combined-modality treatment (e.g., radiation therapy and chemotherapy in Hodgkin's lymphoma) or prolonged therapy with alkylating agents or nitrosoureas (e.g., for multiple myeloma). In general, this form of treatment-related acute leukemia arises in the setting of myelodysplasia and is refractory even to intensive treatment. Treatment with the epipodophyllotoxins has also been associated with the development of acute nonlymphocytic leukemia. This may be the result of a specific gene rearrangement between chromosome 9 and chromosome 11 that creates a new cancer-causing oncogene: ALL-1/AF-9. The peak time of occurrence of secondary acute leukemia in patients with Hodgkin's lymphoma is 5 to 7 years after treatment, with an actuarial risk of 6% to 12% by 15 years. Therefore, a slowly developing anemia in a survivor of Hodgkin's lymphoma should alert the clinician to the possibility of a secondary myelodysplasia or leukemia.

Fortunately, the risk of secondary leukemias in women treated with standard adjuvant therapy for breast cancer (e.g., cyclophosphamide, methotrexate, and fluorouracil) is not much higher than that in the general population. Treatments using higher-than-standard doses of cyclophosphamide (with doxorubicin) or nonstandard drugs (such as mitoxantrone) as adjuvant therapy in breast cancer and high-dose chemotherapy used as preparative therapy for autologous peripheral blood progenitor cell transplant have been associated with increased risk of acute nonlymphocytic leukemia and myelodysplasia.

2. Solid tumors and other malignancies are seen with increased frequency in survivors who have been treated with chemotherapy or radiation therapy. Non–Hodgkin's lymphomas have been reported as a late complication in patients treated for Hodgkin's lymphoma or multiple myeloma. Patients treated with long-term cyclophosphamide are at risk of bladder cancer. Patients who have received mantle irradiation for Hodgkin's lymphoma have an increased risk of breast cancer, thyroid cancer, osteosarcoma, bronchogenic carcinoma, colon cancer, and mesothelioma. In these cases, the second neoplasm is usually in the irradiated field. In general, the risk of solid tumors begins to increase during the second decade of survival after Hodgkin's lymphoma. As a result, young women who have received mantle irradiation for Hodgkin's lymphoma should be screened more carefully for breast cancer, starting at an age earlier than what is advised in standard screening recommendations.

C. Other sequelae

1. Endocrine problems may result from cancer treatment. Patients receiving radiation therapy to the head and neck region may develop subclinical or clinical hypothyroidism. This is a particular risk in patients receiving mantle irradiation for Hodgkin's lymphoma. Biennial assessment of thyroid-stimulating hormone should be undertaken in these patients. Thyroid replacement therapy should be given if the thyroid-stimulating hormone level rises, to decrease the risk of thyroid cancer. Short stature may be a result of pituitary irradiation and growth hormone deficiency.

2. Premature menopause may occur in women who have received certain chemotherapeutic agents (e.g., alkylating agents, procarbazine) or abdominal and pelvic irradiation. The risk is age related, with women older than 30 years at the time of treatment having the greatest risk of treatment-induced amenorrhea and menopause. Early hormone replacement therapy should be considered in such women, if not otherwise contraindicated, to reduce the risk of accelerated osteoporosis and premature heart disease from estrogen deficiency.

3. Gonadal failure or dysfunction can lead to infertility in both male and female cancer survivors during their peak reproductive years. Azoospermia is common, but the condition may improve over time after the completion of therapy. Retroperitoneal lymph node dissection in testicular cancer may produce infertility due to retrograde ejaculation. Psychological counseling should be provided to these patients to help them adjust to these long-term sequelae of therapy. Cryopreservation of sperm before treatment should be considered in men. For women, there are limited means available to preserve ova or protect against ovarian failure associated with treatment. Abdominal irradiation in young girls can lead to loss of pregnancy due to decreased uterine capacity.

4. The musculoskeletal system can be affected by radiation therapy, especially in children and young adults. Radiation may injure the growth plates of long bones and lead to muscle atrophy. Short stature may be a result of direct injury to bone.

Acknowledgment: The author is indebted to Dr. Patricia A. Ganz who contributed to previous editions of this chapter. Most of the section on the late consequences of cancer treatment represents Dr. Ganz's work and has been included verbatim in this revision of the handbook.

SUGGESTED READINGS

Cancer Therapy Evaluation Program. *Common Terminology Criteria for Adverse Events v3.0 (CTCAE)*. *http://ctep.cancer.gov/reporting/ctc.html*. 2003.

Centers for Disease Control and Prevention. *A national action plan for cancer survivorship: advancing public health strategies*. Atlanta: Centers for Disease Control and Prevention, 2004.

Curtis RE, Boice J-D Jr, Stovall M, et al. Risk of leukemia after chemotherapy and radiation treatment for breast cancer. *N Engl J Med* 1992;326:1745–1751.

Ganz PA. A teachable moment for oncologists: cancer survivors, 10 million strong and growing! *J Clin Oncol* 2005;23:5458–5460.

Goldhirsch A, Gelber PD, Simes RJ, et al. Costs and benefits of adjuvant therapy in breast cancer: a quality-adjusted survival analysis. *J Clin Oncol* 1989;7:36–44.

Greene FL, Page DL, Fleming ID, et al. eds. *AJCC cancer staging manual*, 6th ed. New York: Springer-Verlag, 2002.

Hewitt M, Greenfield S, Stovall S. *From cancer patient to cancer survivor: lost in transition.* Washington, DC: Committee on Cancer Survivorship, Improving Care and Quality of Life, Institute of Medicine and National Research Council, 2005.

Hudson MM, Mertens AC, Yasui Y, et al. Health status of adults who are long-term childhood cancer survivors: a report from the childhood cancer survivor study. *JAMA* 2003;290:1583–1592.

van Leeuwen FE, Klokman JW, Hagenbeek A, et al. Second cancer risk following Hodgkin's disease: a 20-year follow-up study. *J Clin Oncol* 1994;12:312–325.

Loescher LJ, Welch-McCaffrey D, Leigh SA, et al. Surviving adult cancers. Part 1: physiologic effects. *Ann Intern Med* 1989;111: 411–432.

Neglia JP, Friedman DL, Yasui Y, et al. Second malignant neoplasms in five-year survivors of childhood cancer: childhood cancer survivor study. *J Natl Cancer Inst* 2001;93:618–629.

Nieman CL, Kazer R, Brannigan RE, et al. Cancer survivors and infertility: a review of a new problem and novel answers. *J Support Oncol* 2006;4:171–178.

Oeffinger KC, Mertens AC, Sklar CA, et al. Prevalence and severity of chronic diseases in adult survivors of childhood cancer: a report from the childhood cancer survivor study. *J Clin Oncol* 2005;23:3s. (Abstract 9).

Oken MM, Creech RH, Tormey DC, et al. Toxicity and response criteria of the Eastern Cooperative Oncology Group. *Am J Clin Oncol* 1982;5:649–655.

Pedersen-Bjergaard J, Sigsgaard TC, Nielsen D, et al. Acute monocytic or myelomonocytic leukemia with balanced chromosome translocations to band 11q23 after therapy with 4-epidoxorubicin and cisplatin or cyclophosphamide for breast cancer. *J Clin Oncol* 1992;10:1444–1451.

Pui CH, Ribeiro RC, Hancock ML, et al. Acute myeloid leukemia in children treated with epipodophyllotoxins for acute lymphoblastic leukemia. *N Engl J Med* 1991;325:1682–1687.

Schagen SB, van Dam FS, Muller MJ, et al. Cognitive deficits after postoperative adjuvant chemotherapy for breast carcinoma. *Cancer* 1999;85:640–650.

Tallman MS, Gray R, Bennett JM, et al. Leukemogenic potential of adjuvant chemotherapy for early-stage breast cancer: the Eastern Cooperative Oncology Group experience. *J Clin Oncol* 1995;13:1557–1563.

Therasse P, Arbuck SG, Eisenhauer EA, et al. New guidelines to evaluate the response to treatment in solid tumors. *J Natl Cancer Inst* 2000;92:205–216.

CHAPTER 3

Selection of Treatment for the Patient with Cancer

Roland T. Skeel

I. Setting treatment goals

A. Patient perspective. Although most often patients come to the physician looking for a medical perspective on what can be done about their cancer, it is critical that physicians and other health care professionals remember that unless we know what the patient's goals are, our ideas and plans of therapy may not address the patient's needs. As a consequence, it is critical for the physician to ask the patient to participate in setting treatment goals because it is the patient who must undergo the rigors of treatment and be willing to abide by its consequences. Whereas the physician's medical recommendations are most commonly accepted, some patients reject them as inappropriate for them for a variety of reasons. Some ask the physician for another recommendation, and others seek the opinion of a second physician. The physician must clearly present the reasons for the treatment recommendations and why they seem to be the best ways to achieve the treatment objective. The physician has the obligation to make a treatment recommendation, but the patient always has the right to reject that advice without fear that the physician will be upset, will dislike the patient, or will refuse to continue to give the patient care.

B. Medical perspective. Before a physician decides on a course of treatment to recommend for a patient with cancer, an achievable medical goal of treatment must be clearly defined. If the goal is to cure the patient of cancer, the strategy of therapy is likely to be different from the strategy chosen if the purpose is to prolong life, or to relieve symptoms. To propose the goal of therapy, the physician must be

- familiar with the natural history and behavior of the cancer to be treated
- knowledgeable about the principles and practice of therapy for each of the treatment modalities that may be effective in that cancer
- well grounded in the ethical principles of the treatment of patients with cancer
- familiar with the theory and use of antineoplastic agents
- informed about the particular therapy for the cancer in question
- aware of the patient's individual circumstances, including stage of disease, performance status, social situation, psychological status, and concurrent illnesses.

Armed with this information and with the treatment goals in mind, the physician can develop a course of treatment, and make a recommendation to the patient.

Components of the treatment plan include the following:

1. Should the cancer be treated at all, and, if so, is the treatment to be designed for cure, prolongation of life, or palliation of symptoms?
2. How aggressive should the therapy be to achieve the defined objective?
3. Which modalities of therapy will be used and in what sequence?
4. How will the treatment efficacy be determined?
5. What are the criteria for deciding the duration of therapy?

II. Choice of cancer treatment modality

A. Surgery. The oldest, most established, and still most effective way to cure most cancers is surgery. Surgery is selected as the treatment if the cancer is limited to one area and if it is anticipated that all cancer cells can be removed without unduly compromising vital structures. If it is believed that the patient can survive the surgery and return to a worthwhile life, surgery is recommended. Surgery is not recommended if the risk of surgery is greater than the risk of the cancer, if metastasis always occurs despite complete removal of the primary tumor, or if the patient will be left so debilitated, disfigured, or otherwise impaired that although cured of cancer, he or she feels that life is not worthwhile. If metastasis regularly (or always) occurs despite complete removal of the primary tumor, the benefits of removal of the gross tumor should be clearly defined before surgery is undertaken.

Most commonly, surgery is reserved for treatment of the primary neoplasm, although at times it may be used effectively to remove isolated metastases (e.g., in lung, brain, liver) with curative intent. Surgery is also used palliatively, such as for decompression of the brain in patients with glioma, or biliary bypass in patients with carcinoma of the pancreas. In nearly all nonhematologic cancers, a surgeon should be consulted to determine the role of surgery in the optimal treatment of the patient.

B. Radiotherapy. Radiotherapy is used for the treatment of local or regional disease when surgery cannot completely remove the cancer or when it would unduly disrupt normal structures or functions. In the treatment of some cancers, radiotherapy is as effective as surgery for eradicating the tumor. In this circumstance, factors such as the anticipated side effects of the treatment, the expertise and experience of local oncologists, and the preference of the patient may influence the choice of treatment.

One determinant of the appropriateness of radiotherapy is the inherent sensitivity of the cancer to ionizing radiation. Some kinds of cancer (e.g., the lymphomas and seminomas) are highly sensitive to radiotherapy. Other kinds (e.g., melanomas and sarcomas) tend to be less sensitive. Such considerations do not preclude the use of radiotherapy, however, and it is helpful to obtain an evaluation by the radiotherapist before initiating treatment so that treatment planning can take into consideration the possible contribution of this modality.

Although radiotherapy is frequently used as the primary or curative mode of therapy, it is also well suited to palliative management of problems such as bone metastases, superior vena cava syndrome, and local nodal metastases. The use of radiotherapy in the management of spinal cord compression and superior vena cava syndrome is discussed in Chapter 30.

C. Chemotherapy. Chemotherapy has as its primary role in the treatment of disease that is no longer confined to one site or region and has spread systemically. In the earliest days of chemotherapy, this interpretation directed its use to diseases that regularly presented in a disseminated form (e.g., leukemia) or after disease recurred following primary management with surgery or radiotherapy. It is now understood that widespread systemic micrometastases commonly occur early in cancer. These metastases are associated with certain predictive factors such as the axillary node metastases of carcinoma of the breast and the large tumor size and poorly differentiated histologic features of sarcomas or the cancer's genetic profile. Therefore, chemotherapy is now applied earlier to treat systemic disease. When this treatment is used for micrometastases, the response of an individual patient cannot be measured, unless the chemotherapy is used as a 'neoadjuvant,' that is, before surgery or radiotherapy. Then tumor response may predict more important end points such as time to treatment failure and survival. More commonly, when the chemotherapy is used as an adjuvant after removal of visible disease, the effectiveness of therapy must be determined by comparing the survival (or disease free survival) of patients who receive therapy with that of similar (control) patients who do not receive therapy for the micrometastases. Chemotherapy also has a role in the treatment of localized or regional disease. These specialized uses are discussed in Chapter 31.

D. Biologic response modifiers. It has long intrigued cancer biologists that cancer does not occur randomly but preferentially selects specific populations: the young, the elderly, the immunosuppressed (certain types of cancer only), and those with a strong family history of cancer. These observations have led cancer biologists to postulate that some kind of biologic control over or proclivity toward the emergence of cancer exists, which some people have and others do not, at least at the time the cancer becomes established. One prime candidate for the mechanism of biologic control of cancer has been immunity. That immunity plays some role in controlling the development of cancer has been clearly demonstrated in animal models and a few, although not most, human neoplasms. Other biologic factors, including those controlled by oncogenes and tumor suppressor genes and their protein products, which affect the cancer cell directly or its environment, are becoming better defined, and are even more important than classic immunity in the development of cancer.

In an attempt to exploit and enhance the biologic control that is presumed to exist to some degree in everyone, or to counteract cancer-promoting factors that facilitate cancer growth, invasion, and metastases, a variety of agents called *biologic response modifiers* have been used in the treatment of cancer. Two classes of biologic response modifiers, the interferons and lymphokines (of which interleukin 2 is an example), have been studied for many years, and there is evidence of their substantial activity in some types of cancer. Related, but separate, are molecular targeted agents that inhibit the activity of abnormally expressed protein products such as the constitutively activated Bcr-Abl tyrosine kinase in chronic myelogenous leukemia or other unique components of the cancer cell. This area of intensive research (as well as Wall Street interest) has begun to reach fruition and is expected to provide an increasingly important, although expensive, contribution to effective cancer therapy.

E. Combined-modality therapy. Neither surgery, radiotherapy, biotherapy, nor chemotherapy alone is appropriate for the treatment of all cancers. Frequently, patients present with cancer in which there is a bulky primary lesion, macroscopically evident regional disease, and presumed microscopic or submicroscopic systemic disease. For this reason, oncologists have turned to a multidisciplinary approach to the treatment of cancer, selecting two or more modalities of therapy for sequential or simultaneous use. This approach requires close cooperation among the surgical oncologist, radiation oncologist, and medical oncologist to provide the patient with the best overall treatment plan. Although combined-modality therapy is neither effective nor desirable for all kinds or stages of cancers, the regular practice of a multidisciplinary approach provides the best opportunity to exploit the advantages of each mode of treatment. "Tumor Boards" often serve as the forum for ensuring that patients will regularly have the benefit of various treatment perspectives.

III. Palliative care. The medical oncologist, who is also an internist, is often seen as the coordinator of cancer treatment. In this role, although the cancer is focused on, the broader perspective of the oncologist as a coordinator of the patient's care—in partnership with the patient—should not become obscured. Decisions about what therapy to use and how aggressively to treat the cancer are critically important to medically sound patient care. Decisions about when to stop active cancer treatment are also vitally important and may be among the most difficult responsibilities for the oncologist. It is critical that oncologists, who provide and profit from therapy, recognize the inherent conflict of interest in their dual role as care givers and drug salespersons.

Quality of life is often enhanced in patients responding to chemotherapy and other cancer treatments; it just as surely deteriorates more rapidly when the tumor does not respond to therapy and the patient experiences the toxicity of treatment along with the pain, fatigue, cachexia, and other symptoms of the cancer. For the 50% of patients with cancer who are not cured, the decision to stop antineoplastic therapy is just as important as the selection of chemotherapeutic regimens earlier in the disease. There comes a time when the best advice a physician can give is for the patient to forgo additional chemotherapy or any other active cancer treatment.

The introduction and rapid acceptance of hospice programs throughout the United States during the last 35 years reflect the need for this kind of care. Hospice programs have effectively addressed the special physical, psychological, social, and spiritual needs of patients approaching the end of life and have provided the unique skills required to maintain the best possible quality of life as long as possible. More recently, acute care hospitals have recognized that they, too, have patients who are at the end of life and need a special focus on the palliative aspects of their care. Yet, too often, physicians are reluctant to "give up" and are unable to recognize or accept when the patient will be helped more by an acknowledgment that active cancer therapy will not improve survival or enhance quality of life.

Oncologists and others caring for patients with cancer who have been trained as acute care physicians can learn specific techniques to enhance the quality of life from those who are experts in palliative care. For example, one might compare the quality of death in hospitalized patients given "maintenance" IV hydration with that of hospice home care patients offered oral fluids and mouth care to assuage thirst. The former method may result in an overhydrated, edematous patient who dies with an uncomfortable-sounding "death rattle" that is disconcerting to family and staff; the latter usually results in a visibly more comfortable patient who is more likely to die with less edema and without as much apparent respiratory distress.

Legitimate questions can also be raised about medical costs toward the end of life that are incurred when physicians give "futile" and "marginal" care. Development of guidelines by physicians and hospitals that define futile care, along with thoughtful consideration of when the therapy that is offered to patients has marginal value, may enable physicians to improve the quality of life for patients and at the same time hold down one component of the rising spiral of health care costs.

SUGGESTED READINGS

Brody H, Campbell ML, Faber-Langendoen K, et al. Withdrawing intensive life-sustaining treatment—recommendations for compassionate clinical management. *N Engl J Med* 1997;336:6.

Emanuel EJ, Patterson WB. Ethics of randomized clinical trials. *J Clin Oncol* 1998;16:365–366.

Jacobson M, O'Malley AJ, Earle CC, et al. Does reimbursement influence chemotherapy treatment for cancer patients? *Health Aff* 2006;25:437–443.

Lundberg GO. American health care system management objectives: the aura of inevitability becomes incarnate. *JAMA* 1993;269: 2254–2255.

Skeel RT. Measurement of quality of life outcomes. In: Berger AM, Portnoy RK, Weissman DE, eds. *Principles and practice of palliative care and supportive oncology*, 2nd ed. Philadelphia: Lippincott Williams & Wilkins, 2002:1107–1122.

Taylor LM, Feldstein ML, Skeel RT, et al. Fundamental dilemmas of the randomized clinical trial process: results of a survey of the 1737 Eastern Cooperative Oncology Group investigators. *J Clin Oncol* 1994;12:1776–1805.

Chemotherapeutic and Biotherapeutic Agents and Their Use

CHAPTER 4

Antineoplastic Drugs and Biologic Response Modifiers: Classification, Use, and Toxicity of Clinically Useful Agents

Roland T. Skeel

I. Classes of drugs. Chemotherapeutic agents are customarily divided into several classes. For two of the classes, the *alkylating agents* and the *antimetabolites*, the names indicate the mechanism of cytotoxic action of the drugs in their class. For *hormonal agents*, the name designates the physiologic behavior of the drug, and for *natural products*, the name reflects the source of the agents. The *biologic response modifiers* include agents that mimic, stimulate, enhance, inhibit, or otherwise alter host responses to the cancer. Several new agents have emerged that affect defined and putative abnormalities in the cancer cell and its environment and can best be classed as *molecularly targeted agents*. Drugs that do not fit easily into other categories are grouped together as *miscellaneous agents*. Data for individual agents are given in Section III of this chapter.

Within each class are several types of agents (Table 4.1). As with the criteria for separating into classes, the types are also grouped according to the mechanism of action, biochemical structure or derivation, and physiologic action. In some instances, these groupings into classes and types are arbitrary, and some drugs seem to fit into either more than one category or none. However, the classification of chemotherapeutic agents in this manner is helpful in several respects. For example, because the antimetabolites interfere with purine and pyrimidine metabolism and the formation of deoxyribonucleic acid (DNA) and ribonucleic acid (RNA), they are all at least cell cycle–specific and in some instances primarily cell cycle

Table 4.1. *(Continued)*

Class and Type	Agents
Luteinizing hormone–releasing hormone agonist	Goserelin, leuprolide, triptorelin
Polypeptide hormone release suppression	Octreotide
Progestin	Megestrol acetate, medroxyprogesterone acetate
Thyroid hormones	Levothyroxine, liothyronine
Molecularly targeted agents	
Gene expression modulators	Retinoids, rexinoids
Interleukin 2 receptor toxin	Denileukin diftitox
Monoclonal antibody	Alemtuzumab, cetuximab, gemtuzumab, ibritumomab tiuxetan, panitumumab, trastuzumab, rituximab, ^{131}I-tositumomab
mTOR kinase inhibitor	Temsirolimus
Proteosome inhibitor	Bortezomib
Receptor tyrosine kinase inhibitors	Dasatinib, erlotinib, gefitinib, imatinib mesylate, lapatinib, semaxanib, sorafenib, sunitinib
Retinoic acid receptor expression modification	Tretinoin (ATRA)
Biologic response modifiers	
Interferons	Interferon α-2a, interferon α-2b
Interleukins	Aldesleukin (interleukin 2), oprelvekin, denileukin diftitox
Myeloid- and erythroid-stimulating factors	Epoetin, filgrastim, sargramostim
Nonspecific immunomodulation	Thalidomide, lenalidomide
Miscellaneous agents	
Adrenocortical suppressant	Mitotane
Bisphosphonates	Pamidronate, zoledronic acid
Cytoprotector (reactive species antagonists)	Amifostine, dexrazoxane, mesna
Methylhydrazine derivative	Procarbazine
Photosensitizing agents	Porfimer
Platelet-reducing agent	Anagrelide
Salt	Arsenic trioxide
Somatostatin analog	Octreotide
Substituted melamine	Altretamine (hexamethylmelamine)
Substituted urea	Hydroxyurea

mTOR, mammalian target of rapamycin.

phase–specific. The nitrosourea group of alkylating agents, on the other hand, contains drugs that are predominantly or entirely cell cycle–nonspecific. Such knowledge can be helpful in planning therapy for tumors when sufficient kinetic information permits a rational selection of agents and when drugs are selected for use in combination.

The classification scheme may also help predict cross-resistance between drugs. Tumors that are resistant to one of the nitrogen mustard types of alkylating agents would therefore be likely to be resistant to another of that same type, but not necessarily to one of the other types of alkylating agents such as the nitrosoureas or the metal salts (e.g., cisplatin). The classification system does not help in predicting multidrug resistance, which may have several phenotypes.

A. **Alkylating agents**

1. **General description** alkylating agents are a diverse group of chemical compounds capable of forming molecular bonds with nucleic acids, proteins, and many molecules of low molecular weight. The compounds either are electrophiles themselves or generate electrophiles *in vivo* to produce polarized molecules with positively charged regions. These polarized molecules can then interact with electron-rich regions of most cellular molecules. The cytotoxic effect of the alkylating agents appears to relate primarily to the interaction between the electrophiles and DNA. This interaction may result in substitution reactions, cross-linking reactions, or strand-breaking reactions. The net effect of the alkylating agent's interaction with DNA is to alter the information coded in the DNA molecule. This alteration results in inhibition or inaccurate replication of DNA, with resultant mutation or cell death. One implication of the mutagenic capability of alkylating agents is the possibility that they are teratogenic and carcinogenic. Because they interact with preformed DNA, RNA, and protein, the alkylating agents are not phase-specific, and at least some are cell cycle–nonspecific.

2. **Types of alkylating agents**

a. **Nitrogen mustards.** These compounds produce highly reactive carbonium ions that react with the electron-rich areas of susceptible molecules. They vary in reactivity from mechlorethamine, which is highly unstable in aqueous form, to cyclophosphamide, which must be biochemically activated in the liver.

b. **Ethylenimine derivatives.** Triethylenethiophosphoramide (thiotepa) is the only compound in this group that has much clinical use. Ethylenimine derivatives are capable of the same kinds of reactions as the nitrogen mustards.

c. **Alkyl sulfonates.** Busulfan is the only clinically active compound in this group. It appears to interact more with cellular thiol groups than with nucleic acids.

d. **Triazines.** Dacarbazine, the only agent of this type, was originally thought to be an antimetabolite because of its resemblance to 5-aminoimidazole-4-carboxamide.

Dacarbazine is now known to act as an alkylator after 5-aminoimidazole-4-carboxamide is cleaved from active diazomethane.

e. Nitrosoureas. Nitrosoureas undergo rapid, spontaneous activation in aqueous solution to form products capable of alkylation and carbamoylation. They are unique among the alkylating agents with respect to not being cross-resistant with other alkylating agents, being highly lipid soluble, and having delayed myelosuppressive effects (6 to 8 weeks).

f. Metal salts. Cisplatin, carboplatin, and oxaliplatin inhibit DNA synthesis probably through the formation of intrastrand cross-links in DNA and formation of DNA adducts. They also react with DNA through chelation or binding to the cell membrane.

B. Antimetabolites

1. General description. Antimetabolites are a group of low-molecular-weight compounds that exert their effect by virtue of their structural or functional similarity to naturally occurring metabolites involved in nucleic acid synthesis. Because they are mistaken by the cell for normal metabolites, they either inhibit critical enzymes involved in nucleic acid synthesis or become incorporated into the nucleic acid and produce incorrect codes. Both mechanisms result in the inhibition of DNA synthesis and ultimate cell death. Because of their primary effect on DNA synthesis, antimetabolites are most active in cells that are actively growing and are largely cell cycle phase–specific.

2. Types of antimetabolites

a. Folic acid analogs. Methotrexate, the dominant member of this group, inhibits the enzyme dihydrofolate reductase. This inhibition blocks the production of reduced N-methylenetetrahydrofolate, the coenzyme in the synthesis of thymidylic acid. Other metabolic processes in which there is one–carbon unit transfer are also affected but are probably of less importance in the cytotoxic action of methotrexate. Ralitrexed (Tomudex) is a quinazoline antifolate that is an inhibitor of thymidylate synthase. Pemetrexed is a multitargeted pyrrolopyrimidine-based antifolate that, when polyglutamated, inhibits dihydrofolate reductase, thymidylate synthase, and glycinamide ribonucleotide formyltransferase.

b. Pyrimidine analogs. These compounds inhibit critical enzymes necessary for nucleic acid synthesis and may become incorporated into DNA and RNA.

c. Purine analogs. The specific site of action for the purine analogs is not as well defined as for most pyrimidine analogs, although it is well demonstrated that they interfere with normal purine interconversions and therefore with DNA and RNA synthesis. Some of the analogs are also incorporated into the nucleic acids. The adenosine deaminase (ADA) inhibitor pentostatin increases the intracellular concentration of deoxyadenosine

triphosphates in lymphoid cells and inhibits DNA synthesis, probably by blocking ribonucleotide reductase.
Among the metabolic alterations is nicotinamide adenine dinucleotide (NAD) depletion, which may result
in cell death. Cladribine accumulates in cells as the
triphosphate, is incorporated into DNA, and inhibits
DNA repair enzymes and RNA synthesis. As with pentostatin, NAD levels are also depleted.

C. **Natural products**
  1. **General description.** The natural products are grou-
     ped together not on the basis of activity but because they are
     derived from natural sources. The clinically useful drugs
     are plant products, fermentation products of various species
     of the soil fungus *Streptomyces*, and bacterial products.
  2. **Types of natural products**
     a. **Mitotic inhibitors.** Vincristine, vinblastine, and
        their semisynthetic derivatives vindesine and vinorel-
        bine are derived from the periwinkle plant (*Catharan-
        thus roseus*), a species of myrtle. They appear to act
        primarily through their effect on microtubular protein
        with a resultant metaphase arrest and inhibition of
        mitosis.
     b. *Podophyllum* **derivatives.** Etoposide and tenipo-
        side, semisynthetic podophyllotoxins derived from the
        root of the May apple plant (*Podophyllum peltatum*),
        form a complex with topoisomerase II, an enzyme that
        is necessary for the completion of DNA replication. This
        interaction results in DNA strand breakage and arrest
        of cells in late S and early G_2 phases of the cell cycle.
     c. **Camptothecins (CPTs).** These agents are analogs
        of CPT, a derivative of the Chinese tree *Camptotheca
        accuminata*. The primary target of the two clinically
        active agents, irinotecan and topotecan, is DNA topoiso-
        merase I.
     d. **Antibiotics.** The antitumor antibiotics are a group
        of related antimicrobial compounds produced by *Strepto-
        myces* species in culture. Their cytotoxicity, which limits
        their antimicrobial usefulness, has proved to be of great
        value in treating a wide range of cancers. All of the clini-
        cally useful antibiotics affect the function and synthesis
        of nucleic acids.
        (1) **Dactinomycin, the anthracyclines (doxoru-
            bicin, daunorubicin, epirubicin, and idaru-
            bicin), and the anthracenedione mitoxantrone**
            cause topoisomerase II–dependent DNA cleavage
            and intercalate with the DNA double helix.
        (2) **Bleomycins** cause DNA strand scission. The
            resulting fragmentation is believed to underlie the
            cytotoxic activity of the drug.
        (3) **Mitomycin** causes cross-links between comple-
            mentary strands of DNA that impair replication.
     e. **Enzymes.** Asparaginase, the one example of this
        type of agent, catalyzes the hydrolysis of asparagine to
        aspartic acid and ammonia and deprives selected ma-
        lignant cells of an amino acid that is essential for their
        survival.

D. Hormones and hormone antagonists

1. General description. The hormones and hormone antagonists that are clinically active against cancer include steroid estrogens, progestins, androgens, corticoids and their synthetic derivatives, nonsteroidal synthetic compounds with steroid or steroid-antagonist activity, hypothalamic–pituitary analogs, and thyroid hormones. Each agent has diverse effects. Some effects are mediated directly at the cellular level by the drug binding to specific cytoplasmic receptors or by inhibition or stimulation of the production or action of the hormones. These agents may also act by stimulating or inhibiting natural autocrine and paracrine growth factors (e.g., epidermal growth factor, transforming growth factors [TGF]-α and -β). The relative roles of the various actions of hormones and hormone antagonists are only partially understood and probably vary among tumor types. For estrogen receptor antagonists such as tamoxifen, which, when bound to the estrogen receptor, ultimately controls the promoter region of genes that affect cell growth, there are a host of modulating factors including approximately 20 receptor-interacting proteins and 50 transcription-activating factors, as well as many response elements. Other effects are mediated through indirect effects on the hypothalamus and its anterior pituitary–regulating hormones. The final common pathway in most circumstances appears to lead to the malignant cell, which has retained some sensitivity to direct or indirect hormonal control of its growth. An exception to this mechanism is the effect of corticosteroids on leukemias and lymphomas, in which the steroids appear to have direct lytic effects on abnormal lymphoid cells that have high numbers of glucocorticoid receptors.

2. Types of hormones and hormone antagonists

a. Androgens may exert their antineoplastic effect by altering pituitary function or directly affecting the neoplastic cell.

b. Antiandrogens inhibit nuclear androgen binding.

c. Corticosteroids cause lysis of lymphoid tumors that are rich in specific cytoplasmic receptors and may have other indirect effects as well.

d. Estrogens suppress testosterone production (through the hypothalamus) in men and alter breast cancer cell response to prolactin.

e. Progestins appear to act directly at the level of the malignant cell receptor to promote differentiation.

f. Estrogen antagonists compete with estrogen for binding on the cytosol estrogen receptor protein in cancer cells. The receptor/hormone complex ultimately controls the promoter region of genes that affect cell growth.

g. Aromatase inhibitors are nonsteroidal inhibitors of the aromatization of androgens to estrogens. Aminoglutethimide is relatively nonselective, having many biochemical sites of inhibition of steroidogenesis. Its use requires corticosteroid replacement. In contrast, the selective aromatase inhibitors such as anastrozole or letrozole primarily block the conversion of adrenally generated androstenedione to estrone by aromatase in peripheral tissues without inhibition of progesterone or corticosteroid synthesis.

h. Hypothalamic hormone analogs, such as the luteinizing hormone–releasing hormone (LHRH) agonists leuprolide or goserelin, can inhibit luteinizing hormone and follicle-stimulating hormone (after initial stimulation) and the production of testosterone or estrogen by the gonads.

i. Thyroid hormones inhibit the release of thyroid-stimulating hormone, thereby inhibiting the growth of well-differentiated thyroid tumors.

E. Molecularly targeted agents

1. General. This is a new classification in oncology that has become possible because of maturation of knowledge about the molecular events that are responsible for the development of cancer. Understanding of the genetic changes in the cancer cell, the downstream molecular events that follow as a consequence, and the mechanisms by which these events regulate cell growth and death has led to a host of possibilities for the control of cancer growth.

2. Tyrosine kinase inhibitors. The first clinical example of this is the signal transduction inhibitor imatinib mesylate, which inactivates the constitutively active fusion product tyrosine kinase arising from the Philadelphia chromosome found in chronic myelogenous leukemia (CML), Bcr-Abl, as well as c-Kit kinase, which is overexpressed in gastrointestinal stromal tumors (GISTs). A second promising target is the epidermal growth factor receptor (EGFR)–associated tyrosine kinase, because of its overexpression in a large variety of cancers. A number of small-molecule inhibitors of its enzymatic activity are in clinical use or are under development. One of these, erlotinib, which inhibits intracellular phosphorylation of the tyrosine kinase associated with EGFR, has demonstrated efficacy in non–small cell lung cancer and pancreatic cancer.

Other receptors such as the vascular endothelial growth factor (VEGF) receptor are stimulated by an increase in VEGF, which in turn is stimulated, among other things, by hypoxia and tumor cell products. The result is to increase angiogenesis and facilitate further tumor growth. Inhibitors of VEGF receptor tyrosine kinases (RTKs) (as well as other receptor tyrosine kinases), such as sunitinib, result in prolonged time to progression in gastrointestinal stromal tumors (GISTs) that have shown progression during prior treatment with imatinib or in patients who are intolerant to imatinib, and renal cell carcinoma.

3. Monoclonal antibodies. Monoclonal antibodies have emerged over the last 10 to 15 years as useful adjuncts to the medical oncologist's armamentarium. These agents, which may be directed at growth factors or their receptors, are derived from murine antibodies, may have varying levels of humanization (chimerism) and may be unconjugated (alemtuzumab, bevacizumab, cetuximab, rituximab, trastuzumab) or conjugated with radionuclides (ibritu-momab tiuxetan, tositumomab) or another toxic moiety (gemtuzumab).

4. Other agents. Other agents affect nuclear activity, such as the binding of all-*trans*-retinoic acid with cytoplasmic proteins, which in turn interact with nuclear retinoic acid receptors (RARs) that affect expression of genes that control cell growth and differentiation.

F. Miscellaneous agents. Miscellaneous agents are listed in Table 4.1. Descriptions of specific agents are found in Section III of this chapter.

II. Clinically useful chemotherapeutic and biologic agents. Section III of this chapter contains an alphabetically arranged description of the chemotherapeutic and biologic agents that are recognized to be clinically useful. Each drug is listed by its generic name, with other common names or trade names included. A brief description is given of the probable mechanism of action, clinical uses, recommended doses, and schedules, precautions, and side effects.

A. Recommended doses: CAUTION. Although every effort has been made to ensure that the drug dosages and schedules given here are accurate and in accord with published standards, readers are advised to check the product information sheet included in the package of each U.S. Food and Drug Administration (FDA)–approved drug. For drugs not yet approved for general use, FDA–National Cancer Institute (NCI) guidelines and any current medical literature should be used to verify recommended dosages, contraindications, and precautions, and to review potential toxicity.

B. Dose selection and designation. The doses are listed using body surface area (square meters) as the base for nearly all the agents included. Adult doses from the literature, which are expressed using a weight base, have been converted by multiplying the milligram-per-kilogram dose by 37 to give the milligram-per-square-meter dose. Doses using a weight base, which have been taken from the pediatric literature, have been converted using a factor of 25. Because many of the drugs are given in combination with other agents, doses most commonly used in popular combinations may also be indicated. These data should not be used as the sole source of information for any of the drugs but rather should be used as a guide to confirm and compare dose ranges and schedules and to identify potential problems. For some agents, the area-under-the-curve (AUC) method of dose calculation seems to be the most reliable for achieving the most accurate dosing and balance between efficacy and toxicity; when that is the standard, the AUC dose is used.

C. Drug toxicity: frequency designation. The designation of the frequency of toxic side effects is indicated as follows (probability of occurrence equals percentage of patients):

1. Universal (90%–100%)
2. Common (15%–90%)
3. Occasional (5%–15%)
4. Uncommon (1%–5%)
5. Rare (<1%)

These designations are meant only to be guides, and the likelihood of a side effect in each patient depends on that patient's physical status, including comorbidities, treatment history, dose, schedule, and route of drug administration, and other concurrent treatment.

D. Dose modification

1. Philosophy. The optimal dose and schedule of a drug are those that give maximum benefit with tolerable toxicity. Most chemotherapeutic agents have a steep dose–response curve; therefore, if no toxicity is seen, as a rule, a higher dose should be given to get the best possible therapeutic benefit. If toxicity is great, however, the patient's life may be threatened or the patient may decide that the treatment is worse than the disease and refuse further therapy. How much toxicity the patient and the physician are willing to tolerate depends on the likelihood that more intensive treatment will make a major therapeutic difference (e.g., cure vs. no cure) and on the patient's physical and psychological tolerance for adverse effects.

The general grading scheme for all toxicity is as follows:

0—None
1—Mild
2—Moderate
3—Severe
4—Life threatening

2. Guidelines

a. Nonhematologic toxicity

(1) Acute effects. Acute drug toxicity that is limited to 1 to 2 days and is not cumulative is not usually a cause of dose modification unless it is of grade 3 or 4, that is, severe or life threatening (see Common Terminology Criteria for Adverse Events v3.0 (CTCAE) at *http://ctep.cancer.gov/reporting/ctc.html* for individual toxicities.) Occasionally, repeating a dose that caused intractable nausea and vomiting or a temperature higher than 40°C (104°F) is warranted, but for most other grade 3 or 4 toxicity, the subsequent doses should be reduced by 25% to 50%. If the acute drug effects (e.g., severe paresthesias or abnormalities of renal or liver function) last longer than 48 hours, the subsequent doses should be reduced by 35% to 50%.

A recurrence of the grade 3 or 4 side effects at the reduced doses would be an indication either to reduce by another 25% to 50% or to discontinue the drug altogether. Non–dose-related toxicity such as anaphylaxis is an indication to discontinue the offending drug. Lesser degrees of hypersensitivity can often be dealt with effectively by increasing the dose of protective agents (such as dexamethasone or diphenhydramine) or slowing the rate of infusion. For some biologic agents, such as trastuzumab, physiologic effects that look like hypersensitivity reactions occur primarily on first or second doses of treatment and diminish with continued treatment.

(2) Chronic effects. Chronic or cumulative toxicity such as pulmonary function changes with bleomycin or decreased cardiac function with doxorubicin is nearly always an indication to discontinue the responsible agent. Chronic or cumulative neurotoxicity due to vincristine, cisplatin, paclitaxel, or other agents may require no dose change, reduction, or discontinuation, depending on the severity of the resultant neurologic dysfunction and the patient's ability to tolerate it.

b. Hematologic toxicity. The degree of myelosuppression and attendant risk of infection and bleeding that are acceptable depend on the cancer, the duration of myelosuppression, the goals of therapy, and the general health of the patient. In addition, one must consider the relative benefit of less aggressive or more aggressive therapy. For example, with acute nonlymphocytic leukemia, remission is unlikely unless sufficient therapy is given to cause profound pancytopenia for at least 1 week. Because there is little benefit with lesser treatment, grade 4 leukopenia and thrombocytopenia are acceptable toxicities in this circumstance. Grade 4 myelosuppression is also acceptable when the goal is cure of a cancer that does not involve the marrow, such as testicular carcinoma. With breast cancer, on the other hand, responses are seen with less aggressive treatment, and prolonged pancytopenia may not be acceptable, particularly if chemotherapy is being used palliatively or in an adjuvant setting in which the proportion of patients expected to benefit from chemotherapy is relatively small and excessive toxicity would pose an unacceptable risk.

With these caveats in mind, the dose modification schemes shown in Tables 4.2 and 4.3 can serve as a guide to reasonable dose changes for drugs whose major toxicity is myelosuppression. Separate schemes are given for the nitrosoureas and for drugs that have more prolonged myelosuppression.

III. Data for clinically useful chemotherapeutic and biologic agents. *Note:* Although every effort has been made to ensure that the drug dosage and schedules herein are accurate and in accord with published standards, users are advised to check the product information sheet included in the package of each FDA-approved drug and FDA-NCI guidelines for drugs that are not yet approved for general use to verify recommended dosages, contraindications, and precautions.

Agents that have not yet been approved by the FDA are included because they either have some demonstrated usefulness or are widely used in investigational studies. As their efficacy and toxicity are more firmly established, it is expected that some will be approved by the FDA for general use, whereas others will remain investigational or be dropped from further study.

Table 4.2. Dose modifications for myelosuppressive drugs with a nadir[a] at less than 3 weeks

Degree of Suppression	ANC (WBC)/µL on Day of Scheduled Treatment[b]		Platelets/µL on Day of Scheduled Treatment	Dose as percentage of immediately preceding cycle
Minimal	$\geq$1,500 ($\geq$3,500)	and	$\geq$100,000	100
Mild	1,200–1,500 (3,000–3,500)	or	75,000–100,000	75
Moderate	1,000–1,200 (2,500–3,000)	or	50,000–75,000	50
Severe	<1,000 (<2,500)	or	<50,000	0 (delay 1 wk)

ANC, absolute neutrophil count; WBC, white blood cell count.

[a]If the nadir of ANC is <1,000/µL and is associated with fever of >38.3°C (101°F) or the nadir of platelets is <40,000/µL, decrease dose by 25% in subsequent cycles. If the dose is already to be reduced on the basis of the ANC or platelet count on the day of treatment as per this table, do not reduce further because of the nadir count.

[b]ANC is the preferred parameter, if available. If counts are rising at the end of a treatment cycle, it is often appropriate to delay 1 wk and then treat according to the dose modification scheme shown here.

Table 4.3. Dose modifications for myelosuppressive drugs[a] with a nadir at 3 weeks or later

Point in Time	ANC (WBC)/μL		Platelets/μL		Dose as Percentage of Immediately Preceding Cycle
I. On day of scheduled treatment[b]	≥1,800(≥3,500)	*and*	≥100,000		Dose modified for nadir only
	<1,800 (<3,500)	*or*	<100,000		0[c]
II. At last nadir	>750	*and*	>75,000		100
	500–750	*or*	40,000–75,000		75
	<500	*or*	<40,000		50
III. After 2-wk delay	≥1,800 (≥3,500)	*and*	≥100,000		Dose modified for nadir only
	1,200–1,800 (2,500–3,500)	*or*	75,000–100,000		75
	<1,200	*or*	<75,000		Continue to hold

ANC, absolute neutrophil count; WBC, white blood cell count.
[a] Nitrosoureas or other agents with prolonged nadir.
[b] ANC is the preferred parameter to use.
[c] Withhold treatment and repeat count in 2 wk. At 2 wk, treat on basis of lowest dose indicated by nadir (II) or delay (III) section of table.

ALDESLEUKIN

Other name. Interleukin 2 (IL-2), Proleukin.

Mechanism of action. Enhances mitogenesis of T cells, natural killer (NK) cells, and lymphokine-activated killer (LAK) cells; augments cytotoxicity of NK and LAK cells; induces interferon-γ.

Primary indication.

1. Renal cell carcinoma.
2. Melanoma.

Usual dosage and schedule. A wide range of doses and routes (IV or SC) have been used. In any of the schedules, therapy may be stopped prematurely for severe constitutional symptoms or for cardiovascular, renal, hepatic, neurologic, pulmonary, or hematologic toxicity.

1. 600,000 IU/kg (22×10^6 IU/m^2) as a 15-min IV infusion every 8 h for up to 14 doses on days 1 to 5. Repeat on days 15 to 19. Repeat cycle in 6 to 12 weeks if the disease is stable or is responding.
2. 18×10^6 IU/m^2/24 h as a continuous IV infusion daily for up to 5 days. Repeat in 4 weeks. Repeat cycle in 4 to 6 weeks if the disease is stable or is responding.
3. 22×10^6 IU/m^2 as a 15-min infusion for 5 consecutive days for 2 successive weeks. Repeat every 3 to 6 weeks as tolerated. In some regimens, it is preceded on day 3 by a single dose of low-dose cyclophosphamide, 350 mg/m^2 IV push.
4. 9×10^6 IU/m^2 daily by continuous IV infusion on days 1 to 4 (96 h), together with chemotherapy (cisplatin, vinblastine, dacarbazine) and interferon in melanoma.

Schedules 1, 2, and 4 require hospitalization. Schedule 3 can be given in an outpatient setting but may require several hours of observation after treatment.

Special precautions. Patients must be carefully monitored after treatment using any of the dosing regimens. Outpatient regimens require that patients have cardiovascular status observed for up to 5 h, particularly after the first several doses. With higher doses, capillary leak syndrome resulting in hypotension, pulmonary edema, myocardial infarction, arrhythmias, azotemia, and alterations in mental status may occur. Intensive care, controlled volume replacement, and intubation may be required. The lower doses can be given in an outpatient setting.

Toxicity. All are dose dependent.

1. *Myelosuppression and other hematologic effects.* Uncommon at lower doses, common, but rarely serious at higher doses. Anemia requiring transfusion is common at higher doses. Thrombocytopenia is common at higher doses.
2. *Nausea, vomiting, and other gastrointestinal effects.*
   a. Anorexia, nausea, vomiting, and diarrhea are common.
   b. Transient liver function abnormalities, including hyperbilirubinemia, and hypoalbuminemia and elevation of the prothrombin time and partial thromboplastin time are common.
   c. Colonic perforations are rare.
3. *Mucocutaneous effects.* Mucositis is occasional to common. Alopecia is uncommon. Pruritic erythematous rash is common.

4. *Cardiovascular effects.*
   a. Arrhythmias are common and dose-related.
   b. Hypotension is dose-related but is occasionally seen with lower-dose schedules.
   c. Myocardial injury is seen primarily with higher-dose schedules.
   d. Pulmonary edema from capillary leak syndrome is common with intensive dose regimens.
   e. Weight gain is common from edema, particularly in more intensive dose regimens.
5. *Neuropsychiatric effects.*
   a. Changes in mental status are common, with dose-related severity.
   b. Dizziness or light-headedness is common.
   c. Blurry vision and other visual disturbances are occasional.
   d. Seizures are uncommon to rare at lower-dose regimens.
6. *Renal function impairment.* Common but reversible. More frequent laboratory abnormalities include creatinine elevation, hypomagnesemia, acidosis, hypocalcemia, hypophosphatemia, hypokalemia, hypouricemia, and hypoalbuminemia.
7. *Fever.* With or without chills—universal and may be severe.
8. *Bacterial infection.* Occasional. Probably related to chemotactic defect induced in granulocytes.
9. *Myalgias and arthralgias.* Occasional to common.
10. *Malaise and fatigue.* Common and dose related.

Prophylaxis of acute toxicity.
1. Acetaminophen, 650 mg PO before therapy and every 6 h for one or two doses for outpatient IL-2 dosing; every 6 h for 3 doses for inpatient IL-2 regimens.
2. Cimetidine, 800 mg PO, or other histamine H_2-receptor antagonist before therapy and daily for duration of treatment.
3. Antiemetics. Granisetron, ondansetron, or other $5HT_3$ antagonist, metoclopramide, and prochlorperazine may be used. Do not use dexamethasone.
4. Meperidine, 25 to 50 mg IV, when chills start after first dose. For subsequent doses, meperidine, 50 mg PO 1.5 h before chills are predicated to start, based on the first treatment.
5. Hydromorphone 0.5 to 1 mg IV, may be substituted for meperidine in patients who tolerate the latter drug poorly.
6. Diphenoxylate with atropine (Lomotil), one tablet up to six times daily for diarrhea.
7. Hydroxyzine, 25 to 50 mg every 6 h for itching.

ALEMTUZUMAB

Other names. Campath, Campath-1H

Mechanism of action. Alemtuzumab is a chimeric (murine and human) monoclonal antibody directed against the CD52 antigen found on the surface of 95% of B and T lymphocytes. It is also expressed in other normal cells found in the peripheral blood and marrow, and some other somatic cells. Cellular cytotoxicity is mediated through complement-mediated lysis, antibody-dependent cellular cytotoxicity (ADCC), and induction of apoptosis.

Primary indications.

1. B-cell chronic lymphocytic leukemia that has previously been treated with alkylating agents and has failed fludarabine therapy.
2. T-cell prolymphocytic leukemia
3. Multiple myeloma
4. Nonmalignant conditions, including rheumatoid arthritis and graft-versus-host disease

Usual dosage and schedule. (Malignant conditions only)

1. Initiation. 3 mg as a 2-h IV infusion daily.
2. Escalation. When infusion-related toxicities are less severe than grade 2, the dose is escalated to 10 mg as a 2-h IV infusion daily. When the 10-mg dose is tolerated, maintenance therapy is initiated.
3. Maintenance. 30 mg as a 2-h IV infusion three times a week on alternate days for 12 weeks.

Infusion-related events (see following text) are ameliorated by pretreatment with antihistamines, acetaminophen, and antiemetics, as well as incremental dose escalation.

Special Precautions. Must not be administered as IV push or bolus dose. Single doses of more than 30 mg and cumulative doses of more than 90 mg/week should not be given. If therapy is interrupted for 7 or more days, the dose initiation and escalation scheme is required to avert toxicity. Alemtuzumab is contraindicated in patients who have active systemic infections, underlying immunodeficiency, or known type I hypersensitivity or anaphylactic reactions to the drug or any of its components.

Toxicity.

1. *Myelosuppression and other hematologic effects.* Lymphopenia is universal. Neutropenia, anemia, and thrombocytopenia are common and are often severe (grade 3 or greater). Opportunistic and other infections, including pneumonia and sepsis, are seen in 10% to 15% of patients. Autoimmune hemolytic anemia and thrombocytopenia are uncommon (1%–2%). Pancytopenia and marrow hypoplasia are uncommon, but may require permanent discontinuation of therapy. Because of the high incidence of opportunistic infections, antiherpes and anti–*Pneumocystis carinii* pneumonia (PCP) prophylaxis is recommended.[1]
2. *Nausea, vomiting, and other gastrointestinal effects.* Nausea and vomiting are common; diarrhea, abdominal pain, and dyspepsia are occasional.
3. *Mucocutaneous effects.* Rash, urticaria, pruritus, and increased sweating are common. Stomatitis is occasional.
4. *Infusion-related events.* Rigors, fever, nausea and vomiting, and rash—including urticaria—are common. Shortness of breath, hypotension, bronchospasm, headache, pruritus, and diarrhea are occasional. Angioedema is uncommon.

---

[1]For PCP prophylaxis: trimethoprim-sulfamethoxazole DS, 1 PO b.i.d. Monday, Wednesday, Friday. If allergic, use Dapsone 100 mg MWF. For herpes zoster prophylaxis: famciclovir 500 mg PO b.i.d. or valacyclovir 500 mg PO t.i.d.

5. *Miscellaneous effects*.
   a. *Respiratory*. Dyspnea, cough, and bronchitis are common. Pneumonia, pharyngitis, bronchospasm, and rhinitis are occasional.
   b. *Cardiovascular*. Hypotension is common, hypertension occasional. Tachycardia and supraventricular tachycardia are occasional, but usually not severe. Syncope is uncommon.
   c. Hypersensitivity reactions to alemtuzumab may occur (2%) and result in hypersensitivity to other monoclonal antibodies.
   d. *Neuropsychiatric*. Insomnia, depression, and somnolence are occasional. Headache, dysesthesias, dizziness, and tremor are occasional .

ALITRETINOIN

Other names. 9-*cis*-retinoic acid, Panretin Gel.
Mechanism of action. Binds to cytoplasmic retinoic acid–binding proteins and is then transported to the nucleus where it interacts with nuclear retinoic acid receptors (RARs). These then affect expression of the genes that control cell growth and differentiation.
Primary indication. AIDS-related cutaneous Kaposi's sarcoma.
Usual dosage and schedule. Apply sufficient gel (0.1%) to cover lesion with a generous coating 2 to 4 times daily, according to individual lesion tolerance. Allow to dry for 3 to 5 min before covering with clothing.
Special Precautions. Women are advised to avoid becoming pregnant because of potential fetal risk. Minimize exposure to ultraviolet rays from sun or sun lamps.
Toxicity.
1. *Myelosuppression and other hematologic effects*. None.
2. *Nausea, vomiting, and other gastrointestinal effects*. None
3. *Mucocutaneous effects*. Skin reactions with erythema, scaling, irritation, redness, rash, or other dermatitis are common. Pruritus, exfoliative dermatitis, or other erosive or draining skin lesions are occasional.
4. *Miscellaneous effects*.
   a. Neurologic complaints of burning or pain are common.
   b. Edema is occasional.

ALTRETAMINE

Other names. Hexamethylmelamine, Hexalen, HXM.
Mechanism of action. Unknown. Although it structurally resembles the known alkylating agent triethylenemelamine, it has some antimetabolite characteristics.
Primary indication. Carcinoma of the ovary, persistent or recurrent after first-line therapy.
Usual dosage and schedule.
1. 260 mg/m^2 PO daily in three or four divided doses after meals and at bedtime for 14 or 21 days every 4 weeks when used as a single agent.

2. 150 to 200 mg/m^2 PO daily in three or four divided doses for 2 out of 3 or 4 weeks when used in combination.

Special precautions. Concurrent altretamine and antidepressants of the monoamine oxidase (MAO) inhibitor class may cause severe orthostatic hypotension. Cimetidine may increase toxicity.

Toxicity.

1. *Myelosuppression and other hematologic effects.* Dose-limiting leukopenia and thrombocytopenia are uncommon, though lesser degrees are common. Anemia is common.
2. *Nausea, vomiting, and other gastrointestinal effects.* Mild-to-moderate nausea, vomiting, and other gastrointestinal effects occur in approximately 30% of patients and are rarely severe. Tolerance may develop.
3. *Mucocutaneous effects.* Alopecia, skin rash, and pruritus are rare.
4. *Miscellaneous effects.*
   a. Peripheral sensory neuropathies are common and may be ameliorated by pyridoxine, but tumor response may be compromised.
   b. Central nervous system (CNS) effects, including agitation, confusion, hallucinations, depression, and parkinsonian-like symptoms are uncommon with recommended intermittent schedule.
   c. Decreased renal function is occasional.
   d. Increased alkaline phosphatase level is occasional.
   e. Diarrhea is occasional.

AMIFOSTINE

Other name. Ethyol.

Mechanism of action. The prodrug, amifostine, is dephosphorylated to an active free thiol metabolite that can reduce the toxic effects of cisplatin. The differential activity between normal and cancer tissues is thought to be related to higher capillary alkaline phosphatase activity and better vascularity of normal tissue. Pretreatment reduces cumulative renal toxicity from cisplatin.

Primary indications.

1. For reduction of cumulative renal toxicity associated with repeated administration of cisplatin in patients with advanced cancer.
2. For reduction of moderate-to-severe xerostomia from radiation of the head and neck where the radiation port includes a substantial portion of the parotid glands.

Usual dosage and schedule.

1. For reduction of cumulative renal toxicity with chemotherapy. 910 mg/m^2 IV over 15 min once daily, starting 30 min before chemotherapy.
2. For reduction of xerostomia from radiation of the head and neck. 200 mg/m^2 administered once daily as a 3-min IV infusion, starting 15 to 30 min before standard-fraction radiation therapy (1.8–2.0 Gy).

Special precautions. To minimize hypotension during the infusion, patients should be adequately hydrated before the amifostine infusion and kept in a supine position during the infusion.

Blood pressure should be monitored every 5 min during the infusion, and thereafter as clinically indicated. Interrupt the infusion if the decrease in systolic pressure is more than 20% to 25% of the baseline systolic pressure.

Toxicity.

1. *Myelosuppression and other hematologic effects.* Not increased by amifostine.
2. *Nausea, vomiting, and other gastrointestinal effects.* Nausea and vomiting are common and may be severe.
3. *Mucocutaneous effects.* Skin rash is rare.
4. *Miscellaneous effects.*
   a. Transient hypotension during the infusion is common. Loss of consciousness may occur, but is usually easily reversed.
   b. Flushing and feeling of warmth are occasional.
   c. Chilling and feeling of coldness are occasional.
   d. Dizziness, somnolence, hiccups, and sneezing are occasional.
   e. Allergic reactions are rare but have included anaphylactic reactions.
   f. Hypocalcemia is rare.
   g. Seizures are rare.

AMINOGLUTETHIMIDE

Other name. Cytadren.

Mechanism of action. Inhibits aromatization and cytochrome P-450 hydroxylating enzymes, thereby blocking the conversion of androgens to estrogens and the biosynthesis of all steroid hormones. This drug causes, in effect, a reversible chemical adrenalectomy.

Primary indication. Adrenocortical carcinoma, ectopic Cushing's syndrome.

Usual dosage and schedule. 1,000 mg PO daily in four divided doses.

Special precautions. Hydrocortisone must be given concomitantly to prevent adrenal insufficiency, particularly if used in breast cancer. Suggested dose is 100 mg PO daily in divided doses for 2 weeks, and then 40 mg PO daily in divided doses.

Toxicity.

1. *Myelosuppression and other hematologic effects.* Leukopenia and thrombocytopenia are rare, and if they occur they resolve rapidly when the drug is stopped.
2. *Nausea, vomiting, and other gastrointestinal effects* are occasional and usually mild.
3. *Mucocutaneous effects.* A morbilliform rash is commonly seen during the first week of treatment, but it usually disappears within 1 week.
4. *Hormonal effects.*
   a. Adrenal insufficiency is common without replacement hydrocortisone in patients with normal adrenal glands.
   b. Hypothyroidism is uncommon.
   c. Masculinization is possible.
5. *Neurologic effects.*
   a. Lethargy is common. Although usually mild and transient, it is occasionally severe.
   b. Vertigo, nystagmus, and ataxia are occasional.

6. *Miscellaneous effects.*
   a. Facial flushing is uncommon.
   b. Periorbital edema is uncommon.
   c. Cholestatic jaundice is rare.
   d. Fever is uncommon.

ANAGRELIDE

Other names. Imidazo(2,1-b)quinazolin-2-one, Agrelin.

Mechanism of action. Mechanism for thrombocytopenia is unknown but may be due to impaired megakaryocyte function. Inhibitor of platelet aggregation but not at usual therapeutic doses.

Primary indication. Uncontrolled thrombocytosis in chronic myeloproliferative disorders, such as essential thrombocythemia, chronic granulocytic leukemia, and polycythemia rubra vera.

Usual dosage and schedule. (Supplied as 0.5- and 1-mg capsules)
1. 0.5 mg PO q.i.d. or 1 mg PO b.i.d. Increase by 0.5 mg/day every 5 to 7 days if no response. Maximum daily dose is 10 mg/day. Maximum single dose is 2.5 mg. Higher doses cause postural hypotension.
2. Alternate dosing schedules:
   a. *Elderly.* 0.5 mg PO daily; increase by 0.5 mg each week.
   b. *Abnormal renal or hepatic function.* 0.5 mg PO b.i.d.

Special precautions. Contraindicated in pregnancy. Use with caution in patients with heart disease. Tachycardia and forceful heartbeat may be exacerbated by caffeine; consumption of caffeine should be avoided for 1 h before and after anagrelide is taken. Use other drugs that inhibit platelet aggregation (such as nonsteroidal anti-inflammatory drugs) with caution. Monitor platelet count every few days during first week, and then weekly until the maintenance dose is reached.

Toxicity.
1. *Myelosuppression.* No White cell count suppression. Anemia is common (36%) but mild. Thrombocytopenic hemorrhage is uncommon (2%).
2. *Nausea and vomiting.* Nausea is occasional (15%), and vomiting is uncommon.
3. *Mucocutaneous effects.* Rash, including urticaria is occasional (8%). Hyperpigmentation is rare. Sun sensitivity is possible.
4. *Miscellaneous effects.*
   a. *Cardiovascular.* Palpitations (26%), forceful heart beat, and tachycardia are common. Congestive heart failure is uncommon, but fluid retention or edema is common (21%). Tachyarrhythmias (including atrial fibrillation and premature atrial beats) are occasional. Angina, cardiomyopathy, or other severe cardiovascular effects are rare, although there are a few more frequent (8%) episodes of chest pain. Drinking alcoholic beverages may cause flushing. Higher than recommended single doses cause postural hypotension. Cardiovascular effects appear to result from vasodilation, positive inotropy, and decreased renal blood flow.
   b. *Neurologic.* Headaches are common (44%) and are occasionally severe; they usually diminish in approximately

2 weeks. Weakness (asthenia) is common (22%). Dizziness is occasional.
c. *Pulmonary*. Infiltrates are rare but are a reason to stop anagrelide and treat with steroids.
d. *Other gastrointestinal*. Diarrhea (26%), gas, and abdominal pain are common; pancreatitis is rare. Lactase supplementation eliminates diarrhea (anagrelide formulated with lactose). Hepatic enzyme elevation is rare, but caution is recommended when there is evidence of hepatic dysfunction.

ANASTROZOLE

Other name. Arimidex.
Mechanism of action. Decreases estrogen biosynthesis by selective inhibition of aromatase (estrogen synthetase).
Primary indications.
1. Carcinoma of the breast—as adjuvant treatment in postmenopausal women with positive or unknown hormone receptors.
2. Carcinoma of the breast that is advanced or metastatic—as first therapy in postmenopausal women with positive or unknown hormone receptors.
3. Carcinoma of the breast that is advanced or metastatic—as second therapy in women with progression following initial response to tamoxifen.
Usual dosage and schedule. 1 mg PO daily.
Special precautions. Potential hazard to fetus if given during pregnancy. Consider obtaining bone mineral density test and treating with calcium and vitamin D, with or without bisphosphonates as clinically indicated.
Toxicity.
1. *Myelosuppression and other hematologic effects*. No dose-related myelosuppression. Thromboembolic events are uncommon (3%).
2. *Nausea and vomiting, other gastrointestinal effects*. Nausea, diarrhea, and constipation are occasional. Vomiting is uncommon.
3. *Mucocutaneous effects*. Rash is occasional. Hot flashes are common (35%). Vaginal dryness and leukorrhea are uncommon.
4. *Miscellaneous effects*.
   a. Asthenia is common. Headache and dizziness are occasional.
   b. Musculoskeletal pain is occasional. Arthralgia is occasional.
   c. Peripheral edema and weight gain are occasional (lower than with megestrol).
   d. Dyspnea and cough are occasional.
   e. Cataracts are occasional (6%).
   f. Decreased bone mineral density with osteoporosis is occasional (11%) and there is increased risk for fractures (10%).
   g. Vaginal bleeding is uncommon, and endometrial cancer is rare (0.2%).

ARSENIC TRIOXIDE

Other name. Trisenox.

Mechanism of action. Although the mechanism is incompletely understood, effects of arsenic trioxide include morphologic changes and DNA fragmentation characteristic of apoptosis and alteration of the fusion protein PML-RAR α.

Primary indications.

1. Remission induction therapy of acute promyelocytic leukemia that is refractory to retinoid and anthracycline therapy and has t(15;17) translocation or *PML/RAR* α gene expression.
2. Maintenance of remission in acute promyelocytic leukemia.

Usual dosage and schedule.

1. *Induction.* 0.15 mg/kg IV over 1 to 2 hours daily until marrow remission. Maximum of 60 doses.
2. *Consolidation.* 0.15 mg/kg IV daily for 25 doses over a period of up to 5 weeks. Consolidation is started 3 to 6 weeks after completion of induction therapy.

Special precautions.

1. *Cardiovascular.* Tachycardia and prolonged QT interval are common. This may lead to complete arteriovenous (AV) block with fatal ventricular arrhythmia. Electrolyte (including magnesium) abnormalities should be corrected before initiation of therapy and patients with prolonged QT intervals should have measures taken to reduce this prolongation before treatment with arsenic trioxide. A QT value greater than 500 millisecond during therapy is an indication to suspend arsenic trioxide treatment and to initiate measures to correct other risk factors that may be contributing to the prolongation of the QT.
2. Acute promyelocytic leukemic differentiation syndrome, similar to that seen with retinoic acid, may be seen and is potentially fatal. This syndrome consists of fever, dyspnea, weight gain, pulmonary infiltrates, and pleural or pericardial effusions with or without leukocytosis. High-dose corticosteroids (e.g., dexamethasone, 10 mg b.i.d.) should be started at the first signs of this syndrome and continued until it subsides.

Toxicity.

1. *Myelosuppression and other hematologic effects.* Anemia, thrombocytopenia, and neutropenia are occasional. Leukocytosis is common. Disseminated intravascular coagulation is occasional and may be severe. Infections and neutropenic fever are occasional.
2. *Nausea, vomiting, and other gastrointestinal effects.* Nausea, vomiting, diarrhea, and abdominal pain are common (>50%). Gastrointestinal bleeding, with or without diarrhea, is occasional (8%). Constipation, anorexia, and other types of abdominal distress are occasional.
3. *Mucocutaneous effects.* Sore throat is common (40%). Dermatitis, pruritus, and ecchymosis are also common. More severe mucocutaneous reactions including local exfoliation, urticaria, and oral blistering are occasional to uncommon. Epistaxis is common (25%). Eye irritation and injection are occasional.
4. *Miscellaneous effects.*
   a. *Cardiovascular.* Tachycardia and prolonged QT interval are common. This may lead to complete AV block with fatal ventricular arrhythmia.

b. Acute promyelocytic leukemic differentiation syndrome, similar to that seen with retinoic acid, may be seen. This consists of fever, dyspnea, weight gain, pulmonary infiltrates, and pleural or pericardial effusions with or without leukocytosis. This syndrome may be fatal.

c. *General and administration site.* Headache and insomnia are common. Edema and pleural effusion are common (though not commonly serious), and general weight gain is occasional. Drug hypersensitivity is uncommon. Injection site edema, erythema, and pain are occasional.

d. *Metabolic.* Hypokalemia, hypomagnesemia, and hyperglycemia are common (45%–50%). Hyperkalemia is occasional to common (18%), as are elevated transaminases, hypocalcemia, and hypoglycemia.

e. *Pulmonary.* Cough and dyspnea are common (>50%). Pleural effusion, hypoxia, wheezing, and asymptomatic auscultatory findings are occasional to common (8%–20%).

f. *Renal.* Renal failure is occasional.

ASPARAGINASE

Other names.   L-asparaginase, Elspar, Kidrolase, pegaspargase, Oncaspar.

Mechanism of action.   Hydrolysis of serum asparagine occurs, which deprives leukemia cells of the required amino acid and inhibits protein synthesis. Normal cells are spared because they generally have the ability to synthesize their own asparagine. Pegaspargase is a chemically modified formulation of asparaginase in which the L-asparaginase is covalently conjugated with monomethoxypolyethylene glycol (PEG). This modification increases its half-life in the plasma by a factor of 4 to approximately 5.7 days and reduces its recognition by the immune system, which allows the drug to be used in patients previously hypersensitive to native L-asparaginase.

Primary indication.   Acute lymphocytic leukemia, primarily for induction therapy.

Usual dosage and schedule.   All schedules are used in combination with other drugs. The schedules listed are only a few of many acceptable dosing schedules.

1. L-asparaginase 6,000 IU/m^2 of body surface area IM on days 4, 7, 10, 13, 16, 19, 22, 25, and 28 of the treatment period.

2. L-*asparaginase.* 1,000 IU/kg/day (= 25–40 IU/m^2) IV for 10 successive days beginning on day 22 of the treatment period.

3. *Pegaspargase.* 2,500 IU/m^2 IM (or IV) once every 14 days, either for first-line acute lymphocytic leukemia or in patients who have developed hypersensitivity to native forms of asparaginase. For IM use, limit volume at single injection site to 2 mL. For IV administration, give over 1 to 2 h in saline or D5W.

Special precautions.   Asparaginase is contraindicated in patients with pancreatitis or a history of pancreatitis. Asparaginase is contraindicated in patients who have had significant hemorrhagic events associated with prior L-asparaginase therapy. Pegaspargase is also contraindicated in patients who have had previous serious allergic reactions, such as generalized urticaria, bronchospasm, laryngeal edema, hypotension, or other unacceptable adverse reactions to prior pegaspargase therapy.

1. Be prepared to treat anaphylaxis at each administration of the drug. Epinephrine, antihistamines, corticosteroids, and life-support equipment should be readily available.

2. Giving concurrently with or immediately before vincristine may increase vincristine toxicity.

3. The IM route is preferred for pegaspargase, because of a lower incidence of hepatotoxicity, coagulopathy, and gastrointestinal and renal disorders as compared with the IV route of administration.

Toxicity.

1. *Myelosuppression and other hematologic effects.* Occasional myelosuppression. CNS thrombosis and other coagulopathy are uncommon.

2. *Nausea, vomiting, and other gastrointestinal effects.* Occasional and usually mild. (See the following text for liver and pancreas effects.)

3. *Mucocutaneous effects.* No toxicity occurs except as a sign of hypersensitivity.

4. *Anaphylaxis.* Mild to severe hypersensitivity reactions, including anaphylaxis, occur in 20% to 30% of patients. Such reaction is less likely to occur during the first few days of treatment. It is particularly common with intermittent schedules or repeat cycles. If the patient develops hypersensitivity to the *Escherichia coli*–derived enzyme (Elspar), *Erwinia*-derived asparaginase may be safely substituted because the two enzyme preparations are not cross-reactive. Note that hypersensitivity may also develop to *Erwinia*-derived asparaginase, and continued preparedness to treat anaphylaxis must be maintained.

   If given IM, asparaginase should be given in an extremity so that a tourniquet can be applied to slow the systemic release of asparaginase should anaphylaxis occur.

   Approximately 30% of patients previously sensitive to L-asparaginase will have a hypersensitivity reaction to pegaspargase, while only 10% of those who were not hypersensitive to the native form will have a hypersensitivity reaction to the PEG-modified drug.

5. *Miscellaneous effects.*

   a. Mild fever and malaise are common and occasionally progress to severe chills and malignant hyperthermia.

   b. Hepatotoxicity is common and occasionally severe. Abnormalities observed include elevations of serum glutamic-oxaloacetic transaminase (SGOT), alkaline phosphatase, and bilirubin; depressed levels of hepatic-derived clotting factors and albumin; and hepatocellular fatty metamorphosis.

   c. Renal failure is rare.

   d. Pancreatic endocrine and exocrine dysfunction, often with manifestations of pancreatitis, occurs occasionally. Nonketotic hyperglycemia is uncommon.

   e. CNS effects (depression, somnolence, fatigue, confusion, agitation, hallucinations, or coma) are seen occasionally.

They are usually reversible following discontinuation of the drug.

AZACITIDINE

Other name. Vidaza.

Mechanism of action. Pyrimidine analog that inhibits methyltransferase, causing hypomethylation of DNA and thereby, it is believed, results in cellular differentiation or apoptosis. May restore normal function of genes that are critical for the control of cellular differentiation and proliferation. Nonproliferating cells are relatively insensitive to azacitidine.

Primary indication. Myelodysplastic syndromes

Usual dosage and schedule. 75 mg/m^2 SC daily for 7 days, repeated every 4 weeks. Dose may be increased to 100 mg/m^2 if no toxicity other than nausea and vomiting. Therapy may be continued so long as the patient improves from the drug.

Toxicity.

1. *Myelosuppression.* Neutropenia, thrombocytopenia, and anemia are common. Febrile neutropenia is four times as common as in patients receiving supportive care. Petechiae or ecchymosis are occasional.

2. *Nausea and vomiting.* Anorexia, nausea, vomiting, and diarrhea or constipation are common. Abdominal pain is occasional.

3. *Mucocutaneous effects.* Pharyngitis and stomatitis are occasional. Skin rash and urticaria are occasional. Pain at the injection site is common.

4. *Neurotoxicity.* Insomnia is common. Lethargy, dizziness, or confusional state are occasional.

5. *Miscellaneous effects.*
   a. *Cardiorespiratory.* Cough and dyspnea are common. Pulmonary edema—uncommon. Edema is occasional. Tachycardia or other more serious cardiac disorders—uncommon.
   b. Fever is common.
   c. Fatigue and weakness are common.
   d. Arthralgias and back pain are occasional.
   e. Hypokalemia is occasional.

BEVACIZUMAB

Other name. Avastin.

Mechanism of action. Binds VEGF and prevents its interaction with its receptors on the surface of endothelial cells. This in turn impairs endothelial cell proliferation and new blood vessel formation, impeding tumor growth and metastasis.

Primary indication.

1. Carcinomas of the colon, rectum, breast, and lung.

Usual dosage and schedule. Five mg/kg IV once every 2 weeks.

Special precautions. Gastrointestinal perforation occurs in up to 4% of patients, and may have a fatal outcome. Impaired wound healing may rarely lead to anastomotic dehiscence. Bevacizumab should not be initiated for at least 28 days following major surgery. The interval between termination of bevacizumab and subsequent surgery should take into account the accumulation ratio of 2.8 (with every 2-week dosing) and the half-life of approximately 20 days. Serious, and in some cases fatal, hemoptysis has occurred in non–small cell lung cancer, with the highest risk appearing in patients with squamous cell histology. Blood pressure monitoring is recommended every 2 to 3 weeks because of the risk of hypertension. Urinary protein should be evaluated before each treatment with a urine dipstick, and if the value is 2+ or greater, the patient should undergo further assessment to rule out severe proteinuria.

Toxicity.

1. *Myelosuppression and other hematologic effects*. Leukopenia is common, but associated primarily with the cytotoxic agents used together with bevacizumab. Thrombocytopenia is uncommon. Minor bleeding, such as epistaxis, is common; severe hemorrhage is not, except for hemoptysis in patients with squamous cell carcinomas of the lung. Thromboembolic events are occasional.

2. *Nausea, vomiting, and other gastrointestinal effects*. Anorexia, nausea, vomiting, and constipation are common. Diarrhea is common, particularly when used with fluorouracil and irinotecan chemotherapy. Abdominal pain is common. Gastrointestinal hemorrhage is occasional.

3. *Mucocutaneous effects*. Dry skin, skin discoloration, stomatitis, and exfoliative dermatitis are occasional to common. Alopecia, skin ulcers, and nail changes are uncommon. Nasal septum perforation is rare.

4. *Immunologic effects and infusion reactions*. Infusion reactions with wheezing and stridor are uncommon.

5. *Miscellaneous effects*.
   a. Fatigue, weakness, and headache are common
   b. *Cardiovascular and respiratory*. Hypertension is common and occasionally is severe (>200/110 mm Hg). Hypotension is occasional. Dyspnea is occasional. Congestive heart failure is uncommon, but risk with anthracyclines is increased (14%). Venous thromboembolic events are increased by approximately 15% compared with chemotherapy not containing bevacizumab.
   c. *Neurologic*. Dizziness is common. Reversible posterior leukoencephalopathy syndrome is rare.
   d. *Metabolic*. Hypokalemia is occasional. Proteinuria is common, but severe proteinuria (>3.5 g/24 h) is uncommon and rarely leads to nephrotic syndrome.

BEXAROTENE (CAPSULES)

Other name. Targretin.

Mechanism of action. A member of the subclass of retinoids (rexinoid) that selectively activates retinoid X receptors (RXRs). These receptors are distinct from RARs, but they also act as transcription factors that regulate the expression of genes that control cellular differentiation and proliferation. The exact mechanism in cutaneous T-cell lymphoma (CTCL) is unknown.

Primary indication. Cutaneous manifestations of CTCL in patients refractory to at least one prior systemic therapy.

Usual dosage and schedule. 300 mg/m^2/day to start as a single oral daily dose taken with a meal. Dosage is adjusted downward by 100 mg/m^2/day decrements for toxicity, or upward to 400 mg/m^2/day if there has been no response but good tolerability after 8 weeks of treatment. Treatment may be continued for up to 2 years.

Special precaution. Avoid use in pregnant women because of marked teratogenic potential.

Toxicity.

1. *Myelosuppression and other hematologic effects.* Mild-to-moderate leukopenia is occasional to common with a time of onset of 4 to 8 weeks. Severe or worse leukopenia is occasional.

2. *Nausea, vomiting, and other gastrointestinal effects.* Mild nausea, abdominal pain, and diarrhea are occasional. Vomiting and anorexia are uncommon.

3. *Mucocutaneous effects.* Skin reactions are occasional to common. They include redness, dryness, and pruritus of the skin and mucous membranes; possible vesicle formation; exfoliative dermatitis; cheilitis; and conjunctivitis. There may also be increased skin photosensitivity (e.g., to sun) and the nails may become brittle. Alopecia is uncommon.

4. *Miscellaneous effects.*
   a. Cataracts and corneal ulcerations or opacities are uncommon.
   b. *Systemic.* Arthralgias, bone pain, and muscle aches are occasional. Fever, chills, and headache (flu syndrome) are occasional.
   c. Hypertriglyceridemia (80%) and hypercholesterolemia (35%–40%) are common. Hypertriglyceridemia is usually more severe. These are reversible with discontinuation of therapy and may be reduced by antilipemic therapy.
   d. *Neurologic.* Headache is common. Lethargy, fatigue, confusion, and mental depression are uncommon; pseudotumor cerebri is rare.
   e. *Gastrointestinal.* Inflammatory bowel disease and pancreatitis (associated with hypertriglyceridemia) are rare.
   f. Hepatotoxicity with increased lactate dehydrogenase (LDH), SGOT, serum glutamic-pyruvic transaminase (SGPT), gamma glutamyl transpeptidase (GGTP), and alkaline phosphatase is occasional.
   g. Hypothyroidism is common, with decreased T$_4$ and thyroid-stimulating hormone (TSH).
   h. Peripheral edema is occasional.
   i. Hypernatremia is rare.

BEXAROTENE (GEL)

Other name. Targretin gel (1%).

Mechanism of action. A member of the subclass of retinoids (rexinoid) that selectively activates retinoid X receptors (RXRs). These receptors are distinct from RARs, but they also act as transcription factors that regulate the expression of genes that control cellular differentiation and proliferation. The exact mechanism in CTCL is unknown.

Primary indication. Cutaneous manifestations of CTCL (Stage IA and IB) in patients who have refractory or persistent disease after other therapies or who have not tolerated other therapies.

Usual dosage and schedule. The gel is applied once every other day for the first week. The frequency is then increased at weekly intervals as tolerated to once daily, twice daily, and up to four times daily, according to individual lesion tolerance. Treatment frequency should be reduced or treatment suspended for severe local irritation.

   Special precautions. Avoid use in pregnant women because of marked teratogenic potential.

Toxicity.

1. *Myelosuppression and other hematologic effects.* Uncommon.
2. *Nausea, vomiting, and other gastrointestinal effects.* Not expected.
3. *Mucocutaneous effects.* Skin reactions are occasional to common. They include pain, redness, dryness, and pruritus of the skin; possible vesicle formation; and exfoliative dermatitis. There may also be increased skin photosensitivity (e.g., to sun).
4. *Miscellaneous effects.*
    a. Hypertriglyceridemia is occasional.
    b. *Neurologic.* Headache and paresthesias are occasional.
    c. *Peripheral edema.* Occasional.

BICALUTAMIDE

Other name. Casodex.

Mechanism of action. A nonsteroidal antiandrogen that is a competitive inhibitor of androgens at the cellular androgen receptor in target tissues, such as the prostate.

Primary indication. Carcinoma of the prostate, often in combination with LHRH agonist.

Usual dosage and schedule. 50 mg PO daily, in the morning or evening.

Special precautions. Rare cases of severe liver injury have been reported. Bicalutamide should be used with caution in patients with moderate-to-severe hepatic impairment.

Toxicity.

1. *Myelosuppression and other hematologic effects.* No myelosuppression. May interact with warfarin, and increase international normalized ratio (INR).
2. *Nausea, vomiting, and other gastrointestinal effects.* Nausea, diarrhea, flatulence, and constipation are occasional; vomiting is uncommon.
3. *Mucocutaneous effects.* Mild skin rash is occasional.
4. *Miscellaneous effects.*
    a. Secondary pharmacologic effects, including breast tenderness, breast swelling, hot flashes (49%), impotence, and loss of libido are common but reversible after cessation of therapy.
    b. Elevated liver function tests are uncommon.
    c. Adverse cardiovascular events are similar to those seen with orchiectomy.
    d. Dizziness or vertigo is occasional.

BLEOMYCIN

Other name. Blenoxane.

Mechanism of action. Bleomycin binds to DNA, causes single- and double-strand scission, and inhibits further DNA, RNA, and protein synthesis.

Primary indications.

1. Testis, head and neck, penis, cervix, vulva, anus, and skin carcinomas.
2. Hodgkin's and non–Hodgkin's lymphomas.
3. Pleural effusions—used as sclerosing agent.

Usual dosage and schedule.

1. 10 to 20 units/m^2 IV or IM once or twice a week *or*
2. 30 units IV push weekly for 9 to 12 weeks in combination with other drugs for testis cancer.
3. 60 units in 50 mL of normal saline instilled intrapleurally.

Special precautions.

1. In patients with lymphoma, a test dose of 1 or 2 units should be given IM before the first dose of bleomycin because of the possibility of anaphylactoid, acute pulmonary or severe hyperpyretic responses. If no acute reaction occurs within 4 h, regular dosing may begin.
2. Reduce dose for renal failure.

Serum creatinine	% of full dose
2.5–4.0	25
4.0–6.0	20
6.0–10.0	10

3. The cumulative lifetime dose should not exceed 400 units because of the dose-related incidence of severe pulmonary fibrosis. Smaller limits may be appropriate for older patients or those with preexisting pulmonary disease. Frequent evaluation of pulmonary status, including symptoms of cough or dyspnea, rales, infiltrates on chest x-ray film, and pulmonary function studies are recommended to avert serious pulmonary sequelae.
4. Glass containers are recommended for continuous infusion to minimize drug instability.
5. High F$_{IO_2}$ (fraction of inspired oxygen) (such as might be used during surgery) should be avoided as it exacerbates lung injury, sometimes acutely.

Toxicity.

1. *Myelosuppression and other hematologic effects.* Significant depression of counts is uncommon. This factor permits bleomycin to be used in full doses with myelosuppressive drugs.
2. *Nausea, vomiting, and other gastrointestinal effects.* Occasional and self-limiting.
3. *Mucocutaneous effects.* Alopecia, stomatitis, erythema, edema, thickening of nail bed, and hyperpigmentation and desquamation of skin are common.
4. *Pulmonary effects.*
   a. Acute anaphylactoid or pulmonary edema–like response is occasional in patients with lymphoma (see Special precautions, in the preceding text).

   b. Dose-related pneumonitis with cough, dyspnea, rales, and infiltrates, progressing to pulmonary fibrosis.
5. *Fever*. Common. Occasionally severe hyperpyrexia, diaphoresis, dehydration, and hypotension have occurred and resulted in renal failure and death. Antipyretics help control fever.
6. *Miscellaneous effects*.
   a. Lethargy, headache, and joint swelling are rare.
   b. IM or SQ injection may cause pain at injection site.

BORTEZOMIB

Other name. Velcade.
Mechanism of action. A reversible inhibitor of the chymotrypsin-like activity of the 26S proteosome, which mediates protein degradation and plays an essential role in intracellular protein regulation and consequent cellular signal transduction pathways and cellular homeostasis.
Primary indications.
1. Multiple myeloma in patients with at least one prior therapy.
2. Mantle cell lymphoma in patients with at least one prior therapy.
Usual dosage and schedule.
1. 1.3 mg/m^2 IV bolus on days 1, 4, 8, and 11, every 3 weeks.
2. After eight cycles, may use 1.3 mg/m^2 IV bolus weekly $\times$ 4, every 5 weeks.
Special precautions. Cardiogenic shock, congestive heart failure, and respiratory insufficiency have been rarely observed. Anaphylaxis has also been observed. Patients with hepatic or renal impairment should be monitored closely.
Toxicity.
1. *Myelosuppression and other hematologic effects*. Anemia, neutropenia, and thrombocytopenia are common; neutropenia is only occasionally severe (grade 3 or 4). Thrombocytopenia is severe in 30% of patients. Disseminated intravascular coagulation has been observed (rare to uncommon).
2. *Nausea and vomiting*. Anorexia, nausea, vomiting, diarrhea, and constipation are common. Dehydration is a concern because of vomiting and diarrhea and may be seen occasionally.
3. *Mucocutaneous effects*. Rash is common (20%).
4. *Neurotoxicity*. Peripheral neuropathy is common, and occasionally (7%) severe. This frequently manifests as paresthesias and dysesthesias. Headache is common.
5. *Immunologic effects*. Hypersensitivity reactions have been seen, including anaphylactic reactions and immune complex–mediated hypersensitivity (rare).
6. *Miscellaneous effects*.
   a. Fatigue and weakness are common.
   b. Arthralgias, muscle cramps, and back pain are occasional.
   c. Fever is common.
   d. *Cardiovascular*. Hypotension is occasional, is seen throughout therapy, and may be orthostatic or not. Peripheral edema is common. Other cardiovascular events during treatment have included severe congestive heart failure, AV block, angina, atrial fibrillation, and flutter—these

    are probably uncommon to rare as a consequence of the drug.
  e. Infiltrative pulmonary disease—rare, but may be severe or fatal.
  f. Hepatitis and pancreatitis have been observed—probably rare.

BUSULFAN

Other names. Myleran, Busulfex.

Mechanism of action. Bifunctional alkylating agent. Its effect may be greater on cellular thiol groups than on nucleic acids.

Primary indications.

1. *Standard doses*. Chronic granulocytic (myelogenous) leukemia.
2. *High doses with stem cell rescue*. Acute leukemia, lymphoma, and chronic granulocytic leukemia.

Usual dosage and schedule.

1. 3 to 4 mg/m^2 PO daily for remission induction in adults until the leukocyte count is 50% of the original level, and then 1 to 2 mg/m^2 PO daily. Busulfan may be given continuously or intermittently for maintenance.
2. High doses with stem cell rescue—consult specific protocols. Not recommended outside research setting. Typical dose is 1 mg/kg PO q6h for 4 consecutive days. Alternative dosing of intravenous form (Busulfex) is 0.8 mg/kg of ideal body weight (or actual if lower) as a 2-h infusion through a central catheter every 6 h for 4 days (16 doses). High-dose therapy requires pretreatment with phenytoin.

Special precautions. Obtain complete blood count weekly while patient is on therapy. If leukocyte count falls rapidly to less than $15,000/\mu L$, discontinue therapy until nadir is reached and rising counts indicate a need for further treatment.

Toxicity.

1. *Myelosuppression and other hematologic effects*. Dose limiting. A fall in the leukocyte count may not begin for 2 weeks after starting therapy, and it is likely to continue for 2 weeks after therapy has been stopped. Recovery of marrow function may be delayed for 3 to 6 weeks after the drug has been discontinued. High-dose therapy requires stem cell rescue (e.g., bone marrow transplantation).
2. *Nausea, vomiting, and other gastrointestinal effects*. Rare.
3. *Mucocutaneous effects*. Hyperpigmentation occurs occasionally, particularly in skin creases.
4. *Pulmonary effects*. Interstitial pulmonary fibrosis is rare and is an indication to discontinue drug. Corticosteroids may improve symptoms and minimize permanent lung damage.
5. *Metabolic effects*. Adrenal insufficiency syndrome is rare. Hyperuricemia may occur when the leukemia cell count is rapidly reduced. Ovarian suppression and amenorrhea are common.
6. *Miscellaneous effects*.
  a. Secondary neoplasia is possible.
  b. Fatal hepatoveno-occlusive disease with high-dose therapy is occasional.
  c. Seizures after high-dose therapy are occasional.

CAPECITABINE

Other name. Xeloda.

Mechanism of action. An orally administered prodrug that is converted to fluorouracil intracellularly. When this is converted to the active nucleotide, 5-fluoro-2-deoxyuridine monophosphate, it inhibits the enzyme thymidylate synthetase and blocks DNA synthesis. The triphosphate may also be mistakenly incorporated into RNA, which interferes with RNA processing and protein synthesis.

Primary indications.
1. Metastatic breast cancer that is resistant to anthracycline- and paclitaxel-containing chemotherapeutic regimens. May also be used in patients in whom anthracyclines are con-traindicated.
2. Colorectal, stomach, pancreas, and biliary carcinomas.
3. As a radiosensitizer in lieu of fluorouracil.

Usual dosage and schedule. Generally taken with water, twice daily (~12 h between doses) within 30 min of a meal. Dose reductions are commonly required, by reducing the daily dose, the number of consecutive daily treatments, or both.
1. 1,000 to 1,250 mg/m^2 orally twice daily for 2 weeks as a single agent, followed by a 1-week rest, given as 3-week cycles.
2. 800 to 1,250 mg/m^2 orally twice daily for 2 weeks when used in combination with other drugs, followed by 1-week rest, given as 3-week cycles.
3. 800 mg/m^2 orally twice daily 5 days per week during radio-therapy as a radiosensitizer.

Special precautions. Patients with moderate renal impair-ment (C$_{Cr}$ 30 to 50 mL/min) require a 25% dosage reduction: diarrhea may be severe and necessitate fluid and electrolyte re-placement. Incidence and severity may be worse in patients 80 years of age or older. Therapy may need to be interrupted and subsequent doses decreased for severe or repeated toxicity. In-crease in prothrombin time (PT) and INR may be seen in patients previously stable on oral anticoagulants. Monitor PT/INR more frequently when patient is on capecitabine.

Toxicity.
1. *Myelosuppression and other hematologic effects.* Common, but when used as a single agent, these are usually mild to moder-ate with anemia predominating. Neutropenia is common when used in combination and may be associated with neutropenic fever.
2. *Nausea, vomiting, and other gastrointestinal effects.* Both nau-sea (45%) and vomiting (35%) are common, but usually not severe. Diarrhea is common (55%); in up to 15% of patients, it is severe to life threatening. Gastrointestinal motility disor-ders, including ileus may be seen, and necrotizing enterocolitis has been reported. Abdominal pain is occasional to common. Anorexia is occasional to common (26%). Hyperbilirubine-mia is common (48%), but only occasionally severe or life threatening.
3. *Mucocutaneous effects.* Hand-and-foot syndrome is common (54%) and may be severe. Dermatitis is also common (27%), as is stomatitis, but it is uncommon that these are severe. Eye irritation and increased lacrimation are occasional.

4. *Miscellaneous effects*.
   a. Fatigue is common.
   b. Paresthesias are occasional.
   c. Fever is occasional.
   d. Headache or dizziness is occasional.
   e. Cardiotoxicity is possible as with any fluorinated pyrimidine.

CARBOPLATIN

Other names. Paraplatin, CBDCA.
Mechanism of action. Covalent binding to DNA.
Primary indication. Ovarian, endometrial, breast, bladder, and lung cancers, and other cancers in which cisplatin is active.
Usual dosage and schedule. AUC (area-under-the-curve) dosing (Calvert formula) is generally preferred.

1. Target AUC is commonly 4 to 6, depending on previous treatment and other drugs to be used. Administration dose (mg) = (target AUC) × ([creatinine clearance] +25). Administration dose is given by IV infusion over 15 to 60 min, and repeated every 4 weeks.
2. Higher doses up to 1,600 mg/m^2 divided over several days have been used followed by stem cell rescue (e.g., bone marrow transplantation).

Special precautions. Much less renal toxicity than cisplatin, so there is no need for a vigorous hydration schedule or forced diuresis. Reduced creatinine clearance reduces carboplatin clearance and increases toxicity.

Anaphylactic-like reactions to carboplatin have been reported and may occur within minutes of carboplatin administration. Infusion reactions may develop after several months of drug tolerance. Epinephrine, corticosteroids, and antihistamines have been employed to alleviate symptoms.

Toxicity.

1. *Myelosuppression and other hematologic effects*. Anemia, granulocytopenia, and thrombocytopenia are common and dose limiting. Red blood cell transfusions or epoetin may be required. Thrombocytopenia may be delayed (days 18–28).
2. *Nausea, vomiting, and other gastrointestinal effects*. Nausea and vomiting are common, but vomiting (65%) is not as frequent or as severe as with cisplatin and can be controlled with combination antiemetic regimens. Liver function abnormalities are common. Gastrointestinal pain is occasional.
3. *Mucocutaneous effects*. Alopecia is uncommon. Mucositis is rare.
4. *Renal tubular abnormalities*. Elevation in serum creatinine or blood urea nitrogen occurs occasionally. More common is electrolyte loss with decreases in serum sodium, potassium, calcium, and magnesium.
5. *Miscellaneous effects*.
   a. Peripheral neuropathy or central neurotoxicity is uncommon.
   b. Allergic reactions are uncommonly seen with rash, urticaria, pruritus, and rarely bronchospasm and hypotension as infusion reactions.

c. Cardiovascular (cardiac failure, embolism, cerebrovascular accidents) effects are uncommon.

d. Hemolytic uremic syndrome is rare.

CARMUSTINE

Other names. BCNU, BiCNU, Gliadel wafer (surgically implantable, biodegradable polymer wafer that releases impregnated carmustine from the hydrophobic matrix after implantation).

Mechanism of action. Alkylation and carbamoylation by carmustine metabolites interfere with the synthesis and function of DNA, RNA, and proteins. Carmustine is lipid soluble and easily enters the brain.

Primary indications.

1. *Systemic therapy.*
   a. Brain tumors.
   b. Hodgkin's and non–Hodgkin's lymphomas.
   c. Melanoma.
2. *Implantable carmustine-impregnated wafer.*
   a. Glioblastoma multiforme.

Usual dosage and schedule.

A. *Systemic therapy.*
   a. 200 to 240 mg/m² IV as a 30- to 45-min infusion every 6 to 8 weeks. Dose is often divided and given over 2 to 3 days. Some recommend limiting the lifetime cumulative dose to 1,000 mg/m² to limit pulmonary and renal toxicities.
   b. Higher doses of up to 600 mg/m² have been used with stem cell rescue (e.g., bone marrow or peripheral blood stem cell transplantation).

B. Implantable carmustine-impregnated wafer: up to 8 wafers, each containing 7.7 mg of carmustine, are applied to the resection cavity surface after removal of the tumor.

Special precautions (systemic therapy). Because of delayed myelosuppression and other hematologic effects (3 to 6 weeks), do not administer the drug more often than every 6 weeks. Await a return of normal platelet and granulocyte counts before repeating therapy. Amphotericin B may enhance the potential for renal toxicity, bronchospasm, and hypotension.

Toxicity.

A. *Systemic therapy.*
   a. *Myelosuppression and other hematologic effects.* Delayed and often biphasic, with the nadir at 3 to 6 weeks; it may be cumulative with successive doses. Recovery may be protracted for several months. High-dose therapy requires stem cell rescue.
   b. *Nausea, vomiting, and other gastrointestinal effects.* Are common, beginning 2 h after therapy and lasting 4 to 6 h.
   c. *Mucocutaneous effects.*
      1. Facial flushing and a burning sensation at the IV site may be due to alcohol used to reconstitute the drug; this is common with rapid injection.
      2. Hyperpigmentation of skin after accidental contact is common.
   d. *Miscellaneous effects.*
      1. Hepatotoxicity is uncommon but can be severe.

2. Pulmonary fibrosis is uncommon at low doses, but its frequency increases at cumulative doses higher than 1,000 mg/m^2.
3. Secondary neoplasia is possible.
4. Renal toxicity is uncommon at cumulative doses of less than 1,000 mg/m^2.
5. With high-dose therapy, encephalopathy, hepatotoxicity, and pulmonary toxicity are common and dose limiting. Hepatoveno-occlusive disease also occurs. (occasional).

B. *Implantable carmustine-impregnated wafer*. Limited toxicity beyond that expected from craniotomy is seen. Serious intracranial infection was seen in 4% of patients, compared with 1% of placebo-treated patients. Brain edema not responsive to steroids may also be seen in a similar percentage of patients. Abnormal wound healing may occur. Remnants of the wafer may be seen for many months after implantation.

CETUXIMAB

Other names. EGFR antibody, C225, Erbitux.

Mechanism of action. EGFR antibody that blocks the ligand-binding site and inhibits proliferation of cells. It is thought to be potentially most useful in those tumors that overexpress EGFR, but correlation with the percentage of positive cells or intensity of EGFR expression is weak.

Primary indications.
1. Carcinoma of head and neck, in combination with radiation therapy or after failure of platinum-based therapy.
2. Colon cancer, usually in combination with irinotecan.

Usual dosage and schedule. 400 mg/m^2 IV loading dose administered over 2 h on day 1. Then 250 mg/m^2 IV maintenance doses administered over 1 h weekly thereafter. May be administered in combination with other agents.

Special precautions. Severe anaphylactoid reactions that include cardiac arrest (2%) may occur. One hour of observation is recommended following a cetuximab infusion. Severe hypomagnesemia is seen in 10% to 15% of patients, and all patients should have magnesium levels monitored throughout the systemic persistence of cetuximab (8 weeks).

Toxicity.
1. *Myelosuppression and other hematologic effects*. Leukopenia and anemia are occasional.
2. *Nausea, vomiting, and other gastrointestinal effects*. Anorexia, nausea, vomiting, diarrhea, and constipation are occasional. Abdominal pain is common.
3. *Mucocutaneous effects*. Acne-like rash is common (76%). Stomatitis is occasional when used alone, but universal when used in combination with radiation therapy.
4. *Miscellaneous effects*.
   a. Asthenia is common; headache and back pain are occasional.
   b. Weight loss, peripheral edema, and dehydration are occasional.

  c. Infusion reactions with allergic or hypersensitivity reactions, fever, chills, or dyspnea are occasional to common (~20%) but may be severe.
  d. Human antichimeric antibodies (HACAs) are uncommon.
  e. Electrolyte depletion, particularly hypomagnesemia, occurs commonly. Hypomagnesemia is occasionally severe.

CHLORAMBUCIL

Other name. Leukeran.
Mechanism of action. Classic alkylating agent, with primary effect on preformed DNA.
Primary indications.
1. Chronic lymphocytic leukemia.
2. Low-grade non–Hodgkin's lymphoma.
Usual dosage and schedule.
1. 3 to 4 mg/m^2 PO daily until a response is seen or cytopenias occur; then, if necessary, maintain with 1 to 2 mg/m^2 PO daily.
2. 30 mg/m^2 PO once every 2 weeks (with or without prednisone 80 mg/m^2 PO on days 1 to 5).
Special precautions. Increased toxicity may occur with prior barbiturate use.
Toxicity.
1. *Myelosuppression and other hematologic effects.* Dose limiting and may be prolonged.
2. *Nausea, vomiting, and other gastrointestinal effects.* May be seen with higher doses but are uncommon.
3. *Mucocutaneous effects.* Rash is uncommon.
4. *Miscellaneous effects.*
   a. Liver function abnormalities are rare.
   b. Secondary neoplasia is possible.
   c. Amenorrhea and azoospermia are common.
   d. Drug fever is uncommon.
   e. Pulmonary fibrosis is rare.
   f. CNS effects including seizure and coma may be seen at very high doses (>100 mg/m^2).

CISPLATIN

Other names. *cis*-Diamminedichloroplatinum (II), DDP, CDDP, Platinol.
Mechanism of action. Similar to alkylating agents with respect to binding and cross-linking strands of DNA.
Primary indications. Usually used in combination with other cytotoxic drugs.
1. Testis, ovary, endometrial, cervical, bladder, head and neck, gastrointestinal, and lung carcinomas.
2. Soft tissue and bone sarcomas.
3. Non–Hodgkin's lymphoma.
Usual dosage and schedule.
1. 40 to 120 mg/m^2 IV on day 1 as infusion every 3 weeks.
2. 15 to 20 mg/m^2 IV on days 1 to 5 as infusion every 3 to 4 weeks.
Special precautions. Do not administer if serum creatinine level is more than 1.5 mg/dL. Irreversible renal tubular damage may occur if vigorous diuresis is not maintained, particularly

with higher doses (>40 mg/m^2) and with additional concurrent nephrotoxic drugs, such as aminoglycosides. At higher doses, diuresis with mannitol with or without furosemide plus vigorous hydration are mandatory.

1. An acceptable method for hydration in patients without cardiovascular impairment for cisplatin doses up to 80 mg/m^2 is as follows:

   a. Have the patient void, and begin infusion of 5% dextrose in half-normal saline with potassium chloride (KCl) 20 mEq/L and magnesium sulfate (MgSO$_4$) 1 g/L (8 mEq/L); run at 500 mL/h for 1.5 to 2.0 L.

   b. After 1 h of infusion, give 12.5 g of mannitol by IV push.

   c. Immediately thereafter, start the cisplatin (mixed in normal saline at 1 mg/mL) and infuse over 1 h through the sidearm of the IV, while continuing the hydration.

   d. Give additional mannitol (12.5–50.0 g by IV push) if necessary to maintain urinary output of 250 mL/h over the duration of the hydration. If patient gets behind on urinary output by more than 1 L or signs or symptoms of congestive heart failure develop, 40 mg of furosemide may be given.

2. For doses more than 80 mg/m^2 a more vigorous hydration is recommended.

   a. Have the patient void, and begin infusion of 5% dextrose in half-normal saline with KCl 20 mEq/L and MgSO$_4$ 1 g/L (8 mEq/L); run at 500 mL/h for 2.5 to 3.0 L.

   b. After 1 h of infusion, give 25 g of mannitol by IV push.

   c. Continue hydration.

   d. After 2 h of hydration, if urinary output is at least 250 mL/h, start the cisplatin (mixed in normal saline at 1 mg/mL) and infuse over 1 to 2 h (1 mg/m^2/min) through the sidearm of the IV, while continuing the hydration.

   e. Give additional mannitol (12.5–50 g by IV push) if necessary to maintain urinary output of 250 mL/h over the duration of the hydration. If patient gets behind on urinary output by more than 1 L or signs or symptoms of congestive heart failure develop, 40 mg of furosemide may be given.

3. For patients with known or suspected cardiovascular impairment (ejection fraction <45%), a less vigorous rate of hydration may be used, provided the dose of cisplatin is limited (e.g., <60 mg/m^2). An alternative is to give carboplatin.

Toxicity.

1. *Myelosuppression and other hematologic effects.* Mild to moderate, depending on the dose. Relative lack of myelosuppression and other hematologic effects allows cisplatin to be used in full doses with moremyelosuppressive drugs. *Anemia* is common and may have a hemolytic component. Anemia is often amenable to epoetin therapy.

2. *Nausea, vomiting, and other gastrointestinal effects.* Severe and often intractable vomiting regularly begins within 1 h of starting cisplatin and lasts for 8 to 12 h. Prolonged nausea, vomiting, and other gastrointestinal effects occur occasionally. Nausea, vomiting, and other gastrointestinal effects may be minimized by the use of a combination antiemetic regimen (see Chapter 27).

3. *Mucocutaneous effects.* None.

4. *Renal tubular damage*. Acute reversible and occasionally irreversible nephrotoxicity may occur, particularly if adequate attention is not given to achieving sufficient hydration and diuresis. Nephrotoxic antibiotics increase risk of acute renal failure.

5. *Ototoxicity*. High-tone hearing loss is common, but significant hearing loss at vocal frequencies occurs only occasionally. Tinnitus is uncommon.

6. *Severe electrolyte abnormalities*. These abnormalities, for example, marked hyponatremia, hypomagnesemia, hypocalcemia, and hypokalemia, may be seen up to several days after treatment.

7. *Anaphylaxis*. May occur after several doses. Responds to epinephrine, antihistamines, and corticosteroids.

8. *Miscellaneous effects*.
   a. Peripheral neuropathies are clinically significant; signs and symptoms are common at cumulative doses more than 300 mg/m^2.
   b. Hyperuricemia is uncommon, and parallels renal failure.
   c. Autonomic dysfunction with symptomatic postural hypotension is occasional.

CLADRIBINE

Other names.   2-Chlorodeoxyadenosine, Leustatin.

Mechanism of action.   Deoxyadenosine analog with high cellular specificity for lymphoid cells. Resistant to effect of ADA. Accumulates in cells as triphosphate, is incorporated into DNA, and inhibits DNA repair enzymes and RNA synthesis. Also results in NAD depletion. Effect is independent of cell division.

Primary indication.   Hairy-cell leukemia, chronic lymphocytic leukemia, Waldenström's macroglobulinemia, and possibly other lymphoid neoplasms.

Usual dosage and schedule.

1. 0.09 mg/kg (3.33 mg/m^2) IV daily as a continuous 7-day infusion.
2. 0.14 mg/kg (5.2 mg/m^2) IV as a 2-h infusion daily for 5 days.
3. 0.14 mg/kg (5.2 mg/m^2) SC daily for 5 days.

Special precautions.   Give allopurinol, 300 mg daily, as prophylaxis against hyperuricemia. Opportunistic infections occur occasionally and should be watched for closely.

Toxicity.

1. *Myelosuppression and other hematologic effects*. Moderate granulocyte suppression is common. Marrow suppression with leukopenia and thrombocytopenia may be prolonged for more than a year. Serious infection is common. Profound suppression of CD4 and CD8 counts is common and often prolonged for more than 1 year. Opportunistic infections, including herpes, fungus, and pneumocystic infection, may occur and should be watched for. Some routinely use prolonged prophylaxis against one or more of these infections, to include acyclovir 400 mg b.i.d. and trimethoprim–sulfamethoxazole, 1 double-strength tablet twice daily on 2 or 3 days a week.

2. *Nausea, vomiting, and other gastrointestinal effects*. Mild nausea with decrease in appetite is common, but no vomiting is expected.

3. *Mucocutaneous effects*. Rash is common. Injection site reactions are occasional.
4. *Miscellaneous effects*.
   a. Fever, possibly due to release of pyrogens from tumor cells, is common.
   b. Fatigue is common. Headache, dizziness, insomnia, myalgia, and arthralgia are occasional.
   c. Edema and tachycardia are occasional.
   d. Cough, shortness of breath, and abnormal breath sounds are occasional.

CLOFARABINE

Other name. Clolar.
Mechanism of action. Clofarabine is a nucleoside analog (an adenine derivative) that is a potent inhibitor of ribonucleotide reductase. Also inhibits DNA polymerases and DNA synthesis. Increases intracellular ara-CTP when used with cytarabine.
Primary indications.
1. Acute lymphoblastic leukemia in children (age 1–21) who have relapsed or are refractory to other therapy.
2. Acute lymphoblastic or acute myelogenous leukemia (AML) in adults.
Usual dosage and schedule.
1. 52 mg/m^2 IV over 2 h daily for 5 consecutive days; may be repeated in 2 to 6 weeks.
2. 40 mg/m^2 IV over 1 h (days 2–6), followed in 4 h by cytarabine 1 g/m^2 IV as a 2-h infusion (days 1–5) in AML in adults.
Special precautions. Capillary leak syndrome or systemic inflammatory response syndrome (SIRS) has been observed with clofarabine administration.
Toxicity.
1. *Myelosuppression and other hematologic effects*. Pancytopenia is common. Febrile neutropenia and documented infections are common.
2. *Nausea, vomiting, and other gastrointestinal effects*. Nausea, vomiting, diarrhea, and abdominal pain are common. Elevation of transaminases is common and may be severe (grade 3–4); jaundice is occasional. Anorexia is common.
3. *Mucocutaneous effects*. Nonspecific dermatitis and pruritus are common. Palmar-plantar erythrodysesthesia is occasional.
4. *Miscellaneous effects*.
   a. Capillary leak syndrome and SIRS may occur following drug administration.
   b. Arthralgia and back pain are occasional.
   c. Creatinine elevations are uncommon to occasional.
   d. Fatigue is common. Lethargy is occasional.
   e. Flushing and hypotension are occasional to common.
      Left ventricular dysfunction is occasional to common.

CORTICOSTEROIDS

Other names. Prednisone, dexamethasone (Decadron), and others.
Mechanism of action. Unknown but apparently related to the presence of glucocorticoid receptors in tumor cells.

Mediated in part by *bcl*-2 gene and promotion of apoptotic cell death.

Primary indications.
1. Acute and chronic lymphocytic leukemia.
2. Hodgkin's and non–Hodgkin's lymphomas.
3. Multiple myeloma.
4. Carcinoma of the breast.
5. Cerebral edema or spinal cord injury (compression).
6. Nausea and vomiting from chemotherapy.

Usual dosage and schedule.
1. *Prednisone.* Dose varies with neoplasm and combination. Typical regimen, *except* for acute lymphocytic leukemia, is as follows.
   a. 40 mg/m^2 PO days 1 to 14 every 4 weeks *or*
   b. 100 mg/m^2 PO days 1 to 5 every 4 weeks.
2. *Prednisone.* For acute lymphocytic leukemia: 40 to 50 mg/m^2 PO daily for 28 days.
3. *Dexamethasone.* For cerebral edema or spinal cord injury: 10 mg IV push, and then 16 to 32 mg PO daily in four divided doses. As signs and symptoms are controlled, gradually reduce to the lowest effective dose.

Special precautions. Monitor for hyperglycemia.

Toxicity.
1. *Myelosuppression and other hematologic effects.* None.
2. *Nausea, vomiting, and other gastrointestinal effects.* No acute nausea and vomiting. Epigastric pain, extreme hunger, and occasional peptic ulceration with bleeding may occur even with short courses. Antacids or inhibitors of acid secretion are recommended as prophylaxis.
3. *Mucocutaneous effects.* Acne; increased risk for oral, rectal, and vaginal thrush. Thinning of skin and striae develop with continuous use.
4. *Suppression of adrenal–pituitary axis.* May lead to adrenal insufficiency when corticosteroids are withdrawn. This problem is not common with intermittent schedules.
5. *Metabolic effects.* Potassium depletion, sodium and fluid retention, diabetes, increased appetite, loss of muscle mass, myopathy, weight gain, osteoporosis, and development of Cushingoid features. Their frequency depends on dose and duration of therapy. Quadriceps weakness is common with prolonged dosing.
6. *Miscellaneous effects.*
   a. CNS effects, including euphoria, depression, and sleeplessness, are common and may progress to dementia or frank psychosis.
   b. Immunosuppression with increased susceptibility to infection is common.
   c. Subcapsular cataracts in patients are uncommon but have been seen even when used for prophylaxis and treatment of drug-induced emesis.

CYCLOPHOSPHAMIDE

Other names. CTX, Cytoxan, Neosar.

Mechanism of action. Metabolism of cyclophosphamide by hepatic microsomal enzymes produces active alkylating metabolites. The primary effect of cyclophosphamide is probably on DNA.

Primary indications.
1. Breast, lung, ovary, testis, and bladder carcinomas.
2. Bone and soft tissue sarcomas.
3. Hodgkin's and non–Hodgkin's lymphomas.
4. Acute and chronic lymphocytic leukemias.
5. Waldenström's macroglobulinemia.
6. Neuroblastoma and Wilms' tumor of childhood.
7. Gestational trophoblastic neoplasms.
8. Multiple myeloma.

Usual dosage and schedule.
1. 1,000 to 1,500 mg/m^2 IV every 3 to 4 weeks *or*
2. 400 mg/m^2 PO days 1 to 5 every 3 to 4 weeks *or*
3. 60 to 120 mg/m^2 PO daily.
4. High-dose regimens (4–7 g/m^2 divided over 4 days) are investigational and should only be used with some kind of stem cell rescue (e.g., bone marrow transplantation) and mesna bladder protection.

Special precautions. Give dose in the morning, maintain ample fluid intake, and have the patient empty the bladder several times daily to diminish the likelihood of cystitis.

Toxicity.
1. *Myelosuppression and other hematologic effects.* Dose limiting. Platelets are relatively spared. Nadir is reached approximately 10 to 14 days after IV dose with recovery by day 21.
2. *Nausea, vomiting, and other gastrointestinal effects.* Frequent with large IV doses; less common after oral doses. Symptoms begin several hours after treatment and are usually over by the next day.
3. *Mucocutaneous effects.* Reversible alopecia is common, usually starting after 2 to 3 weeks. Skin and nails may become darker. Mucositis is uncommon.
4. *Bladder damage.* Hemorrhagic or nonhemorrhagic cystitis may occur in 5% to 10% of patients treated. It is usually reversible with discontinuation of the drug, but it may persist and lead to fibrosis or death. Frequency is diminished by ample fluid intake and morning administration of the drug. Mesna will protect from this effect.
5. *Miscellaneous effects.*
   a. Immunosuppression is common.
   b. Amenorrhea and azoospermia are common.
   c. Inhibition of antidiuretic hormone is only of significance with very large doses.
   d. Interstitial pulmonary fibrosis is rare.
   e. Secondary neoplasia is possible.
   f. Acute and potentially fatal cardiotoxicity occurs with high-dose therapy. Abnormalities include pericardial effusion, congestive heart failure, decreased electrocardiographic (ECG) voltage, and fibrin microthrombi in cardiac capillaries with endothelial injury and hemorrhagic necrosis.

CYTARABINE

Other names. Cytosine arabinoside, ara-C, Cytosar-U, DepoCyt (cytarabine, liposomal for intrathecal use only).

Mechanism of action. A pyrimidine analog antimetabolite that, when phosphorylated to arabinosyl-cytosinetriphosphate (ara-CTP), is a competitive inhibitor of DNA polymerase.

Primary indications.

1. Acute nonlymphocytic leukemia.
2. Meningeal lymphoma or leukemia.

Usual dosage and schedule.

1. *Induction.* 100 mg/m² IV daily as a continuous infusion for 5 to 7 days (in combination with other drugs).
2. *Maintenance.* 100 mg/m² SQ every 12 h for 4 or 5 days every 4 weeks (with other drugs).
3. *Intrathecally.*
   a. 40 to 50 mg/m² of cytarabine, unencapsulated, every 4 days in preservative-free buffered isotonic diluent.
   b. 50 mg of cytarabine, liposomal, repeated in 14 to 28 days.
4. *High dose.*
   a. *Induction.* 2 to 3 g/m² IV over 1 to 2 h every 12 h for up to 12 doses.
   b. *Consolidation.* 3 g/m² IV over 3 h every 12 h on days 1, 3, and 5.

Special precautions. None for standard doses. High dose, give in *1- to 3-h infusion.* Longer infusion enhances toxicity. CNS toxicity is increased in patients with a decreased creatinine clearance. Cytarabine, liposomal (DepoCyt) should be used only intrathecally.

Toxicity (standard dose only).

1. *Myelosuppression and other hematologic effects.* Dose-limiting leukopenia and thrombocytopenia occur, with nadir at 7 to 10 days after treatment has ended, and with recovery during the following 2 weeks, depending on the degree of suppression. Megaloblastosis is common.
2. *Nausea, vomiting, and other gastrointestinal effects.* Common, particularly if the drug is given as a push or rapid infusion.
3. *Mucocutaneous effects.* Stomatitis is seen occasionally.
4. *Miscellaneous effects.*
   a. Flu-like syndrome with fever, arthralgia, and sometimes a rash is occasional.
   b. Transient mild hepatic dysfunction is occasional.

Toxicity (high dose).

1. *Myelosuppression and other hematologic effects.* Universal.
2. *Nausea, vomiting, and other gastrointestinal effects.* Common.
3. *Mucocutaneous effects.* Occasional to common mucositis.
4. *Neurotoxicity.* Cerebellar toxicity is common, particularly in the elderly, but is usually mild and reversible. However, on occasion it has been severe and permanent or fatal.
5. *Conjunctivitis.* Hydrocortisone 2 drops OU q.i.d. for 10 days may ameliorate or prevent keratitis.
6. *Hepatic toxicity with cholestatic jaundice.* Uncommon.
7. *Diarrhea.* Common.

DACARBAZINE

Other names. Imidazole carboxamide, DIC, DTIC-Dome.

Mechanism of action. Uncertain but probably interacts with preformed macromolecules by alkylation. Inhibits DNA, RNA, and protein synthesis.

Primary indications.
1. Melanoma.
2. All soft tissue sarcomas.
3. Hodgkin's lymphoma.

Usual dosage and schedule.
1. 150 to 250 mg/m^2 IV push or rapid infusion on days 1 to 5 every 3 to 4 weeks *or*
2. 400 to 500 mg/m^2 IV push or rapid infusion on days 1 and 2 every 3 to 4 weeks *or*
3. 200 mg/m^2 IV daily as a continuous 96-h infusion.

Special precautions.
1. Administer cautiously to avoid extravasation, as tissue damage may occur.
2. Venous pain along the injection site may be reduced by diluting dacarbazine in 100 to 200 mL of 5% dextrose in water and infusing over 30 min rather than injecting rapidly. Ice application may also reduce pain.

Toxicity.
1. *Myelosuppression and other hematologic effects*. Mild to moderate. This factor allows dacarbazine to be used in full doses with other myelosuppressive drugs.
2. *Nausea, vomiting, and other gastrointestinal effects*. Common and severe but decrease in intensity with each subsequent daily dose. Onset is within 1 to 3 h, with duration up to 12 h.
3. *Mucocutaneous effects*.
   a. Moderately severe tissue damage if extravasation occurs.
   b. Alopecia is uncommon.
   c. Erythematous or urticarial rash is uncommon.
4. *Miscellaneous effects*.
   a. Flu-like syndrome with fever, myalgia, and malaise lasting several days is uncommon.
   b. Hepatic toxicity is uncommon.

DACTINOMYCIN

Other names.   Actinomycin D, act-D, Cosmegen.

Mechanism of action.   Binds to DNA and inhibits DNA-dependent RNA synthesis. Inhibition of topoisomerase II.

Primary indications.
1. Gestational trophoblastic neoplasms.
2. Wilms' tumor, childhood rhabdomyosarcoma, and Ewing's sarcoma.

Usual dosage and schedule.
1. *Children*. 0.40 to 0.45 mg/m^2 (up to a maximum of 0.5 mg) IV daily for 5 days every 3 to 5 weeks.
2. *Adults*.
   a. 0.40 to 0.45 mg/m^2 IV on days 1 to 5 every 2 to 3 weeks.
   b. 0.5 mg IV daily for 5 days every 3 to 5 weeks.

Special precautions.
1. Administer by slow IV push through the sidearm of a running IV infusion, being careful to avoid extravasation, which causes severe soft tissue damage.
2. If given at or about the time of infection with chickenpox or herpes zoster, a severe generalized disease may occur that sometimes results in death.

Toxicity.
1. *Myelosuppression and other hematologic effects.* May be dose limiting and severe. It begins within the first week of treatment, but the nadir may not be reached for 21 days.
2. *Nausea, vomiting, and other gastrointestinal effects.* Severe vomiting often occurs during the first few hours after drug administration and lasts up to 24 h.
3. *Mucocutaneous effects.*
   a. Erythema, hyperpigmentation, and desquamation of the skin with potentiation by previous or concurrent radiotherapy are common.
   b. Oropharyngeal mucositis is potentiated by previous or concurrent radiotherapy.
   c. Alopecia is common.
   d. Moderately severe tissue damage occurs with extravasation.
4. *Miscellaneous effects.*
   a. Mental depression is rare.
   b. Hepatoveno-occlusive disease, worse with higher doses and shorter schedules, for example, single dose of 2.5 mg versus 5 days at 0.5 mg/day.

DARBEPOETIN

Other names.   Aranesp, darbepoetin α.

Mechanism of action.   Darbepoetin is an erythropoiesis-stimulating protein, closely related to erythropoietin, which is produced in Chinese hamster ovary (CHO) cells by recombinant DNA technology. It differs from recombinant human erythropoietin in that it contains five *N*-linked oligosaccharide chains, whereas recombinant human erythropoietin contains three chains. It has the same biologic activity as endogenous erythropoietin, inducing erythropoiesis by stimulating the division and differentiation of committed erythroid progenitor cells.

Primary indications.
1. Anemia from chemotherapy in patients with nonmyeloid malignancies.
2. Anemia from cancer in patients with nonmyeloid malignancies.
3. Anemia associated with chronic renal failure.

Usual dosage and schedule.   Patients with anemia from cancer or chemotherapy:
1. Starting dose of 2.25 μg/kg/week by SC injection, or
2. 500 μg by SC injection every 3 weeks.

Adult patients with chronic renal failure: starting dose of 0.45 μg/kg/week by IV or SC injection.

Dose adjustments of 25% to 40% upward or downward are recommended to keep the hemoglobin below 12.

Special precautions.   Contraindicated in patients with uncontrolled hypertension or known hypersensitivity to albumin or mammalian cell-derived products. Potential for serious allergic or anaphylactic reaction. Rare cases of pure red cell aplasia have been reported.

Toxicity.
1. *Myelosuppression and other hematologic effects.* Myelosuppression is not seen, except for rare cases of pure

red cell aplasia. Thromboembolic complications are uncommon.
2. *Nausea, vomiting, and other gastrointestinal effects.* Diarrhea is occasional.
3. *Mucocutaneous effects.* Uncommon rashes or urticaria. Pruritus is occasional.
4. *Miscellaneous effects.*
   a. *Cardiovascular.* Hypertension may occasionally occur in association with a significant increase in hematocrit; the risk is greatest in patients with preexisting hypertension. Chest pain is uncommon and myocardial infarction is uncommon to rare. Edema is occasional.
   b. *Neurologic.* Seizures, stroke, and transient ischemic attack are rare.
   c. *Musculoskeletal.* Arthralgia and myalgia are occasional.
   d. Influenza-like syndrome is rare to uncommon. Fever alone is occasional.

DASATINIB

Other name. SPRYCEL.
Mechanism of action. Inhibition of multiple RTKs, including BCR-ABL and the SRC family. Believed to bind to multiple conformations of the ABL kinase.
Primary indications.
1. CML in the chronic, accelerated, or blast phase (myeloid or lymphoid) with resistance or intolerance to prior therapy including imatinib.
2. Acute lymphoblastic leukemia (ALL) that is Philadelphia chromosome positive and refractory to prior therapy.
Usual dosage and schedule. 70 mg twice daily. Doses are adjusted up or down in 20-mg increments as needed.
Special precautions. Should not be administered to patients who have or who are at risk for prolonged QT interval.
Toxicity.
1. *Myelosuppression and other hematologic effects.* Neutropenia, thrombocytopenia, and anemia are common in all patients. Bleeding is common and is occasionally severe, but they are seen primarily in the accelerated or blastic phases. Febrile neutropenia is occasional.
2. *Nausea, vomiting, and other gastrointestinal effects.* Nausea and vomiting are common, but rarely severe. Diarrhea is common, but severe diarrhea is uncommon. Abdominal pain is common. Constipation is occasional.
3. *Mucocutaneous effects.* Stomatitis is occasional. Various skin maladies are uncommon.
4. *Neurologic effects.* Peripheral neuropathy is occasional.
5. *Miscellaneous effects.*
   a. *Cardiovascular.* Fluid retention is common and occasionally severe. Pleural and pericardial effusions are uncommon. Severe pulmonary edema is rare. Prolonged cardiac ventricular repolarization (QT prolongation) is uncommon and rarely severe.
   b. *Respiratory.* Dyspnea, cough, and upper respiratory infections are common.
   c. Musculoskeletal pain is common.

d. Fever and fatigue are common.
e. Hypophosphatemia and hypocalcemia are occasional. Abnormal transaminases or elevated bilirubin are uncommon.

DAUNORUBICIN

Other names. Daunomycin, rubidomycin, DNR, Cerubidine.
Mechanism of action. DNA strand breakage mediated by anthracycline effects on topoisomerase II; DNA intercalation; DNA polymerase inhibition.
Primary indication. Acute nonlymphocytic leukemia, acute lymphocytic leukemia.
Usual dosage and schedule.
1. 45 to 60 mg/m^2 IV push on days 1, 2, and 3 as induction therapy for 1 or 2 cycles in combination with other drugs.
2. 45 mg/m^2 IV push on days 1 and 2 every 4 weeks as consolidation therapy for 1 or 2 cycles in combination with other drugs.
Special precautions.
1. Administer over several minutes into the sidearm of a running IV infusion, taking precautions to avoid extravasation.
2. Do not give if patient has significantly impaired cardiac function (ejection fraction <45%), angina pectoris, cardiac arrhythmia, or recent myocardial infarction.
3. Do not exceed cumulative dosage of 550 mg/m^2 (400 mg/m^2 if given previous radiation therapy that has encompassed the heart).
4. Reduce dose if patient has impaired liver or renal function.

Serum bilirubin (mg/dL)		Serum creatinine (mg/dL)	% of full dose
1.2–3.0		—	75
>3.0	or	>3.0	50

Toxicity.
1. *Myelosuppression and other hematologic effects.* Dose-limiting pancytopenia with nadir at 1 to 2 weeks.
2. *Nausea, vomiting, and other gastrointestinal effects.* Nausea and vomiting occur on the day of administration in one half of patients.
3. *Mucocutaneous effects.* Alopecia is common, but stomatitis is rare. Severe local tissue damage may progress to skin ulceration, and necrosis may occur with subcutaneous extravasation.
4. *Cardiac effects.* Potentially irreversible congestive heart failure may occur owing to cardiomyopathy. The incidence is highly dependent on the lifetime cumulative dose, which should not exceed 550 mg/m^2 (400 mg/m^2 if patient was given previous radiotherapy that encompassed the heart). Discontinue drug if there is clinical congestive heart failure or if the ejection fraction falls on the radionuclide angiogram,
   a. to less than 45% *or*
   b. to less than 50% if the total decrease is 10% or more (e.g., falls from 59% to 49%).

If repeat ejection fraction determination shows return of function, drug may be cautiously restarted, but ejection fraction should be measured before each dose. Transient ECG changes are common and are not usually serious.
5. *Miscellaneous effects.*
    a. Red urine caused by the drug and its metabolites is common.
    b. Chemical phlebitis and phlebothrombosis of veins used for injection are common.

DAUNORUBICIN, LIPOSOMAL

Other name. DaunoXome.

Mechanism of action. Daunorubicin, liposomal, which is designed to be protected from removal by the reticuloendothelial system, has a prolonged circulation time compared with unprotected drug. The agent penetrates tumor tissue and releases the active ingredient daunorubicin. The active drug causes DNA strand breakage mediated by anthracycline effects on topoisomerase II; DNA intercalation; and DNA polymerase inhibition.

Primary indication. Kaposi's sarcoma, advanced, human immunodeficiency virus (HIV) associated.

Usual dosage and schedule. 40 mg/m^2 IV over 60 min every 2 weeks.

Special precautions.
1. Must be diluted to a concentration of 1 mg/mL with 5% dextrose for injection. Liposomal doxorubicin should be considered an irritant, and care should be taken to avoid extravasation.
2. Do not give if the patient has significantly impaired cardiac function.
3. Do not exceed a lifetime cumulative dose of 550 mg/m^2 (400 mg/m^2 if the patient was given prior chest radiotherapy). Patients with HIV may experience a decrease in left ventricular ejection fraction and congestive heart failure at lower doses than those without.
4. Reduce or hold dose in patients with impairment of liver function. A 25% dose reduction is recommended if the serum bilirubin is 1.2 to 3 mg/dL. Half the normal dose is recommended in patients with serum bilirubin concentration greater than 3 mg/dL.

Toxicity. Effects that are a result of the liposomal doxorubicin have been somewhat difficult to determine with certainty, because most patients have been on several other agents that can result in other drugs that may cause marrow or other toxicity.
1. *Myelosuppression and other hematologic effects.* Common and dose related. May be severe.
2. *Nausea, vomiting, and other gastrointestinal effects.* Nausea, vomiting, and diarrhea are common.
3. *Mucocutaneous effects.* Alopecia is occasional. Stomatitis is occasional.
4. *Miscellaneous effects.*
    a. Cardiac events, including cardiomyopathy or congestive heart failure may occur and are dose dependent (see Special precautions).
    b. *Infusion reactions.* Acute infusion-associated reactions with back pain, flushing, and tightness in the chest and throat,

alone or in combination, have occurred in approximately 14% of patients treated with liposomal doxorubicin. They usually occur with the first infusion, and are not likely to occur later if the first infusion is given without a reaction. Generally occur during the first 5 min of the infusion and subside with interruption of the infusion. Some patients tolerate restarting at a lower rate of infusion. Most patients are able to continue therapy.
  c. Fatigue is common.
  d. Fever is common.
  e. Pain at the injection site is likely after extravasation.

DECITABINE

Other name. Dacogen.
Mechanism of action. Pyrimidine analog that inhibits methyltransferase, causing hypomethylation of DNA and thus, it is believed, results in cellular differentiation or apoptosis. May restore normal function of genes that are critical for the control of cellular differentiation and proliferation.
Primary indications.
1. Myelodysplastic syndromes.
2. Acute myelogenous leukemia in the elderly.
Usual dosage and schedule. 15 mg/m^2 continuous IV infusion over 3 h, repeated every 8 h for 3 days. This cycle is repeated every 6 weeks for a minimum of four cycles. Therapy may be continued so long as the patient improves from the drug.
Toxicity.
1. *Myelosuppression.* Neutropenia, thrombocytopenia, and anemia are common. Febrile neutropenia is five times as common as in patients receiving supportive care.
2. *Nausea and vomiting.* Nausea, vomiting, and diarrhea or constipation occur in approximately one third of patients. Abdominal pain may be associated.
3. *Mucocutaneous effects.* Stomatitis is occasional. Skin rash is occasional, alopecia is occasional, and urticaria is uncommon.
4. *Neurotoxicity.* Insomnia is common. Lethargy or confusional state are occasional.
5. *Miscellaneous effects.*
  a. Pulmonary edema is uncommon.
  b. Blurred vision is uncommon.
  c. Fever is common; infections are occasional.
  d. Arthralgias and back pain are occasional.
  e. Hypomagnesemia and hypokalemia occur in approximately 25% of patients.
  f. Abnormal liver function tests are uncommon.

DENILEUKIN DIFTITOX

Other name. Ontak.
Mechanism of action. Denileukin diftitox is produced by genetically fusing protein from the diphtheria toxin to IL-2. This stable fusion protein targets cells with receptors for IL-2 on their surfaces, including malignant cells and some normal lymphocytes, resulting in cell death. Efficacy in patients without the CD25 receptor is not known.

Primary indication.   Persistent or recurrent CTCL that expresses the CD25 component of IL-2 receptor.

Usual dosage and schedule.   9 or 18 μg/kg/day (350–700 mg/m²/day) IV over at least 15 min for 5 consecutive days every 21 days.

Special precautions.   Acute hypersensitivity reactions occur commonly. Loss of visual acuity, usually with loss of color vision, usually resulting in permanent visual impairment.

Toxicity.
1. *Myelosuppression and other hematologic effects.* Anemia and lymphopenia are common. Thrombocytopenia is occasional. Thrombotic events are occasional.
2. *Nausea, vomiting, and other gastrointestinal effects.* Nausea, vomiting, and diarrhea are common. Dehydration as a consequence is occasional.
3. *Mucocutaneous effects.* Rashes—including generalized macropapular, petechial, vesicular bullous, urticarial, and eczematous ones—may be seen, with both acute and delayed onset.
4. *Miscellaneous effects.*
   a. Severe infections are common.
   b. Acute hypersensitivity reactions occur commonly, including hypotension, back pain, dyspnea, vasodilation, rash, chest pain or tightness, and tachycardia. Syncope is uncommon; anaphylaxis is rare.
   c. Cardiovascular effects, including hypotension, vasodilation, fluid retention, and tachycardia are common. Hypertension and arrhythmias are occasional.
   d. Respiratory reactions of dyspnea, increase in cough, and pharyngitis are common.
   e. Vascular leak syndrome is common.
   f. Metabolic changes that include hypoalbuminemia, transaminase increase and hypocalcemia are common. Hypokalemia, albuminuria, and increase in creatinine are occasional.
   g. Arterial and venous thromboses are uncommon.
   h. Flu-like symptoms with chills, fever, headache, and weakness are common. Myalgias and arthralgias are occasional.
   i. Loss of visual acuity, usually resulting in permanent visual impairment, uncertain frequency, probably rare to uncommon.

DEXRAZOXANE

Other names.   Zinecard, ICRF-187.

Mechanism of action.   Probably by means of conversion of dexrazoxane intracellularly to a chelating agent that interferes with iron-mediated free radical generation, which is thought to be responsible, in part, for anthracycline-related cardiomyopathy. Appears to protect against myocardial toxicity without impairment of tumor response.

Primary indication.   Prophylaxis of cardiomyopathy in patients who have received a cumulative dose of doxorubicin of 300 mg/m² or greater and who are believed would benefit from continued therapy with this drug.

Usual dosage and schedule.   10 mg of dexrazoxane for every 1 mg of doxorubicin, for example, 600 mg/m² of dexrazoxane for

60 mg/m^2 of doxorubicin. Repeat whenever doxorubicin is to be repeated. Administered as a slow injection or rapid infusion over 15 to 30 min.

Special precautions.   None.

Toxicity.   Most side effects encountered with dexrazoxane administration are likely to be from the concurrent chemotherapeutic regimen.

1. *Myelosuppression and other hematologic effects.* Nadir granulocyte and platelet counts lower than with chemotherapy alone, but duration not prolonged.
2. *Nausea, vomiting, and other gastrointestinal effects.* No increase observed.
3. *Mucocutaneous effects.* No increase observed.
4. *Miscellaneous effects.*
   a. Pain at the injection site is occasional.
   b. Hepatic toxicity is possible.

DOCETAXEL

Other name.   Taxotere.

Mechanism of action.   Enhanced formation and stabilization of microtubules. Antineoplastic effect may result from nonfunctional tubules or altered tubulin–microtubule equilibrium. Mitotic arrest is seen and is associated with accumulated polymerized microtubules.

Primary indication.   Carcinomas of the breast, stomach, lung, ovary, and prostate.

Usual dosage and schedule.

1. 60 to 100 mg/m^2 as a 1-h infusion every 3 weeks.

   Dexamethasone, 8 mg PO b.i.d. for 3 days starting 1 day before docetaxel, should be given before each course of docetaxel to limit the frequency and severity of hypersensitivity reactions and to reduce the severity of fluid retention:

2. 35 mg/m^2 as a 1-h infusion weekly.

   Dexamethasone, 8 mg PO b.i.d. 1 day before and 10 mg IV 30 min before should be given before weeks 1 and 2 of docetaxel to limit the frequency and severity of hypersensitivity reactions. If there are no hypersensitivity reactions in the first 2 weeks, the oral doses given the day before docetaxel may be eliminated.

Special precautions.   Severe hypersensitivity reactions with flushing and hypotension with or without dyspnea occur in approximately 1% of patients (even when premedication is used). Should be used with caution in patients with bilirubin above upper limit of normal (ULN) or other abnormal liver function test results (>1.5 ULN), because of more profound neutropenia.

Toxicity.

1. *Myelosuppression and other hematologic effects.* Severe (grade 4) neutropenia is common and dose related. Many patients have neutropenic fever.
2. *Nausea, vomiting, and other gastrointestinal effects.* Common, but brief; severe episodes are uncommon.
3. *Mucocutaneous effects.* Mild mucositis is common; severe mucositis is uncommon. Alopecia is common. Mild-to-moderate cutaneous reactions such as maculopapular eruptions are

common; severe reactions that may be associated with desquamation, or bullous eruptions occur only occasionally if systemic prophylaxis is used. Mild-to-moderate nail changes are common, but severe oncholysis is uncommon.

4. *Hypersensitivity reactions.* Mild-to-moderate hypersensitivity reactions with flushing, hypotension (or rarely hypertension) with or without dyspnea, and drug fever are occasional; use of the prophylactic regimen recommended. Severe hypersensitivity reactions are uncommon.

5. *Miscellaneous effects.*

   a. Fluid retention syndrome is common and cumulative (more commonly after four courses); can be reduced to occasional frequency (6%) by prophylactic steroids; may limit continuing therapy. May be associated with both pleural and pericardial effusions.

   b. *Neurologic.* Mild and reversible dysesthesias or paresthesias are common; more severe sensory neuropathies are uncommon.

   c. *Hepatic.* Reversible increases in transaminase, alkaline phosphatase, and bilirubin.

   d. *Local reactions.* Reversible peripheral phlebitis.

   e. Mild diarrhea is common; severe diarrhea is rare.

   f. Fatigue, weakness (asthenia), and myalgia are common; arthralgia is occasional.

DOXORUBICIN

Other names. ADR, Adriamycin, Rubex, hydroxyldaunorubicin.

Mechanism of action. DNA strand breakage mediated by anthracycline effects on topoisomerase II; DNA intercalation; DNA polymerase inhibition.

Primary indications.
1. Breast, bladder, liver, lung, prostate, stomach, and thyroid carcinomas.
2. Bone and soft tissue sarcomas.
3. Hodgkin's and non–Hodgkin's lymphomas.
4. Multiple myeloma.
5. Acute lymphocytic and acute nonlymphocytic leukemias.
6. Wilms' tumor, neuroblastoma, and rhabdomyosarcoma of childhood.

Usual dosage and schedule.
1. 60 to 75 mg/m^2 IV every 3 weeks. (Or as 96-h continuous infusion.)
2. 30 mg/m^2 IV on days 1 and 8 every 4 weeks (in combination with other drugs).
3. 9 mg/m^2 IV daily for 4 days as a continuous infusion (in myeloma).
4. 15 to 20 mg/m^2 IV weekly.
5. 50 to 60 mg instilled into the bladder weekly for 4 weeks, then every 4 weeks for six cycles.

Special precautions.
1. Administer over several minutes into the sidearm of a running IV infusion (except when given as a continuous infusion), taking care to avoid extravasation.

2. Do not give if patient has significantly impaired cardiac function (ejection fraction <45%), angina pectoris, cardiac arrhythmia, or recent myocardial infarction.
3. Do not exceed a lifetime cumulative dose of 550 mg/m² (450 mg/m² if patient was given prior chest radiotherapy or concomitant cyclophosphamide) unless there are known risk modifiers, such as continuous infusion, weekly dosing, or cardioprotective dexrazoxane, and serial measurements of cardiac ejection fraction show minimal change and adequate function.
4. Reduce or hold dose if patient has impaired liver function.
   a. For serum bilirubin of 1.2 to 3.0 mg/dL, give one half the normal dose.
   b. For serum bilirubin of more than 3.0 mg/dL, give one fourth the normal dose.

Toxicity.
1. *Myelosuppression and other hematologic effects.* Dose limiting for most patients. Nadir white blood cell (WBC) and platelet counts occur at 10 to 14 days; recovery by day 21.
2. *Nausea, vomiting, and other gastrointestinal effects.* Mild to moderate in approximately one half of patients.
3. *Mucocutaneous effects.*
   a. Stomatitis that is dose dependent.
   b. Alopecia beginning 2 to 5 weeks from start of therapy with recovery following completion of therapy is common.
   c. Recall of skin reaction due to prior radiotherapy is common.
   d. Severe local tissue damage, possibly progressing to skin ulceration and necrosis if subcutaneous extravasation occurs, is common.
   e. Hyperpigmentation of skin overlying the veins used for drug injection in which chemical phlebitis has occurred is common.
4. *Cardiac effects.* Potentially irreversible congestive heart failure may occur owing to cardiomyopathy. The incidence is highly dependent on the lifetime cumulative dose, which should not exceed 550 mg/m². This limit is lower (450 mg/m²) if the patient has received prior chest radiotherapy or is taking cyclophosphamide concomitantly. Weekly schedule and 96-h infusions are less cardiotoxic and higher cumulative doses may be tolerable. Congestive heart failure may be predicted by serial measurement of left ventricular function or endomyocardial biopsy. Discontinue drug if there is clinical congestive heart failure or if the ejection fraction falls on the radionuclide angiogram:
   a. To less than 45% *or*
   b. To less than 50% if the total decrease is 10% or more (e.g., falls from 59% to 49%).

   If repeat ejection fraction determination shows return of function, drug may be cautiously restarted, but ejection fraction determination should be done before each dose. Transient ECG changes are common and are usually not serious.
5. *Miscellaneous effects.*
   a. Red urine caused by the drug and its metabolites is common.

    b. Chemical phlebitis and phlebosclerosis of veins used for injection are common, particularly if a vein is used repeatedly.

    c. Fever, chills, and urticaria are uncommon.

DOXORUBICIN, LIPOSOMAL

Other name. Doxil.

Mechanism of action. Doxorubicin, liposomal, which is designed to be protected from removal by the reticuloendothelial system, has a prolonged circulation time compared with unprotected drug. The agent penetrates tumor tissue and releases the active ingredient doxorubicin. The active drug causes DNA strand breakage mediated by anthracycline effects on topoisomerase II, DNA intercalation, and DNA polymerase inhibition.

Primary indications.

1. Kaposi's sarcoma, advanced, HIV associated.
2. Ovarian and breast carcinomas.
3. Multiple myeloma.

Usual dosage and schedule.

1. 20 mg/m^2 IV infusion at a rate of 1 mg/min for the first dose, then over 30 min for subsequent doses every 3 weeks for Kaposi's sarcoma.
2. 40 to 50 mg/m^2 IV infusion at a rate of 1 mg/min for the first dose, then over 1 h every 4 weeks for ovarian or breast carcinoma when used as a single agent.
3. 40 mg/m^2 IV infusion at a rate of 1 mg/min for the first dose, then over 1 h every 4 weeks for multiple myeloma, together with vincristine and dexamethasone.

Special precautions. Must be diluted in 250 mL of 5% dextrose for injection. Liposomal doxorubicin is not a vesicant but should be considered an irritant. Initial doses should be given at a rate of 1 mg/min to avoid infusion reactions.

Toxicity. Effects that are a result of the liposomal doxorubicin have been somewhat difficult to determine with certainty because most patients have been on several other agents that may cause marrow or other toxicity.

1. *Myelosuppression and other hematologic effects.* Common and dose related. May be severe.
2. *Nausea, vomiting, and other gastrointestinal effects.* Nausea and vomiting are common at the higher doses. Constipation is occasional. Diarrhea is occasional. Anorexia is occasional.
3. *Mucocutaneous effects.* Palmar-plantar erythrodysesthesia is common at the higher doses and is occasionally severe. Stomatitis is common. Alopecia is occasional. Rash is occasional to common.
4. *Miscellaneous effects.*
    a. Cardiac events, including cardiomyopathy or congestive heart failure occur in 5% to 10% of patients treated. This is dose dependent, and not really adequately tested with liposomal doxorubicin.
    b. *Infusion reactions.* Acute infusion-associated reactions with flushing, shortness of breath, facial swelling, headache, chills, back pain, tightness in the chest and throat, or hypotension, alone or in combination, have occurred in approximately 7% of patients treated with liposomal

doxorubicin. They usually occur with the first infusion, and are not likely to occur later if the first infusion is given without a reaction. Most resolve over the course of several hours to a day.
c. Asthenia is occasional.
d. Fever is occasional.
e. Pain at the injection site is likely after extravasation.

EPIRUBICIN

Other names. Ellence, 4'Epi-doxorubicin, EPI.
Mechanism of action. DNA strand breakage, mediated by anthracycline effects on topoisomerase II.
Primary indications.
1. Carcinomas of the breast, esophagus, lung, ovary, and stomach.
2. Hodgkin's and non–Hodgkin's lymphoma.
3. Soft tissue sarcomas.
Usual dosage and schedule.
1. 100 mg/m^2 IV administered through the sidearm of a freely flowing IV infusion, repeated every 3 weeks.
2. 60 mg/m^2 IV days 1 and 8 repeated every 3 weeks.
Special precautions.
1. Take care to avoid extravasation.
2. Do not exceed a lifetime cumulative dose of 900 mg/m^2. (Use a lesser dose for patients with prior chest radiotherapy or prior anthracycline or anthracenedione therapy. 720 mg/m^2 was the maximum cumulative dose in adjuvant studies.)
3. Reduce or hold dose if patient has impaired liver function.
   a. For serum bilirubin of 1.2 to 3.0 mg/dL, give half the normal dose.
   b. For serum bilirubin of more than 3.0 mg/dL, give one fourth the normal dose.
Toxicity.
1. *Myelosuppression and other hematologic effects.* Dose-limiting leukopenia with recovery by day 21.
2. *Nausea, vomiting, and other gastrointestinal effects.* Nausea and vomiting are common. Diarrhea and abdominal pain are occasional.
3. *Mucocutaneous effects.*
   a. Stomatitis that is dose dependent.
   b. Alopecia beginning approximately 10 days after the first treatment with regrowth when cessation of drug treatment occurs is common but not universal (25%–50%).
   c. Flushes, skin and nail hyperpigmentation, photosensitivity, and hypersensitivity to irradiated skin (radiation-recall reaction) have been observed.
   d. Severe local tissue damage possibly progressing to skin ulceration and necrosis is common if subcutaneous extravasation occurs.
4. *Cardiac effects.*
   a. Potentially irreversible congestive heart failure may occur owing to cardiomyopathy. The incidence depends on the lifetime dose, which should not exceed 900 mg/m^2. This limit is lower if patient has received prior chest radiotherapy or prior anthracycline or anthracenedione therapy.

Congestive heart failure may be predicted by serial measurement of left ventricular function or endomyocardial biopsy.
  b. Transient ECG changes are similar in type and frequency to those observed after doxorubicin.
5. *Miscellaneous effects.*
  a. Red-orange urine for 24 h after injection owing to the drug and its metabolites is common.
  b. Urticaria and anaphylaxis have been reported in patients treated with epirubicin; signs and symptoms of these reactions may vary from skin rash and pruritus to fever, chills, and shock.

EPOETIN

Other names. Recombinant human erythropoietin (rHuEPO), EPO, epoetin-α, Epogen, Procrit.

Mechanism of action. Epoetin-α is a recombinant glycoprotein that contains 165 amino acids in a sequence identical to that of endogenous human erythropoietin. It has the same biologic activity, inducing erythropoiesis by stimulating the division and differentiation of committed erythroid progenitor cells.

Primary indications.
1. Anemia from chemotherapy in patients with nonmyeloid malignancies.
2. Anemia associated with malignancy.
3. Anemia associated with chronic renal failure.
4. Anemia associated with zidovudine therapy in HIV-infected patients.

Usual dosage and schedule (in malignancy). 40,000 units SC once weekly. If there is no response after 4 to 8 weeks, the dose may be increased to 60,000 units SC once weekly. If there is no response to this dose, it should be discontinued.

Responders may do well with alternate schedules, such as 80,000 units every other week.

Special precautions.
1. Iron supplementation is beneficial if there is any question of body iron stores. If at any time the hematocrit rises above 40%, hold epoetin injections until the hematocrit falls to 36% or less and reinitiate at a lower dose or a longer interval.
2. Contraindicated in patients with uncontrolled hypertension or known hypersensitivity to albumin or mammalian cell-derived products. Pure red cell aplasia may occur.

Toxicity.
1. *Myelosuppression.* None. Therapeutic effect is an increase in hemoglobin.
2. *Nausea and vomiting.* None.
3. *Mucocutaneous effects.* Rare rashes or hives.
4. *Miscellaneous effects.*
  a. Improved energy level, activity level, and self-rated quality of life scores occur in patients receiving therapy.
  b. Edema is occasional.
  c. Diarrhea is occasional.
  d. A rise in blood pressure occurs in approximately 25% of patients. Hypertension may rarely occur in association with a significant increase in hematocrit; the risk is greatest

in patients with preexisting hypertension. Chest pain is uncommon; edema is occasional.
e. Seizures are rare.
f. Influenza-like syndrome is rare to uncommon. Fever alone is occasional.
g. Thrombotic complications are uncommon.
h. Pure red cell aplasia is rare.

ERLOTINIB

Other name.   Tarceva.
Mechanism of action.   Inhibits intracellular phosphorylation of the tyrosine kinase associated with EGFR.
Primary indications.
1. Non–small cell lung cancer, as monotherapy.
2. Pancreatic cancer (with gemcitabine).
Usual dosage and schedule.
1. 150 mg PO daily, at least 1 h before or 2 h after food. Give with caution if liver impairment is present.
2. 200 mg PO daily when given with gemcitabine or other cytotoxic agents.
Special precautions.   May be associated with interstitial lung disease–like events, manifest by unexplained dyspnea, cough and fever. If this occurs, erlotinib therapy should be discontinued and management of the pulmonary condition instituted. CYP3A4 inhibitors such as ketoconazole increase erlotinib AUC while inducers such as rifampicin decrease erlotinib AUC, resulting in potential increase in toxicity or reduction in efficacy, respectively. Monitor closely for INR elevation in patients taking concomitant warfarin.
Toxicity.
1. *Myelosuppression and other hematologic effects.* Myelosuppression is not an effect of erlotinib. Unexpected INR elevation may occur in patients taking warfarin. Microangiopathic hemolytic anemia with thrombocytopenia is rare.
2. *Nausea, vomiting, and other gastrointestinal effects.* Anorexia, dyspepsia, nausea, vomiting, diarrhea (second most common reason for dose interruption), constipation, and abdominal pain are common. Transaminase elevations are common, and occasionally associated with increased bilirubin, but they are rarely life threatening.
3. *Mucocutaneous effects.* Rash is common (75%) and the most common reason for dose interruption; stomatitis is occasional to common (17%). Keratoconjunctivitis is occasional.
4. *Miscellaneous effects.*
   a. Systemic. Fatigue, weight loss, and edema are common; fever is common, occasionally with rigors.
   b. Bone pain and myalgia are common.
   c. Dyspnea is common, cough is occasional.
   d. Anxiety and neuropathy are occasional.

ESTROGENS

Other names.   Diethylstilbestrol (DES), chlorotrianisene (TACE), DES diphosphate (Stilphostrol), and others.

Mechanism of action. Suppression of testosterone production through negative feedback on hypothalamus.
Primary indication. Prostate carcinoma.
Usual dosage and schedule.
1. DES, 1 to 3 mg PO daily.
2. TACE, 12 to 25 mg PO daily.
Special precautions.
1. Acute fluid retention and pulmonary edema are possible, particularly with high-dose IV therapy (rarely used now).
2. Hypercalcemia may occur with initial therapy.
Toxicity.
1. *Myelosuppression and other hematologic effects.* None.
2. *Nausea, vomiting, and other gastrointestinal effects.* Nausea with possible vomiting is common at the beginning of therapy but diminishes or stops with continued treatment. Severity may be lessened by beginning treatment with doses lower than those recommended. Diarrhea is uncommon.
3. *Mucocutaneous effects.* Darkening of nipples is common.
4. *Miscellaneous effects.*
    a. Peripheral edema due to sodium retention is common, but congestive heart failure occurs in fewer than 5% of patients.
    b. Any patient on estrogens may be at a higher risk than normal for thromboemboli. An increase in cardiovascular deaths has been seen in male patients given DES at 5 mg daily for prostate carcinoma.
    c. Increased bone pain, tumor pain, and local disease flare are associated with both good tumor response and tumor progression.
    d. Feminization with gynecomastia occurs in male patients.

ETOPOSIDE

Other names. Epipodophyllotoxin, VP-16, VP-16-213, VePesid, Etopophos (etoposide phosphate).
Mechanism of action. Interaction with topoisomerase II produces single-strand breaks in DNA. Arrests cells in late S phase or G_2 phase.
Primary indications.
1. Small cell anaplastic and non–small cell lung carcinomas.
2. Stomach carcinoma.
3. Germ cell cancers.
4. Lymphomas.
5. Acute leukemia.
6. Neuroblastoma.
Usual dosage and schedule.
1. 120 mg/m^2 IV on days 1 to 3 every 3 weeks.
2. 50 to 100 mg/m^2 IV on days 1 to 5 every 2 to 4 weeks.
3. 125 to 140 mg/m^2 IV on days 1, 3, and 5 every 3 to 5 weeks.
4. 50 mg/m^2 PO daily for 21 days. Repeat after 1 to 2 weeks' rest.
5. High-dose therapy (750 to 2,400 mg/m^2) is investigational and should only be used with progenitor cell rescue (e.g., bone marrow or peripheral blood stem cell transplantation).
Special precautions.
1. Administer etoposide as a 30- to 60-min infusion to avoid severe hypotension. Monitor blood pressure during infusion.

Etoposide phosphate may be administered as a 5-min bolus infusion.

2. Take care to avoid extravasation.
3. Etoposide must be diluted in 20 to 50 volumes (100 to 250 mL) of isotonic saline before use. Etoposide phosphate vials (100 mg) may be reconstituted in 5 to 10 mL (water, saline, or dextrose) to a concentration of 10 or 20 mg/mL.
4. Decrease dose by 50% for bilirubin levels of 1.5 to 3 mg/dL; decrease by 75% for bilirubin levels of 3 to 5 mg/dL; discontinue drug if bilirubin level is more than 5 mg/dL.
5. Decrease dose by 25% for creatinine clearance rate of less than 30 mL/min.

Toxicity.
1. *Myelosuppression and other hematologic effects.* Dose-limiting leukopenia and less severe thrombocytopenia have a nadir at 16 days with recovery by days 20 to 22.
2. *Nausea, vomiting, and other gastrointestinal effects.* Usually mild-to-moderate nausea and vomiting in approximately one third of patients receiving standard doses; common with high-dose therapy. Anorexia is common. Diarrhea is uncommon.
3. *Mucocutaneous effects.*
   a. Alopecia is common.
   b. Stomatitis is uncommon with standard doses; common with high-dose therapy.
   c. Painful rash may occur with high-dose therapy.
   d. Chemical phlebitis is occasional.
4. *Miscellaneous effects.*
   a. Hepatotoxicity is rare.
   b. Peripheral neurotoxicity is rare.
   c. Allergic reaction is rare.
   d. Hemorrhagic cystitis may occur with high-dose therapy.

EXEMESTANE

Other name. Aromasin.

Mechanism of action. Exemestane is an irreversible, steroidal aromatase inactivator that decreases estrogen biosynthesis by selective inhibition of aromatase (estrogen synthetase) in peripheral tissues.

Primary indications.
1. Carcinoma of the breast in postmenopausal women that has progressed following tamoxifen therapy.
2. Carcinoma of the breast as adjuvant treatment in postmenopausal women with estrogen receptor–positive breast cancer.

Usual dosage and schedule. 25 mg PO once daily after meal.

Special Precautions. Potential hazard to fetus if given during pregnancy.

Toxicity.
1. *Myelosuppression and other hematologic effects.* No dose-related effect. Thromboembolic events are uncommon to rare.
2. *Nausea, vomiting, and other gastrointestinal effects.* Nausea, vomiting, constipation, and diarrhea are uncommon to occasional.
3. *Mucocutaneous effects.* Rash is uncommon.

4. *Miscellaneous effects*.
   a. Fatigue is occasional.
   b. Musculoskeletal pain (arthralgia or bone) is occasional to common.
   c. Headache is occasional.
   d. Peripheral edema, weight gain is occasional.
   e. Dyspnea and cough are uncommon to occasional.
   f. Hot flashes are occasional.
   g. Decreased bone mineral density with osteoporosis is occasional and there is increased risk for fractures.
   h. Hypertension is occasional.

FILGRASTIM

Other names.   Granulocyte colony-stimulating factor, G-CSF, Neupogen.

Mechanism of action.   Promotes growth and differentiation of myeloid progenitor cells. May improve survival and function of granulocytes.

Primary indications.

1. Prophylaxis of granulocytopenia secondary to intensive chemotherapy with a febrile neutropenia rate of greater than 20% or in patients with previous episode of febrile neutropenia.
2. Treatment of granulocytopenia secondary to chemotherapy.
3. Granulocytopenia from primary marrow disorders, such as idiopathic neutropenia and aplastic anemia, and myelodysplastic syndrome.
4. Granulocytopenia associated with acquired immunodeficiency syndrome (AIDS) and its therapy.

Usual dosage and schedule.

1. *Adjunct to chemotherapy*. Commonly 200 to 400 $\mu g/m^2$ (5–10 $\mu g/kg$) SQ daily, starting no sooner than 24 h and no later than 4 days after the last dose of chemotherapy, for 10 to 20 days until the neutrophil count exceeds 10,000/μL after the expected nadir. Because of cost factors, vial size, and comparability of effect with "ballpark" doses, some physicians choose to treat patients weighing less than 75 kg with 300 μg daily and patients weighing more than 75 kg with 480 μg daily.
2. *Other purposes*. 40 to 500 $\mu g/m^2$ SQ, IM, or IV daily. Dose and duration are dependent on the purpose of administration.

Special precautions.   Use with caution in disorders of myeloid stem cells, because it may promote growth of leukemic cells.

Toxicity.

1. *Myelosuppression*. None (leukocytosis).
2. *Nausea and vomiting*. Rare.
3. *Mucocutaneous effects*. Exacerbation of preexisting dermatologic conditions are occasional; pyoderma gangrenosum is rare.
4. *Miscellaneous effects*. Usually mild and short lived.
   a. Bone pain, musculoskeletal symptoms such as cramps, and back or leg pain is common.
   b. Splenomegaly with prolonged use.
   c. Exacerbation of preexisting inflammatory or autoimmune disorders is rare.
   d. Mild elevation of LDH and alkaline phosphatase.

FLOXURIDINE

Other name. FUDR

Mechanism of action. A pyrimidine antimetabolite that, when converted to the active nucleotide, inhibits the enzyme thymidylate synthetase.

Primary indication. Hepatic metastasis of gastrointestinal carcinoma, primary hepatic carcinoma.

Usual dosage and schedule. 4.0 to 6.0 mg/m^2 as a continuous infusion into the hepatic artery daily for 2 weeks, then off for 2 weeks. Administered through continuous infusion pump.

Special precautions.

1. Reduce dose in patients with compromised liver function.
2. Ulcer-like pain or other significant gastrointestinal symptoms are indications to discontinue intra-arterial therapy, as hemorrhage or perforation may occur.

Toxicity.

1. *Myelosuppression and other hematologic effects.* Uncommon.
2. *Nausea, vomiting, and other gastrointestinal effects.* Nausea and vomiting are uncommon unless the hepatic artery catheter has become displaced and the stomach and duodenum are being infused. Abdominal cramps and pain are common if the catheter is displaced and the stomach and duodenum are being infused. Can progress to frank gastritis or duodenal ulcer. Esophagitis, proctitis, and diarrhea may also occur.
3. *Mucocutaneous effects.*
   a. Stomatitis is an early sign of severe toxicity. It progresses from soreness and erythema to frank ulceration, which may become hemorrhagic in a small number of patients.
   b. Partial alopecia is uncommon.
   c. Hyperpigmentation of skin over face, hands, and the vein used for the infusion is occasional.
   d. Maculopapular rash is uncommon.
   e. Sun exposure tends to increase skin reactions.
4. *Miscellaneous effects.*
   a. Neurotoxicity, including headache, minor visual disturbances, and cerebellar ataxia, is rare.
   b. Increased lacrimation is uncommon.
   c. Liver function abnormalities and jaundice are common when given by hepatic arterial infusion. Dose should be reduced during subsequent cycle.
   d. Sclerosing cholangitis when given by hepatic artery infusion is uncommon.

FLUDARABINE

Other names. FAMP, Fludara.

Mechanism of action. Inhibition of DNA polymerase α, ribonucleotide reductase, and DNA primase.

Primary indications.

1. Chronic lymphocytic leukemia (B cell).
2. Macroglobulinemia.
3. Indolent lymphomas.
4. Acute leukemia (in combination).

Usual dosage and schedule. 25 mg/m^2 IV as a 30-min infusion daily for 5 days. Other dose schedules, usually less intensive, have been used, often in combinations with other drugs. Repeat every 4 weeks.

Special precautions. If there is the potential for tumor lysis syndrome, administer allopurinol and ensure good hydration and close clinical monitoring. Transfusion-associated graft-versus-host disease may be seen. Therefore, prior irradiation of blood products for transfusion in patients at risk is recommended. Sometimes fatal cases of autoimmune hemolytic anemia have been reported, and patients should be closely monitored for hemolysis, particularly if there is a prior history of autoimmune hemolysis or immune thrombocytopenia related to chronic lymphocytic leukemia. Not recommended for use in combination with pentostatin because of the high incidence of pulmonary toxicity. Adult patients with moderate impairment of renal function (creatinine clearance 30 to 70 mL/min/1.73 m² should have a 20% dose reduction of fludarabine. It should not be given to patients with severely impaired renal function (creatinine clearance less than 30 mL/min/1.73 m²).

Toxicity.

1. *Myelosuppression and other hematologic effects.* Granulocytopenia and thrombocytopenia are common but appear to become less common in patients whose disease is responding. Infection, particularly pneumonia, is common during initial courses and uncommon after the sixth course. Autoimmune hemolytic anemia.
2. *Nausea and vomiting.* Common (30%) but not usually severe.
3. *Mucocutaneous effects.* Occasional mucositis, rash, no alopecia.
4. *Neurotoxicity.* Uncommon at usual dosage. Somnolence or fatigue, paresthesias, and twitching of extremities may be seen. Severe neurologic symptoms, including visual disturbances, have been common at higher doses than those recommended.
5. *Immune suppression.* Common. Usually seen as a depression in CD4 and CD8 lymphocyte counts. Opportunistic infections may result, and many recommend pneumocystis pneumonia prophylaxis until the CD4 lymphopenia resolves.
6. *Miscellaneous effects.*
   a. Abnormal liver or renal function is rare.
   b. Allergic pneumonitis is occasional to uncommon.
   c. Edema is occasional.
   d. Diarrhea is occasional.
   e. Tumor lysis syndrome is rare.

FLUOROURACIL

Other names. 5-FU, Adrucil, Efudex, Fluoroplex, 5-fluorouracil.

Mechanism of action. A pyrimidine antimetabolite that, when converted to the active nucleotide, inhibits the enzyme thymidylate synthetase and thereby blocks DNA synthesis.

Primary indications.

1. Breast, colorectal, anal, stomach, pancreas, esophagus, liver, head and neck, and bladder carcinomas.
2. Actinic keratosis; basal and squamous cell carcinomas of skin (topically).

Usual dosage and schedule.

1. *Systemic options (alternatives). Other schedules when in combinations.*

  a. 500 mg/m^2 IV on days 1 to 5 every 4 weeks.
  b. 450 to 600 mg/m^2 IV weekly.
  c. 200 to 400 mg/m^2 daily as a continuous intravenous infusion.
  d. 1,000 mg/m^2 daily for 4 days as a continuous IV infusion every 3 to 4 weeks.
  e. Leucovorin 20 mg/m^2 IV is followed by fluorouracil 425 mg/m^2 IV. The combination is given daily for 5 days. Courses are repeated every 4 weeks.
2. *Intracavitary.* 500 to 1,000 mg for pericardial effusion; 2,000 to 3,000 mg for pleural or peritoneal effusions.
3. *Topically.* Apply solution or cream twice daily. Use only 5% strength for carcinomas.

Special precautions.
1. Reduce dose in patients with compromised liver function.
2. Precipitation may occur if leucovorin and fluorouracil are mixed in the same bag.

Toxicity.
1. *Myelosuppression and other hematologic effects.* Dose-limiting with a nadir at 10 to 14 days after the last dose and recovery by 21 days.
2. *Nausea, vomiting, and other gastrointestinal effects.* Nausea and vomiting may occur but are usually not severe. Diarrhea is common with higher doses, continuous infusion, or when used in combination with leucovorin and irinotecan. Esophagitis and proctitis may also occur.
3. *Mucocutaneous effects.*
  a. Stomatitis is an early sign of severe toxicity. It progresses from soreness and erythema to frank ulceration, which becomes hemorrhagic in a small number of patients.
  b. Partial alopecia is uncommon.
  c. Hyperpigmentation of skin over face, hands, and the veins used for infusion is occasional.
  d. Maculopapular rash is uncommon.
  e. Sun exposure tends to increase skin reactions.
  f. "Hand-foot syndrome" with painful, erythematous desquamation and fissures of palms and soles is common with continuous infusion, occasional with other schedules or combinations.
4. *Miscellaneous effects.*
  a. Neurotoxicity, including headache, minor visual disturbances, and cerebellar ataxia is rare.
  b. Increased lacrimation is uncommon.
  c. Cardiac toxicity, including arrhythmias, angina, ischemia, and sudden death is rare. May be more common with continuous infusion and previous history of coronary artery disease.

FLUTAMIDE

Other name. Eulexin.
Mechanism of action. Competitive inhibitor of androgens at the cellular androgen receptor in the prostate cancer cells.
Primary indication. Carcinoma of the prostate, most often in combination with LHRH agonists.
Usual dosage and schedule. 250 mg PO every 8 h.

Special precautions. Serum transaminase levels should be measured before starting treatment with flutamide. Flutamide is not recommended in patients whose serum transaminase values exceed twice the ULN.

Toxicity.

1. *Myelosuppression and other hematologic effects.* None.
2. *Nausea, vomiting, and other gastrointestinal effects.* Nausea and vomiting are uncommon to occasional. Diarrhea, flatulence, and mild abdominal pain are common.
3. *Mucocutaneous effects.* Mild skin rash is occasional.
4. *Miscellaneous effects.*
   a. Secondary pharmacologic effects, including breast tenderness, breast swelling, hot flashes, impotence, and loss of libido, are common but reversible after cessation of therapy.
   b. Elevated liver function tests are uncommon; liver failure is rare, but may be preceded by flu-like symptoms or right upper quadrant pain and tenderness.
   c. Hypertension is occasional.
   d. Adverse cardiovascular events are similar to those seen with orchiectomy.

FULVESTRANT

Other name. Faslodex.

Mechanism of action. An estrogen receptor antagonist that binds to the estrogen receptor in a competitive manner. It downregulates the estrogen receptor protein in human breast cancer cells. *In vitro*, there is reversible inhibition of the growth of tamoxifen-resistant as well as estrogen-sensitive human breast cancer cell lines.

Primary indications.

1. Hormone receptor–positive metastatic breast cancer in postmenopausal women with disease progression following antiestrogen therapy. (There are no efficacy data for premenopausal women with advanced breast cancer.)
2. Hormone receptor–positive metastatic breast cancer in postmenopausal women with disease progression following therapy with a third-generation aromatase inhibitor.

Usual dosage and schedule. 250 mg IM (into the buttock[s]) as either a single 5-mL injection or two concurrent 2.5-mL injections, repeated once monthly.

Special precautions. Safety has not been evaluated in patients with moderate-to-severe hepatic impairment.

Toxicity.

1. *Myelosuppression and other hematologic effects.* Anemia is rare.
2. *Nausea, vomiting, and other gastrointestinal effects.* Nausea is common; vomiting, constipation, diarrhea, and anorexia are occasional.
3. *Mucocutaneous effects.* Rash and increased sweating are occasional.
4. *Miscellaneous effects.*
   a. For the body as a whole, headache, back pain, abdominal pain, injection site pain, and pelvic pain are occasional. Occasional patients also experience a flu-like syndrome or fever.

b. Vasodilation is occasional (18%).
c. Dizziness, insomnia, paresthesias, depression, and anxiety are uncommon to occasional.
d. Pharyngitis, dyspnea, and increased cough are occasional.

GEFITINIB

Other names. Iressa, ZD1839.
Mechanism of action. Selectively inhibits tyrosine kinase activity of the EGFR. EGFR tyrosine kinase inhibition by gefitinib impairs epidermal growth factor–stimulated autophosphorylation and thereby blocks growth signals within the cell.
Primary indication. Carcinoma of the lung.
Usual dosage and schedule.
1. 250 to 500 mg daily.
Special precautions. Diarrhea may be dose limiting and may require discontinuation of the drug.
Toxicity.
1. *Myelosuppression and other hematologic effects.* Uncommon, except for anemia, which is occasional and not dose related.
2. *Nausea, vomiting, and other gastrointestinal effects.* Nausea, vomiting, and diarrhea are common. Diarrhea may be dose limiting. Anorexia, constipation, and abdominal pain are also common but usually not severe.
3. *Mucocutaneous effects.* Acne-like or folliculitis-type rash is common, usually appearing by day 14; frequency and severity are dose related. May be associated with dry skin and itching. Rash usually does not worsen with continued treatment and resolves within a week of discontinuation of the drug. Dry mouth and conjunctivitis are occasional.
4. *Miscellaneous effects.*
   a. Dyspnea is occasional to common.
   b. Asthenia is common.
   c. Headache is occasional.
   d. Somnolence is occasional.
   e. Elevated hepatic transaminases are occasional but may be severe (grade 3 or 4).

GEMCITABINE

Other name. Gemzar.
Mechanism of action. After being metabolized intracellularly to the active diphosphate and triphosphate nucleotides, gemcitabine, a cytidine analog, inhibits ribonucleotide reductase and competes with deoxycytidine triphosphate for incorporation into DNA.
Primary indications.
1. Carcinoma of the pancreas, locally advanced or metastatic.
2. Non–small cell carcinomas of the lung.
3. Carcinomas of breast, biliary tract, bladder, and ovary.
4. Non–Hodgkin's lymphoma.
5. Soft tissue sarcoma.
Usual dosage and schedule.
1. 1,000 mg/m^2 IV over 30 min once weekly for up to 7 weeks when used as a single agent. After 1 week of rest, subsequent

cycles are given once weekly for 3 consecutive weeks out of 4.

2. 1,000 to 1,250 mg/m^2 IV over 30 min once weekly for 2 or 3 successive weeks during each 3- to 4-week cycle, when used in combination regimens.

Special precautions. Prolongation of infusion time beyond 60 min increases toxicity.

Toxicity.

1. *Myelosuppression and other hematologic effects.* Dose related and common.
2. *Nausea, vomiting, and other gastrointestinal effects.* Nausea and vomiting are common, but only occasionally severe. Diarrhea and constipation are occasional to common.
3. *Mucocutaneous effects.* Rash, alopecia, and mucositis are occasional.
4. *Miscellaneous effects.*
   a. Transient elevations of serum transaminases and alkaline phosphatase are common.
   b. Mild proteinuria and hematuria are common.
   c. Hemolytic uremic syndrome is rare (0.25%).
   d. Fever without documented infection is common.
   e. Neurotoxicity: mild paresthesias are occasional.
   f. Dyspnea is occasional.

GEMTUZUMAB OZOGAMICIN

Other name. Mylotarg.

Mechanism of action. Gemtuzumab ozogamicin is a humanized recombinant monoclonal antibody against the CD33 antigen that is conjugated with the cytotoxic antitumor antibiotic calicheamicin. Once bound to the CD33 antigen, the agent is internalized, calicheamicin is released, and its reactive intermediate binds to DNA and causes DNA double-strand breaks and cell death.

Primary indications. Patients with CD33-positive acute non-lymphocytic (myeloid) leukemia in first relapse who are older than 60 and are not considered candidates for other cytotoxic chemotherapy.

Usual dosage and schedule. 9 mg/m^2 as a 2-h IV infusion on days 1 and 15.

Special precautions.

1. Infusion-related events may include fever, nausea, chills, hypotension, shortness of breath, and anaphylaxis. Pretreatment with acetaminophen and diphenhydramine should be given before treatment to lessen these effects, and prior methylprednisolone may also be of benefit.
2. If dyspnea or significant hypotension occurs, the infusion should be interrupted. Anaphylaxis, pulmonary edema, and acute respiratory distress syndrome usually necessitate discontinuation of therapy.
3. Hepatotoxicity, including veno-occlusive disease may occur, even in patients without a history of liver disease or hematopoietic stem cell transplant.
4. Tumor lysis syndrome may occur, particularly when the WBC count is higher than 30,000/μL.

Toxicity.
1. *Myelosuppression and other hematologic effects.* Severe-to-life-threatening granulocytopenia and thrombocytopenia are universal. Severe or worse anemia is common.
2. *Nausea, vomiting, and other gastrointestinal effects.* Anorexia, nausea, vomiting, and diarrhea are common but only occasionally severe.
3. *Mucocutaneous effects.* Rash, local reaction, petechiae, stomatitis, pharyngitis, and rhinitis are occasional to common. Herpes simplex is common. Alopecia is not seen.
4. *Miscellaneous effects.*
   a. Infusion-related events: chills, fever, headache, nausea, and vomiting are common. Hypotension, hypertension, hyperglycemia, and dyspnea are occasional. Hypoxia is uncommon (~5%).
   b. Increased cough, dyspnea, and epistaxis are common. Severe dyspnea or pneumonia is occasional. Pleural effusions, noncardiogenic pulmonary edema, and acute respiratory distress syndrome are rare.
   c. Severe or life-threatening infections are common. These include sepsis, pneumonia, and opportunistic infections.
   d. Hypertension, hypotension, and tachycardia are occasional.
   e. Reversible abnormalities in liver function are common and occasionally severe or life threatening. Fatal liver abnormalities including veno-occlusive disease are rare. Findings that may indicate severe hepatotoxicity include rapid weight gain, right upper quadrant pain, hepatomegaly, ascites, and elevations in liver function test values.

HYDROXYUREA

Other names. Hydrea, Droxia.
Mechanism of action. Interferes with DNA synthesis, at least in part by inhibiting the enzymatic conversion of ribonucleotides to deoxyribonucleotides.
Primary indications.
1. Head and neck carcinomas.
2. Chronic granulocytic (myelogenous) leukemia; acute lymphocytic and acute nonlymphocytic leukemia with high blast counts.
3. Essential thrombocythemia.
4. Polycythemia rubra vera.
5. Prevention of retinoic acid syndrome in acute promyelocytic leukemia.
6. Sickle cell anemia with frequent painful crises.
Usual dosage and schedule.
1. 800 to 2,000 mg/m^2 PO as a single or divided daily dose *or*
2. 3,200 mg/m^2 PO as a single dose every third day (not for leukemias).
3. Starting dose in sickle cell anemia is 15 mg/kg/day, with increments of 5 mg/kg every 12 weeks, so long as the absolute neutrophil count (ANC) is more than 2,000 cells/μl and platelets more than 80,000/μl.
Special precautions. The daily dose must be adjusted for blood count trends. Be careful not to change the dose too often,

because there is a delay in response. Severe cutaneous vasculitic toxicities, including ulcers and gangrene, have been seen, particularly in association with current or prior interferon therapy. Toxic reactions may be more in patients with impaired renal function, such as may be seen in elderly patients.

Toxicity.

1. *Myelosuppression and other hematologic effects.* Occurs at doses of more than 1,600 mg/m² daily by day 10. Recovery is usually prompt. Increased red cell mean corpuscular volume (MCV) is common.

2. *Nausea, vomiting, and other gastrointestinal effects.* Nausea is common at high doses. Other gastrointestinal symptoms are uncommon. Pancreatitis may be seen in patients with HIV disease being treated with didanosine and other antiviral agents.

3. *Mucocutaneous effects.* Stomatitis is rare. Maculopapular rash may be seen. Inflammation of mucous membranes caused by radiation may be exaggerated.

4. *Miscellaneous effects.*
   a. Temporary renal function impairment or dysuria is uncommon.
   b. CNS disturbances are rare.
   c. May be leukemogenic or teratogenic.

IBRITUMOMAB TIUXETAN

Other names.   Zevalin, IDEC-Y2B8.

Mechanism of action.   Ibritumomab is a murine monoclonal anti-CD20 antibody conjugated to tiuxetan that chelates to the pure β-emitting yttrium 90 (⁹⁰Y). The mechanism of action includes antibody-mediated cytotoxicity and cellularly targeted radiotherapy (Radioimmunotherapy [RIT]).

Primary indications.

1. Non–Hodgkin's lymphoma, follicular B cell, CD-20 positive.
2. Rituximab refractory.
3. Relapsed or refractory to other agents, but not rituximab refractory (experimental).

Usual dosage and schedule.   Rituximab, 250 mg/m² is given days 1 and 8, and 90Y-ibritumomab tiuxetan 0.3 to 0.4 mCi/kg IV on day 8. The maximum dose is 32 mCi.

Special Precautions.   Use with caution in patients with greater than or equal to 25% marrow involvement with lymphoma, prior external beam radiotherapy to greater than or equal to 25% of the bone marrow, or a history of human antimouse antibodies (HAMA) or HACA. Because the drug does not emit γ radiation, hospitalization is not required.

Toxicity.

1. *Myelosuppression and other hematologic effects.* Neutropenia and thrombocytopenia are common and related to the radionuclide dose. At the higher end of the dosing, 25% will develop nadir neutrophil counts of less than 500/μl.

2. *Nausea, vomiting, and other gastrointestinal effects.* Low-grade nausea and vomiting are common.

3. *Mucocutaneous effects.* Urticaria and pruritus are occasional.

4. *Miscellaneous effects.*
   a. Immunologic. HAMA or HACA may develop.

b. Infusion-related fever, chills, dizziness, asthenia, headache, back pain, arthralgia, and hypotension are occasional.

IDARUBICIN

Other names. 4-Demethoxydaunorubicin, IDA, Idamycin.

Mechanism of action. DNA strand breakage mediated by anthracycline effects on topoisomerase II or free radicals; DNA intercalation; DNA polymerase inhibition.

Primary indications.

1. Acute nonlymphocytic leukemia.
2. Blast crisis of chronic granulocytic (myelogenous) leukemia.
3. Acute lymphocytic leukemia.

Usual dosage and schedule. 12 to 13 mg/m^2 IV daily for 3 days (usually in combination with cytarabine) during induction; 10 to 12 mg/m^2 IV daily for 2 days during consolidation.

Special precautions. Administer over several minutes into the sidearm of a running IV infusion, taking care to avoid extravasation. Cardiac toxicity may be less than that with daunorubicin. Maximum dose not yet established. Cumulative doses of more than 150 mg/m^2 have been associated with decreased cardiac ejection fraction.

Toxicity.

1. *Myelosuppression and other hematologic effects*. Universal and dose limiting.
2. *Nausea, vomiting, and other gastrointestinal effects*. Nausea, vomiting, and anorexia are common. Diarrhea is occasional to common.
3. *Mucocutaneous effects*. Alopecia is common; mucositis is common but usually not severe.
4. *Hepatic dysfunction*. Common but usually not severe and not clearly due to the idarubicin.
5. *Renal effects*. Common but usually not clinically significant.
6. *Cardiac effects*. Uncommon during induction and consolidation (1%–5%).
7. *Tissue damage*. is probable if infiltration occurs.
8. *Neurologic effects*. Occasional.

IFOSFAMIDE

Other name. Ifex.

Mechanism of action. Metabolic activation by microsomal liver enzymes produces biologically active intermediates that attack nucleophilic sites, particularly on DNA.

Primary indications.

1. Testicular and lung cancers.
2. Bone and soft tissue sarcomas.
3. Lymphoma.

Usual dosage and schedule.

1. 1.2 g/m^2 IV over 30 min or more daily for 5 consecutive days every 3 or 4 weeks, usually with other agents. Mesna 120 mg/m^2 is given just before ifosfamide, then mesna 1,200 mg/m^2 as a daily continuous infusion is given until 16 h after the last dose of ifosfamide.

2. 3.6 g/m^2 IV daily as a 4-h infusion for 2 consecutive days, usu-ally with other agents. Mesna is given at a dose of 750 mg/m^2 IV just before and at 4 and 8 h after the start of the ifosfamide.
3. Higher dosage schedules have been used experimentally with up to 14 g/m^2 being used per course over a 6-day period, with equal or greater doses of mesna.

Special precautions. Must be used with mesna to prevent hemorrhagic cystitis. Mesna dose is at least 20% of the ifos-famide dose (on a weight basis), administered just before (or mixed with) the ifosfamide dose and again at 4 and 8 h after the ifosfamide to detoxify the urinary metabolites that cause the hemorrhagic cystitis. Higher doses of ifosfamide may require higher doses and longer durations of mesna. Neither mesna nor its only metabolite, mesna disulfide, affect ifosfamide or its antineoplastic metabolites. Mesna disulfide is reduced in the kid-ney to a free thiol compound, which then reacts chemically with urotoxic metabolites resulting in their detoxification. Vigorous hydration is also required with a minimum of 2 L of oral or IV hydration daily. Administer as a slow IV infusion over a period of at least 30 min.

Toxicity.
1. *Myelosuppression and other hematologic effects.* Dose limit-ing. Platelets are relatively spared. Granulocyte nadirs are commonly reached at 10 to 14 days, and recovery is seen by day 21. Thrombocytopenia may be seen with higher doses.
2. *Nausea, vomiting, and other gastrointestinal effects.* Common without standard antiemetics.
3. *Mucocutaneous effects.* Alopecia is common; mucositis is rarely seen at standard doses; dermatitis is rare.
4. *Hemorrhagic cystitis.* Common and dose limiting unless a uroprotective agent such as mesna is used. With mesna, the incidence of hemorrhagic cystitis is 5% to 10%, and gross hematuria is uncommon. Increasing the duration of mesna may alleviate the problem during subsequent cycles.
5. *Miscellaneous effects.*
    a. CNS toxicity (somnolence, confusion, depressive psychosis, hallucinations, disorientation, and uncommonly, seizures, cranial nerve dysfunction, or coma) is occasional with doses in lower range, more common with larger doses.
    b. Infertility is common in men and women, as with other alkylating agents.
    c. Renal impairment is occasional to common. Fanconi syn-drome dependent on dose. May be severe acidosis.
    d. Liver dysfunction is uncommon.
    e. Phlebitis is uncommon.
    f. Fever is rare.
    g. Peripheral neuropathy with high-dose therapy is un-common.

IMATINIB MESYLATE

Other names. Gleevec, STI-571 (Signal transduction inhibitor 571).

Mechanism of action. Inhibitor of the constitutively activated Bcr-Abl tyrosine kinase that is created as a consequence of the (9;22) chromosomal translocation and is required for the transforming function and excess proliferation seen in CML. It also inhibits platelet-derived growth factor receptor (PDGF-R) tyrosine kinase and c-Kit tyrosine kinase, the latter being activated in gastrointestinal stromal tumors (GISTs).

Primary indications.
1. CML in chronic phase, accelerated or blast phase of the disease.
2. ALL, Philadelphia chromosome positive.
3. GIST.
4. Dermatofibrosarcoma protuberans (DFSP)
5. Other rare hematologic disorders with susceptible mutations.

Usual dosage and schedule.
1. 400 to 600 mg PO daily in the chronic phase of CML, ALL, GISTs, and other susceptible hematologic disorders.
2. 600 to 800 mg PO daily in the accelerated phase or blast crisis and DFSP.

Toxicity.
1. *Myelosuppression and other hematologic effects.* Moderate neutropenia and thrombocytopenia are common in all phases, but severe neutropenia or thrombocytopenia is uncommon unless patients are in the accelerated phase or blast crisis of CML.
2. *Nausea, vomiting, and other gastrointestinal effects.* Nausea, vomiting, abdominal pain, and diarrhea are common, but it is uncommon that they are severe.
3. *Mucocutaneous effects.* Skin rash is common; pruritus and petechiae are occasional.
4. *Miscellaneous effects.*
   a. Fluid retention and edema are common. Pleural effusion and ascites are occasional.
   b. Musculoskeletal pain or cramps, arthralgia, headache, fever, and fatigue are common, but it is uncommon that they are severe or life threatening.
   c. Dyspnea and cough are occasional.
   d. Elevated liver function tests or serum creatinine are uncommon to rare. Rare cases of severe hepatotoxicity have been seen.
   e. Congestive heart failure is rare. It may be related to imatinib inhibition of Abl, which in turn may be related to mitochondrial function in the heart.

INTERFERON α

Other names. Roferon-A (interferon α-2a, recombinant α-A interferon), Intron A (interferon α-2b, recombinant α-2 interferon).

Mechanism of action. Believed to involve direct inhibition of tumor cell growth and modulation of the immune response of the host, including activation of NK cells, modulation of antibody production, and induction of major histocompatibility antigens.

Primary indications.
1. Melanoma (both as adjuvant and metastatic disease therapy).
2. Renal cell carcinoma.
3. Multiple myeloma.
4. Kaposi's sarcoma, HIV associated.
5. CML.
6. Non–Hodgkin's lymphoma (low grade), mycosis fungoides.

7. Condyloma acuminatum (intralesional).
8. Chronic hepatitis B and C.

Usual dosage and schedule.

1. 3 to 10 million IU IM or SQ in various schedules. Daily dosing is often used for several weeks or months, followed by 3 times a week dosing.
2. As adjuvant therapy for high-risk melanoma, 20 million IU/m^2 IV 5 consecutive days weekly for 4 weeks, then 10 million IU/m^2 SQ three times weekly for 48 weeks.
3. For HIV-related Kaposi's sarcoma, 30 million IU/m^2 SC or IM three times weekly, with dose modifications based on toxicity.

Special Precautions. May cause or aggravate life-threatening or fatal neuropsychiatric, autoimmune, ischemic, and infectious disorders. Patients with persistently severe or worsening signs or symptoms of these conditions should be withdrawn from therapy.

Toxicity.

1. *Myelosuppression and other hematologic effects.* Common but usually mild to moderate and transient, even with continued therapy. Higher doses may be associated (25% of patients receiving the recommended adjuvant therapy for melanoma) with granulocyte counts of less than $750/\mu L$ and consequent increased risk for infection.
2. *Nausea and vomiting and other gastrointestinal effects.* Anorexia and nausea are common, occurring in up to two thirds of all patients, but vomiting is only occasional. Diarrhea or loose stools are occasional to common.
3. *Mucocutaneous effects.* Rash, dryness, or inflammation of the oropharynx, dry skin or pruritus, and partial alopecia is occasional to common.
4. *Flu-like syndrome.* with fatigue, fever, chills, sweating, myalgias, arthralgias, and headache is common to universal, with greater severity at higher doses. Tends to diminish with continuing therapy and acetaminophen.
5. *Neurologic effects.*
   a. Peripheral nervous system: occasional paresthesias or numbness.
   b. CNS toxicity is uncommon at lower doses, but with higher doses there is an increased likelihood of problems, including headache, dizziness, somnolence, anxiety, depression (including suicidal behavior), confusion, hallucinations, cerebellar dysfunction, and emotional lability.
6. *General systemic effects.* Fatigue, anorexia, and weight loss are common with chronic administration.
   a. *Cardiovascular effects.* Mild hypotension is common but rarely symptomatic. Rarely to uncommonly seen hypertension, chest pain, arrhythmias, or other cardiovascular disorders.
   b. *Respiratory effects.* Dyspnea and cough are occasional at higher doses.
7. *Infectious effects.* Exacerbation of herpetic eruptions and nonherpetic cold sores is uncommon.
8. *Miscellaneous effects.* Leg cramps, insomnia, urticaria, hot flashes, coagulation disorders are uncommon. Visual problems, including blurring, diplopia, dry eyes, nystagmus, and photophobia are uncommon.

9. *Metabolic effects and laboratory abnormalities.*
   a. Elevated liver enzymes are common.
   b. Mild proteinuria; increase in serum creatinine is occasional.
   c. Hypercalcemia is occasional.
   d. Hypothyroidism and hyperthyroidism with or without antithyroid antibodies.
   e. Hypertriglyceridemia is rare.
10. Antibody development (binding and neutralizing) occurs more readily with interferon α-2a than with interferon α-2b. The significance of this is not clear, though it may be associated with the development of clinical resistance in some patients.

IRINOTECAN

Other names. Camptosar, CPT-11.

Mechanism of action. Irinotecan, a semisynthetic water-soluble derivative of CPT, is a prodrug for the lipophilic metabolite SN-38, a potent inhibitor of topoisomerase I, an enzyme essential for effective replication and transcription. It binds to the topoisomerase I—DNA cleavable complex, preventing religation after cleavage by topoisomerase I.

Primary indications.
1. Carcinoma of the colon or rectum, esophagus, or stomach.
2. Carcinoma of the lung.

Usual dosage and schedule.
1. 80 to 125 mg/m^2 IV over 90 min weekly for 4 weeks followed by a 2-week rest to complete one cycle when used either as a single agent or in combination with fluorouracil and leucovorin.
2. 180 mg/m^2 IV over 90 min every 2 weeks when used with leucovorin (over 2 h) plus bolus fluorouracil followed by a 22-h infusion of fluorouracil.

   For severe or worse diarrhea (≥ 7 stools over pretreatment), doses should be held. When the diarrhea has improved (≤ 7 stools over pretreatment) treatment may be restarted with doses modified downward by 25 to 30 mg/m^2 during the current and subsequent cycles if there was an increase in stools of seven to nine times per day, and by 50 to 60 mg/m^2 if there was an increase in stools of 10 times or more. Doses are also held during treatment and reduced in the same and subsequent cycles for severe neutropenia (ANC <1,000).

Special precautions.
1. Both early and late diarrhea may occur. That which occurs within 24 h (a cholinergic effect) should be treated with atropine, 0.25 to 1 mg IV. Late diarrhea should be treated promptly with loperamide (up to 2 mg every 2 h until the patient is diarrhea-free for 12 h) and prompt fluid and electrolyte replacement as indicated, if the diarrhea becomes severe (increase of 7 or more stools per day) or there is dehydration or postural hypotension. Consideration should be given to antibiotic therapy, such as with an oral fluoroquinolone, particularly if the patient is neutropenic. A vascular syndrome

characterized by sudden unexpected thromboembolic events has also been described.

2. Dose must be reduced in patients who are homozygous for the UGT1A1*28 allele, a variation of a uridine diphosphate glucuronosyltransferase gene and its corresponding enzyme (UGT1A1) that is responsible for glucuronidation of bilirubin and involved in deactivation of irinotecan's toxic active metabolite SN-38. Testing may be done by the *Invader UGT1A1 Molecular Assay* (Third Wave Technologies).

Toxicity.

1. *Myelosuppression and other hematologic effects.* Neutropenia is common and often severe, particularly in combination therapy; anemia and thrombocytopenia are common, but uncommonly severe, unless homozygous for UGT1A1*28.

2. *Nausea, vomiting, and other gastrointestinal effects.* Nausea and vomiting are common, and are occasionally severe. Early diarrhea is common, but is uncommonly severe. Late diarrhea is common (85%) and is occasionally severe (15%) to life threatening (5–10%). Severe diarrhea may be more common if homozygous for UGT1A1*28. Abdominal cramping is common, occasionally severe. Anorexia is common. Constipation and dyspepsia are occasional. Ileus, colitis, or toxic megacolon are seen rarely.

3. *Mucocutaneous effects.* Alopecia and mucositis are common. Rash and sweating occur occasionally.

4. *Miscellaneous effects.*
   a. Fever is common, rarely severe.
   b. Headache, back pain, chills, and edema are occasional.
   c. Grade 1 to 2 increases in liver function test values are common; it is uncommon for liver function abnormalities to be severe, except in patients with known liver metastasis.
   d. Dyspnea, cough, or rhinitis is occasional to common, but usually not severe.
   e. Insomnia or dizziness is occasional.
   f. Flushing is occasional.
   g. Anaphylactic reactions are rare.

LAPATINIB

Other name. Tykerb.

Mechanism of action. Lapatinib is a dual tyrosine kinase inhibitor with specificity for epidermal growth factor (ErbB1) receptor (EGFR) and ErbB2 (Her2/neu).

Primary indication. Carcinoma of breast that overexpresses the HER2 protein.

Usual dosage and schedule.

1. 1,500 mg PO daily.
2. 1250 mg PO daily with other agents such as capecitabine.

Special precautions. The drug being a new agent, unanticipated adverse effects may emerge with further experience.

Toxicity.

1. *Myelosuppression and other hematologic effects.* Myelosuppression is not an effect of lapatinib. Other EGFR inhibitors may potentiate warfarin and cause unexpected rise in INR.

2. *Nausea, vomiting, and other gastrointestinal effects.* Nausea and diarrhea are common; vomiting dyspepsia, and anorexia are occasional. Other EGFR inhibitors are associated with transaminase elevations and occasionally with increased bilirubin.
3. *Mucocutaneous effects.* Rash is common.
4. *Miscellaneous effects.*
    a. Left ventricular ejection fraction decrease is rare and generally asymptomatic.
    b. Fatigue is common.

LENALIDOMIDE

Other name. Revlimid.
Mechanism of action. Multiple potential mechanisms, including immunomodulatory and antiangiogenic effects. Precise mechanism not delineated.
Primary malignancy indications.
1. Myelodysplastic syndrome, low or intermediate-1 risk, associated with deletion of 5q31 (del 5q).
2. Multiple myeloma.
Usual dosage and schedule. 10 mg PO daily, with dosing interruptions and subsequent dose reduction to 5 mg daily as determined by cytopenias or other toxicity. Renal insufficiency is associated with decreased clearance.
Special precautions. Severe and life-threatening birth defects, primarily phocomelia, may be caused by this analog of thalidomide, a known human teratogen. For this reason, special precautions must be taken to assure that female patients are not pregnant when the drug is started, and that both female and male patients practice strict birth control measures.
Toxicity.
1. *Myelosuppression and other hematologic effects.* Neutropenia and thrombocytopenia are common and dose limiting. Febrile neutropenia is uncommon. Anemia is occasional, and may be autoimmune in nature (uncommon). Hypercoagulability with thromboembolic events, including pulmonary emboli (2%), have been seen in patients treated with lenalidomide combination therapy—uncommon to occasional. Relative benefit of prophylactic anticoagulation or antiplatelet therapy is uncertain, but some form of prophylaxis is generally recommended, particularly in patients with myeloma or in others receiving corticosteroids.
2. *Nausea, vomiting, and other gastrointestinal effects.* Diarrhea is common; constipation is common but less frequent than diarrhea. Nausea is common, but vomiting is only occasional. Abdominal pain is occasional.
3. *Mucocutaneous effects.* Macular rash, dryness of the skin, increased sweating, and pruritus are common. Urticaria is occasional.
4. *Miscellaneous effects.*
    a. Cough, nasopharyngitis, dyspnea, and bronchitis are occasional.
    b. Myalgia, arthralgia, muscle cramps, or limb pain are occasional.

c. Fatigue and fever are common, but rigors are uncommon.
d. Headache and dizziness are occasional. Peripheral neuropathy is uncommon (5%). Insomnia and depression are occasional.
e. Hypothyroidism is occasional.
f. Palpitations, hypertension, chest pain, and peripheral edema are occasional.
g. Hypokalemia and hypomagnesemia are occasional.
h. Birth defects. (See Special precautions in the preceding text.)

LETROZOLE

Other name.   Femara.

Mechanism of action.   Decreases estrogen biosynthesis by selective, competitive inhibition of the aromatase enzyme in peripheral tissues, thereby reducing the conversion of the adrenal androgens testosterone and androstenedione to estradiol and estrone, respectively.

Primary indications.

1. Carcinoma of the breast, advanced or metastatic, that is hormone receptor positive or unknown in postmenopausal women as first-line treatment; or in hormone-responsive post-menopausal women with progression following antiestrogen therapy.
2. Carcinoma of the breast as adjuvant therapy in hormone receptor–positive postmenopausal women.

Usual dosage and schedule.   2.5 mg PO daily.

Special precautions.   Potential hazard to fetus if given during pregnancy. Because of the potential fracture risk, bone density testing and treatment with calcium and Vitamin D with or without bisphosphonates are often used.

Toxicity.

1. *Myelosuppression and other hematologic effects.* No dose-related effect. Thromboembolic events are uncommon to rare.
2. *Nausea, vomiting, and other gastrointestinal effects.* Nausea, vomiting, constipation, and diarrhea are uncommon to occasional.
3. *Mucocutaneous effects.* Rash is uncommon.
4. *Miscellaneous effects.*
   a. Thromboembolic events are uncommon (1.2%) and less than with tamoxifen.
   b. Hot flashes are common and night sweats are occasional.
   c. Musculoskeletal pain (arthralgia or bone) is occasional to common.
   d. Weight increase is occasional.
   e. Fatigue is occasional.
   f. Osteoporosis (occasional) is accelerated, with increase in fracture risk (uncommon).
   g. Headache is uncommon.
   h. Peripheral edema, weight gain is occasional (lower than with megestrol).
   i. Dyspnea and cough are uncommon to occasional.
   j. Hypercalcemia is rare.
   k. Endometrial cancer is rare (0.2%) and less likely than with tamoxifen.

LOMUSTINE

Other name. CCNU, CeeNU.

Mechanism of action. Alkylation and carbamoylation by lomustine metabolites interfere with the synthesis and function of DNA, RNA, and proteins. Lomustine is lipid soluble and enters the brain easily.

Primary indication. Malignant brain tumors.

Usual dosage and schedule. 100 to 130 mg/m^2 PO once every 6 to 8 weeks (lower dose used for patients with compromised bone marrow function). Some recommend restricting cumulative dose to 1,000 mg/m^2 to limit pulmonary and renal toxicity.

Special precautions. Because of delayed myelosuppression (3–6 weeks), do not treat more often than every 6 weeks. Await a return of normal platelet and granulocyte counts before repeating therapy.

Toxicity.

1. *Myelosuppression and other hematologic effects.* Universal and dose limiting. Leukopenia and thrombocytopenia are delayed 3 to 6 weeks after therapy begins and may be cumulative with successive doses.
2. *Nausea, vomiting, and other gastrointestinal effects.* Nausea and vomiting may begin 3 to 6 h after therapy and last up to 24 h.
3. *Mucocutaneous effects.* Stomatitis and alopecia are rare.
4. *Miscellaneous effects.*
   a. Confusion, lethargy, and ataxia are rare.
   b. Mild hepatotoxicity is infrequent.
   c. Secondary neoplasia is possible.
   d. Pulmonary fibrosis is uncommon at doses of less than 1,000 mg/m^2.
   e. Renal toxicity is uncommon at doses of less than 1,000 mg/m^2.

LUTEINIZING   HORMONE–RELEASING   HORMONE (LHRH) ANALOGS

Other names. Leuprolide (Lupron, Lupron depot, Viadur), goserelin (Zoladex depot), triptorelin pamoate (Trelstar depot).

Mechanism of action. Initial release of follicle-stimulating hormone and luteinizing hormone from the anterior pituitary, followed by diminution of gonadotropin secretion owing to desensitization of the pituitary to gonadotropin-releasing hormone (GnRH) and consequent decrease in the respective gonadal hormones. May also have direct effects on cancer cells, at least in cancer of the breast, in which GnRH-binding sites have been demonstrated.

Primary indications.

1. Metastatic prostate carcinoma.
2. Breast carcinoma in premenopausal and perimenopausal women with metastatic disease (goserelin).

Usual dosage and schedule.

1. Leuprolide depot, 7.5 mg IM monthly, 22.5 mg IM every 3 months, or 30 mg IM every 4 months.

2. Goserelin depot, 3.6 mg SC every 4 weeks or 10.8 mg SC every 12 weeks. Use only 3.6-mg implant for breast carcinoma.
3. Triptorelin depot 3.75 mg IM monthly.

Special precautions. Worsening of symptoms may occur during the first few weeks.

Toxicity.

1. *Myelosuppression and other hematologic effects.* Rare, if at all.
2. *Nausea, vomiting, and other gastrointestinal effects.* Anorexia, nausea, vomiting, and constipation are uncommon.
3. *Mucocutaneous effects.* Erythema and ecchymosis at the injection site, rash, hair loss, and itching are uncommon.
4. *Cardiovascular effects.* Congestive heart failure, hypertension, and thrombotic episodes are uncommon. Peripheral edema is occasional.
5. *Miscellaneous effects.*
   a. *CNS*: dizziness, pain, headache, and paresthesias are uncommon.
   b. *Endocrine*: hot flashes are common; decreased libido is common; gynecomastia with or without tenderness is uncommon; impotence is occasional to common.
   c. Bone pain, or "flare," is common on initiation of therapy in patients with bony metastasis. This can be minimized by pretreating with flutamide or another androgen antagonist in men with prostate cancer.
   d. Hypersensitivity reactions with rare angioneurotic edema and anaphylaxis have been reported.

MECHLORETHAMINE

Other names. Nitrogen mustard, HN2, Mustargen.

Mechanism of action. Mechlorethamine is a prototype alkylating agent. Its action involves transfer of the alkyl group to amino, carboxyl, hydroxyl, imidazole, phosphate, and sulfhydryl groups within the cell, altering structure and function of DNA (primarily), RNA, and proteins.

Primary indications.

1. Hodgkin's lymphoma.
2. Malignant pleural and, less commonly, peritoneal or pericardial effusions.
3. CTCLs (topically).

Usual dosage and schedule.

1. 6 mg/m^2 IV on days 1 and 8 every 4 weeks (in MOPP regimen for Hodgkin's disease).
2. 8 to 16 mg/m^2 by intracavitary injection.
3. 10 mg in 60 mL of tap water applied to entire body surface (avoid eyes).

Special precautions.

1. Administer over several minutes into the sidearm of a running IV infusion, taking care to avoid extravasation.
2. Because mechlorethamine is a potent vesicant, extreme care must be exercised while preparing and administering the drug. Gloves and eyeglasses are recommended to protect the preparer. If accidental eye contact should occur, institute copious irrigation with normal saline and follow by prompt ophthalmologic consultation. If accidental skin contact occurs,

irrigate the affected part immediately with water for at least 15 min and follow by 2.6% sodium thiosulfate solution (1/6 M).

3. Mechlorethamine should be used soon after preparation (15–30 min) as it decomposes on standing. It *must not* be mixed in the same syringe with any other drug.

Toxicity.

1. *Myelosuppression and other hematologic effects.* Dose-limiting, with the nadir at approximately 1 week and recovery by 3 weeks.

2. *Nausea, vomiting, and other gastrointestinal effects.* Universal. They usually begin within the first 3 h and last 4 to 8 h.

3. *Mucocutaneous effects.* Severe painful inflammation and necrosis are likely if extravasation occurs. May be ameliorated if 2.6% thiosulfate solution (1/6 M) is instilled into the area to neutralize active drug, and ice packs are applied locally for 6 to 12 h. Maculopapular rash is uncommon.

4. *Miscellaneous effects.*
   a. Phlebitis, thrombosis, or both of the vein used for the injection are common.
   b. Amenorrhea and azoospermia are common.
   c. Hyperuricemia with rapid tumor destruction.
   d. Weakness, sleepiness, and headache are uncommon.
   e. Severe allergic reactions, including anaphylaxis, are rare.
   f. Secondary neoplasms, including myelodysplasia, acute leukemia, and carcinomas are possible.

MELPHALAN

Other names. Phenylalanine mustard, L-sarcolysin, L-PAM, Alkeran.

Mechanism of action. Alkylating agent with primary effect on DNA. Amino acid–type structure may result in cellular transport that is different from other alkylating agents.

Primary indications.

1. Multiple myeloma.
2. Stem cell preparative regimens.

Usual dosage and schedule.

1. 8 mg/m^2 PO on days 1 to 4 every 4 weeks *or*
2. 10 mg/m^2 PO on days 1 to 4 every 6 weeks *or*
3. 3 to 4 mg/m^2 PO daily for 2 to 3 weeks, and then 1 to 2 mg/m^2 PO daily for maintenance.
4. High-dose regimens of 140 to 200 mg/m^2 IV have been used, followed by stem cell rescue (e.g., bone marrow transplantation).
5. 16 mg/m^2 IV every 2 weeks ×4, then every 4 weeks.

Special precautions.

1. Myelosuppression and other hematologic effects may be delayed and prolonged to 4 to 6 weeks. Reduce IV dose by 50% for creatinine more than 1.5 times normal.

2. Use in early myeloma may preclude harvest of sufficient numbers of peripheral stem cells for autologous transplantation.

Toxicity.

1. *Myelosuppression and other hematologic effects.* Dose limiting; nadir at days 14 to 21.

2. *Nausea, vomiting, and other gastrointestinal effects*. Nausea, vomiting, and diarrhea are uncommon at standard doses, but common with high-dose regimens.
3. *Mucocutaneous effects*. Alopecia, dermatitis, and stomatitis are uncommon at standard doses; alopecia and mucositis are common with high-dose regimens.
4. *Miscellaneous effects*.
   a. Acute nonlymphocytic leukemia and myelodysplasia are rare but well documented.
   b. Pulmonary fibrosis is rare.

MERCAPTOPURINE

Other names. 6-Mercaptopurine, 6-MP, Purinethol.
Mechanism of action. A purine antimetabolite that, when converted to the nucleotide, inhibits the formation of nucleotides necessary for DNA and RNA synthesis.
Primary indication. Acute lymphocytic leukemia.
Usual dosage and schedule.
1. 100 mg/m^2 PO daily if used alone.
2. 50 to 90 mg/m^2 PO daily if used with methotrexate.
Special precautions.
1. Decrease dose by 75% when used concurrently with allopurinol.
2. Increase interval between doses or reduce dose in patients with renal failure.
Toxicity.
1. *Myelosuppression and other hematologic effects*. Common but mild at recommended doses.
2. *Nausea, vomiting, and other gastrointestinal effects*. Nausea and vomiting are uncommon. Diarrhea is rare.
3. *Mucocutaneous effects*. Stomatitis may be seen with very large doses. Dry, scaling rash is uncommon.
4. *Miscellaneous effects*.
   a. Intrahepatic cholestasis and mild focal centrolobular necrosis with jaundice are uncommon.
   b. Hyperuricemia with rapid leukemia cell lysis is common.
   c. Fever is uncommon.

MESNA

Other name. Mesnex.
Mechanism of action. Mesna disulfide is reduced in the kidney to a free thiol compound, which then reacts chemically with urotoxic metabolites of ifosfamide or cyclophosphamide, resulting in their detoxification.
Primary indication. Prophylaxis for ifosfamide (or high-dose cyclophosphamide)-induced hemorrhagic cystitis.
Usual dosage and schedule. Mesna dose is at least 20% of the ifosfamide dose (on a weight [mg] basis), administered just before (or mixed with) the ifosfamide dose and again at 4 and 8 h after the ifosfamide to detoxify the urinary metabolites that cause the hemorrhagic cystitis. Higher doses of ifosfamide may require higher doses and longer durations of mesna.
Special Precautions. Contraindicated if patient is sensitive to thiol compounds. Does not prevent or ameliorate any adverse effects of ifosfamide or cyclophosphamide other than hemorrhagic

cystitis. Neither mesna nor its only metabolite, mesna disulfide, affects ifosfamide, cyclophosphamide, or the antineoplastic metabolites.

Toxicity.

1. *Myelosuppression and other hematologic effects.* None.
2. *Nausea, vomiting, and other gastrointestinal effects.* Nausea, vomiting, and diarrhea are occasional. Nausea and vomiting are more commonly from ifosfamide.
3. *Mucocutaneous effects.* Bad taste in the mouth is common.
4. *Miscellaneous effects.*
   a. Headache, fatigue, and limb pain are occasional.
   b. Hypotension or allergic reactions are uncommon to rare.
   c. Gives false positive test for urinary ketones.

METHOTREXATE

Other names. Amethopterin, MTX, Mexate, Folex, Trexall.

Mechanism of action. Inhibition of dihydrofolate reductase, which results in a block of the reduction of dihydrofolate to tetrahydrofolate. This blockage in turn inhibits the formation of thymidylate and purines, and arrests DNA (predominantly), RNA, and protein synthesis.

Primary indications.

1. Bladder, breast, head and neck, gastrointestinal, lung, and gestational trophoblastic carcinomas.
2. Osteosarcomas (high-dose methotrexate).
3. Acute lymphocytic leukemia.
4. Meningeal leukemia or carcinomatosis.
5. Non–Hodgkin's lymphoma.

Usual dosage and schedule.

1. *Gestational trophoblastic carcinoma.* 15 to 30 mg PO or IM on days 1 to 5 every 2 weeks.
2. *Other carcinomas.* 40 to 80 mg/m^2 IV or PO two to four times monthly with a 7- to 14-day interval between doses.
3. *Acute lymphocytic leukemia.* 15 to 20 mg/m^2 PO or IV weekly (together with mercaptopurine).
4. *Osteogenic sarcoma.* Up to 12 g/m^2 with leucovorin rescue (high-dose methotrexate). This usage requires on-site monitoring of methotrexate levels and a high degree of expertise to administer safely.
5. *Intrathecally.* 12 mg/m^2 (not >20 mg) twice weekly.

Special precautions.

1. High-dose methotrexate (>80 mg/m^2) should be administered only by individuals experienced in its use and at institutions where serum methotrexate levels can be readily measured.
2. Intrathecal methotrexate must be mixed in buffered physiologic solution containing no preservative.
3. Avoid aspirin, sulfonamides, tetracycline, phenytoin, and other protein-bound drugs that may displace methotrexate and cause an increase in free drug.
4. Oral anticoagulants, e.g., warfarin, may be potentiated by methotrexate; therefore prothrombin times should be followed carefully.

5. Oral antibiotics may decrease methotrexate absorption; penicillin and nonsteroidal anti-inflammatory drug (NSAIDs) decrease clearance of methotrexate.
6. Monitor use with theophylline.
7. In patients with renal insufficiency, it may be necessary to markedly reduce the dose or discontinue methotrexate therapy.
8. Do not give if patient has an effusion, because of "reservoir" effect.

Toxicity.
1. *Myelosuppression and other hematologic effects.* Occurs commonly, with nadir at 6 to 10 days after a single IV dose. Recovery is rapid.
2. *Nausea, vomiting, and other gastrointestinal effects.* Occasional at standard doses.
3. *Mucocutaneous effects.*
   a. Mild stomatitis is common and a sign that a maximum tolerated dose has been reached. Higher doses may result in confluent or hemorrhagic stomal ulcers and bloody diarrhea.
   b. Erythematous rashes, urticaria, and skin pigment changes are uncommon.
   c. Mild alopecia is frequent.
4. *Miscellaneous effects.*
   a. Acute hepatocellular injury is uncommon at standard doses.
   b. Hepatic fibrosis is uncommon but seen at low chronic doses.
   c. Pneumonitis is rare.
   d. Polyserositis is rare.
   e. Renal tubular necrosis is rare at standard doses.
   f. Convulsions and a Guillain-Barré–like syndrome following intrathecal therapy are uncommon.

MITOMYCIN

Other names. Mitomycin C, Mutamycin.

Mechanism of action. Alkylation and cross-linking by mitomycin metabolites interfere with structure and function of DNA.

Primary indication. Bladder (intravesical), esophagus, stomach, anal, and pancreas carcinomas.

Usual dosage and schedule.
1. 20 mg/m^2 IV on day 1 every 4 to 6 weeks *or*
2. 2 mg/m^2 IV on days 1 to 5 and 8 to 12 every 4 to 6 weeks.
3. 10 mg/m^2 IV on day 1 every 8 weeks in combination with fluorouracil and doxorubicin for stomach and pancreatic carcinomas.
4. 30 to 40 mg instilled into the bladder weekly for 4 to 8 weeks, then monthly for 6 months.

Special precautions. Administer as slow push or rapid infusion through the sidearm of a rapidly running IV infusion, taking care to avoid extravasation. Pulmonary, renal, and hematologic toxicity (microangiopathic anemia and thrombocytopenia) may result from endothelial cell damage.

Toxicity.
1. *Myelosuppression and other hematologic effects.*

a. Myelosuppression is serious, cumulative, and dose limiting. Nadir is reached usually by 4 weeks but may be
delayed. Recovery is often prolonged over many weeks, and
occasionally the cytopenia never disappears.

b. Hemolytic–uremic syndrome is rare, but when it occurs,
may be poorly responsive to plasmapheresis and other
therapies.

2. *Nausea, vomiting, and other gastrointestinal effects*. Nausea
and vomiting are common at higher doses, but severity is
usually mild to moderate.

3. *Mucocutaneous effects*.
   a. Stomatitis and alopecia are common.
   b. Cellulitis is common at injection site if extravasation occurs.

4. *Miscellaneous effects*.
   a. Renal toxicity is uncommon.
   b. Pulmonary toxicity is uncommon but may be severe.
   c. Fever is uncommon.
   d. Secondary neoplasia is possible.

MITOTANE

Other names. *o,p′*-DDD, Lysodren.

Mechanism of action. Suppresses adrenal steroid production, modifies peripheral steroid metabolism, and is cytotoxic to
adrenal cortical cells.

Primary indication. Adrenocortical carcinoma.

Usual dosage and schedule. Begin with 2 to 6 g PO daily
in 3 or 4 divided doses and build to a maximum tolerated daily
dose that is usually 8 to 10 gm, although it may range from 2 to
16 gm. Glucocorticoid and mineralocorticoid replacements during mitotane therapy are necessary to prevent hypoadrenalism.
Cortisone acetate (25 mg PO in the morning and 12.5 mg PO in
the evening) and fludrocortisone acetate (0.1 mg PO in the a.m.)
are recommended.

Special precautions. Patients who experience severe trauma,
infection, or shock should be treated with supplemental corticosteroids. Because of the effect of mitotane on peripheral
steroid metabolism, larger than usual replacement doses may be
necessary.

Toxicity.

1. *Myelosuppression and other hematologic effects*. None.

2. *Nausea, vomiting, and other gastrointestinal effects*. Common
and may be dose limiting.

3. *Mucocutaneous effects*. Skin rash occurs occasionally.

4. *CNS effects*. Lethargy, sedation, vertigo, or dizziness in up to
40% of patients; may be dose limiting.

5. *Miscellaneous effects*. Albuminuria, hemorrhagic cystitis, hypertension, orthostatic hypotension, and visual disturbances
are uncommon.

MITOXANTRONE

Other names. Novantrone, dihydroxyanthracenedione, DHAD,
DHAQ.

Mechanism of action. DNA strand breakage mediated by the
effects of anthracenedione on topoisomerase II.

Primary indications.
1. Acute nonlymphocytic leukemia.
2. Carcinoma of the breast or ovary.
3. Non–Hodgkin's and Hodgkin's lymphoma.

Usual dosage and schedule.
1. 12 to 14 mg/m^2 IV as a 5- to 30-min infusion once every 3 weeks for solid tumors.
2. 12 mg/m^2 IV as a 5- to 30-min infusion daily for 3 days for acute nonlymphocytic leukemia.

Special precautions. Rarely causes extravasation injury if infiltrated. Cardiotoxicity is probably less than that with doxorubicin; but prior anthracycline, chest irradiation, or underlying cardiac disease increases the risk.

Toxicity.
1. *Myelosuppression and other hematologic effects.* Universal.
2. *Nausea, vomiting, and other gastrointestinal effects.* Nausea and vomiting are common but less frequent and less severe than with doxorubicin. Diarrhea is uncommon.
3. *Mucocutaneous effects.* Alopecia is common, but its frequency and severity are less than with doxorubicin. Mucositis is occasional.
4. *Cardiac toxicity.* Probably less than with doxorubicin; there is no clear maximum dose, though the risk appears to increase at 125 mg/m^2 cumulative dose.
5. *Miscellaneous effects.*
   a. Local erythema and swelling with transient blue discoloration if extravasated, but rarely leads to severe skin damage.
   b. Green or blue discoloration of urine.
   c. Phlebitis is uncommon.

NELARABINE

Other name. Arranon.

Mechanism of action. Nelarabine is a prodrug of arabinofuranosylguanine (ara-G), a cytotoxic analog of deoxyguanosine. When converted to triphosphorylated ara-G, it is incorporated into DNA (preferentially into T cells), inducing fragmentation and apoptosis.

Primary indication. T-cell ALL and T-cell lymphoblastic lymphoma that have relapsed or are refractory to at least two prior chemotherapeutic regimens.

Usual dosage and schedule.
1. Adults—1,500 mg/m^2 IV over 2 h on days 1, 3, and 5, repeated every 21 days.
2. Children—650 mg/m^2 IV over 1 h daily for 5 consecutive days, repeated every 21 days.

Special precautions. Close monitoring for neurologic events is recommended, owing to the possibility of severe neurologic complications of therapy. Prophylaxis against tumor lysis syndrome is recommended.

Toxicity.
1. *Myelosuppression and other hematologic effects.* Anemia, neutropenia, and thrombocytopenia are common. Febrile neutropenia is occasional.

2. *Nausea and vomiting and other gastrointestinal effects.* Nausea, vomiting, diarrhea, and constipation are common. Abdominal pain is occasional.
3. *Mucocutaneous effects.* Stomatitis is occasional.
4. *Neurologic effects.*
   a. Headache is occasional.
   b. Somnolence and confusion are occasional.
   c. Peripheral neuropathy is occasional. May range from numbness and paresthesias to motor weakness and paralysis.
   d. Ataxia is occasional.
   e. Insomnia is occasional.
   f. Convulsions and coma are rare.
   g. Leukoencephalopathy and demyelination and ascending peripheral neuropathy are rare.
5. Immune effects and infusion reactions.
6. *Miscellaneous effect.*
   a. Fatigue, weakness, and fever (occasionally with rigors) are common.
   b. Cough, dyspnea, and pleural effusion are common to occasional.
   c. Abnormal liver function test results are occasional.
   d. Hypokalemia, hypomagnesemia, hypocalcemia, and increased creatinine are occasional.
   e. Edema is occasional.
   f. Sinus tachycardia is occasional.
   g. Musculoskeletal pain is occasional.

NILOTINIB

Other names.   Tasigna, AMN107.

Mechanism of action.   Selective inhibitor of the constitutively activated Bcr-Abl tyrosine kinase that is created as a consequence of the (9;22) chromosomal translocation and is required for the transforming function and excess proliferation seen in chronic myelogenous leukemia (CML). *In vitro*, nilotinib is active against many *Bcr-Abl* mutations associated with imatinib resistance.

Primary indications.
1. CML— in chronic, accelerated, or blastic phase—and Philadelphia chromosome–positive acute lymphocytic leukemia in patients resistant or intolerant to imatinib.

Usual dosage and schedule.   600 mg PO daily or 400 mg PO twice daily.

Toxicity.
1. *Myelosuppression and other hematologic effects.* Thrombocytopenia is common. Neutropenia and anemia are occasional.
2. *Nausea, vomiting and other gastrointestinal effects.* Nausea and vomiting are occasional.
3. *Mucocutaneous effects.* Skin rash is common; alopecia, dry skin, and pruritus are occasional.
4. *Miscellaneous effects.*
   a. Abnormal liver function tests, including elevations in bilirubin (primarily unconjugated) are occasional.
   b. Increase in the corrected QT interval by 5 to 15 msec has been seen.
   c. Increase in lipase and amylase are uncommon.

NILUTAMIDE

Other name. Nilandron.

Mechanism of action. Competitive inhibitor of androgens at the cellular androgen receptor in prostate cancer cells. Complements surgical castration.

Primary indication. Metastatic carcinoma of the prostate, in combination with surgical castration or LHRH agonist.

Usual dosage and schedule. 300 mg PO once daily for 30 days, followed by 150 mg PO once daily thereafter.

Special precautions. Should be restricted to patients with normal liver function test values. A routine chest radiograph should be obtained before therapy and any time that the patient reports new exertional dyspnea or worsening of preexisting dyspnea. Inhibits activity of liver cytochrome P-450 isoenzymes and may delay elimination of drugs such as warfarin, phenytoin, and theophylline.

Toxicity.

1. *Myelosuppression and other hematologic effects.* None.
2. *Nausea, vomiting, and other gastrointestinal effects.* Occasional nausea. Constipation is uncommon.
3. *Mucocutaneous effects.* Rash, dry skin, and sweating are uncommon.
4. *Miscellaneous effects.*
   a. Hepatitis is rare (1%).
   b. Interstitial pneumonitis with dyspnea is uncommon (2%). May be higher in patients with Asian ancestry.
   c. Inhibits activity of liver cytochrome P-450 isoenzymes and may delay elimination of drugs such as warfarin, phenytoin, and theophylline.
   d. Hot flashes are common.
   e. Increased liver function test values are uncommon.
   f. Impaired adaptation to darkness is common.

OCTREOTIDE

Other name. Sandostatin, Sandostatin LAR depot.

Mechanism of action. Somatostatin analog that inhibits release of polypeptide hormones, particularly in the pancreas and gut. Slows gastrointestinal transit time. Promotes water and electrolyte absorption, reflecting change from overall secretory to absorptive state.

Primary indications.

1. Carcinoid tumors.
2. Vasoactive intestinal peptide tumors and other amine precursor uptake and decarboxylation tumors.
3. Chemotherapy-induced diarrhea.
4. Acromegaly.

Usual dosage and schedule. 100 to 1,500 μg/day SC, in two to four divided doses. Doses are usually started at the lower end and titrated upward to the best symptomatic improvement. If patients respond favorably to the rapid-acting SC injections, may be maintained on 20 mg IM of the depot preparation by intragluteal injection every 4 weeks. Caution should be used in treating for more than 3 months.

Special precautions. Lower doses indicated if there is severe renal dysfunction (creatinine >5 mg/dL).

Toxicity.

1. *Myelosuppression and other hematologic effects.* None.
2. *Nausea, vomiting, and other gastrointestinal effects.* Nausea abdominal discomfort, bloating, and diarrhea are common, particularly early in early therapy. Vomiting is only occasionally seen. Decreased gall bladder contractility and decreased bile secretion may result in biliary abnormalities. Gallstones develop in less than 2% if treatment is for 1 month or less but can be 25% if treatment is for 1 year or more. Ascending cholangitis and pancreatitis are uncommon to rare.
3. *Mucocutaneous effects.* Local site reactions are occasional; other effects are rare.
4. *Endocrine effects.* Hypoglycemia or hyperglycemia is uncommon; hypothalamic pituitary dysfunction is rare.
5. *Bradycardia* and other conduction abnormalities occur in up to 25% of patients with acromegaly who are treated with octreotide.

OPRELVEKIN

Other names. Neumega, IL-11.

Mechanism of action. Stimulates proliferation of hematopoietic stem cells and megakaryocyte progenitor cells and induces megakaryocyte maturation, resulting in increased platelet production.

Primary indication. Prevention of severe thrombocytopenia after chemotherapy in patients with nonmyeloid malignancies.

Usual dosage and schedule. 50 μg/kg SQ once daily, starting 6 to 24 h after completion of chemotherapy. Continue until the postnadir count is $\geq 50,000/\mu$L. (Treatment for more than 21 days in a row is not recommended.) Next planned cycle of chemotherapy should begin at least 2 days after discontinuation of oprelvekin.

Special precautions. Use with caution in patients with history of atrial arrhythmia or congestive heart failure. Severe allergic reactions, including anaphylaxis, may be seen.

Toxicity.

1. *Myelosuppression and other hematologic effects.* None. Mild decrease in hemoglobin concentration, predominantly due to increase in plasma volume.
2. *Nausea, vomiting, and other gastrointestinal effects.* None.
3. *Mucocutaneous effects.* Occasional rash, particularly at injection site.
4. *Miscellaneous effects.*
   a. *Cardiovascular.* Atrial arrhythmia (flutter or fibrillation) and palpitations are occasional ($\sim$10%), but usually transient. Ventricular arrythmias have been seen (rare).
   b. Syncope is occasional. (Anaphylactic reactions have been observed rarely.)
   c. Fluid retention with edema (renal sodium and water retention) or dyspnea on exertion is common, but usually mild to moderate. Renal failure is rare. May be associated with capillary leak syndrome.

d. Conjunctival injection and mild visual blurring are occasional. Papilledema is rare, but may be more common in children. Caution should be exerted in patients with preexisting papilledema or tumors of the CNS.
e. Asthenia is occasional.
f. Dizziness and insomnia are occasional.

OXALIPLATIN

Other name. Eloxatin.

Mechanism of action. Similar to alkylating agents with respect to binding and cross-linking strands of DNA, forming DNA adducts, and thereby inhibiting DNA replication and transcription.

Primary indications.
1. Carcinoma of the colon and rectum.
2. Carcinoma of the stomach.
3. Non−small cell lung cancer.

Usual dosage and schedule.
1. *Single agent*. 130 mg/m^2 as a 2-h infusion every 3 weeks or 85 mg/m^2 as a 3-h infusion every 2 weeks.
2. *Combination therapy*. 85 to 100 mg/m^2 as a 2-h infusion every 2 weeks in combination with fluorouracil (often as a continuous infusion).

Special precautions. Acute neurosensory and neuromotor symptoms may develop with the infusion. Laryngospasm may be minimized by avoiding cold drinks or food for a few days following treatment. Chronic neurosensory symptoms are dose limiting.

Toxicity.
1. *Myelosuppression and other hematologic effects*. Low grade myelosuppression is common, but grade 3 or 4 granulocytopenia, thrombocytopenia, or anemia is uncommon (~5%). Hemolytic anemia is rare.
2. *Nausea, vomiting, and other gastrointestinal effects*. Nausea, vomiting, and diarrhea are common. Severe diarrhea may lead to hypokalemia. May be worsening of cholinergic syndrome when given with irinotecan. Hepatotoxicity is common with oxaliplatin, in some cases associated with fibrosis or severe veno-occlusive lesions, but grade 3 to 4 toxicity is uncommon.
3. *Mucocutaneous effects*. Alopecia is uncommon. Stomatitis is increased when used with fluorouracil.
4. *Miscellaneous effects*.
   a. Neurotoxicity, consisting of paresthesias and cold-induced dysesthesias in the stocking glove or perioral distribution are common as acute transient changes that begin with the infusion and last for less than one week. Chronic sensory neuropathy, fine motor disturbance, or ataxia is occasional to common with cumulative dosing (cumulative dose dependent), and may last for months. It is occasionally grade 3 to 4.
   b. Laryngospasm may develop during or within 2 h of the infusion and can last up to 5 days. Cold temperatures may induce the spasm, and warm liquids or a hot-pack may ameliorate.

   c. Nephrotoxicity is uncommon.
   d. Ototoxicity is rare.
   e. Anaphylaxis is rare.

PACLITAXEL

Other name.   Taxol, Onxol.

Mechanism of action.   Enhanced formation and stabilization of microtubules. Antineoplastic effect may result from non-functional tubules or altered tubulin–microtubule equilibrium. Mitotic arrest is seen and is associated with accumulated polymerized microtubules.

Primary indications.
1. Carcinomas of the ovary, breast, lung, head and neck, bladder, and cervix.
2. Melanoma.
3. Kaposi's sarcoma, AIDS related.

Usual dosage and schedule.
1. 135 to 225 mg/m^2 as a 3-h infusion every 3 weeks.
2. 135 to 200 mg/m^2 as a 24-h infusion every 3 weeks.
3. 100 mg/m^2 as a 3-h infusion every 2 weeks for the treatment of AIDS-related Kaposi's sarcoma.
4. 80 to 100 mg/m^2 as a 1-h weekly infusion.
5. 30–50 mg/m^2 as a 1-h infusion weekly as a radiosensitizer.

Special precautions.   Anaphylactoid reactions with dyspnea, hypotension (or occasionally hypertension), bronchospasm, urticaria, and erythematous rashes may occur as a result of the paclitaxel itself or the Cremophor vehicle required to make paclitaxel water soluble. Such a reaction is minimized but not totally prevented by pretreatment with antihistamines and corticosteroids and by prolonging the infusion rate (to 24 h). Paclitaxel must be filtered with a 0.2-micron in-line filter.

Standard pretreatment regimen.
1. Dexamethasone, 20 mg IV for doses more than 100 mg/m^2 and 10 mg IV for doses less than 100 mg/m^2, 30 to 60 min before treatment.
2. Diphenhydramine, 50 mg IV 30 to 60 min before treatment.
3. Histamine H$_2$-receptor antagonist, IV 30 to 60 min before treatment (e.g., Cimetidine, 300 mg).

Toxicity.
1. *Myelosuppression and other hematologic effects.* Granulocytopenia is universal and dose limiting; thrombocytopenia is common; anemia is occasional.
2. *Nausea, vomiting, and other gastrointestinal effects.* Common, but usually not severe.
3. *Mucocutaneous effects.* Alopecia is universal; mucositis is occasional at recommended doses.
4. *Hypersensitivity reactions.* Dyspnea, hypotension (or occasionally hypertension), bronchospasm, urticaria, and erythematous rashes are occasionally seen, despite precautions.
5. *Miscellaneous effects.*
   a. Sensory neuropathy is common (30%–35%), and may be progressively worse with time. Recovery may take months to years.
   b. Hepatic dysfunction is uncommon.

   c. Diarrhea is occasional and mild.
   d. Myalgias and arthralgias are common (25%).
   e. Seizures are rare.
   f. Abnormal electrocardiogram is occasional. If there is clinically significant bradycardia, stop the drug. Restart at slower rate when stable.

PACLITAXEL, PROTEIN-BOUND

Other names.   Nanometer albumin-bound paclitaxel (nab-paclitaxel),
Abraxane.

Mechanism of action.   Albumin binding circumvents the requirement for Cremophor vehicle for paclitaxel and its associated toxicity, and exploits albumin receptor–mediated endothelial transport. As with parent compound, intratumor paclitaxel results in enhanced formation and stabilization of microtubules. Antineoplastic effect may result from nonfunctional tubules or altered tubulin–microtubule equilibrium. Mitotic arrest is seen and is associated with accumulated polymerized microtubules.

Primary indications.
1. Metastatic carcinoma of the breast, non–small cell carcinomas of the lung, head and neck, and ovary.
2. Melanoma.

Usual dosage and schedule.
1. 260 mg/m^2 IV over 30 min every 3 weeks.

Special precautions.   Hypersensitivity reactions may occur during the infusion of nab-paclitaxel, but are rare. Premedication, as is used with paclitaxel with Cremophor, is not required.

Toxicity.
1. *Myelosuppression and other hematologic effects.* Granulocytopenia is common and dose limiting; anemia is common as well, but rarely severe. Thrombocytopenia is uncommon. Febrile neutropenia is rare.
2. *Nausea, vomiting, and other gastrointestinal effects.* Nausea and vomiting are occasional to common, but usually not severe. Diarrhea is common, but rarely severe.
3. *Mucocutaneous effects.* Alopecia is universal; mucositis is occasional.
4. *Hypersensitivity reactions.* Uncommon and rarely severe.
5. *Miscellaneous effects.*
   a. Cardiovascular events during the infusion, including hypotension or bradycardia, are uncommon to rare. Late cardiovascular effects are also uncommon. Abnormal ECGs are common, but not associated with symptoms and usually require no intervention. Edema is occasional.
   b. Sensory neuropathy is common and may be progressively worse with time. Recovery may take months to years.
   c. Asthenia is common.
   d. Ocular or visual disturbances are occasional.
   e. Cough and dyspnea are occasional.
   f. Abnormal liver function tests are common, and occasionally severe.
   g. Myalgias and arthralgias are common.
   h. Seizures are rare.

PAMIDRONATE

Other name. Aredia.

Mechanism of action. A bisphosphonate that inhibits osteo-clastic resorption of bone and calcium release induced by tumor cytokines.

Primary indications.
1. Hypercalcemia associated with malignancy.
2. Osteolytic bone metastases of breast cancer.
3. Osteolytic and osteoporotic bone lesions of multiple myeloma.
4. Paget's disease.

Usual dosage and schedule.
1. Multiple myeloma: 90 mg IV as a 4-h infusion every month.
2. Breast cancer: 90 mg IV as a 2-h infusion every 3 to 4 weeks.
3. Hypercalcemia of malignancy: 60 to 90 mg IV as a 4- to 24-h infusion. May be repeated every 1 to 8 weeks, as needed.
4. Paget's disease: 30 mg IV daily as a 4-h infusion on 3 consec-utive days.

Special precautions.
1. Potential for renal tubular damage, particularly if infused more rapidly. Renal clearance parallels creatinine clearance, but adverse effects do not appear to be worse with decreased clearance when given on a monthly basis. Older patients (>75 years) may be more susceptible. Serum electrolytes and renal function should be monitored closely.
2. Osteonecrosis of the jaw has been reported, primarily in asso-ciation with dental procedures such as tooth extraction; such procedures should be avoided during and following bisphos-phonate treatment, if possible.

Toxicity.
1. *Myelosuppression and other hematologic effects*. Rare.
2. *Nausea, vomiting, and other gastrointestinal effects*. Abdomi-nal pain, anorexia, constipation, nausea, vomiting are uncom-mon to occasional.
3. *Mucocutaneous effects*. Infusion site reaction is occasional.
4. *Miscellaneous effects*.
   a. Fatigue is occasional.
   b. Abnormal laboratory reports are occasional (hypocalcemia, hypokalemia, hypomagnesemia, and hypophosphatemia, particularly at the 90-mg dose).
   c. Uveitis, iritis, scleritis, and episcleritis are rare.
   d. Bone pain or generalized pain is occasional.
   e. Osteonecrosis of the jaw is uncommon to rare.

PANITUMUMAB

Other names. Vectibix Epidermal growth factor receptor (EGFR) antibody, rHuMAb-EGFR.

Mechanism of action. Fully humanized EGFR antibody that blocks the ligand-binding site and inhibits proliferation of cells. It is thought to be potentially most useful in those tumors that overexpress EGFR, but correlation with percentage of positive cells or intensity of EGFR expression is lacking.

Primary indication. Colon cancer expressing EGFR.

Usual dosage and schedule. 6 mg/kg (220 mg/m^2) IV over 60 min every 2 weeks.

Special precautions.   Anti-panitumumab antibodies have not been seen, but are possible. Severe hypomagnesemia may be seen, and all patients should have magnesium levels monitored throughout the persistent use of cetuximab (8 weeks).

Toxicity.
1. *Myelosuppression and other hematologic effects.* Leukopenia and anemia are occasional.
2. *Nausea, vomiting, and other gastrointestinal effects.* Anorexia, nausea, vomiting, and diarrhea are occasional. Other chemotherapy-induced diarrhea may be exacerbated. Abdominal pain is common.
3. *Mucocutaneous effects.* Acne-like rash is universal and may be severe. Other skin, mucous membrane, and conjunctival reactions are occasional to common.
4. *Miscellaneous effects.*
   a. Fatigue, headache, and back pain are occasional.
   b. Weight loss, peripheral edema, and dehydration are occasional.
   c. Infusion reactions with allergic or hypersensitivity reactions, fever, chills, or dyspnea are occasional but only rarely severe.
   d. Electrolyte depletion, particularly hypomagnesemia, occurs commonly. Hypomagnesemia is occasionally severe.
   e. Pulmonary fibrosis is rare.

PEGFILGRASTIM

Other names.   Neulasta, Pegylated G-CSF.

Mechanism of action.   Pegfilgrastim is recombinant G-CSF that is conjugated to polyethylene glycol. This delays renal clearance and increases the serum half-life from approximately 3.5 to approximately 15 to 80 h after a single SC injection. Promotes growth and differentiation of myeloid progenitor cells. May improve survival and function of granulocytes.

Primary indication.   Prophylaxis of granulocytopenia and associated infection in patients who are at high risk from chemotherapy for nonmyeloid malignancies.

Usual dosage and schedule.   6 mg SC once (usually on day 2) for each 21- or 28-day chemotherapy cycle. Should not be given between 14 days before and 24 h after each chemotherapy cycle.

Special precautions.
1. Use with caution in disorders of myeloid stem cells as it may promote growth of leukemic cells.
2. The fixed-dose formulation should not be used in infants, children, and others weighing less than 45 kg.

Toxicity.
1. *Myelosuppression and other hematologic effects.* None (leukocytosis with immature forms in the peripheral blood is common).
2. *Nausea, vomiting, and other gastrointestinal effects.* Rare to uncommon.
3. *Mucocutaneous effects.* Exacerbation of preexisting dermatologic conditions is occasional; pyoderma gangrenosum is possible.
4. *Miscellaneous effects.* Usually mild and short lived.

a. Bone pain, musculoskeletal symptoms such as cramps, and back or leg pain are common, somewhat more frequent than in placebo-treated patients and may be severe.
b. Splenomegaly with prolonged use is possible. Splenic rupture is rare.
c. Exacerbation of preexisting inflammatory or autoimmune disorders is rare.
d. Mild elevation of LDH and alkaline phosphatase.
e. Allergic-type reactions may occur, including anaphylaxis (rare).
f. Adult respiratory distress syndrome has been reported in neutropenic patients receiving filgrastim and is possible with pegfilgrastim.

PEMETREXED

Other name. Alimta
Mechanism of action. Interference with folate-dependent metabolic processes, including inhibition of thymidylate synthase, dihydrofolate reductase, and glycinamide ribonucleotide formyltransferase, largely after being converted to polyglutamate forms.
Primary indications.
1. Malignant pleural mesothelioma that is unresectable or not amenable to curative surgery. Given in combination with cisplatin.
2. Non–small cell lung cancer after prior chemotherapy.
Usual dosage and schedule.
1. 500 mg/m^2 IV over 10 min on day 1 of each 21-day cycle. For mesothelioma, it is followed in 30 min by cisplatin 75 mg/m^2 over 2 h.
Special precautions.
1. Folic acid, 400 to 1,000 μg PO 5 times daily, starting 7 days before pemetrexed and continuing for 21 days after the last dose; and 1,000 μg of vitamin B$_{12}$ IM during the week before pemetrexed and every three cycles thereafter must be taken as a prophylactic measure to reduce treatment-related hematologic and GI toxicity.
2. Dexamethasone 4 mg PO twice daily the day before, on the day of, and the day after pemetrexed should be given to reduce skin rash.
3. If creatinine clearance is less than 45 mL/min, give with caution and avoid NSAIDs.
Toxicity.
1. *Myelosuppression.* Anemia is common. Neutropenia and thrombocytopenia are occasional.
2. *Gastrointestinal effects.* Anorexia, nausea, vomiting, and constipation or diarrhea are common. Liver function abnormalities are occasional.
3. *Mucocutaneous effects.* Rash is occasional to common. Stomatitis and pharyngitis are common. Alopecia is occasional.
4. *Neurotoxicity.* Fatigue is common.
5. Immune suppression.
6. *Miscellaneous effects.*
   a. Fever is common.
   b. Serum creatinine elevation is uncommon; renal failure is rare.

c. Myalgia and arthralgia are occasional.
d. Dyspnea and chest pain are common, but may be secondary to underlying condition.
e. Hypersensitivity reactions are occasional, but rarely severe.
f. Thrombosis, embolism, and cardiac ischemia are each uncommon.

PENTOSTATIN

Other names. 2'-Deoxycoformycin, Nipent.

Mechanism of action. Inhibition of ADA, particularly in the presence of adenosine or deoxyadenosine leads to cytotoxicity. Is associated with block of DNA synthesis through inhibition of ribonucleotide reductase. Other effects that may contribute to cytotoxicity include inhibition of RNA synthesis and increased DNA damage.

Primary indication. Hairy-cell leukemia, chronic lymphocytic leukemia, CTCL (mycosis fungoides), other lymphoid neoplasms.

Usual dosage and schedule.

1. 4 mg/m² IV push over 1 to 2 min or diluted in a larger volume over 20 to 30 min. Patients should be given hydration with 500 to 1,000 mL of 5% dextrose in 0.5 N saline or equivalent before pentostatin administration and 500 mL after the drug is given. Repeat every 2 weeks.
2. 2 mg/m² IV every three weeks when used in combination with cyclophosphamide or other agents.

Special precautions.

1. Hydration required to ensure urine output of 2 L daily on the day pentostatin is administered. Patients are often hospitalized for the first drug administration. Allopurinol 300 mg b.i.d. is recommended in patients with a large tumor mass. Sedative and hypnotic drugs should be used with caution or not at all because CNS toxicity may be potentiated. Dose reduction or discontinuation is needed for renal impairment (creatinine clearance <50 mL/min).
2. Should not be used in combination with fludarabine because of a high probability of severe or fatal pulmonary toxicity.

Toxicity.

1. *Myelosuppression.* Common but severity variable.
2. *Nausea, vomiting, and other gastrointestinal effects.* Nausea and vomiting are common but usually not severe. Diarrhea is occasional. Hepatic dysfunction is occasional at recommended doses.
3. *Mucocutaneous effects.* Mucositis is rare; skin rashes and pruritus are occasional to common.
4. *Pulmonary.* Cough is common and dyspnea is occasional. Higher doses or use in combination of fludarabine may lead to severe pulmonary toxicity.
5. *Miscellaneous effects.*
   a. Fatigue is common.
   b. Chills and fever are common.
   c. Infections, probably related both to myelosuppression and lymphocytopenia are occasional.
   d. Renal insufficiency is rare at usual doses.

e. Neuropsychiatric effects. High doses may cause serious neurologic and psychiatric symptoms, including seizures, mental confusion, irritability, and coma.

f. Cough or other respiratory problems are occasional.

PROCARBAZINE

Other names. Matulane, Natulan.

Mechanism of action. Uncertain but appears to affect preformed DNA, RNA, and protein.

Primary indications.

1. Hodgkin's and non–Hodgkin's lymphomas.
2. Brain tumors.
3. Melanoma.

Usual dosage and schedule. 60 to 100 mg/m² PO daily for 7 to 14 days every 4 weeks (in combination with other drugs).

Special precautions. Many food and drug interactions are possible, although their clinical significance may be low.

Drug or food	Possible result
Ethanol	Disulfiram-like reactions: nausea, vomiting, visual disturbances, headache
Sympathomimetics, tricyclic antidepressants, tyramine-rich foods (cheese, wine, bananas)	Hypertensive crisis, tremors, excitation, angina, cardiac palpitations
CNS depressants	Additive depression

Toxicity.

1. *Myelosuppression and other hematologic effects.* Pancytopenia is dose limiting. Recovery may be delayed.
2. *Nausea, vomiting, and other gastrointestinal effects.* Nausea is frequent during first few days until tolerance develops. Diarrhea is uncommon.
3. *Mucocutaneous effects.*
   a. Stomatitis is uncommon.
   b. Alopecia, pruritus, and drug rash are uncommon.
4. *CNS effects.* Paresthesias, neuropathies, headache, dizziness, depression, apprehension, nervousness, insomnia, nightmares, hallucinations, ataxia, confusion, convulsions, and coma have been reported with varying frequency.
5. *Miscellaneous effects.*
   a. Secondary neoplasia is possible.
   b. Visual disturbances are rare.
   c. Postural hypotension is rare.
   d. Hypersensitivity reactions are rare.
   e. There is a strong potential for teratogenesis.

PROGESTINS

Other names. Medroxyprogesterone acetate (Provera, Depo-Provera), hydroxyprogesterone caproate (Delalutin), megestrol acetate (Megace).

Mechanism of action.   Mechanisms of antitumor effects or for appetite stimulation are not clear.
Primary indications.
1. Appetite stimulation.
2. Endometrial carcinoma.
Usual dosage and schedule.
1. As *appetite stimulant*. Megestrol acetate 800 mg PO daily.
2. As *antineoplastic*.
   a. Megestrol acetate 80 to 320 mg PO daily.
   b. Medroxyprogesterone acetate 1,000 to 1,500 mg IM weekly or 400 to 800 mg PO twice weekly.
   c. Hydroxyprogesterone caproate 1,000 to 1,500 mg IM weekly.
Special precautions.   Acute local hypersensitivity or dyspnea due to oil in IM preparations is uncommon.

Hypercalcemia with initial therapy is occasional, particularly in patients with bone metastasis.
Toxicity.
1. *Myelosuppression and other hematologic effects*. None.
2. *Nausea, vomiting, and other gastrointestinal effects*. Rare.
3. *Mucocutaneous effects*. Mild alopecia or skin rash is uncommon.
4. *Miscellaneous effects*.
   a. Mild fluid retention is occasional to common.
   b. Mild liver function abnormalities is occasional; intrahepatic cholestasis may occur.
   c. Menstrual irregularities are common.
   d. Increased appetite and weight gain are common.

RALOXIFENE

Other name.   Evista.
Mechanism of action.   A selective estrogen receptor modulator that inhibits estrogen effects by competing with estrogen for binding on the cytosol estrogen receptor protein in normal and cancer cells. The receptor–hormone complex ultimately controls the promoter region of genes that affect cell growth. Effects may manifest as estrogen agonistic (bone) or antagonistic (breast and uterus), depending on the tissue and other modifying factors.
Primary indications.
1. Prevention of osteoporosis in postmenopausal women.
2. Prevention of invasive breast cancer in postmenopausal women at increased risk. (No apparent decrease in ductal or lobular *in situ* carcinomas.)
Usual dosage and schedule.   60 mg PO daily.
Special precautions.   Contraindicated in women with active or past history of venous thromboembolic events, including deep vein thrombosis, pulmonary embolism, and retinal vein thrombosis. May cause fetal harm if administered to a pregnant woman.
Toxicity.
1. *Myelosuppression and other hematologic effects*. Uncommon and mild.
2. *Nausea, vomiting, and other gastrointestinal effects*. Uncommon.

3. *Mucocutaneous effects*. Rash, sweating, and vaginitis are uncommon.
4. *Miscellaneous effects*.
    a. Thromboembolic events, including deep vein thrombosis, pulmonary embolism, and retinal vein thrombosis, are rare. Lower risk than with tamoxifen.
    b. Leg cramps are uncommon to occasional.
    c. Hot flashes are common.
    d. Lowers total cholesterol and low-density lipoprotein cholesterol.
5. *Carcinogenesis*. Risk for endometrial carcinoma is rare (0.5%) and lower than with tamoxifen (0.75%).

RALTITREXED

Other name. Tomudex.
Mechanism of action. Raltitrexed is a quinazoline antifolate that is a direct specific inhibitor of thymidylate synthase, which thereby blocks the conversion of uridylate to thymidylate and consequent DNA synthesis.
Primary indication. Advanced colorectal carcinoma in patients in whom fluorouracil regimens are not tolerated or are inappropriate.
Usual dosage and schedule. 3 mg/m^2 IV over 15 min every 3 weeks.
Special precautions. Dose must be reduced for renal insufficiency. For creatinine clearance of 55 to 65 mL/min, give 75% dose; for 25 to 54 mL/min, give 50% dose; for <25 mL/min, give no raltitrexed.
Toxicity.
1. *Myelosuppression and other hematologic effects*. Common, but severe or worse less than 5% of the time.
2. *Nausea, vomiting, and other gastrointestinal effects*.
    a. Nausea, vomiting, and diarrhea are common and occasionally severe.
    b. Asymptomatic increases in hepatic transaminases are occasional.
    c. Abdominal pain is common.
3. *Mucocutaneous effects*. Mucositis is occasional and rarely severe. Skin rash is occasional
4. *Miscellaneous effects*.
    a. Asthenia and fever are common, but usually mild to moderate, although a more severe flu-like syndrome is occasional.
    b. Weight loss and dehydration are occasional.
    c. Arthralgia is uncommon.
    d. Headache is occasional.

RITUXIMAB

Other name. Rituxan.
Mechanism of action. Rituximab is a genetically engineered chimeric (murine and human) monoclonal antibody directed against the CD20 antigen found on the surface of normal cells and in high copy number on malignant B lymphocytes (but not stem cells). The F$_{ab}$ domain of rituximab binds to the CD20 antigen on B lymphocytes and B-cell non–Hodgkin's lymphomas,

and the F_c domain recruits immune effector functions to mediate B-cell lysis.

Primary indications.
1. Non–Hodgkin's B-cell lymphoma that is low grade or follicular, CD20 positive, as a single agent or in combination or sequence with cytotoxic chemotherapy.
2. Non–Hodgkin's lymphoma, diffuse large B-cell, CD20 positive, in combination or sequence with cytotoxic chemotherapy.
3. Other B-cell non–Hodgkin's lymphomas.
4. Chronic lymphocytic leukemia, usually in combination or sequence with cytotoxic chemotherapy.

Usual dosage and schedule. 375 mg/m^2 given as a slow IV infusion, initially at a rate of 50 mg/h. If hypersensitivity or other infusion-related events do not occur, escalate in 50-mg/h increments to a maximum of 400 mg/h. Usually takes 4 to 6 h to infuse initial therapy. Interrupt or slow down the infusion rate for infusion-related events. As a single agent, often given once weekly for four to eight doses; in combination with cytotoxic chemotherapy, often given on day 1 or 2 of each cycle of chemotherapy. Premedication with acetaminophen and diphenhydramine may attenuate infusion-related symptoms. Corticosteroids should not be used for premedication.

Special precautions.
1. An infusion-related set of symptoms consisting of fever and chills, with or without true rigors, occurs commonly during the first infusion. Other hypersensitivity symptoms including nausea, urticaria, fatigue, headache, pruritus, bronchospasm, dyspnea, sensation of swelling in tongue or throat, rhinitis, vomiting, hypotension, flushing, and pain at disease sites may also be seen. Rarely infusion-related events result in a fatal outcome. Fatal reactions have followed a symptom complex that includes hypoxia, pulmonary infiltrates, acute respiratory distress syndrome, myocardial infarction, ventricular fibrillation, and cardiogenic shock. Hypersensitivity reactions generally start within 30 to 120 min of starting the infusion. Most will resolve with slowing down or interruption of the infusion and with supportive care, including IV saline, diphenhydramine, and acetaminophen. Severe reactions will additionally require aggressive cardiorespiratory support including oxygen, epinephrine, vasopressors, corticosteroids, and bronchodilators and may preclude additional treatment with rituximab. The rate of infusion events decreases from 80% during the first infusion to 40% during subsequent infusions.
2. Abdominal pain, bowel obstruction, and perforation have been seen in patients receiving rituximab in combination with chemotherapy.
3. Hepatitis B reactivation with related fulminant hepatitis and other viral infections has been reported.

Toxicity.
1. *Myelosuppression and other hematologic effects.* Uncommon. However, B-cell depletion occurs in 70% to 80% of patients, with decreased immunoglobulins in a minority of patients. Infectious events occur in approximately 30% of patients treated with rituximab, but only uncommonly are they severe.

2. *Nausea, vomiting, and other gastrointestinal effects.* Nausea is common (23%) but rarely severe. Vomiting and diarrhea are occasional. Bowel obstruction and perforation are rare.
3. *Mucocutaneous effects.* Pruritus, rash, urticaria, and night sweats are occasional. Severe mucocutaneous reactions including Stevens–Johnson syndrome, lichenoid dermatitis, vesiculobullous dermatitis, and toxic epidermal necrolysis are rare but have been reported from 1 to 13 weeks following rituximab exposure.
4. *Miscellaneous effects.*
   a. Infusion-related hypersensitivity reaction (may include fever, chills, headache, myalgia, weakness, nausea, urticaria, pruritus, throat irritation, rhinitis, dizziness, and hypertension) is common but usually resolves with interrupting or slowing the rate of the infusion and administration of supportive therapy; see Special precautions in the preceding text.
   b. Myalgia and arthralgia are occasional. Rarely, a serum sickness–like reaction may be seen that requires corticosteroid therapy.
   c. Hypotension is occasional but rarely severe. Chest pain, bronchospasm, tachycardia, increased cough, edema, and postural hypotension are uncommon. Severe though potentially fatal cardiac events, including angioedema, arrhythmia, and angina are rare.
   d. Renal failure, possibly requiring dialysis, has been seen, particularly in association with tumor lysis syndrome in patients with high tumor cell burden. May also be seen if used in combination with cisplatin.
   e. Hepatitis B reactivation with related fulminant hepatitis is rare.
   f. Dizziness and anxiety are occasional.
   g. Progressive multifocal leukoencephalopathy is rare.

SARGRAMOSTIM

Other names.   Granulocyte macrophage colony–stimulating factor, GM-CSF, Leukine.

Mechanism of action.   Promotes growth and differentiation of myeloid progenitor cells. May improve survival and function of granulocytes, eosinophils, monocytes, and macrophages. Induces release of secondary cytokines (IL-1 and tumor necrosis factor).

Primary indications.
1. Myeloid reconstitution after peripheral blood or bone marrow progenitor cell transplantation.
2. Neutrophil recovery following chemotherapy in acute myelogenous leukemia.
3. Mobilization of peripheral blood progenitor cells (PBPC).
4. Granulocytopenia from primary marrow disorders, such as myelodysplastic syndrome or aplastic anemia.
5. Granulocytopenia associated with AIDS and its therapy.

Usual dosage and schedule.
1. *Myeloid reconstitution after autologous stem cell transplantation.* 250 μg/m^2 IV daily as a 2-h infusion beginning 2 to 4 h after the autologous stem cell infusion and not less than 24 h after the last dose of chemotherapy or less than 12 h after the

last dose of radiotherapy. Continue for 21 days or until the absolute neutrophil count reaches 20,000/μL.

2. *Bone marrow transplantation failure or engraftment delay.* 250 μg/m² daily for 14 days as a 2-h IV infusion. If there is no marrow recovery, may be repeated in 7 days at same or higher dose (500 μg/m²). Dose and duration are dependent on the response.

3. *Mobilization of PBPC.* The recommended dose is 250 μg/m²/day administered IV over 24 h or SC once daily. Dosing should continue at the same dose through the period of PBPC collection.

4. *Neutrophil recovery following chemotherapy in acute myelogenous leukemia.* 250 μ/m²/day administered intravenously over a 4-h period starting 4 days following the completion of induction chemotherapy and continuing until the ANC is more than 1,500 cells/μL for 3 consecutive days or a maximum of 42 days.

5. *Aplastic anemia, myelodysplastic syndrome, and AIDS.* Doses may be much lower (50–100 μg/m² SQ or IM daily).

Special precautions. Flushing, tachycardia, dyspnea, and nausea occur commonly with the first dose of IV therapy; do not infuse over less than 2 h; longer infusion may help.

Toxicity.

1. *Myelosuppression and other hematologic effects.* None (leukocytosis).

2. *Nausea, vomiting, and other gastrointestinal effects.* Occasional.

3. *Mucocutaneous effects.* Rash is uncommon; exacerbation of preexisting dermatologic conditions is occasional; mild local reactions at injection site is common.

4. *Miscellaneous effects.* Usually mild and short lived at standard doses, but with increasing dose, may be more severe.
   a. Bone pain, musculoskeletal symptoms such as cramps, and back or leg pain are common.
   b. Pericarditis, fluid retention, and venous thrombosis are dose related and uncommon at standard doses.
   c. Flu-like symptoms (fever, chills, aches, headache) are occasional at standard doses, but common at higher doses.

SORAFENIB

Other names. Nexavar.

Mechanism of action. Inhibition of multiple tyrosine kinases and serine/threonine kinases within tumor cells and tumor vasculature resulting in decreased tumor cell proliferation and reduction of tumor angiogenesis.

Primary indication. Renal cell carcinoma.

Usual dosage and schedule. 400 mg PO twice daily either without food or with a moderate fat meal.

Special precautions. Increased risk of bleeding compared with placebo. In patients also taking warfarin, sorafenib may increase the prothrombin time and INR, resulting in increased risk of bleeding.

Toxicity.

1. *Myelosuppression and other hematologic effects.* Lymphopenia is common; anemia, neutropenia, and thrombocytopenia

are occasional; various bleeding events (including epistaxis, gastrointestinal hemorrhage, respiratory tract hemorrhage, hematomas) are common but only rarely life threatening.

2. *Nausea, vomiting, and other gastrointestinal effects.* Diarrhea is common (33%); nausea and vomiting are occasional to common (10%–20%); anorexia and constipation are occasional. Increased amylase and lipase are common and transient increases in transaminases are occasional. Clinical pancreatitis is uncommon.

3. *Mucocutaneous effects.* Hand–foot skin reaction is common (30%). Alopecia is common (27%). Pruritus is occasional to common (19%). Other skin changes are rare to uncommon.

4. *Miscellaneous effects.*
   a. Hypertension, usually mild to moderate, is occasional. Hypertensive crisis is rare.
   b. Fatigue is common.
   c. Sensory neuropathy is occasional (13%).
   d. Hypophosphatemia is common (45%) (unknown etiology).

STREPTOZOCIN

Other names. Streptozotocin, Zanosar.

Mechanism of action. Inhibition of DNA synthesis, possibly by interference with pyridine nucleotide synthesis. Streptozocin appears to have some specificity for neoplastic pancreatic endocrine cells. Glucose moiety attached to nitrosourea appears to diminish myelotoxicity.

Primary indications.

1. Pancreatic islet cell and pancreatic exocrine carcinomas.
2. Carcinoid tumors.

Usual dosage and schedule.

1. 1.0 to 1.5 g/m^2 IV weekly for 6 weeks followed by 4 weeks of observation.
2. 1.0 g/m^2 IV on days 1 and 8 in combination with fluorouracil and mitomycin. Repeat every 4 weeks.
3. 500 mg/m^2 IV on days 1 to 5 every 6 weeks.

Special precautions.

1. A 30- to 60-min infusion is recommended to reduce local pain and burning around the vein during treatment.
2. Avoid extravasation.
3. Have 50% glucose available to treat sudden hypoglycemia.

Toxicity.

1. *Myelosuppression and other hematologic effects.* Uncommon and mild.
2. *Nausea, vomiting, and other gastrointestinal effects.* Nausea and vomiting are common and severe. May become progressively worse over a 5-day course of therapy.
3. *Mucocutaneous effects.* Uncommon.
4. *Nephrotoxicity.* Renal toxicity is common. Although it is not clearly dose related, it may limit continued drug use in individual patients. Proteinuria, glucosuria, azotemia, and hypophosphatemia, if persistent or severe, are indications to discontinue therapy. Hydration may ameliorate the problem.
5. *Miscellaneous effects.*

   a. Hypoglycemia: in patients with insulinoma, hypoglycemia may be severe (although transient) owing to a burst of insulin release.

   b. Hyperglycemia is uncommon in healthy persons or diabetic patients, as normal β cells are usually insensitive to streptozocin's effect.

   c. Transient mild hepatotoxicity is occasional.

   d. Second malignancies are possible.

SUNITINIB

Other names. Sutent, Sunitinib malate.

Mechanism of action. Inhibition of multiple RTKs, including PDGF-Rs, VEGF receptors, and several forms of the mutation-activated stem cell factor receptor (Kit) with consequent inhibition of tumor cells expressing dysregulated target RTKs and tumor angiogenesis. Metabolized primarily by the cytochrome P-450 enzyme allele, CYP3A4.

Primary indications.

1. GIST that has shown progression during prior treatment with imatinib or in patients who are intolerant to imatinib.
2. Renal cell carcinoma.

Usual dosage and schedule. 50 mg PO daily for 4 weeks followed by a 2-week rest, with incremental dose reductions or increase (12.5 mg/day) based on tolerability.

Special precautions. Dose reduction should be considered when administered concurrently with strong CYP3A4 inhibitors. Dose increase should be considered when administered concurrently with strong CYP3A4 inducers.

Toxicity.

1. *Myelosuppression and other hematologic effects.* Myelosuppression and lymphopenia are common, but it is uncommon to rare for them to be of high grade (3 or 4). Bleeding is occasional, with possible tumor-related hemorrhage. Venous thromboembolic events are uncommon.
2. *Nausea, vomiting, and other gastrointestinal effects.* Diarrhea, nausea, vomiting, dyspepsia, anorexia, and abdominal pain are common. Rare fatal gastrointestinal complications, including perforation, have been seen. Hepatic and pancreatic enzyme elevations and other liver function abnormalities are occasional to common.
3. *Mucocutaneous effects.* Stomatitis and altered taste are common. Skin discoloration is common. Rash and hand-foot syndrome are occasional. Alopecia is uncommon.
4. *Miscellaneous effects.*

   a. Congestive heart failure with decrease in left ventricular ejection fraction to below the lower limit of normal is occasional.

   b. Hypertension is common, but severe hypertension is uncommon.

   c. Adrenal insufficiency is possible, based on animal studies.

   d. Fatigue is common. Asthenia, headache, arthralgia, myalgia, oral pain, and back pain are occasional.

   e. Cough and dyspnea are occasional.

f. Renal function abnormalities (low grade) are occasional. Hypo- and hyperkalemia, hypo- and hypernatremia, and hypophosphatemia are occasional.
g. Hypothyroidism is uncommon.
h. Edema is occasional.

TAMOXIFEN

Other name. Nolvadex.

Mechanism of action. Tamoxifen is a selective estrogen receptor modulator that inhibits estrogen effects by competing with estrogen for binding on the cytosol estrogen receptor protein in cancer cells. This complex is probably transported into the nucleus, where it affects nucleic acid function. It also has effects on cellular growth factors, epidermal growth factors, and TGF-α and TGF-β.

Primary indications.

1. Breast carcinoma.
   a. Metastatic tumors in postmenopausal or premenopausal women with estrogen receptor–positive (or unknown) tumors.
   b. Adjuvant therapy in women with estrogen receptor–positive (or progesterone—receptor–positive) tumors after primary therapy. Optimal duration of therapy for most women is probably limited to 5 years.
   c. Breast cancer prevention in very high–risk women.
2. Melanoma, in combination with other drugs (controversial).

Usual dosage and schedule. 20 mg PO as single daily dose.

Special precautions. Hypercalcemia may be seen during initial therapy.

Toxicity.

1. *Myelosuppression and other hematologic effects.* Uncommon and mild.
2. *Nausea, vomiting, and other gastrointestinal effects.* Nausea occurs early in the course of therapy in up to 20% of patients but abates rapidly as therapy is continued. Diarrhea is occasional.
3. *Mucocutaneous effects.* Cataracts and other eye toxicities have been observed, but effects due to drug are uncommon. Skin rash and pruritus vulvae are uncommon. May cause increase or marked decrease in vaginal secretions and result in difficult or painful intercourse.
4. *Miscellaneous effects.*
   a. Hot flashes are common.
   b. Vaginal bleeding and menstrual irregularity are uncommon to occasional.
   c. Lassitude, headache, leg cramps, and dizziness are uncommon.
   d. Peripheral edema is occasional.
   e. Increased bone pain, tumor pain, and local disease flare (associated both with good tumor response as well as with tumor progression) are occasional.
   f. Slowed progression of osteoporosis.
   g. Reduction in serum cholesterol with favorable changes in lipid profile.
   h. Thromboembolic phenomena are rare.
   i. Liver function test abnormalities are occasional.

5. *Carcinogenesis.* Uterine carcinomas are rare (two to four times the predicted incidence in adjuvant trials).

TEMOZOLOMIDE

Other name. Temodar.

Mechanism of action. Undergoes rapid conversion to the reactive substituted imidazole carboxamide, MTIC. This compound is believed to be active primarily through alkylation (methylation) of DNA at the O^6 and N^7 positions of guanine.

Primary indication.

1. Glioblastoma, concurrently with radiotherapy and as maintenance after radiotherapy.
2. Anaplastic astrocytoma that is refractory to nitrosoureas.
3. Melanoma.
4. Metastatic carcinomas to the brain.

Usual dosage and schedule.

1. 150 to 200 mg/m² PO on an empty stomach daily for 5 days every 28 days.
2. 75 mg/m² PO on an empty stomach daily during radiation therapy for up to 7 weeks.

Special precautions. Contraindicated in patients with a hypersensitivity to dacarbazine (DTIC), because both drugs are metabolized to MTIC. Preventive treatment for pneumocystis jiroveci pneumonia (PCP) is required when temozolomide is administered with radiotherapy.

Toxicity.

1. *Myelosuppression and other hematologic effects.* Myelosuppression with anemia, thrombocytopenia, and neutropenia, is common and dose dependent, but only occasionally is it severe.
2. *Nausea, vomiting, and other gastrointestinal effects.* Nausea and constipation are occasional to common, but usually not severe. Vomiting is occasional as is anorexia. Abdominal pain is uncommon.
3. *Mucocutaneous effects.* Rash and pruritus are occasional. Alopecia is common.
4. *Miscellaneous effects.*
   a. Headache, fatigue, asthenia, and fever are common (20–65%).
   b. Peripheral edema is occasional.
   c. Neurologic symptoms are common on temozolomide, but it is difficult to distinguish whether the symptoms are from the drug or the disease. Common findings are convulsions, hemiparesis, dizziness, abnormal coordination, amnesia, or insomnia. Occasional findings are paresthesias, somnolence, paresis, incontinence, ataxia, dysphasia, gait abnormality, myalgias, and confusion. Diplopia or other visual abnormalities are occasional.
   d. Anxiety and depression are occasional.

TEMSIROLIMUS

Other names. TEMSR, CCI-779.

Mechanism of action. After temsirolimus complexes with the immunophilin FKBP12, the complex inhibits mTOR (mammalian target of rapamycin) kinase activity. mTOR, as a master regulator of cell physiology, is involved in regulation of cell growth and angiogenesis, and changes that are induced downstream from mTOR as a consequence of the temsirolimus inhibition lead to cell cycle arrest at the G_1 phase.

Primary indications. Renal cell carcinoma.

Usual dosage and schedule. 25 mg IV weekly.

Toxicity.

1. *Myelosuppression and other hematologic effects.* Anemia and thrombocytopenia are common.
2. *Nausea, vomiting, and other gastrointestinal effects.* Anorexia, nausea, and vomiting are common. Diarrhea is common.
3. *Mucocutaneous effects.* Mucositis is common. Maculopapular rash or acne are common. Nail disorders are common.
4. Immune effects and infusion reactions.
5. *Miscellaneous effects.*
   a. Asthenia is common.
   b. Hyperglycemia is common and occasionally severe.
   c. Hypophosphatemia is occasional and may be severe.
   d. Hypertriglyceridemia is common and may be severe.
   e. Dyspnea is occasional.
   f. Taste perversion is common.

TENIPOSIDE

Other names. VM-26, Vumon.

Mechanism of action. Topoisomerase II–mediated double-strand DNA breaks. Causes cell cycle transit delay through S phase and arrest at late S/G_2.

Primary indications.

1. Acute lymphocytic leukemia.
2. Neuroblastoma.
3. Non–Hodgkin's lymphomas.

Usual dosage and schedule.

1. 165 mg/m² IV over 30 to 60 min twice weekly for eight to nine doses (with cytarabine).
2. 250 mg/m² IV over 30 to 60 min weekly for 4 to 8 weeks (with vincristine and prednisone).

Special precautions.

1. Hypersensitivity reactions usually resolve with interruption of the infusion and often can be prevented with diphenhydramine and hydrocortisone pretreatment. Hypotension is alleviated by prolonging the infusion time. It is a possible vesicant.
2. See package insert for IV preparation and administration equipment requirements.

Toxicity.

1. *Myelosuppression and other hematologic effects.* Common and dose limiting.
2. *Nausea, vomiting, and other gastrointestinal effects.* Nausea, vomiting, and diarrhea are common.
3. *Mucocutaneous effects.* Alopecia and mucositis are common.
4. *Miscellaneous effects.*
   a. Hepatic and renal dysfunction are rare.
   b. Hypersensitivity reactions with urticaria and flushing are occasional. Anaphylaxis is uncommon.
   c. Hypotension is related to drug infusion rate but should be seen only occasionally at the recommended dose schedules.
   d. Secondary leukemias are uncommon.
   e. Chemical phlebitis is uncommon.

THALIDOMIDE

Other name.   Thalomid.

Mechanism of action.   Multiple potential mechanisms, including inhibition of VEGF, inhibition of TNF-α, direct inhibition of G1 growth and promotion of apoptosis, expansion of NK cells, and costimulation of T cells.

Primary indications.
1. Multiple myeloma.
2. Myelodysplastic syndrome.

Usual dosage and schedule.   A starting dose of 50 to 100 mg once daily in the evening. The dose is escalated weekly by 50 to 100 mg until the maximum dose specified, commonly 400 mg daily.

Special precautions.   Severe and life-threatening birth defects, primarily phocomelia, can be caused by taking even a single 50-mg dose. For this reason, special precautions must be taken to ensure that female patients are not pregnant when the drug is started, and that both female and male patients practice strict birth control measures. Deep venous thrombosis is enhanced by corticosteroids.

Toxicity.
1. *Myelosuppression and other hematologic effects.* None to minimal myelosuppression. Occasional deep venous thrombosis.
2. *Nausea, vomiting, and other gastrointestinal effects.* Constipation is common.
3. *Mucocutaneous effects.* Macular rash, usually involving trunk, is common. Alopecia is uncommon. Rare severe or life-threatening epidermal damage.
4. *Miscellaneous effects.*
   a. Dose-dependent somnolence and dizziness are common. Tolerance usually develops to the sedative effects. Dizziness may be related to hypotension and can be minimized by adequate hydration and avoidance of rapid postural changes.
   b. Peripheral neuropathy is common (25%) with chronic therapy. Occasional patients develop myalgia, tremor, or muscle spasms.
   c. Fatigue is common.
   d. Headache is occasional.
   e. Edema is occasional to common.
   f. Hypothyroidism is occasional.
   g. Birth defects. (see Special precautions in the preceding text.)
   h. Hypercoagulability with deep venous thrombosis is occasional.

THIOTEPA

Other name.   Triethylenethiophosphoramide, Thioplex.

Mechanism of action.   Alkylating agent similar to mechlorethamine.

Primary indications.
1. Superficial papillary carcinoma of urinary bladder.
2. Malignant peritoneal, pleural, or pericardial effusions.
3. Neoplastic meningeal infiltrates.

Usual dosage and schedule.
1. 12 mg/m^2 IV bolus every 3 weeks in combination with vinblastine and doxorubicin for breast cancer.

2. 30 to 60 mg in 40 to 50 mL water instilled into the bladder and retained for 1 h. Dose is repeated weekly for 3 to 6 weeks, then every 3 weeks for 5 cycles.
3. 25 to 30 mg/m^2 in 50 to 100 mL saline solution as a single intracavitary injection. Dose may be repeated as tolerated, monitoring through blood counts.
4. 10 to 15 mg intrathecally.
5. High-dose therapy using 500 to 1,000 mg/m^2 over 3 days has been used followed by stem cell rescue (e.g., bone marrow transplantation).

Special precaution.   Dose should be reduced in patients with impaired renal function, as the drug is primarily excreted in the urine.

Toxicity.
1. *Myelosuppression and other hematologic effects.* Dose limiting. Pancytopenia and sepsis may follow intravesical or intracavitary administration. Nadir counts are reached in 1 to 2 weeks; recovery by 4 weeks is usual.
2. *Nausea, vomiting, and other gastrointestinal effects.* Uncommon.
3. *Mucocutaneous effects.* Uncommon. Thiotepa is *not* a vesicant. Hyperpigmentation of skin occurs at high doses.
4. *Miscellaneous effects.*
   a. Local pain, dizziness, headache, and fever are uncommon.
   b. Secondary neoplasms are possible.
   c. Amenorrhea and azoospermia are common.
   d. CNS effects with high-dose therapy.

TOPOTECAN

Other name.   Hycamtin.

Mechanism of action.   Topotecan, a semisynthetic derivative of CPT, is a potent inhibitor of topoisomerase I, an enzyme essential for effective replication and transcription. It binds to the topoisomerase I–DNA cleavable complex, preventing religation after cleavage by topoisomerase I.

Primary indications.
1. Ovarian carcinoma.
2. Carcinoma of the cervix.
3. Small cell and non–small cell carcinoma of the lung.

Usual dosage and schedule.
1. As a single agent, 1.5 mg/m^2 IV as a 30-min infusion daily, five times every 3 weeks.
2. In combination with cisplatin, 0.75 mg/m^2 IV as a 30-min infusion daily, three times every 3 weeks.

Special precautions.   None.

Toxicity.
1. *Myelosuppression and other hematologic effects.* Leukopenia is universal and dose limiting. Anemia and thrombocytopenia are common and occasionally severe. Febrile neutropenia is occasional to common.
2. *Nausea, vomiting, and other gastrointestinal effects.* Nausea and vomiting and diarrhea are common, but usually mild. Other gastrointestinal symptoms, including constipation and abdominal pain, occur occasionally.

3. *Mucocutaneous effects.* Alopecia is common; stomatitis is occasional but usually mild; skin rash is rare.
4. *Miscellaneous effects.*
   a. Fever, headache, fatigue, and weakness are common (15% to 25%) but rarely severe.
   b. Microscopic hematuria is occasional.
   c. Dyspnea occurs occasionally, but it is uncommon for it to be severe.
   d. Infection as a consequence of severe leukopenia is common.

TOREMIFENE

Other name. Fareston.

Mechanism of action. A selective estrogen receptor modulator that inhibits estrogen effects by competing with estrogen for binding on the cytosol estrogen receptor protein in cancer cells. The receptor–hormone complex ultimately controls the promoter region of genes that affect cell growth.

Primary indication. Metastatic carcinoma of the breast in postmenopausal women with estrogen receptor—positive (or unknown) tumors.

Usual dosage and schedule. 60 mg PO daily.

Special precautions. Uncertain whether it has any carcinogenic effect on endometrium as has been observed with tamoxifen. May result in increased prothrombin time in patients taking warfarin (Coumadin). Cytochrome P-450 3A4 enzyme inhibitors, such as phenobarbital, phenytoin, and carbamazepine increase the rate of toremifene metabolism, lowering the concentration in the serum.

Toxicity.
1. *Myelosuppression and other hematologic effects.* Uncommon and mild.
2. *Nausea, vomiting, and other gastrointestinal effects.* Minimal nausea is common early in treatment; vomiting is occasional.
3. *Mucocutaneous effects.* Dry eyes and cataracts are rare. May cause an increase or decrease in vaginal secretions, which may result in difficult or painful intercourse.
4. *Miscellaneous effects.*
   a. Hot flashes are common.
   b. Sweating is occasional.
   c. Vaginal bleeding and menstrual irregularity are occasional.
   d. Hypercalcemia is uncommon.
   e. Thromboembolic phenomena are rare.

^{131}I-TOSITUMOMAB

Other name. Bexxar.

Mechanism of action. ^{131}I-Tositumomab is a murine Ig-2a monoclonal anti-CD20 antibody radiolabeled with iodine-131 (^{131}I), an emitter of both β and γ radiation. The mechanism of action includes antibody-mediated cytotoxicity and cellularly targeted radiotherapy (radioimmunotherapy [RIT].)

Primary indications.
1. Non–Hodgkin's lymphoma, chemotherapy refractory, CD-20 positive, low grade or transformed low grade.

2. Non–Hodgkin's lymphoma, follicular, as initial treatment (investigational).

Usual dosage and schedule.

1. Before dosimetric and therapeutic doses, patients are premedicated with acetaminophen, 650 mg and diphenhydramine, 50 mg. A saturated solution of potassium iodide, two to three drops orally three times daily, is given, beginning 24 h before the dosimetric dose and continuing for 14 days after the therapeutic dose to prevent uptake of ^{131}I by the thyroid.

2. *Dosimetric dose.* 450 mg of unlabeled tositumomab is given as a 1-h infusion followed by a 20-min infusion of 5 mCi (35 mg) of ^{131}I tositumomab to determine the patient-specific activity (mCi) of radiolabeled tositumomab to deliver a therapeutic dose of 65 to 75 cGy 7 to 15 days later.

3. *Therapeutic dose.* 450 mg of unlabeled tositumomab is given as a 1-h infusion followed by a 20-min infusion of patient-specific (in mCi) activity labeled to 35 mg of tositumomab. (Median 90 mCi, range ∼50–200 mCi.)

Special precautions. Use with caution in patients with more than 25% marrow involvement with lymphoma, prior external beam radiotherapy to more than 25% of the bone marrow, or a history of HAMA or HACA. A saturated solution of potassium iodide, two to three drops orally three times daily, is given beginning 24 h before the dosimetric dose and continuing for 14 days after the therapeutic dose to prevent uptake of ^{131}I by the thyroid.

Toxicity.

1. *Myelosuppression and other hematologic effects.* Myelosuppression is universal, with approximately 35% to 65% of patients having grade 3 or 4 thrombocytopenia or neutropenia. These nadir counts occur at a median of 4 to 7 weeks, last for 3 weeks, with recovery to baseline by 10 to 12 weeks after drug administration. Febrile neutropenia is common in previously treated patients, but not when used as initial therapy.

2. *Nausea, vomiting, and other gastrointestinal effects.* Nausea is common; vomiting, abdominal pain, and anorexia are occasional.

3. *Mucocutaneous effects.* Pruritus, rash, and sweating are occasional.

4. *Miscellaneous effects.*

   a. *Immunologic.* HAMA or HACA is common, and associated with influenza-like syndrome. Hypersensitivity reactions are occasional and may range from mild allergic reactions or injection site reactions to anaphylaxis and serum sickness.

   b. Infusion-related fever, chills, dizziness, asthenia, wheezing or coughing, nasal congestion, headache, back pain, arthralgia, and hypotension are common, more with dosimetric dose than with therapeutic dose. Most commonly, these are self-limited and mild to moderate in severity.

   c. Fatigue or asthenia is common.

   d. *Cardiorespiratory.* Cough, dyspnea, and edema are occasional; hypotension and vasodilatation are uncommon.

   e. Thyroid suppression is occasional despite prophylaxis with potassium iodide.

   f. Myelodysplasia and secondary leukemia are uncommon.

TRASTUZUMAB

Other names. Humanized anti-Her2 antibody, Herceptin.

Mechanism of action. A recombinant humanized monoclonal antibody that targets the extracellular domain of the human EGFR protein, Her2 (p185^{Her2}).

Primary indications.
1. Carcinoma of the breast that has overexpression of Her2/neu (c-erbB-2), either in advanced disease or as adjuvant therapy.
2. Other carcinomas that exhibit overexpression of Her2.
3. Usual dosage and schedule. 4 mg/kg IV loading dose over 90 min, then 2 mg/kg IV over 30 min weekly.

Special precautions.
1. During the first infusion, and occasionally during later infusions, a systemic symptom complex similar to that seen with other human monoclonal antibodies is common. Severe hypersensitivity reactions, and pulmonary adverse events have been reported, but are uncommon to rare. These events include anaphylaxis, angioedema, bronchospasm, hypotension, hypoxia, dyspnea, pulmonary infiltrates, pleural effusions, noncardiogenic pulmonary edema, and acute respiratory distress syndrome. A more common symptom complex consists of mild-to-moderate chills, fever, asthenia, pain, nausea, vomiting, and headache. These latter symptoms are generally well managed by temporary slowing or interruption of the infusion and administration of acetaminophen, diphenhydramine, and meperidine.
2. Cardiac dysfunction (cardiac symptoms or an asymptomatic decrease in ejection fraction of 10% or greater) occurs in approximately 7% of patients treated with trastuzumab alone but in 28% of patients treated with trastuzumab plus anthracycline and in 11% of patients treated with trastuzumab plus paclitaxel. In most cases, this improves with symptomatic therapy. Severe disability or death from cardiac dysfunction occurs in approximately 1% of patients. Extreme caution should be exercised in treating patients with preexisting cardiac dysfunction.

Toxicity.
1. *Myelosuppression.* Uncommon.
2. *Nausea, vomiting, and other gastrointestinal effects.* Nausea and vomiting are common with the first infusion. Diarrhea is also common.
3. *Mucocutaneous effects.* A rash is occasional to common, and may be associated with urticaria or pruritus.
4. *Miscellaneous effects.*
   a. Mild-to-moderate chills, fever, asthenia, pain, and headache are common, primarily during the first infusion.
   b. Cardiac dysfunction occurs in approximately 7% of patients treated with trastuzumab alone, but in 28% of patients treated with trastuzumab plus anthracycline and in 11% of patients treated with trastuzumab plus paclitaxel. In most cases, this improves with symptomatic therapy.
   c. Chest pain, back pain, dyspnea, and cough are occasional to common.
   d. Peripheral edema is occasional.

TRETINOIN

Other names. All-*trans*-retinoic acid, t-RNA, ATRA, Vesanoid, Retin-A.

Mechanism of action. Binds to cytoplasmic retinoic acid–binding proteins and is then transported to the nucleus where it interacts with nuclear RARs. These then affect expression of the genes that control cell growth and differentiation. In acute promyelocytic leukemia, which characteristically has a chromosomal translocation, t(15:17), abnormal messenger ribonucleic acid (mRNA) transcripts are seen for RAR-α, the gene for which is on chromosome 17.

Primary indication. Acute promyelocytic leukemia for induction of remission.

Usual dosage and schedule. 45 mg/m^2 PO daily (divided into 2 doses at least 6 h apart in the morning and 6 h later) until 30 days after complete remission is documented, up to a maximum of 90 days. Therapy is usually initiated concurrently with anthracycline.

Special precautions. Avoid use in pregnant women because of marked teratogenic potential. Advise patient to avoid pregnancy by using two reliable contraceptive methods simultaneously. Retinoic acid acute promyelocytic (RA-APL) syndrome (see following text) may require mechanical ventilation and dexamethasone 10 mg every 12 h at the first signs of fever with respiratory distress until resolution of the acute symptoms (often several days). Continuation of retinoid therapy is controversial.

Toxicity.

1. *Myelosuppression and other hematologic effects.* Myelosuppression is rare. Forty percent of patients develop leukocytosis, which increases the risk of RA-APL syndrome. Disseminated intravascular coagulation is common (26%).
2. *Nausea, vomiting, and other gastrointestinal effects.* Nausea and vomiting, abdominal pain, diarrhea, anorexia, and constipation are common, but usually not severe. Gastrointestinal hemorrhage is occasional to common and may be severe. Inflammatory bowel disease is rare.
3. *Mucocutaneous effects.* Universal, particularly at doses at higher end of range. They include redness, dryness, and pruritus of the skin and mucous membranes; increased sweating; possible vesicle formation; peeling of the skin of the palms and soles; cheilitis; and conjunctivitis. There may also be increased skin photosensitivity (e.g., to sun) and the nails may become brittle. Alopecia is uncommon.
4. *Retinoic acid syndrome.* High fever, respiratory distress, weight gain, diffuse pulmonary infiltrates, pleural or pericardial effusions with the possibility of impaired myocardial contractility, and hypotension, with or without concomitant leukocytosis, are common in patients with acute promyelocytic leukemia (25%) (see Chapter 19).
5. *Miscellaneous effects.*
   a. *Cardiovascular.* Arrhythmias, flushing, hypotension, hypertension, and phlebitis are occasional. Cardiac failure,

cardiac arrest, pulmonary hypertension, and other more severe cardiovascular problems are uncommon.
   b. Cataracts and corneal ulcerations or opacities are uncommon.
   c. *Musculoskeletal.* Arthralgias, bone pain, muscle aches are occasional to common; skeletal hyperostosis is common at higher doses (80 mg/m²/day).
   d. *Hypertriglyceridemia.* Mild-to-moderate elevations are common; marked elevations (>5 times normal) are uncommon; hypercholesterolemia occurs to a lesser degree.
   e. *Neurologic.* Headache is common; paresthesias, dizziness, and visual disturbances are occasional; lethargy, fatigue, and mental depression are uncommon; pseudotumor cerebri is rare.
   f. Hepatotoxicity with increased LDH, SGOT, SGPT, GGTP, alkaline phosphatase is common.
   g. Hyperhistaminemia with shock is rare.
   h. Renal insufficiency is occasional.
   i. Fever, malaise, shivering, and edema are common.

VALRUBICIN

Other name. Valstar.

Mechanism of action. Valrubicin, a semisynthetic analog of doxorubicin, penetrates into cells where its metabolites inhibit the incorporation of nucleosides into nucleic acids, causes chromosomal damage, and arrests cell cycle in G2. A principal mechanism of valrubicin metabolites is DNA strand breakage mediated by anthracycline effects on topoisomerase II.

Primary indication. Intravesical therapy of BCG-refractory carcinoma *in situ* (CIS) of the urinary bladder in patients for whom immediate cystectomy would be associated with unacceptable morbidity or mortality.

Usual dosage and schedule. 800 mg, diluted in 75 mL of normal saline, intravesically once a week for 6 weeks. Retain in bladder for 2 h before voiding.

Special Precautions. Should not be administered if there is any question about perforation of the bladder or integrity of bladder mucosa.

Toxicity.
1. *Myelosuppression and other hematologic effects.* Uncommon, unless bladder rupture or perforation occurs, in which case severe neutropenia can be expected 2 weeks after administration.
2. *Nausea, vomiting, and other gastrointestinal effects.* Uncommon.
3. *Mucocutaneous effects.* Rash is uncommon.
4. *Miscellaneous effects.*
   a. *Local reactions.* Frequency, dysuria, urgency, bladder spasm, hematuria, and bladder pain are common. Urinary incontinence and cystitis are occasional. Local burning symptoms associated with the procedure, urethral pain, pelvic pain, and gross hematuria are uncommon to rare.

b. *Body as a whole*. Abdominal pain, asthenia, back pain, chest pain, fever, headache, and malaise are uncommon.

VINBLASTINE

Other name. VLB, Velban.

Mechanism of action. Mitotic inhibition with reversible metaphase arrest due to action on microtubular and spindle contractile proteins.

Primary indications.

1. Hodgkin's and non–Hodgkin's lymphomas.
2. Testicular, gestational trophoblastic, kidney, and breast carcinomas.

Usual dosage and schedule.

1. 4 to 18 mg/m^2 IV weekly.
2. 6 mg/m^2 IV on days 1 and 15 in combination with doxorubicin, bleomycin, and dacarbazine for lymphomas.
3. 4.5 mg/m^2 IV on day 1 every 3 weeks, in combination with doxorubicin and thiotepa for breast cancer.

Special precautions. Administer as a slow push, taking care to avoid extravasation.

Toxicity.

1. *Myelosuppression and other hematologic effects*. Dose-related leukopenia occurs with a nadir at 4 to 10 days and recovery in 7 to 10 days. Severe thrombocytopenia is uncommon.
2. *Nausea, vomiting, and other gastrointestinal effects*. Common but not usually severe.
3. *Mucocutaneous effects*.
   a. Extravasation may lead to severe inflammation, pain, and tissue damage. Local infiltration with 1 to 6 mL of hyaluronidase (150 units/mL) may help.
   b. Mild alopecia is common.
   c. Stomatitis is occasionally severe.
4. *Miscellaneous effects*.
   a. Neurotoxicity manifested by (1) constipation, adynamic ileus, and abdominal pain if very high doses are used; or (2) paresthesias, peripheral neuropathy, and jaw pain with lower doses.
      Neurotoxicity is less frequent with vinblastine than with vincristine.
   b. Transient hepatitis is uncommon.
   c. Depression, headache, convulsions, and orthostatic hypotension are rare.

VINCRISTINE

Other names. VCR, Oncovin, Vincasar.

Mechanism of action. Mitotic inhibition with reversible metaphase arrest due to drug action on microtubular and spindle contractile proteins.

Primary indications.

1. Hodgkin's and non–Hodgkin's lymphomas.
2. Acute lymphocytic leukemia.
3. Multiple myeloma.
4. Wilms' tumor, neuroblastoma, rhabdomyosarcoma, and Ewing's sarcoma of childhood.
5. Breast carcinoma.

Usual dosage and schedule.
1. 1 to 2 mg/m^2 (maximum 2.0–2.4 mg) IV weekly.
2. 0.4 mg/day as a continuous IV infusion on days 1 to 4.

Special precautions.
1. Administer as a slow IV push, taking care to avoid extravasation.
2. Because neurotoxicity is cumulative, neurologic evaluation should be done before each dose and therapy withheld if severe paresthesias, motor weakness, or other severe abnormalities occur. Underlying neurologic problems accentuate vincristine's effect.
3. Reduce dose if liver disease is significant.
4. Stool softeners or high-fiber or bulk diets may avert severe constipation.

Toxicity.
1. *Myelosuppression and other hematologic effects.* Mild and rarely of clinical significance.
2. *Nausea, vomiting, and other gastrointestinal effects.* Nausea and vomiting are not seen unless paralytic ileus occurs. Constipation is common.
3. *Mucocutaneous effects.* Severe local inflammation if extravasation occurs. Alopecia is common.
4. *Neurotoxicity.* Is dose dependent and dose limiting. Mild paresthesias and decreased deep tendon reflexes are to be expected. More extensive peripheral neuropathies, severe constipation, or ileus are indications to reduce or hold therapy. Autonomic dysfunction with orthostatic hypotension or urinary retention may be seen.
5. *Miscellaneous effects.*
   a. Uric acid nephropathy due to rapid tumor cell lysis and release of uric acid is always a potential problem when therapy is first given.
   b. Syndrome of inappropriate antidiuretic hormone is rare.
   c. Jaw pain is uncommon.

VINDESINE

Other names. VDS, Eldisine.

Mechanism of action. Mitotic inhibition with reversible metaphase arrest due to action on microtubule and spindle contractile protein.

Primary indications.
1. Lung, breast, and esophageal carcinomas.
2. Hodgkin's and non–Hodgkin's lymphomas.
3. Melanoma.

Usual dosage and schedule.
1. 2 to 4 mg/m^2 IV bolus (over 2–3 min) weekly for induction, then every 2 weeks.
2. 1.5 mg/m^2/day for 5 to 7 days as a continuous infusion.

Special precautions. Take care to avoid extravasation, as the agent is a vesicant.

Toxicity.
1. *Myelosuppression and other hematologic effects.* Leukopenia is common but not usually severe.
2. *Nausea, vomiting, and other gastrointestinal effects.* Occasional and mild.
3. *Mucocutaneous effects.* Alopecia is common. Rash is rare.

4. *Neurotoxicity.* Dose dependent and cumulative, and includes constipation, paralytic ileus, paresthesia, myalgias, and weakness. Severity is intermediate between vincristine and vinblastine. Cranial neuropathy may manifest as jaw pain.
5. *Miscellaneous effects.*
   a. Chills and fever are occasional.
   b. Phlebitis is occasional.
   c. Confusion and lethargy are rare.

VINORELBINE

Other name. Navelbine.
Mechanism of action. Binds to tubulin, and depolymerizes microtubules causing mitotic inhibition, similar to other vinca alkaloids. Lower affinity for axonal microtubules is associated with lower neurotoxicity.
Primary indications.
1. Metastatic carcinoma of the breast.
2. Non–small cell carcinoma of the lung.
Usual dosage and schedule.
1. 30 mg/m^2 IV as 6- to 10-min rapid infusion weekly when used with a single agent or with cisplatin.
2. 20 to 25 mg/m^2 IV as a 6- to 10-min rapid infusion in various schedules, when used with other myelotoxic agents.
Special precautions. Administer infusion through the side arm of a freely flowing IV, taking care to avoid extravasation. Reduce dose by 50% for serum bilirubin levels of 2.1 to 3 mg/dL and by 75% for bilirubin levels of more than 3 mg/dL.
Toxicity.
1. *Myelosuppression and other hematologic effects.* Granulocytopenia is common and dose limiting, with nadir at 7 to 10 days. Thrombocytopenia is uncommon. Anemia is occasional to common.
2. *Nausea, vomiting, and other gastrointestinal effects.* Nausea and vomiting are common, but usually mild to moderate. Diarrhea occurs occasionally.
3. *Mucocutaneous effects.* Alopecia, mild diarrhea, and stomatitis are occasional. Severe local inflammation can occur with extravasation.
4. *Miscellaneous effects.*
   a. Neurotoxicity: cumulative but reversible constipation and decreased deep tendon reflexes are occasional; paresthesias are uncommon.
   b. Erythema, pain, and skin discoloration at injection site are common; phlebitis at injection site is occasional.

VORINOSTAT

Other name. Zolinza.
Mechanism of action. Inhibits histone deacetylases (HDACs), which are overexpressed in some cancer cells. Accumulation of acetylated histones following vorinostat exposure induces cell cycle arrest or apoptosis in some transformed cells *in vitro*.

Primary indication.
1. Cutaneous T-cell lymphoma with progressive, persistent, or recurrent skin disease after two other systemic therapies.

Usual dosage and schedule. 400 mg PO daily with food. May be reduced to 300 mg daily or 5 days weekly if the higher dose is not tolerated.

Special precautions. Patients should drink at least 2 L of fluid daily to prevent dehydration from vomiting and diarrhea. Deep venous thrombosis and pulmonary embolism (5%) have been reported. Serum chemistries (including potassium, magnesium, calcium, glucose, and creatinine) and platelets should be monitored every 2 weeks during the first 2 months of treatment. Severe thrombocytopenia and gastrointestinal bleeding may occur with concomitant use with other HDAC inhibitors, such as valproic acid.

Toxicity.
1. *Myelosuppression and other hematologic effects*. Thrombocytopenia is common; anemia and neutropenia are occasional. Increased prothrombin time and INR may be seen with concomitant use of warfarin with vorinostat.
2. *Nausea, vomiting, and other gastrointestinal effects*. Anorexia, nausea, and diarrhea are common. Vomiting, constipation, and weight loss are occasional.
3. *Mucocutaneous effects*. Alopecia is occasional to common.
4. *Miscellaneous effects*.
   a. *Blood chemistry abnormalities*. Hypercholesterolemia, hypertriglyceridemia, hyperglycemia, and increased creatinine are common and may be severe (grade 3 or higher).
   b. *Cardiovascular*. QTc prolongation on the electrocardiogram is uncommon. Edema is occasional.
   c. *Neuromuscular*. Fatigue is common. Headache, muscle spasms, and dizziness are occasional.

ZOLEDRONIC ACID

Other name. Zometa.

Mechanism of action. A bisphosphonate that inhibits osteoclastic resorption of bone and calcium release induced by tumor cytokines.

Primary indications.
1. Hypercalcemia associated with malignancy.
2. Bone metastases from breast cancer, prostate cancer (after progression on hormonal therapy) and from other solid tumors in conjunction with standard antineoplastic therapy.
3. Osteolytic and osteoporotic bone lesions of multiple myeloma.

Usual dosage and schedule.
1. Hypercalcemia of malignancy: 4 mg IV as a 15-min infusion. May be repeated every 1 to 8 weeks, as needed.
2. Multiple myeloma or metastatic bone lesions: 4 mg IV as a 15-min infusion every 3 to 4 weeks.

Special precautions.
1. Do not infuse over less than 15 min. Potential for renal tubular damage, particularly if infused more rapidly. The risk of adverse reactions, particularly renal adverse reactions may

be greater in patients with impaired renal function. Dose adjustments are not necessary so long as serum creatinine is less than 4.5 mg/dL. Use caution when administered concurrently with aminoglycosides. Serum creatinine should be monitored before each treatment.

2. Osteonecrosis of the jaw has been reported, primarily in association with dental procedures such as tooth extraction; such procedures should be avoided during and following bisphosphonate treatment, if possible.

Toxicity.

1. *Myelosuppression and other hematologic effects.* Rare.
2. *Nausea, vomiting, and other gastrointestinal effects.* Abdominal pain, anorexia, constipation, nausea, and vomiting are uncommon to occasional.
3. *Mucocutaneous effects.* Infusion site reaction is occasional.
4. *Miscellaneous effects.*
   a. Flu-like syndrome with fever, chills, skeletal aches and pains are occasional.
   b. Hypocalcemia and hypomagnesemia are occasional, but grade 3 or 4 abnormalities are uncommon to rare.
   c. Increase of the serum creatinine of 0.5 mg/dL above baseline is occasional, but elevation to more than 3 times ULN is uncommon.
   d. Hypophosphatemia less than 2 mg/dL is occasional, but does not appear to have serious consequences or require treatment.
   e. Osteonecrosis of the jaw uncommon to rare.
   f. Conjunctivitis or other ocular abnormalities are rare.
   g. Potential bronchoconstriction in aspirin-sensitive patients.

SUGGESTED READINGS

Chabner B, Longo DL. *Cancer chemotherapy and biotherapy: principles and practice*, 4th ed. Philadelphia: Lippincott Williams & Wilkins, 2005:1000

Dorr RT, Van Hoff DD, eds. *Cancer chemotherapy handbook*. Norwalk: Appleton & Lange, 1994:1020.

National Cancer Institute Cancer Therapy Evaluation Program. *Common Terminology Criteria for Adverse Events v3.0 (CTCAE)*. at *http://ctep.cancer.gov/reporting/ctc.html*, 2003.

Perry MC. *The chemotherapy source book*. Philadelphia: Lippincott Williams & Wilkins, 2001:1024.

Tannock IF, Hill RP, eds. *The basic science of oncology*. New York: McGraw-Hill, 1998:539.

CHAPTER 5

High-Dose Chemotherapy and Hematopoietic Stem Cell Transplantation in Hematologic Malignancies

Roberto Rodriguez and Chatchada Karanes

The clinical practice of bone marrow transplantation was not widely used in the United States until the early 1970s although the first successful allogeneic hematopoietic stem cell transplantation (HCT) occurred in 1959. Earlier data demonstrated that allogeneic HCT can cure patients with leukemia and aplastic anemia and there was evidence supporting the concept of graft-versus-leukemia (GVL) effect. Subsequently, high-dose chemotherapy and autologous HCT have produced durable remission in non–Hodgkin's lymphoma (NHL), Hodgkin's lymphoma (HL) and multiple myeloma. The availability of hematopoietic growth factors in mid-1980 resulted in increasing numbers of autologous HCT in hematologic malignancies and later in breast, ovarian, and testicular cancer.

During the last 10 years, the number of transplants performed has grown exponentially. According to the Center for International Blood and Marrow Transplant Research (CIBMTR), 485 transplant centers worldwide performed 16,900 transplantations in 2003, of which 6,900 were autologous transplantations. Since 2000, there has been slowdown in the growth of both autologous and allogeneic transplants. The drop in autotransplants was due to a decrease in their use for breast cancer. The successful treatment of chronic myelogenous leukemia (CML) with imatinib has significantly decreased the numbers of patients receiving allogeneic HCT for this disease. However, the use of allogeneic transplants for other indications continues to increase. In the last 10 years, criteria for the transplantation of hematopoietic stem cells (HSCs) have changed dramatically. These include the concept of tandem autologous transplant in multiple myeloma, reduced-intensity regimens for patients with impaired organ function, or older patients who would not be able to tolerate a full myeloablative conditioning regimen, and the use of donor lymphocytes to eradicate minimal residual diseases. Choices of stem cell sources now include marrow, peripheral blood stem cells (PBSCs), and umbilical cord blood (UCB). Newer immunosuppressive drugs are available for prevention and treatment of graft-versus-host disease (GVHD), resulting in less morbidity and mortality during the post-transplant period. With improved supportive care, the indications for transplantation continue to increase. Selected groups of patients can receive high-dose therapy (HDT) with HCT as outpatients.

Clinical trials during the last 30 years have demonstrated that high-dose chemotherapy with or without the addition of radiation therapy can result in improved response and overall survival (OS) rates for patients with various malignant and nonmalignant diseases. High-dose chemotherapy enables the clinician to exploit the steep dose−response curves observed with many chemotherapeutic agents. The line representing log kill of malignant cells remains linear or slightly curvilinear for many chemotherapeutic agents, particularly for the alkylating agents. Most of the alkylating agents can be dose-escalated 4- to 10-fold; some alkylators such as thiotepa can be escalated 30-fold when supported with HCT. Most nonalkylating agents cannot be dose-escalated more than twofold; some exceptions include cytarabine, etoposide, mitoxantrone, and paclitaxel. Improved supportive modalities including antibiotics, antiemetics, and hematopoietic cytokines and the availability of a variety of blood products have improved the safety of HDT. However, hematopoietic progenitor cells (HPCs) derived from bone marrow, peripheral blood, or cord blood are required to rescue the patient from myeloablative therapy. Therefore, the clinician can continue to escalate the doses of chemotherapy or radiation therapy beyond marrow toxicity to the next level of toxicity, the nonhematologic dose-limiting toxicity.

Although dose escalation is possible with hematopoietic stem cell rescue, not all malignancies can be cured with this treatment modality. In some diseases, the doses necessary to achieve complete tumor cell kill exceed the nonmarrow lethal doses of chemotherapy or radiation therapy. In other malignancies, dose escalation beyond the marrow lethal dose results in only modest increases in cell kill. Metastatic melanoma, non−small cell lung cancer, and colon cancer are examples of malignancies that HDT with hematopoietic stem cell rescue cannot cure.

Even with dose intensification, many patients ultimately experience disease relapse, which probably results from either failure to eradicate residual tumor cells or, in the case of autotransplantation, the reinfusion of hematopoietic stem cells (HSCs) containing contaminating tumor cells. With the use of molecular techniques, the latter has been proved to be the case in some hematologic diseases such as acute myelogenous leukemia (AML) and low-grade lymphoma. It is clear that performing the transplant early in the course of the disease results in better outcome. The role of graft manipulation such as purging or CD34 selection is rarely used for autologous transplantation. Patients with significant marrow involvement should be considered for allogeneic stem cell transplantation.

Allogeneic transplantation provides a source of HSCs that is devoid of contaminating tumor cells. Growing clinical experience supports an immunotherapeutic (graft-versus-tumor) effect of the donor immune system to eradicate minimal residual disease after transplant. This immunoreactivity can be exploited following nonmyeloablative HCT for residual disease or at the time of disease relapse by donor lymphocyte infusions (DLIs), inducing complete remission in many hematologic malignancies. Unfortunately, transplant-related morbidity and mortality remain problematic because of GVHD and prolonged immunosuppression.

I.   Scientific background

A. High-dose therapy (HDT) rationale.
The cytocidal effect of chemotherapy in cell culture and animal models follows first-order kinetics. Each treatment kills a set fraction of cancer cells, irrespective of the starting number. The degree of kill in these experimental systems is dose dependent. Tumor cell viability decreases in a logarithmic manner, with a linear increase in drug dose. A modest escalation in the dose may result in a much higher fractional kill of tumor cells. Sublethal chemotherapy selects for and encourages development of resistant cells. The use of several chemotherapeutic agents in combination with different mechanisms of action inhibits the development of resistance. In addition, combinations of agents selected for nonoverlapping extramedullary dose-limiting toxicities should be used in maximal doses. Therefore, the optimal approach uses the highest possible doses of non−cross-resistant agents with steep dose−response curves as early as possible in the patient's disease course to achieve the highest tumor cell kill and reduce the development of drug resistance. Eradication of tumor (cure) usually requires an 8- to 12-log kill of cancer cells. A complete clinical remission can be obtained with as little as a 4-log cell kill and a partial remission (50% tumor cytoreduction) with as little as a 1- or 2-log kill. Complete remissions are the surrogate short-term markers of potentially successful therapy.

The dosages of many active agents are limited by myelosuppression, even with the use of hematopoietic growth factors. The use of hematopoietic stem cell support allows for increased dosage and combination therapy with agents that would normally produce an unacceptable degree of myelosuppression.

B. Graft-versus-tumor effect.
The eradication of leukemia after allogeneic HCT results both from the cytotoxic chemoradiotherapy administered before transplant and the immunologic mechanisms. The first clinical demonstration of graft-versus-leukemia (GVL) activity was observed after allogeneic HCT for advanced leukemia, in which the probability of leukemic relapse was found to be significantly lower in those patients who developed acute and/or chronic graft-versus-host disease (GVHD). Analysis of patients with leukemia treated with either allogeneic unmodified HCT, allogeneic T-cell−depleted HCT, or syngeneic HCT showed that the risk of relapse was lowest for patients who received allogeneic unmodified HCT and developed acute and/or chronic GVHD. However, GVHD is not a prerequisite for GVL activity. With current approaches to allogeneic HCT, however, it has not been possible to separate the beneficial GVL (or graft-versus-cancer) effect from deleterious GVHD. The association of GVL activity with GVHD has implicated donor T cells reacting with minor histocompatibility antigens expressed by recipient cells as major contributors to the GVL effect. Other effector mechanisms such as natural killer cells may also contribute to GVL activity either directly or as a consequence of inflammation induced by allogeneic T cells.

Three important clinical applications in stem cell transplantation have evolved from GVL effect. The first application is the use of donor lympholyte infusion (DLI) to treat patients with post-transplant leukemic relapse. Patients with CML showed best responses to DLI followed by low-grade lymphoma, mantle cell lymphoma, and chronic lymphocytic leukemia (CLL). AML, intermediate-grade lymphoma, multiple myeloma, HL, renal cell carcinoma, and breast cancer show intermediate sensitivity. Acute lymphoblastic leukemia (ALL) and high-grade lymphoma are insensitive to GVL effect. The second application is the use of nonmyeloablative or reduced-intensity allogeneic conditioning regimens in older and less fit patients. With this approach, low doses of irradiation and chemotherapy, which alone are not sufficient to eradicate tumors, are administered to facilitate graft acceptance, and tumor regression is induced by donor immune cells. The third application is the tandem stem cell transplant using nonmyeloablative allogeneic HCT after reduction of tumor burden by autologous transplants. Several clinical trials using autologous HCT followed by allogeneic HCT in multiple myeloma, low-grade NHL, and HL are in progress.

II. Indications for HDT with hematopoietic stem cell transplantation

   A. Disease. During the last 15 years, the indications for HDT and HCT have changed markedly. The most common indications for allogeneic and autologous transplants differ (Fig. 5.1). For acute and chronic leukemias, myelodysplastic syndromes (MDSs), and nonmalignant diseases (aplastic anemia, immune deficiencies, inherited metabolic disorders), allogeneic transplantation is the predominant approach. Autotransplants are most commonly used for multiple myeloma, non-Hodgkin's lymphoma (NHL), and Hodgkin's lymphoma (HL) and less commonly for AML, neuroblastoma, and breast cancer. Fifteen years ago, autologous transplants were performed almost exclusively for NHL and HL. In 2003, multiple myeloma was the most common indication for autologous transplants, followed by NHL, HL, and AML. The use of autotransplants performed in solid tumors are decreasing due to low efficacy in these diseases and the availability of potentially less toxic and more effective therapy using newer classes of antineoplastic agents. Although most allogeneic transplantations continue to be performed for acute and chronic leukemias, there has been a recent increase in allogeneic transplantations for immunodeficiency disorders, inherited disorders of metabolism, thalassemia, and sickle cell diseases. New data using autologous and allogeneic HCT in autoimmune diseases are encouraging.

   B. Stem cell sources. Bone marrow was used as the only source of stem cells until the mid-1980s. The introduction of hematopoietic growth factors has made it possible to mobilize the stem cells from the bone marrow into the peripheral blood, resulting in the ability to collect large numbers of stem cells through apheresis and accelerate the engraftment. Currently, PBSCs are the major stem cell source of all autologous transplants. Traditionally, allogeneic transplants use bone marrow grafts. From 1997 to 2004, there was a steady increase in

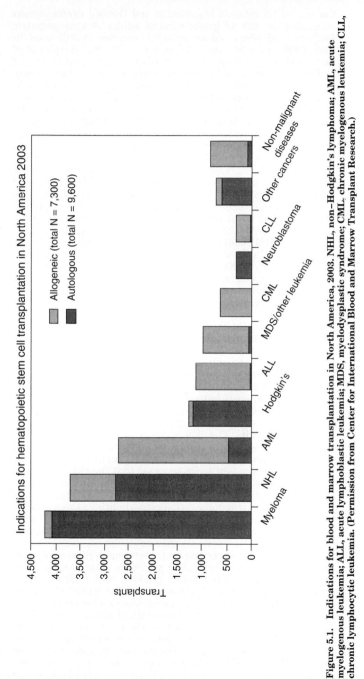

Figure 5.1.   Indications for blood and marrow transplantation in North America, 2003. NHL, non-Hodgkin's lymphoma; AML, acute myelogenous leukemia; ALL, acute lymphoblastic leukemia; MDS, myelodysplastic syndrome; CML, chronic myelogenous leukemia; CLL, chronic lymphocytic leukemia. (Permission from Center for International Blood and Marrow Transplant Research.)

the use of peripheral blood stem cell (PBSC) grafts, which accounted for 70% of grafts used in adults. Among pediatric recipients 20 years old or younger, marrow is still used in 61%, PBSC in 30%, and cord blood in 9%. For recipients of unrelated stem cell sources, cord blood is now used in 34% of recipients 20 years old or younger whereas cord blood is only used in 4% of adult recipients. In addition to differences in their stem cell content, transplants from the three sources differ in the composition and state of activation of immune cells. As a consequence, bone marrow, UCB, and PBSC transplants have different kinetics of hematologic recovery, the most rapid engraftment being observed with PBSCs and the slowest with UCB. Stem cell source also confers different risks for developing GVHD. PBSC transplants show similar incidence of acute GVHD and a possible increase in chronic GVHD compared with bone marrow. UCB transplants have a favorably low risk of GVHD even in one or two antigen-mismatched transplants. Stem cell dose is an independent factor in transplants from any source, determining engraftment rate, transplant-related mortality (TRM), and risk of leukemic relapse. Higher marrow and PBSC cell dose correlated with improved transplant outcome, although PBSC dose of 8 million CD34 cell dose/kg of recipient body weight resulted in increased GVHD. An understanding of the impact of stem cell source and dose is essential to obtain optimum conditions for a successful outcome after transplant.

III.   Patient eligibility

A. Host factors. Autologous transplants can be conducted safely in patients up to 75 years of age if they have adequate performance status, physiologic organ function, and HSCs. There had been a trend of increasing transplant recipient age since 1996. According to CIBMTR data, 60% of autologous transplant recipients between 2001 and 2004 are older than 50 years and 10% of them are older than 60 years. Nineteen percent of patients undergoing allogeneic transplantation are older than 50 years. The risk of death after allogeneic HCT depends on the underlying disease, stage of disease at the time of transplantation, type of conditioning regimen, and donor type. The Seattle transplant team reported that the risk for overall grade 4 toxicity and nonrelapse mortality among nonmyeloablative and ablative allogeneic HCT increased in direct relation to increasing pretransplantation comorbidities as assessed by Charlson comorbidity score. In their series, the 1-year nonrelapse mortality was 20% in nonablative patients compared with 32% in ablative patients. Although nonmyeloablative patients had a higher pretransplantation comorbidity score, were older, and had more often failed preceding ablative transplantation, they experienced fewer grade 3 to 4 toxicities than ablative patients. For allogeneic transplantation, the usual upper age limit is 60 years, although some centers perform human leukocyte antigen (HLA)–identical sibling transplants in selected patients up to 60 to 65 years old. For unrelated or mismatched related donors, the usual age limit is 60 years depending on the recipient performance status and comorbid illness. For both autologous and allogeneic transplants, patients must meet a minimum physiologic organ function. Common criteria include pulmonary function test results (forced vital capacity, forced expiratory volume, and corrected diffusing capacity) more than 50% of predicted, cardiac function results with a left ventricular ejection fraction more than 40% to 45%, no active infections, liver function test results less than two to four times normal, performance status more than 60% on the Karnofsky scale of less than 2 on the Eastern Cooperative Oncology Group scale, and serum creatinine level of less than 2 mg/dL. In certain diseases, patients with impaired renal function could also be considered for autotransplantation (e.g., multiple myeloma patients treated with high-dose melphalan).

B. Disease factors. In general, patients with malignant disease should show at least a partial response (PR) to standard-dose chemotherapy before being considered for HDT with hematopoietic stem cell transfusion (HSCT). Practicing hematologists and oncologists should refer high-risk patients early for transplant evaluation. This allows adequate time to identify matched related or unrelated donors for allogeneic stem cell transplant candidates or in case of autologous transplantation, it enables patients to avoid exposure to stem cell toxic treatment before autologous stem cell collections. A recommended timing for HCT referral to transplant centers is shown in Table 5.1.

IV.   Chemotherapeutic agents for dose-intensive strategies. Agents are chosen for dose intensification based on the steepness and linearity of their dose–response curve, the absence of nonhematologic toxicity that prevents dose escalation (preferably allowing a 5- to 10-fold dose escalation over conventional doses), and, when combined with other agents, a synergistic antitumor effect with a minimum of overlapping nonhematologic toxicity. The doses of alkylating agents are often reduced by 20% to 40% when combined as compared with use as a single agent in high-dose conditioning regimens. Therefore, the choice of chemotherapeutic agents is arbitrary, based largely on anecdotal data and a matter of personal experience and preference. Extramedullary toxicities of the most commonly used conditioning agents are listed in Table 5.2. In most cases, drug doses are limited by gastrointestinal toxicity (mucositis, diarrhea) or major organ toxicity (e.g., heart, lung, kidney, or central nervous system [CNS]). When combining drugs in a conditioning regimen, particular attention must be given to overlapping toxicities. Pre-existing renal or hepatic insufficiency or both may seriously reduce drug clearance. This can result in higher drug levels and further end-organ toxicity.

A. Alkylating agents

    1. BCNU (carmustine) is a nitrosourea with clinical activity against a number of tumors. It is formulated in 10% alcohol solution, which may account for the hypotension seen during or shortly after administration. BCNU, which undergoes spontaneous hydrolysis, should be protected from light and is usually administered as a 2-hour infusion. At high dose, pulmonary and hepatic toxicity are dose limiting. Nonhematologic toxicities are delayed and cumulative. BCNU doses exceeding 300 mg/m^2 are associated with acute or late pneumonitis in at least 20% of patients.

Table 5.1.   Recommended timing for transplant consultation

AML	• High-risk AML including — Antecedent hematologic disease (e.g., myelodysplasia) — Treatment-related leukemia — Induction failure • CR1 with poor-risk cytogenetics • CR2 and beyond
ALL	• High-risk ALL including — Poor-risk cytogenetics (e.g., Philadelphia chromosome–positive, 11q23) — High WBC (>30,000–50,000) at diagnosis — CNS or testicular leukemia — No CR within 4 weeks of initial treatment — Induction failure • CR2 and beyond
Myelodysplastic syndromes	• Intermediate-1, intermediate-2 or high IPSS score which includes — >5% marrow blasts — Other than good risk cytogenetics (good risk includes 5q- or normal) — >1 lineage cytopenia
Chronic myelogenous leukemia	• No hematologic or minor cytogenetic response 3 months post–imatinib initiation • No complete cytogenetic response 6 to 12 months post–imatinib initiation • Disease progression • Accelerated phase • Blast crisis (myeloid or lymphoid)
Non–Hodgkin's lymphoma	• Follicular lymphoma — Poor response to initial treatment — Initial remission duration <12 months — Second relapse — Transformation to diffuse large B-cell lymphoma • Diffuse large B-cell lymphoma — At first or subsequent relapse — CR1 for patients with high or high-intermediate IPI risk — No CR with initial treatment • Mantle cell lymphoma — Following initial therapy

Table 5.1. (*Continued*)

Hodgkin's lymphoma	• No initial CR • First or subsequent relapse
Multiple myeloma	• After initiation of therapy • At first progression

AML, acute myelogenous leukemia; CR, complete response; ALL, acute lymphoblastic leukemia; WBC, white blood cell; CNS, central nervous system; IPSS, Internal Prognostic Scoring System; IPI, International Prognostic Index.

Patients should be informed to monitor exercise tolerance; if tolerance diminishes, further evaluation should be performed (chest radiograph, arterial blood gas, pulmonary diffusion capacity). If drug-induced pneumonitis is confirmed, prednisone should be started with a taper over 2 to 3 months. BCNU is also occasionally associated with an increased incidence of veno-occlusive disease.

2. Busulfan (Myleran [PO], Busulfex [IV]) has a more marked effect on myeloid cells than on lymphoid cells and can cause prolonged aplasia. The major nonhematologic toxicities are veno-occlusive disease of the liver, pneumonitis, and mucositis. Busulfan rapidly enters the CNS and may cause seizures. Patients should receive prophylactic phenytoin (with doses sufficient to achieve therapeutic levels) before initiation of high-dose busulfan, and the phenytoin should be continued for 24 hours after the final dose. Busulfan is available in oral and, recently, in IV formulation. The IV formulation is dissolved in polyethylene glycol and N,N-dimethylacetamide to a final concentration of 6 mg/mL. The usual adult dose of Busulfex is 0.8 mg/kg of ideal body weight or adjusted body weight, whichever is lower, administered as a 2-hour infusion through a central venous catheter every 6 hours for 4 days. Ninety-three percent of patients achieve an area under the curve (AUC) below the target of 1,500 μmol/L/minute with no dosage adjustments. If vomiting occurs within 30 minutes of an oral administration or if pill fragments are present in the emesis, most institutions repeat the dose. Busulfan is well absorbed after oral administration, exhibits low protein binding, and is metabolized through conjugation with glutathione to form a thiophenium ion. At a given dose, there is considerable variability in the systemic exposure of oral busulfan, typically expressed as AUC or average concentration at steady state. Relative to that in adolescents and adults, patients younger than 4 years have an increased apparent oral clearance of busulfan and a higher conjugation rate of busulfan with glutathione in the enterocyte. An increased risk of serious hepatic veno-occlusive disease has been reported when the AUC level exceeds 1,500 μmol/L/minute. Busulfan administration through the IV route ensures complete bioavailability and reliable systemic drug exposure with more predictable blood levels and less veno-occlusive disease.

Table 5.2. Toxicity of common chemotherapeutic agents

Drug (Dose)	Extramedullary Dose-Limiting Toxicity	Other Toxicities
BCNU (carmustine) ($300-600$ mg/m^2)	Interstitial pneumonitis	Renal insufficiency, encephalopathy, N/V, VOD
Busulfan ($12-16$ mg/kg)	Mucositis, VOD	Seizures, rash, N/V, hyperpigmentation, pneumonitis
Cyclophosphamide ($120-200$ mg/kg)	Cardiomyopathy	Hemorrhagic cystitis, SIADH, N/V, interstitial pneumonitis
Cytarabine (ara-C) ($4-36$ g/m^2)	CNS ataxia, mucositis	Pulmonary edema, conjunctivitis rash, fever, hepatitis
Cisplatin ($150-180$ mg/m^2)	Renal insufficiency, peripheral neuropathy	Renal tubular acidosis, hypomagnesemia, hypokalemia, ototoxicity
Carboplatin ($600-1,500$ mg/m^2)	Ototoxicity, renal insufficiency	Hepatitis, hypomagnesemia, hypokalemia, peripheral neuropathy
Etoposide ($600-2,400$ mg/m^2)	Mucositis	N/V, hepatitis, fever, pneumonia
Ifosfamide ($12-16$ g/m^2)	Encephalopathy, renal insufficiency	Hemorrhagic cystitis
Melphalan ($140-200$ mg/m^2)	Mucositis	N/V, hepatitis, SIADH, pneumonitis
Mitoxantrone ($30-75$ mg/m^2)	Cardiomyopathy	Mucositis
Paclitaxel (Taxol) ($500-775$ mg/m^2)	CNS, ataxia, peripheral neuropathy	Anaphylaxis, mucositis
Thiotepa ($500-800$ mg/m^2)	Mucositis	Intertriginous rash, N/V, hyperpigmentation
Fludarabine ($90-180$ mg/m^2)	CNS visual disturbances, peripheral neuropathy	N/V, tumor lysis syndromes, immunosuppression

N/V, nausea/vomiting; VOD, veno-occlusive disease; SIADH, syndrome of inappropriate antidiuretic hormone; CNS, central nervous system.

3. Cyclophosphamide (Cytoxan) is probably the most widely used chemotherapeutic agent for dose intensification. Cyclophosphamide requires activation in the liver, but there is no evidence that the P-450 system necessary for that activation is saturated at the doses used in intensification. Clearance of cyclophosphamide increases quickly after the first dose, and there is considerable interpatient variability in plasma concentrations with repeated dosing. Total doses as high as 5,000 to 7,000 mg/m^2 divided over 1 to 4 days can be safely administered as 1- to 2-hour infusions each day. Aggressive hydration (hyperhydration) and diuresis or administration of mesna as an uroprotectant is necessary to prevent hemorrhagic cystitis (also used for ifosfamide). The dose-limiting toxicities are cardiac and pulmonary. The cardiac effect, some degree of which occurs in up to 25% of patients, is a potentially fatal hemorrhagic myocarditis that may occur acutely or within days or may manifest as heart failure or pericardial effusions as long as 3 to 4 weeks after completion of treatment. The risk of cardiac toxicity is not cumulative, and repeated doses are tolerated in the patients who recover. This toxicity occurs most often in patients who receive more than 200 mg/kg (>7,500 mg/m^2), are older than 50 years, and have a previous history of congestive heart failure. The pulmonary toxicity of cyclophosphamide consists of proliferation of atypical type II pneumocytes with fibrosis. It usually manifests clinically within 4 to 6 weeks of therapy as progressive dyspnea, nonproductive cough, hypoxia, and interstitial radiographic changes. Even at high doses, cyclophosphamide is not myeloablative, and its antitumor effect as a single agent is limited. In autologous transplant, cyclophosphamide, alone or in combination with hematopoietic growth factors, is often used for PBSC mobilization. In allogeneic transplantation, cyclophosphamide is included predominantly as an immunosuppressive agent owing to its lymphocytotoxic effects.

4. Ifosfamide, a closely related analog of cyclophosphamide, is also a prodrug that must undergo hepatic metabolism. As with cyclophosphamide, hyperhydration, and protection with mesna are required to prevent hemorrhagic cystitis. Unlike cyclophosphamide, the dose-limiting toxicity of ifosfamide is toxic encephalopathy manifested as lethargy, confusion, seizures, or stupor. Renal toxicity may also manifest as metabolic acidosis due to accumulation of metabolic by-products resulting in proximal renal tubular acidosis. No definite antitumor advantage of ifosfamide over cyclophosphamide has yet been established.

5. Melphalan alkylates target tissues after spontaneous formation of a (nitrogen) mustard-type reactive intermediate *in vivo*. It is administered rapidly in two daily doses of 70 to 100 mg/m^2 or one dose of 140 to 200 mg/m^2. Because less than 15% of the intact drug is excreted renally, melphalan can be administered safely in patients with renal insufficiency. The dose-limiting toxicities are gastrointestinal toxicity (mucositis, diarrhea) and, less commonly, hepatitis and pneumonitis.

6. Platinum compounds (cisplatin, carboplatin) covalently bind to deoxyribonucleic acid (DNA) bases and disrupt DNA function. Cisplatin can be escalated only two- to threefold owing to renal and neurologic toxicity. Cisplatin must be reconstituted in a chloride-containing solution to minimize spontaneous hydrolysis. Aggressive hydration and diuresis with normal saline loading and maintenance of good urine output are required to avoid renal tubular toxicity. Magnesium wasting commonly leads to hypocalcemia and hypokalemia. Peripheral neuropathy and high-frequency hearing loss are potential long-term side effects. Carboplatin has less renal and neurologic toxicities; myelosuppression and hepatic and gastrointestinal (mucositis and diarrhea) toxicities are more common with carboplatin. Some clinicians use the AUC (Calvert formula) of 20 to 28 for target drug dosing of carboplatin in high-dose preparative regimens.

7. Thiotepa has one of the steepest dose–response curves of all the alkylating agents and is not cross-resistant with cyclophosphamide. It has therefore been included in many different dose-intensity regimens. Thiotepa penetrates the blood–brain barrier better than most alkylating agents. Mucositis is the dose-limiting toxicity, with CNS toxicity being observed only at very high doses. It may increase the risk of hepatic veno-occlusive disease when used with other agents known to have that toxicity.

B. Nonalkylating and less commonly used agents

1. Cytarabine is an analog of deoxycytidine and has multiple effects on DNA synthesis. It is used in high doses for the treatment of leukemia and in some regimens for NHL. At high doses, cytarabine causes neurologic toxicity, manifested by cerebral and cerebellar dysfunction. Renal dysfunction increases the risk of neurotoxicity substantially. This toxicity may present as dysarthria, gait disturbances, dementia, and coma. These toxicities are usually reversible but may be fatal. If neurologic symptoms develop, the cytarabine should be stopped immediately. Another rare but life-threatening complication is noncardiogenic pulmonary edema. Pulmonary symptoms, when they develop, are often fatal. Cytarabine conjunctivitis is responsive to topical steroids, which should be used prophylactically.

2. Etoposide is a topoisomerase II inhibitor that shows synergism with platinum compounds. It has high single-agent activity in the treatment of leukemia, lymphomas, and testicular cancer. Its primary nonhematologic toxicities are mucositis, liver toxicity, and hypotension from the lipid formulation if administered rapidly.

3. Paclitaxel is a taxane that stabilizes microtubules, leading to mitotic arrest. It has activity against breast and ovarian cancers. One phase I study reported a maximum tolerated dose of 725 mg/m^2. At higher doses, unacceptable CNS, renal, mucosal, and pulmonary toxicities were observed. Peripheral neuropathy was tolerable and not associated with motor weakness. Because paclitaxel is eliminated through hepatic metabolism, hepatic insufficiency can prolong elimination and increase toxicity.

4. Fludarabine is a nucleotide analog of adenine arabinoside and inhibits DNA synthesis by inhibiting DNA polymerase α, ribonucleotide reductase, and DNA primase. The drug is converted rapidly to the active metabolite 2-fluoro-ara-A when given IV. The half-life is approximately 10 hours. The drug is eliminated through the kidneys; 23% of the active drug is excreted unchanged in the urine. Therefore, it should be administered cautiously in patients with renal insufficiency. It produces lymphocytopenia and substantial immunosuppression and is approved for the treatment of B-cell chronic lympholyte leukemia (CLL). Owing to its immunosuppression, it is used in combination with alkylating agents or low-dose total-body irradiation (TBI) to enhance engraftment of allogeneic hematopoietic progenitors. At this time, it is available only in IV formulation; the oral form is in clinical trials. The dose recommended for CLL is 25 mg/m^2/day IV over 30 minutes for 5 days; however, the dosage used for conditioning in nonmyeloablative HSCT varies from 25 to 50 mg/m^2 over 30 minutes once a day for 3 to 5 days. Once reconstituted, the drug should be used in 8 hours owing to a lack of antimicrobial preservative. The dose-dependent toxicities include myelosuppression and immunosuppression. Visual disturbances and CNS symptoms have been reported at very high doses.

V. Total-body irradiation (TBI). TBI is an integral component of several conditioning regimens, particularly for hematologic malignancies requiring allogeneic or autologous transplantation. It has been used since the earliest days of bone marrow transplantation for both immunosuppression (prevention of allograft rejection) and antitumor effect. However, the therapeutic ratio of TBI is small. The usual dosage of TBI is 10 to 14 Gy given in twice- or thrice-daily doses over 3 to 4 days (e.g., 2 Gy b.i.d. for 3 days). Fractionation (and hyperfractionation) substantially reduces the risk of both interstitial pneumonitis and veno-occlusive disease of the liver. Above that dose, pulmonary, hepatic, and gastrointestinal toxicities become limiting and life threatening with little therapeutic gain. Acute and chronic toxicities with TBI are summarized in Table 5.3.

VI. Preparative regimens. The regimens used for dose intensification are largely empiric, and few have been compared in randomized trials. Important issues such as optimum combination or doses, the benefit of an "induction" regimen immediately preceding intensification, and the benefit of repeated cycles of dose intensity have shown benefit only in multiple myeloma and possibly HL. TBI-based regimens result in more regimen-related toxicity and are used for NHL, ALL, HL, AML, and multiple myeloma. Examples of commonly employed preparative regimens are shown in Tables 5.4 and 5.5.

A. Allogeneic transplant–myeloablative regimen. Standard myeloablative preparative regimens must provide effective antitumor activity and suppress host immunity to prevent graft rejection. Commonly used cytotoxic agents include TBI, cyclophosphamide, busulfan, cytarabine, and etoposide. Immunosuppression is necessary for allogeneic HCT to prevent graft-versus-host diseases (GVHD) and graft rejection.

Table 5.3. Total-body irradiation–associated acute and chronic toxicities

System	Acute Symptoms and Signs	Acute Onset	Chronic Symptoms and Signs	Onset and incidence
Gastrointestinal	Nausea and vomiting, diarrhea	24–48 h	—	—
Hepatic	Veno-occlusive disease	6–21 days	—	—
Mucosal tissues	Parotitis, decreased lacrimation, sore throat, mucositis	24–48 h	Sicca syndrome, cataracts	20% with fractionation at 0.5 to 3–4 years
Endocrine	Acute pancreatitis, steroid-induced hyperglycemia	7–21 days	Gonadal failure Hypothyroidism Delayed bone growth	>90% 40%–50%
Pulmonary, renal	Pneumonitis	1–3 months	Pulmonary fibrosis Bone marrow transplantation nephropathy	Uncommon
Skin, second malignancies	Erythema, alopecia	5–10 days	Secondary leukemia Solid tumors	5%–10% 2% at 10 years, 7% at 15 years

Table 5.4. Common preparative regimens for high-dose therapy with total-body irradiation

Drug	Total Dose	Daily Dose	Schedule (Day)[a]	Indications	Autologous or Allogeneic
Single–cytotoxic drug regimens					
Cyclophosphamide	120 mg/kg	60 mg/kg	−5, −4	Leukemia, NHL	Both
TBI	1,200 cGy	200 cGy b.i.d.	−3, −2, −1	aplastic anemia	
Etoposide	60 mg/kg	60 mg/kg	−3	Leukemia, NHL	Allogeneic
TBI	1,320 cGy	120 cGy t.i.d.	−7, −6, −5, −4		
Cytarabine (ara-C)	36 g/m²	3 g/m² b.i.d.	−9, −8, −7, −6, −5, −4	Leukemia, NHL	Allogeneic
TBI	1,200 cGy	200 cGy b.i.d.	−3, −2, −1		
Melphalan	140 mg/m²	140 mg/m²	−4	Leukemia, multiple	Both
TBI	1,200 cGy	200 cGy b.i.d.	−3, −2, −1	myeloma	

(continued)

Table 5.4. *(Continued)*

Drug	Total Dose	Daily Dose	Schedule (Day)[a]	Indications	Autologous or Allogeneic
Combination–cytotoxic drug regimens					
Cytarabine (ara-C)	18 g/m^2	3 g/m^2 b.i.d.	$-8, -7, -6$	Leukemia, NHL	Allogeneic
Cyclophosphamide	90 mg/kg	45 mg/kg	$-5, -4$		
TBI	1,200 cGy	200 cGy b.i.d.	$-3, -2, -1$		
Etoposide	60 mg/kg	60 mg/kg	-4	Leukemia, NHL	Both
Cyclophosphamide	120 mg/kg	60 mg/kg	$-3, -2$		
TBI	1,320 cGy	120 cGy t.i.d.	$-8, -7, -6, -5^b$		
Thiotepa	10 mg/kg	5 mg/kg	$-5, -4$	Leukemia, NHL	Allogeneic
Cyclophosphamide	120 mg/kg	60 mg/kg	$-3, -2$		
ATG	120 mg/kg	30 mg/kg	$-5, -4, -3, -2$		
TBI	1,375 cGy	125 cGy t.i.d.	$-9, -8, -7, -6^b$		
Fludarabine	90 mg/m^2	30 mg/m^2	$-4, -3, -2$	Leukemia, NHL	Allogeneic
TBI	200 cGy	200 cGy once	-1		

TBI, total-body irradiation; NHL, non–Hodgkin's lymphoma; ATG, antithymocyte globulin.
[a]Day 0 is day of transplantation, day -5 is 5 days before transplantation, etc.
[b]TBI given twice on this day.

Table 5.5. Common preparative regimens for high-dose therapy without total-body irradiation

Drug	Total Dose	Daily Dose	Schedule (Day)	Indications	Autologous or Allogeneic
"Big" BU/CY					
Busulfan	16 mg/kg	1 mg/kg q.i.d.	$-9, -8, -7, -6$	Leukemia, NHL	Allogeneic
Cyclophosphamide	200 mg/kg	50 mg/kg	$-5, -4, -3, -2$		
"Little" BU/CY					
Busulfan	16 mg/kg	1 mg/kg q.i.d.	$-7, -6, -5, -4$	Leukemia, NHL, myeloma, breast cancer	Both
Cyclophosphamide	120 mg/kg	60 mg/kg	$-3, -2$		
CPB "STAMP I"					
Cisplatin	165 mg/m^2	55 mg/m^2	$-6, -5, -4$	Breast cancer	Autologous
Cyclophosphamide	5,625 mg/m^2	1,875 mg/m^2	$-6, -5, -4$		
BCNU	600 mg/m^2	600 mg/m^2	-3		
TC					
Thiotepa	500 mg/m^2	125 mg/m^2	$-7, -6, -5, -4$	Breast cancer	Autologous
Cyclophosphamide	6 g/m^2	1.5 g/m^2	$-7, -6, -5, -4$		
CBV					
BCNU	300–600 mg/m^2	300–600 mg/m^2	-6	HL	Autologous
Etoposide	900–2,400 mg/m^2	300–800 mg/m^2	$-6, -5, -4$		
Cyclophosphamide	6–7.2 g/m^2	1.5–1.8 g/m^2	$-6, -5, -4, -3$		

(continued)

Table 5.5. *(Continued)*

Drug	Total Dose	Daily Dose	Schedule (Day)	Indications	Autologous or Allogeneic
BEAM					
BCNU	300 mg/m^2	300 mg/m^2	−6	HL, NHL	Autologous
Etoposide	800 mg/m^2	200 mg/m^2	−5, −4, −3, −2		
Cytarabine	$800–1,600 \text{ mg/m}^2$	$200–400 \text{ mg/m}^2$	−5, −4, −3, −2		
Melphalan	140 mg/m^2	140 mg/m^2	−1		
ICE					
Ifosfamide	16 g/m^2	4 g/m^2	−6, −5, −4, −3	NHL, testicular cancer	Autologous
Carboplatin	1.8 g/m^2	600 mg/m^2	−6, −5, −4		
Etoposide	1.5 g/m^2	500 mg/m^2 b.i.d.	−6, −5, −4		
BEAC					
BCNU	300 mg/m^2	300 mg/m^2	−6	NHL, HL	Autologous
Etoposide	800 mg/m^2	200 mg/m^2	−5, −4, −3, −2		
Cytarabine	800 mg/m^2	200 mg/m^2	−5, −4, −3, −2		
Cytoxan	140 mg/kg	35 mg/kg	−5, −4, −3, −2		
MEL					
Melphalan	200 mg/m^2	100 mg/m^2	−3, −2	Multiple myeloma	Autologous
MCC					
Mitoxantrone	75 mg/m^2	25 mg/m^2	−8, −6, −4	Ovarian cancer	Autologous
Carboplatin	AUC 28	1/5 total dose	−8, −7, −6, −5, −4		
Cytoxan	120 mg/m^2	40 mg/m^2	−8, −6, −4		

CBDA/VP				
Carboplatin	2.25 g/m²	750 mg/m²	$-6, -5, -4$	Autologous
Etoposide	2.1 g/m²	700 mg/m²	$-6, -5, -4$	
Fludarabine	90 mg/m²	30 mg/m²	$-6, -5, -4$	Allogeneic, reduced intensity
Cyclophos-phamide	2,250 mg/m²	750 mg/m²		NHL
Fludarabine	150 mg/m²	30 mg/m²	$-6, -5, -4, -3, -2$	Allogeneic, reduced intensity
Melphalan	140 mg/m²	70 mg/m²	$-3, -2$	Leukemia
Fludarabine	180 mg/m²	30 mg/m²	$-10, -9, -8, -7, -6, -5$	Allogeneic, reduced intensity
				Leukemia
Busulfan	8 mg/kg	4 mg/kg	$-6, -5$	Allogeneic, reduced intensity
				NHL
ATG	40 mg/kg	10 mg/kg	$-4, -3, -2, -1$	Allogeneic, reduced intensity
				MDS

ATG, antithymocyte globulin; MDS, Myelodysplastic syndromes; HL, Hodgkin's lymphoma; NHL, non-Hodgkins lymphoma; BCNU, carmustine.

The combined toxicity of preparative regimen and GVHD prophylaxis in these patients increases early morbidity and mortality in the first month of transplant compared with those receiving autologous HCT. The treatment-related mortality of 10% to 30% depends on diagnosis, disease stage, patient age, and donor type. In this model, it has been thought that myeloablation was necessary to create a marrow space, although immunosuppression prevented rejection and GVHD.

B. Reduced-intensity–nonmyeloablative regimens. Increasing recognition of the role of graft-versus-tumor effect has shifted the emphasis from delivery of myeloablative therapy aiming at maximum tumor destruction to optimizing engraftment, thereby providing the platform for further adoptive immunotherapy with DLI. This has resulted in the emergence of new concepts and procedures that allow replacement of the patient bone marrow and immune system with that of the donor by a transplant procedure with markedly reduced intensity of the preparative regimen. The true nonmyeloablative regimen used low-dose TBI of 200 cGy alone or in combination with fludarabine or fludarabine plus cyclophosphamide. This type of preparative regimen provides sufficient immunosuppression to allow engraftment of allogeneic blood progenitor cells without causing profound neutropenia and severe organ toxicity of myeloablative radiochemotherapy. It is suitable only for patients in remission or with more indolent disease, because it takes several weeks to achieve full donor T-cell chimerism to result in graft-versus-tumor effect. To maintain the continued presence of donor cells following nonmyeloablative transplant, it is occasionally necessary to give the recipient posttreatment infusions of additional donor T cells. This is referred to as *donor lymphocyte infusion (DLI)*. However, DLI also carries a significant risk of GVHD development. There are several approaches to improving the safety of DLI, including selective removal of the alloreactive T cells and/or induction of tolerance in the donor lymphocytes to the recipient tissues to prevent GVHD. Such an approach is used in the follow-up phase of treatment for patients who need DLI to further consolidate/maintain the presence of the donor hematopoietic cells. Immunosuppressive agents used in this type of transplant are combinations of oral cyclosporine or tacrolimus with mycophenolate mofetil (MMF) (Table 5.6), avoiding the debilitating oral mucositis from the use of methotrexate as in conventional stem cell transfusion (SCT). This approach reduces the toxicity of the transplant procedure and makes it possible to treat debilitated patients and possibly extend the use of transplantation to older patients (55 to 70 years old) who are not presently eligible for HCT procedures. Other possible indications include treatment of nonmalignant disorders and induction of tolerance for solid organ transplantation. The procedure can be performed in an outpatient setting. Although a potentially lower level of inflammatory cytokines may be present after nonmyeloablative therapies, fatal GVHD still occurs.

C. Reduced-intensity conditioning–myeloablative regimens. These regimens result in more myelosuppression than does a true nonmyeloablative regimen. They are used more frequently because most patients still have active disease

Table 5.6. Common graft-versus-host disease (GVHD) prophylactic drugs, mechanism of action, toxicity, dosage, target serum levels, and usual combination regimens

Drug	Mechanism of Action (see Fig. 5.1)	Toxicity	Dosage, Schedule	Target Serum Level	Usual Combinations
CSA	Calcineurin inhibitor	Hypertension, azotemia, tremors, TTP, hyperlipidemia, hyperglycemia, CNS	3–5 mg/kg/day, from day –3 or day –1 until day +100, taper over 3 months	100–300 ng/mL	CSA/MTX, CSA/MMF
FK-506	Calcineurin inhibitor	Same as CSA	0.002–0.03 mg/kd/day, schedule as CSA	5–10 ng/mL	FK-506/MTX, FK-506/sirolimus
MTX	Dihydrofolate reductase inhibitor	Mucositis, cytopenias, liver	5–15 mg/m² days 1, 3, 6, ±11	NA	CSA/MTX, FK-506/MTX, CSA/MMF/MTX
MMF	IMPDH inhibitor	Cytopenias, nausea, diarrhea, bowel perforation	30–45 mg/kg/day, day 0 to day +28, tapered variably	NA	CSA/MMF, CSA/MMF/MTX
Sirolimus	mTOR inhibitor	Thrombocytopenia, TTP, hyperlipidemia	12 mg PO loading dose, day –3; 4 mg PO/day, day –2 to 100, tapered over 3 months	3–12 ng/mL	FK-506/sirolimus

CSA, cyclosporine-A; TTP, thrombotic thrombocytopenic purpura; CNS, central nervous system; MTX, methotrexate; MMF, mycophenolate mofetil; FK-506, tacrolimus; NA, not applicable; IMPDH, inosine monophosphate dehydrogenase; mTOR, mammalian target of rapamycin.

that requires rapid eradication of the underlying diseases. These regimens are usually fludarabine-based combinations, with melphalan 140 to 200 mg/m^2 or busulfan. Some groups have added alemtuzumab for additional immunosuppression. In this setting, complete chimerism is rapidly achieved and antitumor responses can be expected immediately. Regimen-related mortality has been lower than expected for a high-risk population, between 30% and 40% 1 year post-transplant. These regimens may be selected for more aggressive malignancies where cytoreduction is expected to contribute to eradicating the disease.

D. Autologous transplant. In autologous transplant, non–cross-resistant cytotoxic agents with nonoverlapping extramedullary toxicities are often combined. Combination regimens of two or more agents are generally more effective than single-agent regimens; many of the newer regimens rely on the synergistic effect of alkylating agents with agents such as topoisomerase inhibitors. Immunosuppression is not required.

VII. Type of hematopoietic cell transplant

A. Allogeneic transplant is used mostly for the treatment of leukemia and other hematologic malignancies. Less than 5% of allogeneic transplants are used for nonmalignant diseases such as aplastic anemia, immunodeficiency syndromes, or hemoglobinopathies. Most adult allogeneic transplants now use PBSC more often than marrow donation from an HLA-identical sibling, unrelated donors, and mismatched family donors. Until recently, donors were identified by serologic phenotype testing for class I and class II major histocompatibility complex molecules HLA-A, -B, and -DR on lymphocytes. Mendelian inheritance predicts a 25% likelihood of identifying an HLA-identical sibling donor within a family; another 5% of patients have a one-antigen–mismatched family donor. Through the efforts of the National Marrow Donor Program (NMDP), 5 million volunteer donors and more than 45,000 unrelated cord blood units (CBUs) are available for patients without matched family members. Because of HLA polymorphism, most transplant centers now perform high-resolution HLA typing that includes HLA-C, -DRB1, and -DQ; occasionally, HLA sequence–based typing is required to confirm compatibility for both class I and class II HLA antigens. This is particularly important in evaluating potential unrelated donors. With the use of this technology, an acceptable match can be identified in 80% of white patients in the NMDP. Minorities have less chance of finding suitable unrelated donors. However, cord blood transplant is another alternative for patients who cannot find suitable unrelated donors. Most pediatric patients should be able to find one or two antigen-mismatched CBUs with adequate cell dose for transplant. The pilot data using double cord blood transplants for children and adults showed consistent engraftment for most patients. Transplantation-related mortality (TRM) rates range from 20% to 30% in HLA-identical sibling transplant recipients and are significantly higher in recipients of mismatched unrelated grafts and haploidentical grafts (40%–45%) compared with recipients of matched unrelated marrow grafts (23%). Therefore, patients who lack a closely matched family donor should be offered a phenotypically matched unrelated donor if available.

1. GVHD prophylaxis. GVHD is a serious complication after allogeneic HCT, accounting for approximately half of nonrelapse mortality causes, whereas graft rejection is uncommon (<10%). GVHD, engraftment, and graft-versus-tumor reactions are mediated by donor T cells; therefore, removing T cells from the graft (T-cell depletion) can prevent GVHD at the expense of more frequent graft failure and relapse. There is growing evidence that different T-cell subsets mediate these processes and identifying them has been considered the "Holy Grail" of HCT. Standard drugs used for GVHD prophylaxis have been cyclosporine and methotrexate, which had been shown in a randomized trial to be more effective in GVHD prevention than cyclosporine alone. Later data on tacrolimus, a newer calcineurin inhibitor, has been shown to have equal or better activity than cyclosporine and has been adopted by many, along with methotrexate, as a preferred combination. The addition of corticosteroids has not been shown to improve rates of acute GVHD, and may increase opportunistic infections. Recently, new immunosuppressive drugs have been tested in this setting. MMF is an IMPDH (inosine monophosphate dehydrogenase) inhibitor, inhibiting the *de novo* synthesis of purines; in contrast to other cells, lymphocytes are dependent on the *de novo* pathway for purine synthesis, thereby being selectively affected by MMF. The combination of cyclosporine and MMF is synergistic in animal models and has been used with success in nonmyeloablative transplants as GVHD prophylaxis; however, high rates of GVHD with this regimen were seen in conventional transplants and unrelated donor transplants. Sirolimus, an oral immunosuppressive drug that inhibits the mammalian target of rapamycin (mTOR), a critical step in the activation of T cells, has been shown to have promising GVHD prevention activity when combined with tacrolimus; this regimen has been associated with a greater risk of thrombotic microangiopathy thrombotic thrombocytopenic purpura/hemolytic uremic syndrome (TTP/HUS). A large national randomized study in patients receiving sibling transplants will compare this combination with tacrolimus plus methotrexate, considered by most to be the best standard prophylaxis. Table 5.6 lists the most commonly used immunosuppressive drug and their side effects.

2. Umbilical cord blood (UCB) transplantation. Transplantation of UCB was successfully performed for the first time in 1988 to treat a boy with Fanconi's anemia. Transplantation of unrelated UCB permits a greater degree of HLA mismatching without an unacceptably high incidence of GVHD. Graft characteristics known to allow rapid donor engraftment in recipients of conventional allografts include cell dose, CD34 content, and HLA matching. The higher primary graft failure rates and delayed donor myeloid recovery in UCB recipients are due to the low graft HSC dose, which include up to 10-fold fewer nucleated and CD34 cells as compared with adult donor grafts.

UCB graft variables that have a predictive value for time to donor myeloid engraftment include cryopreserved and reinfused total nucleated graft cell content, CD34 content, and infused colony-forming units (CFUs). Most of the published results on cord blood transplant focus primarily on pediatric patients with hematologic malignancies. Donor myeloid engraftment is delayed compared with conventional allogeneic grafts, and ranges from 22 to 30 days. The probability of donor engraftment ranges from 65% to 88%. Acute GVHD of grades II–IV has ranged from 35% to 40%, despite most receiving grafts being disparate at two or more HLA loci. High peritransplant mortality is attributed in part to delayed donor myeloid recovery. Transplant outcomes for patients allografted with related UCB has been similar or slightly better compared with unrelated UCB grafts. Data regarding cord blood transplant in adults is limited. Initially, a minimum cryopreserved UCB cell dose of 1×10^7 nucleated cells/kg recipient body weight was suggested but a high (>40%) day 100 mortality led to a higher minimum dose more than 2×10^7/kg. The majority of adult UCB recipients have received grafts mismatched at two or more HLA loci. Cord blood transplant is now accepted as an alternative stem cell source in pediatric patients with hematologic malignancies. Two recent large European and North American retrospective studies describe transplants of UCB or bone marrow from unrelated donors in adults with acute leukemia. Multivariate analysis showed UCB to yield lower risks of grade II–IV acute GVHD, but neutrophil recovery was significantly delayed. The incidence of chronic GVHD, TRM, and relapse- and leukemia-free survival were not significantly different in the two groups.

Barker and coinvestigators at the university of Minnesota had conducted a phase I clinical trial testing the safety of combined transplantation of two partially HLA-matched UCB in adult recipients using myeloablative conditioning in order to overcome the cell–dose barrier. All 21 evaluable patients engrafted at a median of 23 days (range, 15–41 days). At day 21, engraftment was derived from both donors in 24% of patients and a single donor in 76% of patients, with one unit predominating in all patients by day 100. An advantage of cord blood over adult marrow for allogeneic transplantation is that the cells are readily available in cord blood banks, are routinely typed for HLA antigens and ABO blood groups, and are tested for infectious agents. This reduces the time required to search for and identify a suitable donor, which is crucial for patients in desperate need of a transplant. The age and weight of the recipient are not obstacles, as long as the unit of cord blood contains more than 2×10^7 nucleated cells/kg of the recipient's weight at the time of collection. A simultaneous search of registries of bone marrow donors and cord blood banks for appropriate matches and adequate cell numbers should be initiated for patients without related family donors. The final choice of the source of stem cells must take into account the degree of HLA identity, the availability of the donor, the urgency of transplantation, and the number of cells in the unit of cord blood.

B. Autologous transplants and the number of centers performing them are increasing at a striking rate. Currently, most centers use autologous PBSCs as the source of HPCs to support high-dose therapy (HDT). With the advent of PBSCs and hematopoietic growth factors, the duration of marrow aplasia has been significantly shortened compared with that of autologous bone marrow transplants. Randomized trials have demonstrated that the use of PBSCs has resulted in fewer infectious complications, shorter hospitalizations, and lower costs. Many centers are performing autologous transplants in the outpatient setting.

    1. Autologous peripheral stem cell collection. PBSCs are collected by a process called *leukapheresis*. This is usually coordinated with the transplantation center's blood bank. Patients require insertion of a large-bore central venous catheter before initiation of apheresis. PBSCs are collected after mobilization by hematopoietic growth factors (e.g., granulocyte colony-stimulating factor (G-CSF) or granulocyte–macrophage colony-stimulating factor [GM-CSF]) with or without chemotherapy. Although cyclophosphamide (1.5 to 2 g/m^2) is the most common single chemotherapeutic agent reported in stem cell mobilization regimens, a number of other agents have been used either alone or in combination with cyclophosphamide or with other agents. Several investigators have found that the infusion of at least 2.5×10^6 CD34$^+$ cells/kg resulted in timely hematopoietic recovery. In addition, more recently it was observed that the infusion of at least 5.0×10^6 CD34$^+$ cells/kg was consistently associated with more predictable and rapid recovery, particularly of platelets. Most patients reach their target CD34$^+$ cell goal within two to five collections. However, in heavily pretreated patients, this minimum requirement is often difficult to achieve. AMD3100, a new selective CXCR4 (CXC chemokine receptor 4) antagonist, rapidly mobilizes CD34$^+$ cells from marrow to peripheral blood in 6 to 8 hours with minimal side effects. The addition of a single dose of AMD3100 to G-CSF produces consistent mobilization of CD34$^+$ cells in particularly poor mobilizers. More patients receiving AMD3100 reached their CD34$^+$ cell dose targets with fewer leukapheresis procedures. Clinical trials to optimize the use of AMD3100 for stem cell mobilization are ongoing.

VIII. Hematopoietic growth factors and cytokines after HCT

    A. Hematopoietic myeloid growth factors shorten the time to bone marrow or PBSC engraftment after high-dose chemotherapy. They act by binding to specific cell surface receptors, stimulating proliferation, differentiation, commitment, and selected end-cell functions. Two commercially available hematopoietic growth factors are G-CSF (filgrastim) and GM-CSF (sargramostim). For HPC mobilization with growth factors alone, most clinicians start the growth factor on day 1, with initiation of apheresis on day 5. For chemotherapy plus growth factor mobilization, the growth factor administration begins the day after completion of the chemotherapy, and apheresis commences when the peripheral blood CD34 count is more than 20 cells/μL or white blood cell count is more than 1,000. After transplantation, the growth factors are usually started after hematopoietic stem cell infusions; growth factor support is continued daily until the absolute neutrophil count is more than 3,000 for a minimum of 1 day.

B. Erythropoietin is not routinely used during the post-transplant period. It has been shown to accelerate the red cell engraftment in patients receiving ABO incompatible grafts.

C. Palifermin, a recombinant human keratinocyte growth factor, when given on three consecutive days before conditioning regimen and repeated daily for 3 days after HCT, has shown significant reductions in grade 4 oral mucositis, patient-reported soreness of mouth and throat, reductions in the use of opioid analgesics, and the use of total parenteral nutrition.

IX.   Toxicities. Toxicities of dose-intensive regimens can be formidable and life threatening. They vary considerably with the different preparative regimens, type of transplant (autologous versus allogeneic, related versus unrelated versus mismatched), and the patient's physiologic organ function and performance status. Some of the toxicities associated with transplant preparative regimens are outlined in Tables 5.2 and 5.3. As indicated, some of the toxicities are acute, whereas others are chronic. Stomatitis, esophagitis, and diarrhea can be severe with some regimens. Hepatic, renal, or pulmonary toxicities can occur in 20% to 30% of patients. Most patients require blood product support in the peri-transplant period. Central venous catheter infections or thrombosis can be problematic. Most centers use prophylactic antibiotics to prevent bacterial, viral, and fungal infections. Guidelines for the post-transplant care are covered at the end of the chapter.

A. Graft-versus-host diseases (GVHD). GVHD may occur in two different forms, known as *acute* and *chronic GVHD*, arbitrarily defined as occurring before and after 100 days post-transplant, respectively. Acute GVHD is characterized by rash, diarrhea, and elevated liver enzymes in varying degrees; chronic GVHD resembles some autoimmune disorders, frequently presenting as dry eye, lichenoid changes of the mouth and skin, sclerodermatous changes of the skin, and elevated liver enzymes. GVHD occurs in approximately 50% of all patients, varying in severity from not requiring treatment to fatal, and being more common in the elderly, in unrelated or mismatched transplants, using peripheral blood cells as opposed to bone marrow, and when donors are multiparous women.

B. Treatment of GVHD. The standard treatment for newly diagnosed acute GVHD is with prednisone or methylprednisolone, 1 to 2 mg/kg/day for 1 week, tapered gradually over several weeks/months, depending on the response. Most patients will respond to this approach; however, approximately 20% of patients will be refractory; to improve on these results, a national study is currently investigating, in a randomized fashion, the concurrent use of steroids in four different combinations as up-front therapy for acute GVHD: MMF, denileukin diftitox (Ontak), pentostatin, or etanercept. To date, no single drug or antibody has been proved of benefit in steroid-refractory acute GVHD, the mortality remaining very high. Numerous new immunosuppressive drugs and monoclonal antibodies are currently in trial, based on encouraging pilot data. Examples include purine analogs (pentostatin), antibodies targeting T-cell alloreactivity (anti CD-3 antibodies; costimulatory molecule inhibitors such as CTLA-4 and anti-CD154; anti IL-2 receptor/CD25 such as denileukin diftitox (Ontak) and daclizumab; anti-adhesion molecule antibodies such as S-1-P receptor antibodies), and anti–tumor necrosis factor (anti-TNF) antibodies such as etanercept.

The initial treatment of chronic GVHD is also with prednisone, usually with a calcineurin inhibitor. The adjunct use of MMF in that setting is currently being tested in a multicenter study. Second-line therapy has not been proved to be of benefit, but similar drugs used as in acute GVHD are being tested.

X.   Response and long-term outcomes. With a few exceptions, the goal of HDT with HSCT is to cure or substantially prolong good-quality survival. The short-term surrogate marker for improved survival or cure is complete remission. Partial remission rarely translates into important increases in survival and represents only a 1- to 3-log kill of malignant cells. Therefore, partial remission rates have little meaning in dose-intensive regimens. Less than 50% of patients with advanced malignancy obtain durable remissions with current dose-intensive regimens, stimulating major research efforts to eradicate minimal residual disease after transplantation.

A. Leukemia

1. Acute myelogenous leukemia (AML). The risk of relapse in AML varies according to the cytogenetic risk.

a. HCT is generally not recommended for patients in first complete remission with *cytogenetic favorable subtypes of AML* where the relapse probability is 35% or less. This applies to most patients with the so-called *core binding factor leukemias*—AML t(8 ; 21), AML inv(16), and acute promyelocytic leukemias with t(15 ; 17). In these conditions, the risk of procedure-related death (approximately 10%–20%) does not outweigh the potential benefit of the transplant. In the favorable-risk category, it seems **reasonable to reserve the option of an allogeneic HCT for an eventual relapse**.

b. For patients with **intermediate or poor cytogenetic risk**, the risk of leukemic recurrence after first remission is approximately 50% to 80%. Furthermore, the chance of salvage after the leukemia recurs is low. When applied as first-line postremission therapy, **allogeneic HCT represents the best option for prevention of relapse** in these patients. The low rate of relapse has been confirmed in all studies comparing allogeneic and autologous HCT but has not translated into a consistent survival advantage. When there is an HLA-matched sibling donor, allogeneic HCT should be recommended for patients in this group up to 60 to 65 years of age. With the use of reduced-intensity regimen, some investigators have raised the upper age limit to 65 to 70 years. Allogeneic HCT provides the best antileukemic effect with a probability of a 3-year survival of 61% when performed in CR1 and 48% in CR2 patients. **c.** For patients who received autologous HCT, 3-year survival probabilities in first remission were 62% in those younger than 20 years and 48% among those older than 20 years. Corresponding survival probabilities after transplantation in second remission were 48% ± 8% and 37% ± 4%. It is recommended that those patients going on to autologous HCT should receive prior intensive chemotherapy as the best method of *in vivo* purging. PBSCs collected after consolidation therapy for autologous transplants indicate a very low mortality rate and faster engraftment. For patients with unfavorable cytogenetic risk, allogeneic HCT from either a family matched donor or an unrelated donor is recommended. Recent data from a randomized EORTC/GIMEMA AML-10 trial comparing allogeneic versus autologous HCT in first remission AML showed that performing early allo-HCT led to better overall results than auto-HCT, especially for younger patients or those with bad/very bad risk cytogenetics. The role of reduced-intensity regimens before allogeneic transplantation is under active investigation; preliminary results suggest similar survival compared with conventional regimens, albeit in older and sicker patients, underscoring the lower toxicity of these regimens. Recently, a nonmyeloablative regimen of total lymphoid irradiation (TLI) and antithymocyte globulin (ATG) developed at Stanford showed very promising results for patients with AML in first remission, with very low rates of GVHD, TRM, and relapse. Larger studies are under way to confirm these results. Dose intensity may still be important in some instances (such as higher tumor burden at transplantation); one retrospective analysis showed less relapse with a reduced-intensity/myeloablative regimen compared with a truly nonmyeloablative regimen.

2. Acute lymphoblastic leukemia (ALL) is curable in 60% to 75% of affected children but in only 20% to 30% of adults. Even in high-risk patients, there are no clinical trials proving that early transplant is beneficial if complete remission is achieved with standard induction therapy. Because of the rarity of ALL in adults, few institutions have enough patients for randomized trials properly analyzed according to risk factors (e.g., CNS leukemia, high white blood cell count at presentation, male gender, hepatosplenomegaly, Philadelphia chromosome–positive [Ph+] cytogenetics, immunophenotype). Most clinicians agree, even without substantial clinical trial data, that patients with Ph+ ALL should proceed to transplant in the first complete remission. Patients who undergo transplant to consolidate the first complete remission have a 50% leukemia-free survival rate as compared with 40% in the second complete remission and beyond and 20% in relapse using HLA-identical sibling donors; again, lower rates are observed with alternative donors. Reduced-intensity regimens for ALL have been rarely reported, but a higher rate of relapse is likely, given the low GVL effect for this disease. The outcome of autologous transplantation in ALL is inferior to that of allogeneic transplants.

3. Chronic myelogenous leukemia (CML) is no longer the most common indication for allogeneic transplantation since the introduction of imatinib mesylate as a first-line therapy for CML patients. The IRIS study has shown that at 42 months, 84% of newly diagnosed CML patients treated with imatinib achieved complete cytogenetic remission (CCR) with progression-free survival (PFS) of 94%. Progression to accelerated phase or blast crisis had occurred in 6.1%, whereas 6.9% of patients had lost complete hematologic response or major cytogenetic response. Although the overall rate of progression had peaked in the second year of therapy (7.6%), the incidence of progression to advanced phase was practically constant over the years, at an average of 2% per year. Analysis of the IRIS study showed that the Sokal score (which is based on age, spleen size, and platelet and peripheral blood blast count) is well correlated with the likelihood of achieving a CCR of 91% for low-, 84% for intermediate-, and 69% for high-risk patients.

Currently, there is a debate as to whether any subgroup of patients with newly diagnosed chronic phase CML should be treated by HCT as primary therapy. It has been suggested that patients classified as "poor risk" by Sokal and good risk for allografting should be transplanted without preceding treatment with imatinib. The same has been suggested for children regardless of their Sokal score. As HCT in accelerated phase or blast crisis carries a much poorer prognosis than in chronic phase, early detection of relapse is critical. However, even meticulous monitoring will not always detect relapse early, as some patients have progressed directly to accelerated phase or blast crisis, even from CCR. Therefore, patients with a low-risk transplant option, for example, young patients with an HLA-matched sibling donor, should be informed that according to currently available data, imatinib does not eradicate leukemia, that life-long therapy is required, and that there is small risk of progression to advanced phase even in those with an excellent response and sometimes without advance warning. Most patients are now referred for transplantation after the disease has transformed to accelerated and blast crisis. Although alternative Abl kinase inhibitors show promising activity, these patients should be offered allogeneic HCT. Our recommendation is to perform HLA typing of the sibling and search for unrelated donors early in patients with high-risk Sokal score or in patients who do not achieve major cytogenetic response after 12 months of 400 mg of imatinib.

4. Chronic lymphocytic leukemia. A significant number of patients with newly diagnosed CLL are relatively young with up to 20% being younger than 55 years. Although the overall median survival for these patients is approximately the same (10 years) as for the older cohort, they are far more likely to die as a result of CLL, particularly in the presence of adverse prognostic features. These are advanced clinical stage, extensive marrow involvement, high lymphocyte count and short doubling time, CD38 positivity, and adverse genetic abnormalities (del 11q, del 17p, and/or unmutated status of the variable region of the immunoglobulin [Ig] heavy-chain gene). Approximately 60% of younger patients with CLL have progressive disease and this group has a median survival of 5 years from therapy. Autologous hematopoietic cell transplantation (HCT) is feasible in young patients with CLL and results in long-lasting clinical and molecular remissions. The transplantation-related mortality (TRM) rate is less than 10%, with complete response (CR) rates of approximately 80%; a risk-matched case–control study revealed a prolongation of survival compared with conventional therapy. However, these results have never been confirmed in prospective randomized studies, and it is becoming evident that most patients attaining complete remissions after autograft will eventually experience relapse. Previous studies have examined autologous transplantation used as salvage therapy. There are also concerns about the ability to mobilize adequate numbers of progenitor cells in patients with CLL, particularly after fludarabine therapy. The UK Medical Research Council (MRC) assessed the response to fludarabine as a first-line chemotherapeutic agent, evaluated the feasibility of progenitor cell mobilization after this treatment, and safety and efficacy of autologous stem cell transplantation in CLL patients younger than 60 years with newly diagnosed stage B, C, and progressive stage A disease. The initial response rate to fludarabine in 115 patients was 82%. Stem cell mobilization was attempted in 88 patients and was successful in 59 (67%). Overall, 65 of 115 patients (56%) entered into the study proceeded to autologous transplantation. The early TRM rate was 1.5%. The number of patients in complete remission after transplantation increased from 37% to 74%, and 63% who were not in complete remission at the time of their transplantation achieved a complete remission after transplantation. The 5-year overall and disease-free survival (DFS) rates from transplantation were 77.5% and 51.5% respectively. Sixteen of 20 evaluable patients achieved a molecular remission on a polymerase chain reaction (PCR) for Ig heavy-chain gene rearrangements in the first 6 months following transplantation. Allogeneic SCT for CLL is associated with significant morbidity and mortality, both from regimen-related toxicity and from GVHD and infection. Despite this, there is evidence that patients who survive can have long-term disease control. The Seattle Group has recently reported on 64 patients diagnosed with advanced CLL treated with nonmyeloablative conditioning with (n = 53) or without (n = 11) fludarabine, who also received a transplant from related (n = 44) or unrelated (n = 20) donors. The overall response rate in 61 evaluable patients was 67% (50% CR). The 2-year incidence of relapse/progression was 26%, whereas the 2-year relapse rate and nonrelapse mortality rate were 18% and 22%, respectively. Although the number is small, unrelated transplants resulted in higher CR and lower relapse rates than related transplants, suggesting more effective GVL activity. We recommend allogeneic transplantation with myeloablative conditioning for patients younger than 50 years. In patients between 50 and 65 years of age and in all those relapsing after an autologous transplantation, an allogeneic stem cell transplantation with a reduced-intensity conditioning regimen is offered.

B. Lymphoma

   1. Hodgkin's lymphoma. The use of autologous HCT (auto-HCT) for relapsed Hodgkin's lymphoma (HL) is now considered the standard of care. Two randomized trials showed significant benefit in freedom from treatment failure (FFTF) for auto-HCT over conventional therapy for relapsed disease. The results of these trials, together with improved tolerability of the procedure, have resulted in the recommendation of auto-HCT at the time of first relapse for even the most favorable patients. The lack of a survival benefit in these randomized trials has been attributed to patients in the nontransplant arm undergoing transplant at the time of second relapse. Investigators for the German Hodgkin Study Group (GHSG) and European Group for Blood and Marrow Transplantation (EBMT) reported on 161 patients with relapsed HL randomized to standard-dose Dexa-BEAM or high-dose BEAM and transplantation with HSCs (BEAM-HCT). Of the 117 patients with chemosensitive relapse, there was a significant improvement in 3-year FFTF for patients undergoing auto-SCT compared with 4 cycles of Dexa-BEAM (55% vs. 34%, $p = 0.019$). Three-year FFTF was significantly better for patients treated with BEAM-HCT, regardless of whether first relapse occurred *early* (<12 months) (41% vs. 12% $p = 0.007$) or *late* (>12 months) (75% vs. 44%, $p = 0.02$). A variety of preparative regimens have been reported; the BEAM, CBV, and BEAC regimens listed in Table 5.5 are the most commonly employed. In patients receiving nitrosoureas (e.g., BCNU), the clinician must pay particular attention to respiratory symptoms (dry cough, shortness of breath, hypoxia, and interstitial infiltrates on chest radiograph) 4 to 12 weeks after transplant because these symptoms are suggestive of BCNU pulmonary toxicity, a potentially fatal complication that can be reversed with prompt initiation of corticosteroids. Allogeneic HCT has been used in the past for patients relapsed after autologous HCT. A recent review of International Bone Marrow Transplant Registry/Autologous Blood and Marrow Transplant Registry (IBMTR/ABMTR) data identified 114 patients (79 NHL, 35 HD) who underwent a conventional allo-HCT (1990–1999) after failing an auto-HCT. The PFS rates at 1, 3, and 5 years of 32%, 25%, and 5%, respectively, with no difference in HL and NHL, and TRM was 21% at 100 days. The EBMT collected data on 94 patients who received reduced-intensity conditioning with allogeneic HCT (RIC-allo) for HL. Approximately 50% had failed previous autograft. Three-year OS, PFS, and TRM rates were 45%, 35%, and 18%, respectively. The only significant prognostic factor for OS and DFS was chemosensitive disease, with a median survival of less than 1 year for patients with resistant disease, although the median had not yet been reached at 2 years in patients with sensitive relapse. The role of tandem auto-HCT as well as tandem auto-HCT followed by reduced-intensity HCT is under investigation. There was a continuing risk of relapse or secondary AML and MDS for 12 years after autologous bone marrow transplant, whereas there were no cases of secondary AML/MDS or relapses beyond 3 years after allogeneic bone marrow transplant.

2. **Non–Hodgkin's lymphoma (NHL)**
   a. **Diffuse large B-cell lymphoma (DLBCL).** Autologous HCT remains the standard of care for patients with relapsed DLBCL following CHOP or similar chemotherapy, provided the disease is sensitive to second-line chemotherapy. Although there are few data to confirm the benefit of this approach in patients relapsing after rituximab-based therapy, it is likely to remain the standard. Early studies of HDT and SCT demonstrated the importance of chemosensitivity as a predictive factor for outcome after transplantation. Other favorable factors identified in many studies include initial remission duration of more than 12 months and the absence of bulky disease at the time of SCT. Poor outcome with less than 20% OS and PFS was reported in patients with age adjusted International Prognostic Index (aaIPI) score of 2 or 3 at the time of auto-HCT. Therefore, for those patients with high aaIPI scores at the time of relapse, and for those with chemorefractory disease at the time of relapse, other alternative therapy should be considered due to poor survival after auto-HCT. Commonly used second-line regimens used before auto-HCT for relapsed DLBCL include DHAP, ESHAP (etoposide, methylprednisone, cisplatin), mini-BEAM (carmustine, etoposide, cytarabine, melphalan), and ICE (ifosfamide, carboplatin, etoposide). These regimens produce CR rates of 25% to 35%. The addition of rituximab to ICE (R-ICE) increases the CR rate to 53% compared with 27% for patients treated with ICE in a previous study. The PFS after transplantation was noted to be slightly longer in patients treated with R-ICE compared with historical patients receiving ICE (54% vs. 43% at 2 years) although this did not reach statistical significance. The pilot data using high-dose yttrium 90 (^{90}Y)-ibritumomab tiuxetan in combination with high-dose BEAM and auto-HCT is effective and did not delay engraftment in patients with CD20$^+$ NHL. Allogeneic transplantation does not appear to be superior to autologous transplantation in treating intermediate-grade lymphomas. Although fewer relapses are observed after allogeneic transplant, presumably because of a graft-versus-lymphoma effect, the TRM offsets the lower relapse rate. The use of reduced-intensity regimen in NHL has increased the 1-year OS rate after allo-HCT from 23% to 67% in one study. This strategy is particularly appealing for patients who have failed previous autologous transplants,

given a very high nonrelapse mortality of more than 70% for these patients after conventional preparative regimens. A high rate of relapse of close to 50% after reduced-intensity regimens has been reported in two retrospective analyses of aggressive lymphomas, with disease sensitivity predicting for better outcome. These data provide limited insight into the potency of the GVL effect in this setting, and it remains unclear if reducing the intensity of the regimen compromises disease control. A more encouraging report with the non-myeloablative regimen of fludarabine/TBI from the Seattle Consortium for aggressive lymphomas suggests that patient selection (chemosensitive disease) may be important for successful transplantation for those patients.

b. Low-grade NHL. Chemotherapy at conventional doses for the treatment of patients with recurrent follicular NHL is likely to produce consecutive remissions of shorter duration each time. Several phase II studies suggest that salvage treatment followed by consolidation with auto-HCT can result in prolonged disease-free survival (DFS). Freedman and colleagues reported the largest single-institution experience. A total of 153 patients were treated with auto-HCT using autologous bone marrow purged *in vitro* with anti–B-cell monoclonal antibody. At a median follow-up of 5 years (range 2–13 years), the estimated 8-year DFS and OS were estimated as 42% and 66%, respectively. All trials suggested an improved median duration of PFS compared with historic controls treated with conventional chemotherapy and prolonged PFS in a fraction of patients. However, recurrence rate of more than 50% is generally observed. The German Low-Grade Lymphoma Study Group randomized patients younger than 60 years with chemosensitive indolent NHL (mostly follicular NHL) in first partial or complete remission to auto-HCT versus maintenance interferon (IFN) therapy. At a median follow-up period of 4.2 years, 27.2% relapses were observed in the auto-HCT study arm versus 60.3% in the IFN arm. The 5-year PFS was also significantly better in the auto-HCT arm (67% vs. 33%). The exact role of allo-HCT in follicular NHL is difficult to define. Allotransplant was initially used in patients thought not to be candidates for auto-HCT because of extent of disease or marrow involvement. Several retrospective studies suggest that allo-HCT is associated with a very low relapse rate and might be a curative treatment for follicular lymphoma (FL). Results from the registry data demonstrate that allogeneic bone marrow transplantation is associated with high morbidity and mortality, attributable largely to GVHD. In this patient population, however, the probability of relapse appears low, with a 50% DFS rate 5 years after transplant. This approach has the advantage of the absence of contaminating tumor cells and a graft-versus-lymphoma effect. These observations, along with cases of disease regression after DLI and withdrawal of immunosuppression, suggest a powerful GVL effect for low-grade lymphomas. Therefore, reduced-intensity regimens are an appealing strategy for these patients, and initial clinical experience confirms this, with low relapse rates (0%−21%) and treatment-related mortality (5%−30%) in single institution and registry series.

c. Mantle cell lymphoma. One area of controversy is mantle cell lymphomas. These are aggressive intermediate-grade lymphomas with a median survival of approximately 2 years using conventional therapy. There is currently no definite evidence of a survival advantage using autologous or allogeneic transplant for primary refractory disease, relapsed disease, or after the second complete remission. Few single-institution data reported event-free survival of 36% to 48% at 3 to 4 years. Blastic morphology and heavily pretreated patients are associated with worse prognosis. Few investigators reported encouraging results with the use of rituximab after auto-HCT or using an intensive-chemotherapeutic regimen, hyper-CVAD, cytarabine, and methotrexate to induce molecular remission followed by auto-HCT. Because most patients with mantle cell lymphoma relapse even after HDT, current emphasis is focused on post-transplant immunotherapy to eradicate minimal residual disease. This includes low-dose IL-2, IFNs, idiotype-specific vaccines, and dendritic cell vaccines, and intensification of the preparative regimen with radioimmunoconjugates.

The literature is limited regarding allogeneic transplantation for mantle cell lymphoma. Conventional myeloablative regimens have led to long-term survival for this disease, usually in the setting of chronic GVHD, suggesting a GVL effect. Reduced-intensity regimens for this disease have been associated with lower toxicity but the long-term disease control is still unknown.

C. Plasma cell dyscrasias

1. Multiple myeloma is an incurable B-cell malignancy that constitutes 10% of all hematologic malignancies. The treatment of multiple myeloma is rapidly evolving. Before the use of thalidomide and dexamethasone as initial treatment, the standard therapy with VAD or melphalan and prednisone resulted in a median survival of 30 to 36 months. It has been shown previously in two randomized trials that high-dose therapy (HDT) plus autologous transplant compared with standard therapy resulted in improved DFS and overall survival (OS). The use of tandem autologous transplant early in the management of multiple myeloma using total therapy I by the Arkansas group produced a CR rate of 41% and OS of 79 months. The IFM94 trial was the first randomized trial comparing single and tandem auto-HCT in multiple myeloma. The 7-year probability of event-free survival doubled from 10% to 20% with a concomitant improvement of OS from 21% to 42%. The data indicate that tandem auto-HCT improves PFS with a variable effect on OS. Two trials suggest that the second procedure provides the most benefit in patients not achieving a CR, near complete response (nCR), or very good PR (>90% reduction in serum monoclonal protein). Melphalan 200 mg/m^2 is considered standard high-dose regimen for auto-HCT in myeloma as a regimen with multiple chemotherapy and TBI produced more toxicity without increasing antitumor benefit. Post-transplant use of IFN after auto-HCT did not demonstrate an advantage of PFS or OS. The use of thalidomide and alternative agent, lenalidomide, post-AHCT is under investigation. Allogeneic transplant, in contrast, may be curative in 20% to 25% of patients but is associated with extremely high TRM rates, approaching 40% to 50% in most reports. There is no advantage of allo-HCT compared with auto-HCT. The French and Spanish group recently reported the use of reduced-intensity regimen allo-HCT performed after auto-HCT as a consolidation measure and showed higher response rate with allo-HCT compared with second auto-HCT but the TRM was greater, leading to comparable survival rates in the two groups.

2. Primary amyloidosis is a plasma cell dyscrasia associated with light-chain deposition in one or more organ systems. With standard therapy, the median survival time is 18 to 24 months, but it is less than 1 year for patients with cardiac amyloidosis. Recent reports from Boston University and the Mayo Clinic indicate that HDT with autotransplantation can effect high remission rates and improve survival rates. Changes in organ function and performance status at 1 year post-auto-HCT correlated with hematologic response. Improvement in at least one organ function was seen in 66% of patients with hematologic response. Improvements in cardiac, renal, liver, and neurologic symptoms were observed. Further improvements were seen after 1 year.

D. Myelodysplastic syndrome (MDS). MDS is a clonal disorder of HPCs. There is no effective standard therapy for this disorder. Allogeneic transplantation can produce long-term disease-free survivors: approximately 40% of patients younger than 40 years but only 15% to 20% of patients older than 40 years. The analysis of MDS transplants reported to the EBMT showed both the estimated DFS and risk at 3 years to be 36% for patients transplanted with stem cells from matched siblings. Age and stage of disease had independent prognostic significance for DFS, survival, and TRM. Patients transplanted at an early stage of disease had a significantly lower risk of relapse than patients transplanted at more advanced stages. The estimated DFS at 3 years was 25% for patients with voluntary unrelated donors, 28% for patients with alternative family donors, and 33% for patients autografted in first complete remission. The relapse rate is lowest for nonidentical related donors and highest in autologous recipients. For patients younger than 55 years with MDS, allo-HCT offers the best effective treatment. The data using a reduced-intensity regimen are encouraging but need long-term follow-up.

E. Myelofibrosis. With conventional therapies being often ineffective, with a median survival of 3 to 5 years, myelofibrosis has the worst prognosis of all the chronic myeloproliferative diseases. Recently, a report on 55 patients younger than 55 years with myelofibrosis who underwent allo-HCT indicated that 48% of the recipients of an HLA-identical transplant survived event-free at 5 years. Nevertheless, the 1-year TRM in this study was 27% in spite of the relatively young age (median 42 years) of the patients receiving transplants. Further, a recent follow-up from this same group of investigators noted only a 14% 5-year OS in a subgroup of transplant recipients older than 45 years compared with 62% for younger patients.

F. Other diseases in which HDT with transplantation has reported efficacy include aplastic anemia and MDSs. Aplastic anemia has a guarded prognosis because of the risk of infection and fatal hemorrhage. The 1-year survival rate for severe aplastic anemia is less than 20%. Allogeneic transplantation results in a long-term survival rate ranging from 50% to 90%. Favorable prognostic factors are younger age (<16 years), no prior transfusions, short interval from diagnosis to transplant, and no evidence of infection. The preparative regimen consists of immunosuppressive agents: cyclophosphamide alone or with antithymocyte globulin or with TBI. Patients who do not have a compatible sibling donor may be considered for a matched unrelated donor transplantation. Approximately 15% to 30% of patients survive with engraftment.

A new arena of clinical interest is autoimmune diseases. Although published predominantly in case reports, there appears to be clinical improvement or stabilization in disease parameters after HDT with autologous transplant for multiple sclerosis, systemic lupus erythematosus, scleroderma, and rheumatoid arthritis. Preparative regimens focus on immunosuppression with cyclophosphamide with TBI or antithymocyte globulin.

XI. Guidelines for long-term care of hematopoietic-cell transplantation survivors. Patients who survive HCT remain at greater risk than the average populations for certain diseases, most notably related to immune and endocrine dysfunction, and second malignancies. The magnitude of the problem is greater after allogeneic transplantation than after autologous transplantation, because of slower immune reconstitution and GVHD, which should be cared for by physicians knowledgeable with this complication.

A. Immune dysfunction. Understanding immune reconstitution after HCT is essential to anticipate and prevent specific infections. Risks of potential complications after stem cell transplantation correlate with immune system recovery. For practical purpose, the following are recommendations by the Center of Disease Control and Prevention together with the Infectious Disease Society of America and American Society of Blood and Marrow Transplantation. Risks of complications and treatment guidelines vary according to period after and type of stem cell transplant.

B. Pre-engraftment period (days 0–30). During the first month post-transplant, neutropenia and injury of mucosal barriers frequently lead to bacteremia, herpes simplex reactivation, and candidemia. Common bacterial organisms include mouth and gut organisms (e.g., *Streptococcus viridans*, gram-negative rods). Prophylactic antimicrobials help reduce some of these infections but emergence of resistant organisms must be considered; randomized studies proving conclusively the value of such strategies are scant.

C. Early postengraftment period, autologous transplants (after day 30) Immunologic function usually recovers rapidly after the first month post-transplantation, and prophylactic antimicrobials are not recommended except for patients with lymphoma who remain at risk for *Pneumocystis jiroveci* (formerly carinii) pneumonia (PCP) and should receive prophylaxis, preferably with trimethoprim/sulfamethoxazole, for approximately 6 months. Reactivation of Varicella zoster is common for several months after transplant; routine use of acyclovir prophylaxis is common despite lack of solid data.

D. Early postengraftment period, allogeneic transplants (days 30–100). Patients usually remain close to the transplant center during the second and third months post-transplant. Cytomegalovirus (CMV) reactivation is common during this period and is treated preemptively with ganciclovir (or foscarnet in resistant cases) when weekly screening tests become positive. Patients begin PCP prophylaxis during this time, and remain on it until immunosuppressive drugs are discontinued. Zoster and fungal prophylaxis are frequently given but data to support this practice is scant.

E. Late postengraftment period, allogeneic transplants (days >100) (Table 5.7). Patients may return closer home during this period, and local oncologists will routinely care for them. Cellular and humoral immunity defects may not fully recover for 2 years or longer following allogeneic transplant, even in the absence of immunosuppressive drugs. These defects are more pronounced in the presence of GVHD; pneumococcal sepsis remains a leading cause of death in these patients, and prophylactic antibiotics (usually daily penicillin and twice or thrice weekly trimethoprim–sulfamethoxazole) are recommended. Similarly, fevers should be treated promptly with empiric antibiotics pending culture results. Prophylactic Ig may be useful in patients who have hypogammaglobulinemia (IgG level <400 mg/dL) and recurrent respiratory infections. Fungal and viral infections are also frequent causes of death in patients with chronic GVHD; prophylactic antifungals and acyclovir are frequently given in this setting with few studies showing benefit. Patients should be re-immunized with inactivated vaccines (*Haemophilus influenzae* type B conjugate, polyvalent pneumococcal polysaccharide, diphtheria and tetanus toxoid, influenza virus, inactivated polio, and hepatitis B in patients at risk) beginning at 1 year post-transplant, and with live attenuated vaccines (measles, mumps, and rubella) at 2 months post-transplant, as long as chronic GVHD is not present.

F. Endocrine dysfunction. Hypothyroidism and hypogonadism are common complications after fractionated total-body irradiation (FTBI)-based conditioning regimens; screening for these problems is recommended 1 year post-transplant and as clinically indicated. Osteoporosis, avascular necrosis, and diabetes are common with steroid use; bone

Table 5.7. Guidelines for long-term management after hematopoietic stem cell transplantation (HCT) (>day 100 post-HCT)

Complication	Risk Factor	Prevention/Screening	Treatment	Duration of Prophylaxis /Screening
PCP	Lymphoma (auto), allo-HCT	TMP/SMT 1 tablet PO b.i.d. 2 day/week[a]	TMP/SMT	6 months or active GVHD
Varicella zoster	Auto- and allo-HCT	Acyclovir 400 mg PO b.i.d.	Acyclovir 800 mg PO 5×/day or 10 mg/kg IV 3×/day if systemic	6–12 months or active GVHD on steroids
Invasive fungal infections	GVHD, steroids	Unknown (azols commonly prescribed)	Azols, amphotericins or echinocandins	Unknown (active GVHD?)
Encapsulated organisms, respiratory infections	GVHD, splenectomy, hy-pogammaglobulinemia	TMP/SMT and/or Pen-V-K 250 mg PO b.i.d. Pooled γ-globulin if IgG <400 mg/dL	Based on susceptibility	Active GVHD or lifetime after splenectomy
Hypothyroidism	Radiation	TSH	Thyroid hormone	Annual
Hypogonadism	Radiation	FSH, LH, estrogen (women), testosterone (men)	Testosterone (men); Gynecology consult (women)	Annual for women and p.r.n. for men
Osteoporosis	Steroids, radiation	Bone densitometry	Bisphosphonates, calcium, and vitamin D	1 year and p.r.n.

Graft dysfunction (cytopenias)	Low cell dose, rejection, relapse, drugs, GVHD (infections, GVHD (platelets), ABO mismatch (red cells only), MDS after auto	CBC, platelet counts, bone marrow examination, call TC (chimerism analysis, rule out relapse and MDS after auto	Transfusions and/or growth factors; decision regarding second transplant or drug therapy per TC	Monthly first year, q3 months second year, q6 months ×5 year and yearly thereafter
Skin sensitivity, GVHD flare, skin cancer	Sun exposure	High-SPF sunscreen; physical examination; biopsy in selected cases	Call TC, usually steroids needed	p.r.n.
Dry eye	GVHD	Schirmer's test	Lubrication, punctual plugs, ophthalmologic evaluation	p.r.n.
cataracts	Steroids, radiation	Ophthalmologic examination	Surgery	1 year and p.r.n.
Dry mouth/ulcers,	GVHD	Dental hygiene, culture to rule out HSV, Candida	Saliva substitutes and stimulants; treat super-infection, call TC for topicals	p.r.n.
Interstitial pneumonitis (autologous)	BCNU, radiation	Chest x-ray, bronchoscopy	Start solumedrol 1 mg/kg/day, call TC	p.r.n., usually occurs within 3 months post-HCT

(continued)

Table 5.7. *(Continued)*

Complication	Risk Factor	Prevention/Screening	Treatment	Duration of Prophylaxis /Screening
Bronchiolitis obliterans	GVHD	PFT, high-resolution CT scan, lung biopsy in selected cases	Bronchodilators, call TC (steroids needed)	Day 100 and 1 year
Liver dysfunction	GVHD, hepatitis, iron overload, drugs	LFTs, hepatitis serologis, ferritin, ultrasound; call TC	Iron chelation if iron overload, anti-virals,[b] ursodeoxycholic acid, call TC	LFT q month ×1 year, q3 months second year, others p.r.n.
Vulvovaginal dryness/dyspareunia	GVHD, low estrogen levels	Physical examination, estrogen levels, rule out super-infection	Lubricants, topical estrogens/steroids, gynecology consult	p.r.n.
Joint stiffness, skin thickening	GVHD	Physical examination	Stretching exercises, emollients; call TC for topicals	p.r.n.

PCP, *Pneumocystis jiroveci (carinii)* pneumonia; TMP/SMT, trimethoprim–sulfamethoxazole; GVHD, graft-versus-host disease; TC, transplant center; IgG, immunoglobulin G; TSH, thyroid stimulating hormone; FSH, follicle stimulating hormone; LH, luteinizing hormone; CBC, complete blood counts; MDS, myelodysplastic syndrome; SPF, sun protection factor; HSV, herpes simplex virus; PFT, pulmonary function test; CT, computed tomography; LFT, liver function test.

[a] Atovaquone 750 mg b.i.d. or dapsone 100 mg/day for sulfa contraindication.

[b] Interferon is usually contraindicated.

density scanning should be performed at 1 year and as clinically indicated thereafter. Stress doses of steroids should also be given during acute illness for such patients.

G. Other organ dysfunction. Poor graft function is uncommon after autologous transplants; patients with grafts with low CD34 cell counts and who are heavily pretreated are at risk and may require transfusions and/or growth factors beyond 1 month; myelodysplasia should be ruled out in that setting. Allogeneic transplant recipients may have graft dysfunction from low cell dose, immunologic rejection (rare), drugs, infections (viral), GVHD (thrombocytopenia) and donor/recipient ABO mismatch (red cells only). Consultation with transplant physicians is recommended; growth factor support may be beneficial, but bone marrow biopsies are recommended to assess chimerism status and rule out relapse and myelodysplasia. Exacerbations of **skin GVHD** may occur after sun exposure in patients with GVHD and often require escalation of immunosuppression; high-SPF sunscreens and avoidance of direct sunlight are recommended. **Oral cavity dryness and ulceration** are common in chronic GVHD; twice yearly dental assessments and cleanings are recommended; exacerbations of GVHD should be discussed with transplant centers, and are usually managed with increased dose steroids, treatment of super-infections, and topical immunosuppressants. **Ocular problems** are also common, including cataracts after fractionated TBI-based regimens, and ocular sicca with chronic GVHD; in addition to aggressive lubrication with artificial tears and immunosuppressant, ophthalmologic evaluation is recommended for symptomatic patients. **Pulmonary complications** are most often related to regimen toxicity, most notably interstitial pneumonitis from BCNU and radiation, which should be treated promptly with steroids; idiopathic pneumonitis and bronchiolitis obliterans are serious complications that usually occur in the setting of GVHD and are usually managed with steroids and inhaled bronchodilators in coordination with transplant and pulmonary physicians. **Liver dysfunction** is also common in the setting of chronic GVHD; viral hepatitis and iron overload should be ruled out and managed accordingly. **Hypertension** is common with calcineurin inhibitors (CI); general guidelines to treat hypertension may be used in this setting. **Azotemia** may occur with CI and dose adjustments should be discussed with transplant centers. **Vaginal dryness** with discomfort may occur with GVHD and should be managed with lubricants, topical estrogens (if levels are low) and topical immunosuppressants.

H. Second cancers. The risk of secondary solid tumors is three times higher after allogeneic transplant than in control populations; risk factors include prior radiation, immunosuppression, and chronic GVHD. All types of malignancies have been described, but skin cancers and oral mucosa squamous cell carcinomas are most common. Avoidance of tobacco and excessive sunlight exposure are recommended. Yearly clinical assessments and other routine screening tests should be performed; the value of earlier and more frequent screening in this population is unclear. Secondary leukemia and myelodysplasia is more common after autologous transplant, with an incidence of 5% to 10%, being highest in patients exposed to alkylators, etoposide, and radiation.

XII. Future directions. The field of hematopoietic cell transplantation is evolving rapidly. Its use in the past had focused on hematologic malignancies and marrow failure. We are now starting to use stem cell transplantation to treat several autoimmune diseases and hemoglobinopathies. Indications for HCT in hematologic malignancies are also changing rapidly because of several new classes of new drugs with different mechanisms that now target molecular changes and result in better control of malignant cells. The preclinical studies showing ability of adult hematopoietic cells, umbilical cord blood, and embryonic stem cells to differentiate into osteoblasts, chondroblasts, myocytes, and neurons will potentially lead us to apply stem cell transplant in several areas of regenerative medicine in the future.

SUGGESTED READINGS

Attal M, Harousseau J-L, Facon T, et al. Single versus double autologous stem-cell transplantation for multiple myeloma. *N Engl J Med* 2003;349:2495–2502.

Barker JN, Weisdorf DJ, DeFor TE, et al. Rapid and complete donor chimerism in adult recipients of unrelated donor umbilical cord blood transplantation after reduced intensity conditioning. *Blood* 2003;102:1915–1919.

De Witte T, Hermans J, Vossen J, et al. Haematopoietic stem cell transplantation for patients with myelodysplastic syndromes and secondary leukaemias: a report on behalf of the Chronic Leukaemia Working Party of the European Group for Blood and Marrow Transplantation. *Br J Haematol* 2000;110:620–630.

Filipovich AH, Stone JV, Tomany SC, et al. Impact of donor type on outcome of bone marrow transplantation for Wiskott—Aldrich syndrome: collaborative study of the International Bone Marrow Transplant Registry and the National Marrow Donor Program. *Blood* 2001;97:1598–1603.

Freedman AS, Gribben JG, Neuberg D, et al. High dose therapy and autologous bone marrow transplantation in patients with follicular lymphoma during first remission. *Blood* 1996;88:2780–2786.

Giralt S, Estey E, Albitar M, et al. Engraftment of allogeneic hematopoietic progenitor cells with purine analog-containing chemotherapy: harnessing graft-versus-leukemia without myeloablative therapy. *Blood* 1997;89:4531–4536.

Gluckman E. Hematopoietic stem-cell transplants using umbilical-cord blood. *N Engl J Med* 2001;344:1860–1861.

Goldman J. Implications of imatinib mesylate for hematopoietic stem cell transplantation. *Semin Hematol* 2001;38(Suppl 8):28–34.

Guardiola P, Anderson JE, Bandini G, et al. Allogeneic stem cell transplantation for agnogenic myeloid metaplasia: a European Group for Blood and Marrow Transplantation, Societe Francaise de Greffe de Moelle, Gruppo Italiano per il Trapianto del Midollo Osseo, and Fred Hutchinson Cancer Research Center Collaborative Study. *Blood* 1999;93:2831–2838.

Guglielmi C, Arcese W, Dazzi F, et al. Donor lymphocyte infusion for relapsed chronic myelogenous leukemia: prognostic relevance of the initial cell dose. *Blood* 2002;100(2):397–405.

Hahn T, Wolff S, Czuczman M, et al. The role of cytotoxic therapy with hematopoietic stem cell transplantation in the therapy of diffuse large cell B-cell non-Hodgkin's lymphoma: an evidence-based review. *Biol Blood Marrow Transplant* 2001;7:308–331.

Kernan NA, Bartsch G, Ash RC, et al. Retrospective analysis of 462 unrelated marrow transplants facilitated by the National Marrow Donor Program (NMDP) for treatment of acquired and congenital disorders of the lymphohematopoietic system and congenital metabolic disorders. *N Engl J Med* 1993;328:593–602.

Khouri IF, Saliba RM, Giralt SA, et al. Nonablative allogeneic hematopoietic transplantation as adoptive immunotherapy for indolent lymphoma: low incidence of toxicity, acute graft versus host disease, and treatment related mortality. *Blood* 2001;98:3595–3599.

Körbling M, Anderlini P. Peripheral blood stem cell versus bone marrow allotransplantation: does the source of hematopoietic stem cells matter? *Blood* 2001;98:2900–2908.

Lenz G, Dreyling M, Schiegnitz E, et al. Myeloablative radiochemotherapy followed by autologous stem cell transplantation in first remission prolongs progression-free survival in follicular lymphoma - results of a prospective randomized trial of the German Low-Grade Lymphoma Study Group (GLSG). *Blood* 2004;104: 2667–2674.

de Lima M, Anagnostopoulos A, Munsell M, et al. Nonablative versus reduced-intensity conditioning regimens in the treatment of acute myeloid leukemia and high risk myelodysplastic syndrome: dose is relevant for long term disease control after allogeneic hematopoietic stem cell transplantation. *Blood* 2004;104:865–872.

Milligan DW, Fernandes S, Dasgupta R, et al. Results of the MRC pilot study show autografting for younger patients with chronic lymphocytic leukemia is safe and achieves a high percentage of molecular responses. *Blood* 2005;105:397–404.

Nademanee A, Forman S, Molina A, et al. A phase 1/2 trial of high-dose yttrium-90-ibritumomab tiuxetan in combination with high-dose etoposide and cyclophosphamide followed by autologous stem cell transplantation in patients with poor-risk or relapsed non-Hodgkin lymphoma. *Blood* 2005;106:2896–2902.

Philip T, Guglielmi C, Hagenbeek A, et al. Autologous bone marrow transplantation as compared with salvage chemotherapy in relapses of chemotherapy-sensitive non-Hodgkin's lymphoma. *N Engl J Med* 1995;333:1540–1545.

Rizzo JD, Wingard JR, Tichelli A, et al. Recommended screening and preventive practices for long-term survivors after hematopoietic cell transplantation: joint recommendations of the European Group for Blood and Marrow Transplantation, the Center for International Blood and Marrow Transplant Research, and the American Society of Blood and Marrow Transplantation. *Biol Blood Marrow Transplant* 2006;12(2):138–151.

Rocha V, Labopin M, Sanz G, et al. Acute Leukemia Working Party of European Blood and Marrow Transplant Group; Eurocord-Netcord Registry. Transplants of umbilical-cord blood or bone marrow from unrelated donors in adults with acute leukemia. *N Engl J Med* 2004;351:2276–2285.

Schmitz N, Pfistner B, Sextro M, et al. Aggressive conventional chemotherapy compared with high-dose chemotherapy with autologous haemopoietic stem-cell transplantation for relapsed chemosensitive Hodgkin's disease: a randomised trial. *Lancet* 2002;359:2065–2071.

Socie G, Curtis RE, Deeg HJ, et al. New malignant diseases after allogeneic marrow transplantation for childhood acute leukemia. *J Clin Oncol* 2000;18:348–357.

Sorror ML, Maris MB, Storer B, et al. Comparing morbidity and mortality of HLA-matched unrelated donor hematopoietic cell transplantation after nonmyeloablative and myeloablative conditioning: influence of pretransplant comorbidities. *Blood* 2004;104:961–968.

Van Besien K, Loberiza FR, Bajorunaite R, et al. Comparison of autologous and allogeneic hematopoietic stem cell transplantation for follicular lymphoma. *Blood* 2003;102:3521–3529.

Zittoun RA, Mandelli F, Willemze R, et al. Autologous or allogeneic bone marrow transplantation compared with intensive chemotherapy in acute myelogenous leukemia. *N Engl J Med* 1995;332:217–223.

SECTION III

Chemotherapy of Human Cancer

CHAPTER 6

Carcinomas of the Head and Neck

Harlan A. Pinto

The management of patients with advanced head and neck cancer is challenging because optimal outcome requires intensive and specialized evaluation, coupled with coordinated multimodality treatment, supportive care, and rehabilitation. The use of chemotherapy to treat head and neck cancer is especially challenging because there is a narrow therapeutic index, high rates of moderate to severe side effects, and only modest benefits for most patients. Nevertheless, successful management plans can be particularly rewarding, because great suffering can be ameliorated and combined modality treatment plans may allow for less disfigurement while maintaining cure as a goal for many patients.

This chapter focuses on the squamous cell carcinomas that arise from the mucosa that lines the aerodigestive tract from the lip to the esophagus and trachea. Squamous cell carcinomas that arise in this upper aerodigestive region account for approximately 5% of the new cancers seen in the United States annually. This chapter will not discuss the chemotherapy for the melanomas, lymphomas, sarcomas, major or minor salivary gland cancers, and thyroid or esophagus cancers that arise in this region.

Improvements in radiotherapy, surgery, and medical therapy often occur in isolation as we use the scientific method to isolate and test one factor at a time. In this setting the treatment options and variations in combined modality therapy have proliferated. This has underscored the need for careful patient selection, because the supportive care needs and interventions have expanded as the complexity of treatments have increased. Adverse effects in one aspect sometimes compromises improvement in another aspect of outcome. Balancing these outcomes that conflict is a major challenge to progress. In this context, quality of life has become an important focus of study but may be difficult to apply to an individual patient. This complexity means that selection of an optimal treatment plan to arrive at the best possible outcome

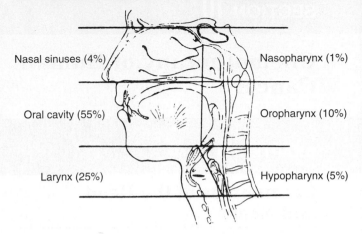

Nasal sinuses (4%)

Nasopharynx (1%)

Oral cavity (55%)

Oropharynx (10%)

Larynx (25%)

Hypopharynx (5%)

Figure 6.1. Anatomic divisions of the head and neck. Percentages indicate the relative frequencies of carcinoma in these regions.

for a specific patient should be individualized and be based on the expertise of the entire treatment team.

Understanding head and neck cancer begins with understanding the aerodigestive anatomy. A cross-sectional view of the anatomic regions and the relative frequency of cancer occurring in each area are shown in Fig. 6.1. The relationship of the anatomic structures to normal functions such as breathing, chewing, swallowing, speaking, and physical interactions related to intimacy is reflected in the anatomic recognition of site and subsite within each region. Table 6.1 lists the major sites within each of the anatomic subdivisions. Many cancers involve more than one subsite and some overlap adjacent sites. This fact has led to the use of regional terms, which can obscure factors about specific cancers that make them unsuitable for optimal outcome in regard to a specific treatment plan for surgery or radiotherapy.

I.   Common and divergent characteristics. Despite this complexity of the anatomy, squamous carcinomas of the head and neck are often considered together because they share cell type, epidemiology and risk factors, natural history, and the need for head and neck surgeons to participate in optimal evaluation and management. Male predominance (3:1), heavy tobacco and alcohol use, and onset in late middle age describe a typical patient. The median age at diagnosis ranges from 55 to 67 years, depending on the site, with nasopharynx and tonsil cancer diagnosed at a younger age and oral cavity and larynx cancer diagnosed at an older age. A relatively new phenomenon of younger patients without the characteristic history of alcohol and tobacco use has been associated with infection with human papillomavirus (HPV). Identification of this population has prognostic implications in that their risk of death from the cancer is 60% to 80% less than that of those who are HPV negative.

Patterns of spread are also similar for head and neck cancers, with detectable local extension to adjacent structures and

Table 6.1.   Upper aerodigestive tract sites

Region	Area	Site
Oral cavity	—	Lip
		Oral tongue
		Upper gum
		Lower gum
		Floor of mouth
		Hard palate
		Cheek mucosa
		Vestibule of mouth
		Retromolar area
Pharynx	Nasopharynx	Superior wall
		Posterior wall
		Lateral wall
		Anterior wall
	Oropharynx	Base of tongue
		Soft palate
		Uvula
		Tonsil, tonsillar fossa, and pillar
		Valleculae
		Lateral wall of oropharynx
	Hypopharynx	Pyriform sinus
		Postcricoid region
		Hypopharyngeal aspect of aryepiglottic fold
		Posterior wall of hypopharynx
Larynx	Supraglottis	Suprahyoid epiglottis
		Infrahyoid epiglottis
		Laryngeal aspect of aryepiglottic folds
		Arytenoid
		Ventricular band (false cords)
	Glottis	True vocal cords
		Anterior commissure
		Posterior commissure
	Subglottis	Subglottis
Nasal cavity and paranasal sinuses	Nasal cavity	Septum
		Floor
		Lateral wall
		Vestibule
	Maxillary sinus	Anteroinferior
		Superoposterior
	Ethmoid sinus	
	Frontal sinus	
	Sphenoid sinus	

lymphatic spread to regional lymph nodes occurring in many cases. For carcinomas of the oral cavity, oropharynx, and larynx, spread below the clavicle is unusual; however, pulmonary metastases are more frequent than bone or hepatic metastases. Direct extension to the mandible or the skull base may occur at diagnosis or recurrence. Most recurrences occur within 18 months of primary treatment, 90% within 2 years. Patients who are not cured usually die from the cancer within 3 to 4 years of diagnosis. The 5-year relative survival rate currently for all cases is approximately 58%, and those who succumb to the cancer generally suffer local, regional, and distant failure in equal proportions. The manifestations of end-stage disease are typified by inanition, cachexia, aspiration, respiratory difficulty due to trouble with secretions or obstruction, fistulas, oral or neck ulceration, edema of the mucosal structures or face, and pain. Among survivors, the risk of second primary head and neck, lung, and esophagus tumors is a perplexing problem.

The differences among carcinomas of the head and neck relate mostly to site, with nasopharynx cancer representing a distinct clinicopathologic entity with unique demographics, etiologic associations, and high susceptibility to radiotherapy and chemotherapy. Cancers that develop at particular sites manifest different presenting symptoms, such as hoarseness with early vocal cord cancer, pain with anterior tongue cancer, and sore throat or dysphagia with pharynx or supraglottic larynx cancer. Cancers at different sites also show clinically important differences in the development of bilateral lymph node or hematogenous metastasis, and comprehensive treatment plans take those differences into account.

II.   Primary treatment. A detailed discussion of the specific treatment options for each site and stage, and how one selects a specific treatment for a particular patient is beyond the scope of this chapter. However, a process that identifies and clarifies the goal(s) of treatment and reflects input from the patient and the treatment team members—head and neck surgeon, radiation oncologist, and medical oncologist—can yield a consensus assessment. In most cases, such a consensus can be reached and the role of chemotherapy will be clearly defined.

   A. Small lesions without regional extension are generally treated with surgery or radiation. The choice is usually related to the anticipated functional impact of the surgical deformity in relation to the expected complications of radiation. Secondary considerations of surgical risk for patients with significant comorbidities and compliance with daily radiotherapy treatments for patients with suboptimal social supports may be determinative.

   B. Larger primary cancers and those with clinically detectable spread to lymph nodes at diagnosis are usually treated with a combination of surgery and radiation, chemotherapy and radiation, or surgery, radiation, and chemotherapy. Disease that is unresectable at the outset rarely becomes resectable and most often will benefit from a combination of chemotherapy and radiation.

   C. Combined modality treatment plans have as their goal improved outcome (decreased local, regional, or distant failure rates, improved survival) or decreased morbidity. How best to combine chemotherapy, radiation and surgery, and the optimal regimen for generalized use has been the focus of clinical research for the past three decades. Only recently have the benefits of combined modality treatment from these multidisciplinary efforts been realized. The addition of chemotherapy concurrently to radiation therapy results in up to a 4% to 8% absolute improvement in survival—a 12% to 19% reduction in the risk of death, whether in definitive or postoperative settings. It has been more difficult to reproducibly demonstrate a survival benefit for induction chemotherapy. Although substantial progress has been made in improving end results for early stage lesions at many sites and in decreasing the morbidity and deformity from treatment, the outcome for tumors in advanced stages remains poor. For Stage III disease, the 3- to 5-year survival rate is 25% to 60%. For Stage IV disease, long-term survival ranges of 10% to 30% have been reported.

The good news is that many regimens and approaches yield similar results, which enables individualized patient care. This ability to individualize patient care, however, adds complexity and may lead to differences of opinion because the initial treatment is dependant on individual patient factors integrating site, stage, general health status, comorbidity, and goals of care.

III.   Staging. Pretreatment determination of disease extent is the starting point for the care of patients with head and neck cancers.

   A. TNM (Tumor, node, and metastases) classification. The American Joint Committee on Cancer (AJCC) TNM staging system integrates clinical and pathologic information on site, size, and functional consequences of the primary tumor (T), the size, number, and location of regional lymph nodes (N), and the presence of detectable distant metastases (M). The stage groupings identify patients with similar prognosis despite differences in disease extent represented by combinations of the TNM components. Table 6.2 shows the AJCC sixth edition TNM criteria and stage grouping for oral cavity cancers. Each disease site within the head and neck region has its own criteria and so reference to these prognostic groups is an essential part of the staging process. The TNM criteria for head and neck cancer recognize the adverse prognosis conferred by initial extent of disease that precludes complete surgical resection.

   B. Stage grouping. The stage grouping for head and neck cancers is shown in Table 6.3. Stages I and II are determined by the size of the tumor in the absence of nodal involvement or distant metastases. Stage III includes both large tumors and tumors of any size with early regional node involvement. Stage IV lesions may be huge with local extension or may be of any size with distant metastatic disease. This stage grouping has been applied to each tumor site to demonstrate gradations in prognosis.

IV.   Chemotherapy. Chemotherapy has many roles in the treatment of head and neck cancer, and the selection of agents and regimens are tailored to the specific role. Chemotherapy is often used to palliate patients with locally recurrent or metastatic

Table 6.2.   TNM Staging System for Carcinomas of the Oral Cavity

Primary tumor

TX	Primary tumor cannot be assessed
T0	No evidence of primary tumor
Tis	Carcinoma *in situ*
T1	Tumor 2 cm or less in greatest dimension
T2	Tumor >2 cm but not more than 4 cm
T3	Tumor >4 cm in greatest dimension
T4a	Tumor invades adjacent structures, e.g., through cortical bone, into deep extrinsic muscle of the tongue, maxillary sinus, skin of face
T4b	Tumor invades masticator space, pterygoid plates, or skull base and/or encases internal carotid artery.

Regional nodal status

NX	Regional lymph nodes cannot be assessed
N0	No regional lymph node metastasis
N1	Metastasis in a single ipsilateral node 3 cm or less in greatest dimension
N2a	Metastasis in a single ipsilateral node >3 cm but not more than 6 cm in greatest dimension
N2b	Metastasis in multiple ipsilateral nodes, none >6 cm in greatest dimension
N2c	Metastasis in bilateral or contralateral lymph nodes, none >6 cm in greatest dimension
N3	Metastasis in a lymph node >6 cm in greatest dimension

Distant metastasis

MX	Distant metastasis cannot be assessed
M0	No distant metastasis
M1	Distant metastasis

disease, and it is frequently used as a radiation sensitizer in simultaneous chemoradiation programs, either as initial treatment or following surgery. Less frequently, chemotherapy is used before radiation or surgery as initial treatment in a "neoadjuvant" or "induction" role or as a single adjuvant modality after surgery or radiation.

The benefits of chemotherapy are always considered in relation to the expected chemotherapy-related adverse effects. Chemotherapy added to radiotherapy clearly improves outcome in patients with nasopharynx cancer, unresectable disease, and in patients with resected tumors and adverse pathologic findings. Recently, improvements in supportive care have allowed for the development of more intensive and complex chemotherapeutic regimens. Although antitumor responses have improved, other measures of benefit are more difficult to demonstrate consistently. The routine use of more intensive and complex regimens necessitates careful patient selection and aggressive supportive care interventions. A commitment to aggressively

**Table 6.3. Stage Grouping
for Carcinomas of the Oral
Cavity, Pharynx,
Hypopharynx, Larynx, and
Paranasal Sinuses**

Stage	Groups
0	Tis, N0, M0
I	T1, N0, M0
II	T2, N0, M0
III	T3, N0, M0
	T1 or T2 or T3, N1, M0
IVa	T4a, N0 or N1, M0
	T1–4a, N2, M0
IVb	T4b, any N, M0
	Any T, N3, M0
IVc	Any T, any N, M1

manage toxicity goes hand in hand with the use of regimens that have substantial rates of severe or life-threatening side effects.

A. Predictive factors. The top three predictive factors for antitumor response include stage group, performance status, and prior treatment. Table 6.4 lists factors identified as having a positive or negative influence on the response to chemotherapy.

1. Stage group. Small tumors with minimal regional node involvement respond more reliably (completely) to chemotherapy compared with larger tumors with extensive large regional nodes. Response rates are lowest for pulmonary or visceral metastases.

2. Performance status. Poor performance status shifts the balance toward increased toxicity, and the ability to deliver treatment is often compromised. Excellent performance status facilitates treatment and is correlated positively with response and survival. Because intensive and complex regimens select patients with excellent performance status, they may appear to represent an improvement.

3. Prior treatment. Head and neck cancers previously treated with surgery or radiation or both respond less frequently than patients treated initially with chemotherapy. This marked difference has fueled enthusiasm for neoadjuvant treatment programs. The failure to respond to radiation and a rapid recurrence after radiation have also been shown to affect response rates adversely.

4. Human papillomavirus–associated cancers. These squamous cell cancers have a better outcome.

B. Patient assessment. The initial assessment focuses on disease extent and treatment goals; that process will determine the role of chemotherapy and thereby the suitable regimens and chemotherapeutic agents. Chemotherapeutic drugs used

Table 6.4. Factors Prognostic for Response to Chemotherapy

Favorable	Unfavorable
Stage III	Stage IV
No metastasis	Pulmonary metastasis
ECOG performance status 0–1 (Karnofsky performance status 70 or more)	ECOG performance status 2–3 (Karnofsky performance status 60 or less)
No weight loss	Weight loss
Normal immune mechanism	Impaired delayed hypersensitivity
Prior surgery	Prior irradiation
Long disease-free interval	Short disease-free interval
No prior chemotherapy	Prior chemotherapy
Combination chemotherapy	Single-agent chemotherapy
Poorly differentiated tumor	Well-differentiated tumor
Nasopharynx	Other sites
Age <70 year	Age >70 year

ECOG, Eastern Cooperative Oncology Group.

in head and neck cancer affect the bone marrow, kidneys, peripheral nerves, mucosal integrity, and fertility. A careful medical history, systems review, physical examination, and complete laboratory evaluation are the next steps, and will help define areas of special concern for particular patients. Evaluation of the patient's (1) ability to perform self-care functions related to hydration and nutrition, (2) pain management, and (3) type and extent of social support is also essential. Attention to nutritional support is required from the outset as many patients have undergone a period of impaired nutrition during the diagnostic and staging process. Education on self-care as well as caregiver education is especially important if toxicity is to be minimized and successfully managed. The oncologist must evaluate and monitor several specific systems initially and during treatment:

1. Bone marrow function. Chronic alcoholism, malnutrition, and tumor-related weight loss contribute to a significant incidence of folate deficiency and decreased bone marrow reserve in many patients. Careful evaluation of baseline anemia or thrombocytopenia calls for proactive plans to carefully monitor and support granulocytes, red cell mass, and platelets.

2. Pulmonary function. Current or distant heavy smoking increases the likelihood of chronic obstructive pulmonary disease (COPD) and chronic bronchitis, leading to an increased risk of pulmonary infection during treatment. Impaired pulmonary reserve coupled with a propensity for aspiration related to tumor effects on swallowing or the clearing of secretions make it important to assess, monitor, and assist with airway issues and respiratory complaints.

Smoking cessation, mucolytics, home suction, nasogastric or gastrostomy tube feedings, and tracheostomy and tracheostomy care are all important adjuncts. Taxanes, cetuximab, tyrosine kinase inhibitors, and bleomycin may lead to acute or chronic pulmonary toxicity; therefore careful baseline assessment and monitoring is indicated.

3. Renal function. Platinum compounds are first-line agents for most patients with head and neck cancer. Adequate baseline renal function, hydration and continued monitoring of renal function is needed to administer these agents safely and prevent renal failure. Methotrexate is also a useful agent, and renal impairment causes decreased excretion and prolonged exposure of normal tissues, resulting in increased toxicity.

4. Hepatic function. The presence of cirrhosis, whether related to alcoholism or viral hepatitis, can complicate management, as it can impair the ability to accomplish forced hydration by leading to third-space accumulations of ascites or edema. Cytopenias may accompany congestive splenomegaly, and baseline diuretic use may exacerbate treatment-related electrolyte abnormalities.

5. Neuropathy. Significant peripheral or autonomic neuropathy may complicate alcoholism or diabetes, and may need careful assessment and monitoring related to the use of platinum compounds and taxanes, especially in combination. Occupational, recreational, and age-related hearing loss occur commonly, and a baseline hearing test is often indicated if cisplatin is to be included in the treatment plan.

6. Fertility. All chemotherapeutic agents may impair fertility either temporarily or permanently. For men who wish to ensure their reproductive capacity, sperm donation should be accomplished promptly. For women, induced ovulation and harvest and preservation of ova may delay chemotherapy and radiation, and for such patients it may be preferable to favor a treatment plan that begins with surgery.

7. Concomitant drugs. Antihypertensives, diuretics, and drugs used for glycemic control all need careful assessment, monitoring, and adjustment during therapy as patients undergo chemotherapy for head and neck cancer. Nausea, vomiting, anorexia, and limited oral intake often lead to substantial dehydration and weight loss, making hypotension a common occurrence during therapy. The use of glucocorticoids as an adjunct to antiemetics and to prevent anaphylactic reactions, coupled with irregular feeding patterns make glycemic control elusive. It is best to emphasize careful monitoring to avoid hypoglycemia, rather than focus on hyperglycemia that is not metabolically (homeostatically) significant.

C. Chemotherapeutic agents. Table 6.5 lists the response rates for chemotherapeutic agents primarily derived from studies palliating recurrent head and neck cancer. Treatment of recurrent or metastatic head and neck cancer with chemotherapy has been shown to improve survival compared with best supportive care, and single agents or combinations can lead to antitumor responses in 20% to 50% of patients. Median

Table 6.5. Response Rate for Single Chemotherapy Agents in Recurrent Head and Neck Cancer

Agent	Response Rate
Methotrexate	10%–50%
Cisplatin	9%–40%
Carboplatin	22%
Paclitaxel	40%
Docetaxel	34%
Fluorouracil	17%
Bleomycin	21%
Ifosfamide	23%
Vinorelbine	20%
Irinotecan	21%
Cetuximab	12%
Gefitinib	10%
In nasopharynx cancer	
Gemcitabine	13%–37%
Capecitabine	23%
Doxorubicin	39%

survival is 6 to 9 months and seems most related to performance status, disease extent, and prior therapy rather than the regimen selected.

1. Cisplatin. Cisplatin is the backbone of many head and neck cancer regimens. There is little enthusiasm for its use as a single agent to treat recurrent disease, because the single-agent response rate is comparable to other drugs in this clinical setting, and the supportive care needs and toxicity may be higher than with other single agents. Significant acute and delayed nausea and vomiting require aggressive antiemetics including serotonin subtype 3 (5-hydroxytryptamine-3 [5-HT3]) receptor antagonists (ondansetron, granisetron, dolasetron, palonosetron), glucocorticoids (dexamethasone or methlyprednisolone), and neurokinin 1 (NK-1) receptor antagonists (aprepitant) for optimum control. These antiemetics have made outpatient high-dose cisplatin feasible for most patients. Cisplatin 60 to 100 mg/m^2 IV given once every 3 weeks preceded by 1 to 2 L of hydration, mannitol 12.5 to 25 g, and 1 to 2 L of postcisplatin hydration with mannitol and/or furosemide 10 to 20 mg to maintain urine output is a standard regimen. Adequate replacement of potassium, magnesium, and sodium losses is needed, and monitoring with hydration as needed for 1 or 2 days after outpatient administration can avoid the serious cycle of nausea and vomiting leading to dehydration, electrolyte abnormalities, and renal failure. The total dose can be divided over 3 to 5 days and is better tolerated by some patients, but it does not alter the need for aggressive antiemetics and hydration.

2. Carboplatin. Carboplatin is easier to administer than cisplatin because there is no requirement for forced hydration, and less nausea and vomiting, less renal toxicity, ototoxicity, and neuropathy. Dosing incorporates renal function by use of the Calvert formula where the calculated dose in milligrams equals the (creatinine clearance +25) multiplied by an area under the curve (AUC) factor of 5 or 6. Response rates comparable to single-agent cisplatin are reported but myelosuppression, in particular thrombocytopenia, can be dose limiting. This is less suitable for ulcerated mucosa or neck lesions where bleeding may already be a management issue.

3. Paclitaxel. Paclitaxel 175 to 250 mg/m^2 over 3 hours every 3 weeks with filgrastim (G-CSF) support is an aggressive standard single-agent dose. A response rate of 15% to 40% has been reported but enthusiasm is limited because of the risk of neutropenia and neuropathy. Premedication with glucorticoids (dexamethasone 10–20 mg) 12 hours, 6 hours, and immediately before paclitaxel administration, together with histamine H_1- and H_2-receptor antagonists (diphenhydramine 50 mg and cimetidine 300 mg or famotidine 20 mg) are used to minimize anaphylactic reactions.

4. Docetaxel. Docetaxel 75 to 100 mg/m^2 IV over 1 hour every 3 weeks or docetaxel 30 to 40 mg/m^2 IV over 1 hour weekly for 4 of 5 weeks or 3 of 4 weeks may be used. Dexamethasone 8 mg twice a day for 3 days—1 day before, on the treatment day, and on the day following docetaxel infusion—generally controls allergic reactions and fluid accumulations. Marrow suppression may require filgrastim support with the higher doses. Caution must be exercised when administering to patients with fluid accumulation or any hepatic dysfunction. Neuropathy may be lower than with paclitaxel but asthenia may be greater with the high-dose regimen.

5. Methotrexate. Methotrexate doses of 40 to 60 mg/m^2 IV weekly given over 15 minutes is a convenient standard single-agent treatment. Response rates and survival are comparable to combination therapy. Dose escalation can increase response rates but is accompanied by increased toxicity and does not improve survival. Minimal to moderate nausea and few significant acute side effects make this a well-tolerated and easily monitored treatment. Careful assessment of renal function, nutritional status, and volume status, are important however, because renal impairment, folate deficiency, and third-space fluid collections (pleural effusions, ascites, edema) can lead to severe toxicity. Responses may occur after 1 or 2 weeks of treatment but usually require 4 to 8 weeks of treatment so patience is needed before abandoning this regimen. Mucositis and bone marrow suppression are the most common side effects encountered. Leucovorin 10 mg PO q6 hours × 6 or more doses starting 24 hours after methotrexate can help ameliorate these problems when they develop in responding patients who continue treatment.

6. Fluorouracil. Fluorouracil is well tolerated and has comparable activity to cisplatin and other single agents.

It is most often given as a 4- or 5-day continuous infusion. Common side effects include mucositis, diarrhea, and bone marrow suppression. The drug is a vascular irritant at high concentrations and therefore, for prolonged infusions, a central venous catheter or access device is customary. Although suitable for use as a single agent, it is most often used in combination with other drugs.

7. Ifosfamide. Ifosfamide 1,000 mg/m^2/day IV over 2 hours × 4 days every 3 to 4 weeks yields response rates of 20% to 40%. The need for uroprotection with mesna 200 mg/m^2 before and 400 mg/m^2 after ifosfamide makes this a cumbersome single-agent regimen to administer. Bone marrow toxicity can be significant and often requires filgrastim support.

8. Bleomycin. Bleomycin is useful in head and neck cancer because of antitumor activity comparable to other agents without associated myelosuppression or nausea. Bleomycin 10 to 30 units/m^2 IM or IV can be given weekly, every 2 weeks, or 5 days a month. Mucositis is commonly seen and responses are often very brief. Pulmonary toxicity is a significant problem when cumulative doses reach the range (400 units) in which responses typically occur.

9. Gemcitabine. Gemcitabine 1,000 mg/m^2 weekly has activity in nasopharynx cancer and is well tolerated. Bone marrow toxicity is the major adverse effect.

10. Cetuximab. Cetuximab is a monoclonal antibody that binds to epidermal growth factor receptors, which are overexpressed in more than 90% of head and neck squamous cell carcinomas. The standard regimen begins with a loading dose of Cetuximab 400 mg/m^2 IV given over 2 hours followed by weekly doses of 250 mg/m^2 IV over 1 hour. Responses of up to 10% have been observed among cisplatin-resistant patients. Skin rash and diarrhea are the common side effects. Allergic reactions are preventable in most cases with diphenhydramine 50 mg premedication. Interstitial pneumonitis is rare but can be life threatening or fatal. Cisplatin-based combinations with cetuximab have reported a higher response rate compared with single-agent cisplatin.

11. Tyrosine kinase inhibitors. Erlotinib 150 mg orally once a day and gefitinib 250 to 500 mg orally once a day have been shown to result in a response rate of 10% among patients who have failed prior cisplatin chemotherapy. The high dose of gefitinib appears to be more active than the lower dose in head and neck cancer, and although no longer commercially available, gefitinib remains under active investigation in combination with other agents and radiation therapy. Other tyrosine kinase inhibitors are also under investigation.

12. Anthracyclines. Doxorubicin and mitoxantrone are useful in nasopharynx cancer, which is very responsive to multiple agents; many patients are younger with good performance status so that they often tolerate and respond to multiple sequential treatment regimens. These agents have utility in that setting.

13. Vinca alkaloids. Vincristine and vinblastine have low single-agent response rates and are generally not used. Vinorelbine 30 mg/m² weekly is reported to produce 8 to 16% response rate.

D. Combination chemotherapy. The basic principle of combination chemotherapy is to combine agents with complementary or synergistic mechanisms of action and non-overlapping toxicity for improved antitumor response and outcome. Many chemotherapy combinations have been tested in head and neck cancer and have come to be utilized for the palliation of recurrent and metastatic disease, in simultaneous chemoradiation treatment programs, and in neoadjuvant treatment regimens. In general, response rates are improved with combinations but survival has not been shown to be better than that obtained with several single agents. Toxicity is usually greater, and therefore combination therapy is most appropriate for patients with an Eastern Cooperative Oncology Group (ECOG) performance status of 0 or 1. The goal of treatment and the clinical setting help select the most appropriate regimen for the particular patient. Simpler regimens are often favored; however, patient factors frequently make the most effective of the simpler drug regimens problematic. The most commonly used combinations used are listed in Table 6.6. Selected regimens for palliation, neoadjuvant therapy, or concurrent chemoradiotherapy are shown in Table 6.7.

1. Cisplatin and fluorouracil. Cisplatin 75 to 100 mg/m² is given intravenously over 1 to 4 hours on day 1 and fluorouracil 600 to 1,000 mg/m²/day is given as a 96-to 120-hour continuous infusion for 4 or 5 days. Forced hydration, aggressive antiemetics, and close monitoring for electrolyte abnormalities, mucositis, dehydration, and cytopenias are needed. Recently, it had been appreciated that significant rates of neutropenia accompany this regimen and that these patients may benefit from filgrastim and prophylactic antibiotics. When this regimen is used during or after prior radiotherapy, only 4 days (96 hours of continuous infusion) of fluorouracil are used because of enhanced mucosal and skin toxicity in that setting.

Table 6.6. Response Rate for Combination Chemotherapy Agents in Recurrent Head and Neck Cancer

Agents	Approximate Response Rate
Cisplatin/fluorouracil	25%–40%
Carboplatin/fluorouracil	26%
Cisplatin/paclitaxel	28%–35%
Cisplatin/docetaxel	42%
Cisplatin/cetuximab	26%
Methotrexate/bleomycin/cisplatin	48%
Paclitaxel/ifosfamide/carboplatin	55%
In nasopharynx cancer	
Gemcitabine/paclitaxel	41%

Table 6.7. Selected Drug Treatment Programs in Head and Neck Cancer

Intent	Suitability	Scheme
Palliation	Any prior treatment	Either Cisplatin 20 mg/m^2 IV on days 1–5 *or* cisplatin 100 mg/m^2 day 1
		and
		fluorouracil 800–1000 mg/m^2/day as 24-h infusion on days 1–4 by ambulatory infusion pump
		or
		carboplatin AUC 5–6 on day 1 *and*
		fluorouracil 800–1000 mg/m^2/day as 24-h infusion on days 1–4 by ambulatory infusion pump
		or
		paclitaxel 135 mg/m^2 IV day 1 and cisplatin 75 mg m^2
		or
		docetaxel 75 mg/m^2 day 1 *and* cisplatin 75 mg/m^2 day 1
		Cycle repeats in 3–4 weeks
		Paclitaxel 175 mg/m^2 as 3-h infusion on day 1 with steroid premedication and carboplatin AUC 6 on day 1
		Cycle repeats in 4 weeks
		Methotrexate 40–60 mg/m^2 IV weekly *or*
	Prior treatment and contraindications to combination drugs	paclitaxel 175–200 mg/m^2 IV every 3 weeks with steroid premedication, *or*
		docetaxel 75–100 mg/m^2 over 1 h with steroid premedication every 3 weeks or
		docetaxel weekly 35 mg/m^2 day 1 on 3 of 4 weeks.
		Cycles repeat every 28 days
	Refractory to cisplatin	Cetuximab 400 mg/m^2 IV day 1 then 250 mg/m^2/week
Concurrent radiotherapy	Advanced stage, no prior treatment	Daily radiation therapy together with either:
		cisplatin 100 mg/m^2 IV on day 1 with induced diuresis, repeat day 22, 43, *or*

Table 6.7.   **(*Continued*)**

Intent	Suitability	Scheme
		carboplatin 70 mg/m² on day 1–4 *and*
		fluorouracil 600 mg/m²/day as 24-h infusion on day 1–4 by ambulatory infusion pump; repeat days 23, 43
		or
		hydroxyurea 1,000 mg PO Q 12 h for 11 doses *and*
		fluorouracil 1,000 mg/m²/day as 24-h infusion on days 1–4 by ambulatory infusion pump
		or
		twice a day radiotherapy with either
		cetuximab 400 mg/m² day 1 then 250 mg/m² weekly
		or
		cisplatin 12 mg/m² IV on days 1–5 with induced diuresis, repeat days 35–40 *and*
		fluorouracil 600 mg/m²/day as 24-h infusion on days 1–5 by ambulatory infusion pump; repeat days 35–40
Neoadjuvant (Induction) chemotherapy	Advanced stage, no prior treatment, concomitant chemoradiation contraindicated	CF Cisplatin 100 mg/m² IV on day 1 with induced diuresis *and* fluorouracil 1,000 mg/m²/day as 24-h infusion on days 1–5 Cycle repeats in 3–4 weeks *or* TPF Docetaxel 75 mg/m² day 1 cisplatin 100 mg/m² day 1, fluorouracil 1000 mg/m²/day as 24-h infusion days 1–4 (96 h)

2.   Carboplatin and fluorouracil. Carboplatin 300 mg/m² IV on day 1 and fluorouracil 1,000 mg/m²/day by continuous infusion for 4 days are used for recurrent disease with responses and survival comparable to cisplatin and fluorouracil. For simultaneous chemoradiation in oropharynx cancer, carboplatin 70 mg/m² IV daily for 4 days and fluorouracil 600 mg/m² daily by continuous infusion (96 hours) for 4 days is a standard regimen. These regimens predate the use of the Calvert formula but roughly correspond to an AUC of 5 and AUC of 1.25 respectively.

3.   Cisplatin and paclitaxel. Cisplatin 60 mg/m² IV and paclitaxel 135 to 175 mg/m² IV every 3 weeks were found to be equivalent to fluorouracil regimens in patients with recurrent disease. The lower dose of paclitaxel was better tolerated. Careful monitoring for neuropathy is needed.

4. Carboplatin and paclitaxel. Carboplatin AUC 6 and paclitaxel upto 175 mg/m^2 given every 3 weeks is a widely utilized combination regimen with similar results.

5. Cisplatin and docetaxel. Cisplatin 75 mg/m^2 IV and docetaxel 75 mg/m^2 IV each on day 1 every 3 weeks. Frequent neutropenia is seen in this regimen.

6. Cisplatin, methotrexate, and bleomycin is an older combination regimen found to have superior response compared with methotrexate. Cisplatin-induced renal impairment can lead to profound toxicity if methotrexate excretion is prolonged.

7. Paclitaxel and gemcitabine. This non-cisplatin combination is useful in patients with recurrent nasopharynx cancer, most of whom are heavily pretreated with cisplatin.

8. Paclitaxel, ifosfamide, and carboplatin is a three-drug regimen with high activity and is well tolerated but requires good performance status of patients and filgrastim support.

E. Chemotherapy as a radiation sensitizer. Simultaneous chemoradiation was first demonstrated to be beneficial in nasopharynx cancer. It has subsequently been shown to improve survival among other patients with unresectable disease, to positively contribute to organ preservation in advanced larynx cancer, and to improve outcome following surgery where a positive margin, spread through the lymph node capsule, and multiple positive nodes are found. As indicated in the preceding text in Section II, the addition of chemotherapy concurrently to radiation therapy results in up to a 4% to 8% absolute improvement in survival—a 12% to 19% reduction in the risk of death, whether in definitive or postoperative adjuvant settings. Simultaneous chemoradiation is also effective in treating paranasal sinus cancer (by either intra-arterial or intravenous route) where surgery is not recommended. Although many regimens have been tested in these various settings, the high-dose cisplatin regimen has been most consistently effective. A variety of radiotherapy treatment programs have been tested with chemotherapy, therefore it is also important to clarify what radiotherapy regimen will be utilized when selecting chemotherapy for concomitant treatment.

1. Cisplatin 100 mg/m^2 IV over 1 to 4 hours every 21 days during radiation. This regimen has been shown to be effective in improving survival compared with radiotherapy alone in nasopharynx cancer, for organ preservation in larynx cancer, and as adjuvant chemoradiation for patients with adverse prognostic factors after surgery. The Radiation Therapy Oncology Group (RTOG) demonstrated 83% organ preservation rate in larynx cancer, and the European Organization for Research and Treatment of Cancer (EORTC) and RTOG demonstrated a benefit when cisplatin was given with postoperative radiation for patients with positive margins, extracapsular lymph node extension or multiple involved nodes. Weekly regimens using lower-dose cisplatin have yielded conflicting results.

2. Carboplatin and fluorouracil. For simultaneous chemoradiation in oropharynx cancer, carboplatin 70 mg/m² IV daily for 4 days and fluorouracil 600 mg/m² daily for 4 days by continuous infusion (96 hours) is a standard regimen.

3. Cetuximab 400 mg/m² IV day 1 as a loading dose followed by 250 mg/m² IV weekly during radiation is an effective radiosensitizer. Most patients are treated with twice-a-day radiation or a concomitant boost radiation schedule. There is improved survival as compared with radiation alone. This regimen has a very good toxicity profile.

4. Cisplatin and fluorouracil. Cisplatin 60 to 75 mg/m² IV day 1 and fluorouracil 600 to 1,000 mg/m² daily for 4 days by continuous 96-hour infusion is a standard regimen with single fraction or hyperfractionated radiation. Mucosal toxicity is significant.

5. Hydroxyurea and fluorouracil (HFX). The combination of hydroxyurea 1,000 mg orally every 12 hours for 11 doses and fluorouracil 800 mg/m² daily for 5 days given as a 120-hour intravenous infusion repeated every 14 days for 5 cycles concomitantly with radiotherapy for 5 days every 14 days is an effective non-cisplatin regimen. This regimen significantly prolongs treatment time as treatment including radiotherapy is administered every other week. It may be feasible for selected patients.

6. Cisplatin and paclitaxel. Cisplatin 20 mg/m² weekly and paclitaxel 30 mg/m² weekly during standard fractionated radiation.

7. Paclitaxel. Paclitaxel 20 to 40 mg/m² given over 1 hour weekly during radiotherapy has been tested. Mucosal toxicity, which may be delayed, is dose limiting.

8. Paclitaxel, hydroxyurea, and fluorouracil (THFX) may be given on alternating weeks during simultaneous chemoradiation. This is an active non-platinum regimen found to be effective but requiring breaks in radiotherapy and aggressive supportive care. It is feasible but complex.

F. Neoadjuvant chemotherapy. Response rates are much higher for patients who have had no prior treatment than for those who have been treated with prior surgery, radiation, or both. Therefore the development of combination regimens for use in induction or neoadjuvant treatment programs continues to attract interest.

The initial demonstration that organ preservation could be accomplished by substituting chemotherapy for surgery led to widespread adoption of neoadjuvant approaches. In particular, this approach was demonstrated to be comparable to surgery in patients who would require total laryngectomy for larynx cancer, hypopharynx cancer, or functionally morbid oropharynx cancer. Treatment for 6 to 9 weeks (two to three cycles) is usually given to induce an antitumor response. Partial and complete responders can be treated with radiotherapy or chemoradiotherapy. Surgery can be integrated for nonresponders and those with persistent or recurrent disease. Only regimens containing cisplatin and fluorouracil have been found to improve survival. This strategy is equivalent to surgery and radiation in resectable larynx and hypopharynx cancer where total laryngectomy is the recommended surgical option. Simultaneous cisplatin and radiotherapy is superior for organ preservation but not for survival in larynx cancer. Simultaneous chemoradiotherapy also appears to be superior for unresectable disease. Separating chemotherapy and radiation may be appropriate for selected patients who may not tolerate the simultaneous regimens well, but simultaneous regimens are currently preferred when feasible. Taxanes added to cisplatin and fluorouracil appear to be more active. Current investigational approaches are exploring neoadjuvant chemotherapy followed by chemoradiation in an attempt to improve survival outcome by maximizing chemotherapy to reduce distant metastases.

   1. Cisplatin and fluorouracil. Cisplatin 100 mg/m^2 IV on day 1 and fluorouracil 1,000 mg/m^2 as a 24-hour continuous IV infusion on days 1 to 5 every 21 days for three cycles. This is the standard regimen for neoadjuvant chemotherapy.

   2. Docetaxel, cisplatin, and fluorouracil. Docetaxel 75 mg/m^2 IV on day 1, cisplatin 100 mg/m^2 IV on day 1, and fluorouracil 1,000 mg/m^2 IV daily on days 1 to 4 (96 hour continuous infusion) every 3 weeks for 3 cycles. This regimen requires prophylactic fluoroquinolone antibiotics.

   3. Paclitaxel, cisplatin, and fluorouracil. Paclitaxel 175 mg/m^2 IV on day 1, cisplatin 100 mg/m^2 IV on day 2, and fluorouracil 500 mg/m^2 daily for 5 days by continuous infusion (120 hours) every 3 weeks for 3 cycles.

   4. Paclitaxel, ifosfamide, and carboplatin. Paclitaxel 175 mg/m^2 IV on day 1, ifosfamide 1,000 mg/m^2 IV on days 1 to 3 (with intravenous mesna 200 mg/m^2 IV before and 400 mg/m^2 IV after ifosfamide), and carboplatin IV at AUC 6. This is repeated every 3 to 4 weeks for two to four cycles. Filgrastim is recommended, given the 9% risk of febrile neutropenia.

   5. Carboplatin and paclitaxel. Carboplatin IV at AUC 2 on day 1 and paclitaxel 135 mg/m^2 IV on day 1 weekly for 6 weeks is a simple outpatient regimen with acceptable response rate. Neutropenia is seen in 18% of patients, but febrile neutropenia is uncommon.

G. Adjuvant chemotherapy. Adjuvant chemotherapy is part of the standard regimen for nasopharynx cancer. Patients are given two or three cycles of cisplatin 80 mg/m^2 IV and fluorouracil 1,000 mg/m^2 daily for 4 days by continuous infusion following initial chemoradiation using cisplatin as a single agent. It is poorly tolerated and has not been isolated by testing apart from the initial simultaneous chemoradiation. Several older phase III studies of adjuvant chemotherapy showed no benefit, although these studies were limited by small sample size, as well as by poor tolerance and compliance with therapy.

   Adjuvant chemoradiation is indicated for high-risk patients after surgery as previously discussed.

V.   Supportive care

   A. Support systems. The head and neck cancer patient population includes many older people who are often socially isolated because of the behavioral effects of chronic alcohol abuse;

many live alone, are separated from family, and have few social or monetary resources. These patients need a primary caregiver to be in the house or nearby. Even among patients with extensive social supports and resources, it is difficult to comply with the prescribed multimodality treatment and self-care regimens for nutrition, mouth or wound care, pain control, and antiemetics. Depression and hopelessness, coupled with moderate to severe treatment-related symptoms often test the patient's commitment to the initial treatment goals, and inadequate social supports tend to exacerbate this problem. Early evaluation by a trained social worker, who can assist with counseling and problem solving, and facilitate hospital and community-based support services is essential. The American Cancer Society's support groups and patient assistance programs, Alcoholics Anonymous, and other social care organizations should be enlisted as part of the treatment team.

B. Nutrition. Adequate nutrition is an essential component of any medical management plan. A poor nutritional state is associated with impaired healing, increased toxicity of treatment, an impaired sense of well-being, and fatigue. Tumor location, surgical or radiation-related treatment effects, chemotherapy, and progressive cancer all lead to symptoms that can cause impaired nutrition. Patients with head and neck cancer often experience dysphagia, odynophagia, dysguesia, xerostomia, poor dentition, mucositis, nausea, vomiting, and anorexia at some point during the illness. These symptoms may be persistent and compromise nutrition by preventing adequate oral feeding. Early consultation with a clinical nutritionist is usually helpful, coupled with the setting of clear calorie goals and strategies for reaching those goals. For most patients, a goal of 2,000 to 2,500 kcal/day or more is needed to maintain weight and re-establish nutritional homeostasis. Reinforcing the nutrition plan with the patient and caregiver is essential. Many patients prefer to blend home foods into a form they can manage, whereas others prefer the prepared liquid nutritional supplements, which are a convenient alternative that greatly facilitates reaching the recommended calorie goals by providing a balanced source of calories in a relatively small volume. Endoscopically or percutaneously placed gastrostomy tubes greatly facilitate enteral feeding when patients are unable to take adequate calories or hydration by mouth. Several of the intensive chemoradiation programs rely on gastrostomy tube feeding and hydration and the long-term impact on swallowing function may be substantial and requires further study. Among patients who are cured, frequently the time and effort needed to eat limit adequate caloric intake. For patients undergoing palliative chemotherapy or supportive care only, adequate nutrition enhances well-being.

C. Mouth care. Mouth care is an important part of the support for patients undergoing treatment for head and neck cancer. Tumor involvement and the effects of surgery, radiation, or chemotherapy can all cause problems that can be helped by mouth care intervention.

Initial dental evaluation is important if prosthetics will be required after surgery, and dental procedures should be performed before radiotherapy in patients who will receive radiation. Mucositis due to chemotherapy and radiation is a major problem and requires frequent monitoring and recognition of treatable problems that may develop such as herpes virus reactivation and superinfection with candida or pathogenic bacteria. Salt and soda mouthwashes, sucralfate mouthwashes, and a variety of mouthwash mixtures, some that contain topical anesthetics, (but not chlorhexidine) may be used to promote optimum oropharyngeal hygiene, decrease inflammation, and treat pain (see Chapter 27-III). Clinical trials of palifermin—a keratinocyte growth factor effective in preventing oral mucositis in patients receiving high dose chemotherapy and total-body radiotherapy for hematologic malignancies—are under way and show promise in ameliorating mucositis in patients with head and neck cancer undergoing chemoradiation. Radiation-induced bone necrosis or tumor-related fistulas need to be cleaned or debrided and occasionally packed with toothpaste or other material to promote comfort. Metronidazole 500 mg three times a day can improve tumor odor that is distressing to both the patient and caregivers.

A common problem during and after radiotherapy is dry mouth—xerostomia. Sugarless gum or lozenges, artificial saliva, and pilocarpine 5 to 10 mg orally t.i.d. or cevimiline 30 mg orally t.i.d. are remedies acceptable to many patients. Amifostine, a thiophosphate compound that can protect normal tissues against chemotherapy and radiation side effects, has been shown to decrease radiation-related acute and chronic xerostomia in patients with head and neck cancer. It is given intravenously at a dose of 200 mg/m^2/day as a slow IV push 15 to 30 minutes before each fraction of radiotherapy. Side effects include nausea requiring 5HT-3 serotonin receptor antagonists, hypotension, and allergic reactions. These factors and the demonstration of only modest long-term benefits have limited its routine use. Subcutaneous dosing has been investigated.

D. Aspiration pneumonia. Many patients suffer from dry mouth, whereas others have copious or thick mucoid secretions and suffer from an inability to clear them because of anatomic factors. Such patients benefit from mucolytics, such as guanifensin, and portable suction machines.

These patients frequently suffer episodes of aspiration pneumonia. Fever, tachycardia, tachypnea, rales, and infiltrates in the lung are usual findings but sometimes microaspiration can simulate pulmonary metastasis. Awareness of this propensity, focusing on a careful history, and comprehensive evaluation followed by treatment with steroids, antibiotics, or both will usually manage the acute problem. A swallowing evaluation may lead to speech and swallowing therapy. Nevertheless, feeding by gastrostomy tube or laryngectomy may be the only solution if the aspiration episodes are frequent or life threatening.

E. Granulocytopenia and infection. Combination chemotherapeutic regimens have an increased risk of granulocytopenia, and patients with head and neck cancer often have multiple risk factors for developing febrile neutropenia. Pulmonary, oropharyngeal, and IV access line infections are common in this patient population and mortality is high when granulocytopenia is present. Prophylactic filgrastim or pegfilgrastim should be administered to those with intermediate or high-risk patient factors such as age above 65, poor nutritional status, extensive prior chemotherapy, open wounds, COPD, and low baseline hemoglobin. If fever develops, evaluation with appropriate cultures and treatment with broad-spectrum antibiotics should be instituted promptly (see Chapter 28).

F. Anemia. Anemia is uncommon during chemoradiation for head and neck cancer but is more frequent during treatment for recurrent disease and in neoadjuvant regimens. One clinical trial found decreased survival when erythropoietin was used to achieve a target hemoglobin of 15 g/dL. Transfusion and erythropoietin can ameliorate fatigue and other symptoms related to anemia associated with hemoglobin levels below 12 g/dL.

G. Hypothyroidism. Weakness, apathy, listlessness, and weight loss may develop insidiously in patients subjected to thyroid irradiation or resection. Estimates are as high as 25% to 50% for radiation doses above 6,000 cGy. Such symptoms may mistakenly be construed as suggesting disease relapse. Monitoring for this phenomenon should continue indefinitely.

H. Hypercalcemia. Hypercalcemia is a common manifestation of late-stage recurrent tumor and is usually caused by parathyroid hormone related protein (PTHrp). It may be precipitated by dehydration but up to 23% of patients with advanced recurrent head and neck cancers will manifest hypercalcemia before death. In most such patients, it is mild and easily controlled with hydration, saline diuresis, or bisphosphonate therapy (see Chapter 30). If patients have advanced disease without the hope of substantial palliation, comfort care is a reasonable choice.

VI. Cancer prevention. Many patients who are cured of head and neck cancer survive to develop second primary cancers of the head and neck or lung, related in part to a field cancerization effect of tobacco and alcohol exposure. Smoking cessation and abstinence from alcohol are important adjuncts to the care of these patients.

Isotretinoin (13-*cis*-retinoic acid) can reverse oral premalignancy; a high dose of 1 to 2 mg/kg was shown to prevent second primary cancers in patients with head and neck cancer but lower, more tolerable doses were ineffective. Tobacco control is the single most important preventive effort under way. The control of HPV infections may lead to decreases in tumors associated with this virus.

SUGGESTED READINGS

Adelstein DJ, Li Y, Adams GL, et al. An intergroup phase III comparison of standard radiation therapy and two schedules of concurrent chemoradiotherapy in patients with unresectable squamous cell head and neck cancer. *J Clin Oncol* 2003;21:92–98.

Al-Sarraf M, LeBlanc M, Giri PG, et al. Chemoradiotherapy versus radiotherapy in patients with advanced nasopharyngeal cancer: phase III randomized Intergroup study 0099. *J Clin Oncol* 1998;16:1310–1317.

Bernier J, Cooper JS, Pajak TF, et al. Defining risk levels in locally advanced head and neck cancers: a comparative analysis of concurrent postoperative radiation plus chemotherapy trials of the EORTC (#22931) and RTOG (# 9501). *Head Neck* 2005;27:843–850.

Bonner JA, Harari PM, Giralt J, et al. Radiotherapy plus cetuximab for squamous-cell carcinoma of the head and neck. *N Engl J Med* 2006;354(6):567–578.

Brizel DM, Albers ME, Fisher SR, et al. Hyperfractionated irradiation with or without concurrent chemotherapy for locally advanced head and neck cancer. *N Engl J Med* 1998;338:1798–1804.

Cohen EE. Role of epidermal growth factor receptor pathway-targeted therapy in patients with recurrent and/or metastatic squamous cell carcinoma of the head and neck. *J Clin Oncol* 2006;24:2659–2665.

Cooper JS, Pajak TF, Forastiere AA, et al. Postoperative concurrent radiotherapy and chemotherapy for high-risk squamous-cell carcinoma of the head and neck. *N Engl J Med* 2004;350:1937–1944.

Denis F, Garaud P, Bardet E, et al. Final results of the 94-01 French Head and Neck Oncology and Radiotherapy Group randomized trial comparing radiotherapy alone with concomitant radiochemotherapy in advanced-stage oropharynx carcinoma. *J Clin Oncol* 2004;22:69–76.

Department of Veterans Affairs Laryngeal Cancer Study Group. Induction chemotherapy plus radiation compared with surgery plus radiation in patients with advanced laryngeal cancer. *N Engl J Med* 1991;324:1685–1690.

Fakhry C, Gillison ML. Clinical implications of human papillomavirus in head and neck cancers. *J Clin Oncol* 2006;24:2606–2611.

Forastiere AA, Ang K, Brizel D, et al. Head and neck cancers. *J Natl Compr Canc Netw* 2005;3(3):316–391.

Forastiere AA, Goepfert H, Maor M, et al. Concurrent chemotherapy and radiotherapy for organ preservation in advanced laryngeal cancer. *N Engl J Med* 2003;349:2091–2098.

Forastiere AA, Metch B, Schuller DE, et al. Randomized comparison of cisplatin plus fluorouracil and carboplatin plus fluorouracil vs. methotrexate in advanced squamous-cell carcinoma of the head and neck: A Southwest Oncology Group study. *J Clin Oncol* 1992;10:1245–1251.

Forastiere AA, Trotti A, Pfister DG, et al. Head and neck cancer: recent advances and new standards of care. *J Clin Oncol* 2006;24:2603–2605.

Garden AS, Harris J, Vokes EE, et al. Preliminary results of Radiation Therapy Oncology Group 97-03: a randomized phase II trial of concurrent radiation and chemotherapy for advanced squamous cell carcinomas of the head and neck. *J Clin Oncol* 2004;22:2856–2864.

Gibson MK, Li Y, Murphy B, et al. Randomized phase III evaluation of cisplatin plus fluorouracil versus cisplatin plus paclitaxel in advanced head and neck cancer (E1395): an intergroup trial of the Eastern Cooperative Oncology Group. *J Clin Oncol* 2005;23:3562–3567.

Greene FL, Page DL, Fleming ID, et al. eds. *AJCC cancer staging manual*, 6th ed. New York: Springer-Verlag, 2002.

Hitt R, Lopez-Pousa A, Martinez-Trufero, et al. Phase III study comparing cisplatin plus fluorouracil to paclitaxel, cisplatin, and fluorouracil induction chemotherapy followed by chemoradiotherapy in locally advanced head and neck cancer. *J Clin Oncol* 2005;23:8636–8645.

Kim JG, Sohn SK, Kim DH, et al. Phase II study of concurrent chemoradiotherapy with capecitabine and cisplatin in patients with locally advanced squamous cell carcinoma of the head and neck. *Br J Cancer* 2005;93:1117–1121.

Lefebvre J-L, Chevalier D, Luboinski B, et al. Larynx preservation in pyriform sinus cancer: preliminary results of a European Organization for Research and Treatment of Cancer phase III trial. *J Natl Cancer Inst* 1996;88:890–899.

Piccirillo JF, Lacy PD, Basu A, et al. Development of a new head and neck cancer-specific comorbidity index. *Arch Otolaryngol Head Neck Surg* 2002;128:1172–1179.

Pignon JP, Bourhis J, Domenge C, et al. on behalf of the MACH-NC Collaborative Group. Chemotherapy added to locoregional treatment for head and neck squamous-cell carcinoma: three meta-analyses of updated individual data. *Lancet* 2000;355:949–955.

Pfister DG, Laurie SA, Weinstein GS, et al. American Society of Clinical Oncology clinical practice guideline for the use of larynx-preservation strategies in the treatment of laryngeal cancer. *J Clin Oncol* 2006;24:3693–3704.

CHAPTER 7

Carcinoma of the Lung

Sophie Sun and Joan H. Schiller

Carcinoma of the lung is responsible for more than 165,000 deaths each year in the United States. This represents one third of all deaths due to cancer and more than the number of deaths due to breast, colon, and prostate cancers combined. Lung cancer consists of four major histologic types: adenocarcinoma, squamous cell carcinoma, large cell carcinoma, and small cell carcinoma. Because of the unique biologic features of small cell lung cancer (SCLC), its staging and treatment differ radically from those of the other three types of lung cancer, which are collectively called *non–small cell lung cancer* (NSCLC). Therefore, these two groups are addressed in two separate sections.

I. **Etiology.** Lung cancer is predominantly a disease of smokers. Eighty-five percent of lung cancer occurs in active or former smokers, and an additional 5% of cases are estimated to occur as a consequence of passive exposure to tobacco smoke. Tobacco smoke causes an increased incidence of all four histologic types of lung cancer, although adenocarcinoma (particularly the bronchoalveolar variant) is also found in nonsmokers. Other risk factors for lung cancer include exposure to asbestos or radon. Familial factors such as polymorphisms in carcinogen-metabolizing hepatic enzyme systems may also play a role in determining an individual's propensity to develop lung cancer.

II. **Molecular biology.** Numerous genetic changes have been associated with lung tumors. Most common among these include activation or overexpression of the *myc* family of oncogenes in SCLC and NSCLC and of the *K-ras* oncogene in NSCLC, particularly adenocarcinoma. Inactivation or deletion of the *p*53 and retinoblastoma tumor suppressor genes and a tumor suppressor gene on chromosome 3p (the *FHIT* gene) have been found in 50% to 90% of patients with SCLC. Abnormalities of *p*53 and 3p have been associated with 50% to 70% of cases of NSCLC. The *K-ras* mutation is more frequently found in smokers, those with adenocarcinoma, and those with poorly differentiated tumors. It is also associated with poor prognosis.

Recently, abnormalities in the epidermal growth factor (EGF) pathway have been identified, making this pathway an attractive target for anticancer therapy. The epidermal growth factor receptor (EGFR) is frequently expressed or overexpressed in NSCLC tumors. Binding of ligand to the EGFR causes dimerization of the receptor, which in turn activates tyrosine kinase on the intracellular domain of the receptor. Autophosphorylation of the receptor induces a cascade of intracellular events leading to cell proliferation, inhibition of apoptosis, angiogenesis, and invasion, all resulting in tumor growth and spread. Inhibition of the EGFR pathway leads to apoptosis and tumor regression in preclinical models. Hence, the EGFR, ligands, and signaling pathway have become active targets for anticancer therapy. Agents targeting this pathway include EGFR tyrosine kinase inhibitors such as gefitinib and erlotinib; monoclonal antibodies to EGFR, which block ligand binding to EGFR (e.g., cetuximab); and antisense oligonucleotides, which inhibit the expression of EGFR by base-pair hybridization with its messenger ribonucleic acid. Mutations and overexpression of the receptor have been described and may predict response to therapy. Of the EGFR inhibitors, gefitinib and erlotinib have been the most studied and are discussed in the subsequent text.

III. Screening. Three U.S. randomized screening studies in the 1980s failed to detect an impact on mortality of screening high-risk patients with chest radiography or sputum cytology, although earlier-stage cancers were detected in the screened groups. Since then, however, low-dose spiral computed tomography (CT) has emerged as a possible new tool for lung cancer screening. Spiral CT is CT imaging in which only the pulmonary parenchyma is scanned, thereby negating the use of IV contrast medium and the necessity for the presence of a physician. This type of scan can usually be done quickly (within one breath) and involves low doses of radiation. In a nonrandomized controlled study from the Early Lung Cancer Action Project, low-dose CT was shown to be more sensitive than chest radiography in detecting lung nodules and lung cancer at an early stage. However, despite these promising results, it is unclear whether screening with spiral CT will result in a reduction in lung cancer mortality. Concerns include issues related to lead-time bias, length-time bias, and "overdiagnosis". In addition, in some geographic regions, such as the Midwest United States, the incidence of benign nodules is extremely high, making the cost of the test with subsequent follow-up testing very expensive. To help resolve the issue, the National Cancer Institute has recently completed a large randomized controlled trial (the Lung Screening Study), involving approximately 50,000 participants over several years, and results are awaited.

IV. Non–small cell lung cancer

A. Histology. Although histologic differences (adenocarcinoma vs. large cell carcinoma vs. squamous cell carcinoma) among the NSCLCs affect their natural history and presentation, these differences are of relatively little importance in determining patient management, with two possible exceptions. First, bronchioalveolar carcinoma, a disease which presents in two forms (nodular and diffuse) tends to occur in younger women who have never smoked, which is a subgroup of patients that is more likely to derive benefit from EGFR inhibitors. Secondly, patients with squamous cell carcinoma are more likely to develop hemoptysis with bevacizumab, a monoclonal antibody to vascular endothelial growth factor (VEGF) (Section IV.D.3.c).

B. Staging. The prognosis and treatment of NSCLC are dependent primarily on the stage of disease at the time of diagnosis. The current TNM definitions and staging system are shown in Table 7.1 and 7.2. Items of note: a pulmonary nodule within the same lobe of the primary is staged as T4, whereas if it is in a different lobe, it is M1; a bloody or exudative pleural effusion is T4 even if it is cytology negative. Patients with "wet" stage IIIB NSCLC have a prognosis similar to those

Table 7.1. TNM definitions

Primary tumor (T)

TX | Tumor proved by the presence of malignant cells in bronchopulmonary secretions but not visualized roentgenographically or bronchoscopically or any tumor that cannot be assessed, as in a retreatment staging

T0 | No evidence of primary tumor

Tis | Carcinoma *in situ*

T1 | A tumor that is ≤3 cm in the greatest dimension, surrounded by lung or visceral pleura and without evidence of invasion proximal to a lobar bronchus at bronchoscopy

T2 | A tumor >3 cm in the greatest dimension or a tumor of any size that either invades the visceral pleura or has associated atelectasis or obstructive pneumonitis extending to the hilar region. At bronchoscopy, the proximal extent of demonstrable tumor must be within a lobar bronchus or at least 2 cm distal to the carina. Any associated atelectasis or obstructive pneumonitis must involve less than an entire lung

T3 | A tumor of any size with direct extension into the chest wall (including superior sulcus tumors), diaphragm, or the mediastinal pleura or pericardium without involving the heart, great vessels, trachea, esophagus, or vertebral body or a tumor in the main bronchus within 2 cm of the carina without involving the carina

T4 | A tumor of any size with invasion of the mediastinum or involving the heart, great vessels, trachea, esophagus, vertebral body, or carina, or presence of malignant pleural effusion; a satellite nodule within the same lobe

Nodal involvement (N)

N0 | No demonstrable metastasis to regional lymph nodes

N1 | Metastasis to lymph nodes in the peribronchial or the ipsilateral hilar region or both, including direct extension

N2 | Metastasis to ipsilateral mediastinal lymph nodes or subcarinal lymph nodes or both

N3 | Metastasis to contralateral mediastinal lymph nodes, contralateral hilar lymph nodes, ipsilateral or contralateral scalene or supraclavicular lymph nodes

Distant metastasis (M)

MX | Cannot be assessed

M0 | No distant metastasis

M1 | Distant metastasis, including pulmonary nodule not in the same lobe as the primary tumor

Table 7.2. 1997 Revisions to the international staging classification for lung cancer

Stage	TNM Subset	5-year Survival Rate (%)	
		Clinical Stage	Pathologic Stage
IA	T1, N0, M0	61	67
IB	T2, N0, M0	38	57
IIA	T1, N1, M0	34	55
IIB	T2, N1, M0	24	39
	T3, N0, M0		
IIIA	T3, N1, M0	9	25
	T1–3, N2, M0		
IIIB	T4, any N, M0	13	23
	Any T, N3, M0		
IV	Any T, any N, M1	1	—

From Mountain CF. Revisions in the international system for staging lung cancer. *Chest* 1997;111:1710–1717.

patients with metastatic disease, and are therefore often included in "advanced" NSCLC trials, whereas "dry" stage IIIB patients are usually included in "locally advanced" trials.

C. Pretreatment evaluation. The diagnosis of lung cancer is usually made by bronchial biopsy or percutaneous needle biopsy. Although the disease is usually discovered on chest radiographs, a CT scan of the chest is necessary to evaluate the extent of the primary disease, mediastinal extension, or lymphadenopathy, and the presence or absence of other parenchymal nodules in patients in whom surgical resection is a consideration. CT of the upper abdomen is performed to look for asymptomatic hepatic or adrenal metastases. (The latter should be distinguished from benign adrenal adenomas.) Bone scans should be obtained for the patient with bone pain, chest pain, or an elevated calcium or alkaline phosphatase level. Head CT or magnetic resonance imaging is not routinely done in the absence of central nervous system (CNS) signs or symptoms.

Mediastinal nodal metastasis is a critical factor in determining tumor resectability. Mediastinoscopy has long been considered the gold standard for mediastinal staging and has been recommended for mediastinal lymph nodes greater than 1 cm on CT scan. Recently, however, positron emission tomography (PET), a metabolic imaging scan using [^{18}F]fluorodeoxyglucose, has been developed as a useful complementary tool for staging. PET scans are more sensitive and specific than CT scans and could therefore potentially save patients with advanced disease, either within or outside the chest, from unnecessary invasive procedures. However, it is not yet clear as to whether PET scanning can replace mediastinoscopy, as the scan can be falsely positive in inflammatory processes and falsely negative in lung tumors with low metabolic activity such as bronchoalveolar carcinoma or carcinoid tumors.

Pulmonary function testing is necessary before definitive surgery. Increased postoperative morbidity is associated with a predicted postoperative 1-second forced expiratory volume of less than 800 to 1,000 mL, a preoperative maximum voluntary ventilation less than 35% of that predicted, a carbon monoxide diffusing capacity less than 60% of that predicted, and an arterial oxygen pressure (Po_2) of less than 60 mm Hg or a carbon dioxide pressure (Pco_2) of more than 45 mm Hg.

D. Management

    1. *Early stage NSCLC*

        a. Stage I disease. Lobectomy is the primary treatment for stage I NSCLC, with cure rates of 60% to 80%. In patients with medical contraindications to surgery but with adequate pulmonary function, high-dose radiotherapy results in cure in approximately 20% of patients. Patients with T2, N0 (stage IB) disease do not fare as well as those with T1, N0 (stage IA) cancers. Adjuvant (postoperative) chemotherapy has been of interest because a meta-analysis in 1995 showed a borderline statistically significant survival benefit with surgery and chemotherapy as compared with surgery alone ($p = 0.07$). Recent randomized clinical trials using adjuvant platinum-based doublet chemotherapy have demonstrated significant survival advantage in early stage patients (Table 7.3). A Cancer and Leukemia Group B trial (CALGB 9633) of patients with completely resected stage IB NSCLC randomized patients to four cycles of adjuvant carboplatin plus paclitaxel or observation. In a reported preliminary planned interim analysis, adjuvant chemotherapy was associated with a significant improvement in 4-year overall survival (71% vs. 59%). A recently published National Cancer Institute of Canada trial (NCIC JBR.10) of patients with stages IB and II (excluding T3, N0) NSCLC randomly assigned to surgery alone or followed by four cycles of cisplatin and vinorelbine reported a 15% absolute improvement in overall survival at 5 years (69% vs. 54%) in patients with stages IB to IIIA disease, favoring the chemotherapy arm.

        The evidence for adjuvant chemotherapy for patients with resected stage IA disease is less clear. A Japanese trial of stage I NSCLC patients (73% stage IA; 27% stage IB) randomized patients to an oral 5-fluorouracil derivative (tegafur plus uracil, UFT) versus surgery alone. The results showed a modest but significantly improved 5-year survival in the UFT group (88% vs. 85%). However, in subgroup analysis, the improved 5-year survival was observed with stage IB patients (5-year survival 85% vs. 74%) with no difference in stage IA disease (5-year survival 89% vs. 90%). UFT is currently not available in North America. Given these data, it is reasonable to offer adjuvant platinum-based doublet chemotherapy to patients with completely resected stage IB disease and with good performance status until more definitive

Table 7.3. Randomized studies of adjuvant chemotherapy for resected non–small cell lung cancer

Trial	Patient Population (Stage)	No. of Patients	Chemotherapeutic Regimen		Absolute Overall Survival Benefit
CALGB 9633 (2004)	IB	344	Carboplatin	AUC 6, on day 1	12% (4-year)
			Paclitaxel	200 mg/m² IV on day 1 every 3 weeks × four cycles	
NCIC JBR.10 (2005)	IB, II	482	Cisplatin	50 mg/m² IV on days 1, 8 every 4 weeks × 4 cycles	15% (5-year)
			Vinorelbine	25 mg/m² IV weekly × 16	
ANITA (2005)	IB, II, IIIA	840	Cisplatin	100 mg/m² IV on day 1 every 4 weekly × four cycles	9% (5-year)
					8% (7-year)
			Vinorelbine	30 mg/m²/weeks IV × 16	
IALT (2004)	I, II, IIIA	1867	Cisplatin	80 mg/m² IV on days 1, 22, 43, 64	5% (4-year)
				100 mg/m² IV on days 1, 29, 57	
			(options)	100 mg/m² IV on days 1, 29, 57, 85	
				120 mg/m² IV on days 1, 29, 71	
			Vindesine	3 mg/m² IV weekly days 1–29, then every 2 weeks after days 43 until last cisplatin	
			or		
			Vinblastine	4 mg/m² IV weekly days 1–29, then every 2 weeks after days 43 until last cisplatin	
			or		
			Vinorelbine	30 mg/m² IV weekly day 1 to last cisplatin	
			or		
			Etoposide	100 mg/m² IV on days 1–3 with each cisplatin	

CALGB, Cancer and Acute Leukemia Group B; NCIC, National Cancer Institute of Canada; ANITA, Adjuvant Navalbine International Trialist Association; IALT, International Adjuvant Lung Cancer Trial results are reported. Additional studies are needed for stage IA disease before adjuvant therapy can be routinely recommended for this group of patients.

Patients with resected stage I NSCLC are at high risk for the development of second lung cancers (~2%–3% per year). Neither vitamin A nor its derivatives, β-carotene or *cis*-retinoic acid, have been found to have any benefit in chemoprevention, and contrary to predictions, may even be deleterious. Other agents, such as selenium, are under investigation.

b. Stage II disease. Surgical resection is a standard component of the treatment for stage II NSCLC. The subset of T3, N0 disease has a natural history and treatment strategy different from those of stage III N2 disease and has therefore been moved to stage II. Patients with peripheral chest wall invasion should undergo resection of the involved ribs and underlying lung. Chest wall defects are then repaired with chest wall musculature or Marlex mesh and methylmethacrylate. Postoperative radiotherapy is often given. Five-year survival rates as high as 50% have been reported.

Recent randomized trials have demonstrated a role for adjuvant chemotherapy after resection for patients with stage II NSCLC (Table 7.3). One of the first positive trials published in 2004 by the International Adjuvant Lung Cancer Trial (IALT) Collaborative Group randomly assigned patients with completely resected NSCLC (pathologic stage I to IIIA) to surgery alone or surgery plus three to four cycles of a cisplatin-containing doublet. The choice of doublet (cisplatin plus either etoposide, vinblastine, vinorelbine, or vindesine) and the use of adjuvant thoracic radiotherapy was decided at the level of each participating institution. The study demonstrated an improvement in overall survival of 5% (45% vs. 40%) at 5 years in favor of chemotherapy. The results of the Adjuvant Navelbine International Trialist Association (ANITA) trial (ANITA) trial have provided further support for adjuvant chemotherapy. In this study, patients with stage IB to IIIA NSCLC were randomized to surgery alone as compared with cisplatin plus vinorelbine for four cycles. In a preliminary report, overall survival was significantly improved at 5 years (51% vs. 43%), although the survival benefit was restricted to patients with stage II and IIIA disease. These data, in combination with the results of the NCIC trials detailed in the preceding text, have led to the recommendation to **offer patients adjuvant platinum-based chemotherapy following complete resection of pathologic stage IB, II, and IIIA NSCLC.**

2. Locally advanced (stage IIIA and IIIB) disease. Treatment of locally advanced NSCLC is one of the most controversial issues in the management of lung cancer. Interpretation of the results of clinical trials involving patients with locally advanced disease has been clouded by a number of issues including changing diagnostic techniques,

different staging systems, and heterogeneous patient populations that may have disease that ranges from "nonbulky"
stage IIIA (clinical N1 nodes, with microscopic N2 nodes
discovered only at the time of surgery or mediastinoscopy)
to "bulky" N2 nodes (enlarged adenopathy clearly visible
on chest radiographs or multiple nodal level involvement)
to clearly inoperable stage IIIB disease.

   a. "Nonbulky" stage IIIA disease. The optimal treatment for "nonbulky" stage IIIA is controversial. Current
investigational efforts are directed at identifying the
optimal combined-modality approach, involving treatments directed at local control of the disease (surgery or
radiotherapy) and micrometastatic disease (chemotherapy). Possibilities include surgery followed by adjuvant chemotherapy; preoperative chemotherapy plus
surgery; or chemotherapy plus radiotherapy.

   The primary treatment of stage II and early stage
IIIA (clinical N0 or N1) disease is surgical resection.
However, even with a complete resection, the cure rate
is disappointing, prompting investigation of adjuvant
chemotherapy and radiotherapy. Postoperative radiotherapy has been shown to reduce local recurrences
after resection of stage II or III squamous cell carcinoma of the lung but does not prolong survival. **Randomized studies with adjuvant cisplatin-based
doublet chemotherapy have confirmed an overall
survival benefit of 5% to 15% at 5 years and this is
now routinely offered to good performance status
patients with resected stage II or IIIA NSCLC.**

   Although patients with N2 disease are also usually
treated with combined chemoradiation therapy, there
have been studies looking at the role of surgery in
this disease. Two small positive randomized studies
involving more than 40 patients, compared surgery
with or without preoperative chemotherapy in this patient population. In a European study, preoperative
chemotherapy (mitomycin, ifosfamide, and cisplatin for
three courses) followed by surgery was compared with
surgery without preoperative chemotherapy in patients
with stage IIIA disease. All patients also received postoperative mediastinal radiotherapy after surgery. The
median survival time was 26 months for 30 patients
receiving preoperative chemotherapy plus surgery compared with 8 months for 30 patients treated with surgery
alone.

   Investigators at the M.D. Anderson Cancer Center
randomized patients to surgery or three cycles of cyclophosphamide, etoposide, and cisplatin followed by
surgery and three cycles of postoperative chemotherapy.
The median survival time of the 32 patients randomized
to the surgery-alone group was 14 months compared
with 21 months in the 28 patients randomized to the
combined-modality arm.

   In a larger randomized trial, French investigators
compared preoperative mitomycin, ifosfamide, and cisplatin plus surgery with surgery alone in 355 patients

with resectable stage I (except T1, N0), stage II, and stage IIIA (including N2 disease). The difference in median survival between two arms was not statistically significant (37 vs. 26 months; $p = 0.15$). However, subset analysis suggested a survival advantage of neoadjuvant chemotherapy for N0 to N1 but not N2 disease.

Trimodality therapy has also been explored in a randomized intergroup trial, where patients with advanced stage IIIA disease receive 45 Gy of induction radiotherapy plus two cycles of cisplatin and etoposide and are subsequently randomized to surgery or boost radiotherapy plus an additional two cycles of chemotherapy. In a planned second interim analysis, there was significant improvement in progression-free survival at 5 years for the trimodality arm (22% vs. 11%; $p = 0.017$) and although there was a trend for better 5-year overall survival with trimodality therapy, this was not significant (27% vs. 20%; $p = 0.10$). There were greater treatment-related mortalities in the surgery arm compared with the chemoradiation-alone arm (8% vs. 2%), with most deaths occurring in patients undergoing pneumonectomy. The role of trimodality therapy for stage IIIA NSCLC remains controversial because of treatment-related morbidity and mortality, particularly for patients requiring right-sided pneumonectomy.

Several studies have shown, in subset analysis, that those patients receiving neoadjuvant therapy who subsequently have their N2 nodes "cleared" with preoperative therapy do better than those who do not. This has prompted some investigators to give preoperative treatment and then resample the N2 nodes. If positive, the thorax is closed and patients go on to receive "definitive chemoradiation." However, if the nodes have turned negative, the patient goes on to have definitive surgery. Of note, patients undergoing a right pneumonectomy following chemoradiation have a mortality rate of up to 20% in some series.

As of this writing, there is no level 1 evidence to recommend neoadjuvant chemotherapy over adjuvant chemotherapy, although several theoretical reasons for doing so include the fact that patients are more likely to tolerate preoperative chemotherapy over postoperative chemotherapy. Results from randomized studies are awaited.

b. Pancoast tumors. Pancoast tumors are upper-lobe tumors that adjoin the brachial plexus and are frequently associated with Horner syndrome or shoulder and arm pain; the latter is due to rib destruction, involvement of the C8 or T1 nerve roots, or both. Treatment consists of a combined-modality approach with radiotherapy and surgery. Five-year survival rates range from 25% to 50%. Combined preoperative chemotherapy and radiotherapy is being studied.

c. "Bulky" stage IIIA (N2) and stage IIIB with no pleural effusion. "Bulky" stage IIIA and IIIB are generally considered unresectable, with the treatment consisting of combined chemoradiation or, in the case of stage IIIB with malignant pleural effusion, chemotherapy alone.

Chemotherapy plus radiation therapy. Chemotherapy plus radiotherapy is the treatment of choice for patients with "bulky" or inoperable stage IIIA or IIIB disease without pleural effusion. Numerous randomized studies have demonstrated an improvement in median and long-term survival with chemotherapy plus by radiation therapy versus radiotherapy alone. Active areas of investigation include proper sequencing of thoracic radiation therapy and chemotherapy (concurrent vs. sequential), choice of chemotherapy, fractionation, and treatment fields.

A randomized Japanese trial reported a 3-month survival advantage with concurrent chemoradiation over a sequential approach. Initial reports from a confirmatory randomized Radiation Therapy Oncology Group trial also showed a trend in favor of concurrent cisplatin and vinblastine with radiation over sequential chemoradiation, albeit with more toxicities, making concurrent chemoradiation therapy the treatment of choice for good performance status patients.

Chemotherapy can be given in full "systemic" doses with radiotherapy, in weekly "radiosensitizing" doses, or a combination of both. One of the most commonly used chemotherapeutic regimens for stage III NSCLC is carboplatin in combination with paclitaxel (Table 7.4). Although single-agent weekly carboplatin has not resulted in a survival benefit when given with radiotherapy, weekly doses of paclitaxel 50 mg/m^2 and carboplatin AUC 2 with concurrent radiation have proved promising in randomized phase II studies.

Other areas of investigation include the role of "standard" systemic doses of chemotherapy either before or after concurrent weekly radiosensitizing chemotherapy with radiotherapy. In a phase III trial, the CALGB did not show a survival benefit when induction chemotherapy was given before weekly low-dose chemoradiation therapy compared with weekly low-dose chemoradiation therapy alone. However, a randomized phase II Southwest Oncology Group (SWOG) trial showed promising results with standard dose chemoradiation therapy (cisplatin and etoposide) followed by docetaxel. These results need to be confirmed in phase III studies.

3. Stage IV disease. Chemotherapy improves survival in patients with metastatic NSCLC (~10% 1-year survival rate in untreated patients vs. 30% to 35% 1-year survival rate with treatment). Goals for treatment should include palliation of symptoms and a modest improvement in survival.

The principal factors predicting response to chemotherapy and survival are performance status and extent of disease. Patients with a poor performance status (Eastern Cooperative Oncology Group [ECOG] performance status of 2 to 4) are less likely to respond to treatment and

Table 7.4. Chemotherapeutic regimens for concurrent chemoradiation for stage III *non–small cell lung cancer*

Induction Chemotherapy (Concurrent with Radiation)		Consolidation Chemotherapy	
EP			
Etoposide	50 mg/m² days 1–5, 29–33	Etoposide	50 mg/m² IV on days 1–5 every 3 weeks × two cycles
Cisplatin	50 mg/m² days 1, 8, 29, 36	Cisplatin	50 mg/m² IV on days 1, 8 every 3 weeks × two cycles
EP followed by docetaxel			
Etoposide	50 mg/m² days 1–5, 29–33	Docetaxel	75–100 mg/m² IV every 3 weeks × three cycles
Cisplatin	50 mg/m² days 1, 8, 29, 36		Starting 4–6 weeks after induction therapy
Carboplatin plus paclitaxel			
Carboplatin	AUC 2 weekly	Carboplatin	AUC 6, on days 1 every 3 weeks × two cycles
Paclitaxel	50 mg/m² over 1 h weekly	Paclitaxel	200 mg/m² IV on days 1 over 3 h every 3 weeks × two cycles

EP, etoposide and platinum (cisplatin); AUC, area under the curve.

they tolerate the therapy poorly, although recent subset retrospective analysis have suggested that performance status 2 patients may also enjoy a modest benefit in survival with treatment. Favorable prognostic factors include no weight loss, female sex, normal serum lactic dehydrogenase level, and no bone or liver metastases.

a. First-line chemotherapy. Chemotherapy for patients with metastatic NSCLC and a good performance status should be a chemotherapeutic regimen consisting of two drugs. A meta-analysis of large randomized trials indicated that there is a small but significant survival advantage with platinum-based therapy compared with best supportive care. Whereas best supportive care resulted in median survival rates of 4 to 5 months and 1-year survival rates of 5% to 10%, current third-generation regimens with paclitaxel and docetaxel, gemcitabine, vinorelbine, and irinotecan have yielded median survivals of 8 to 9 months and 1-year survivals of 35% to 40%. In addition, randomized studies have shown an improvement in symptoms and quality of life compared with patients treated with best supportive care.

b. Choice of chemotherapy. Numerous randomized studies have failed to show a major advantage of one new doublet regimen over another. The common chemotherapeutic regimens for NSCLC are shown in Table 7.5.

Although a direct comparison of cisplatin-based therapies and carboplatin-based therapies is limited, meta-analysis has suggested that cisplatin may have a small benefit in terms of survival over carboplatin, albeit with a different toxicity profile. Whereas this small difference may be of limited clinical consequence for patients with metastatic disease, it may be more important in the adjuvant setting, where cure is the goal.

Table 7.5. Common chemotherapeutic regimens for metastatic non–small cell lung cancer

Cisplatin plus vinorelbine

Cisplatin	100 mg/m^2 IV on day 1
Vinorelbine	25 mg/m^2 weekly
	Repeat cycle every 4 weeks

Carboplatin/paclitaxel plus bevacizumab[a]

Carboplatin	AUC of 6 on day 1
Paclitaxel	225 mg/m^2 IV on day 1 over 3 h
	Repeat cycle every 3 weeks
Bevacizumab[a]	15 mg/kg IV every 3 weeks until progression

Cisplatin/carboplatin plus gemcitabine

Cisplatin	100 mg/m^2 IV on day 1
Gemcitabine	1,000 mg/m^2 IV on days 1, 8, and 15
	Repeat each cycle every 4 weeks

or

Cisplatin	80 mg/m^2 IV on day 1
Gemcitabine	1,250 mg/m^2 IV on days 1 and 8
	Repeat each cycle every 3 weeks

or

Carboplatin	AUC of 5 on day 1
Gemcitabine	1,000 mg/m^2 IV on days 1 and 8
	Repeat each cycle every 3 weeks

Cisplatin/carboplatin plus docetaxel

Cisplatin	75 mg/m^2 IV on day 1
Docetaxel	75 mg/m^2 IV on day 1
	Repeat each cycle every 3 weeks

or

Carboplatin	AUC of 6 on day 1
Docetaxel	75 mg/m^2 IV on day 1
	Repeat each cycle every 3 weeks

AUC, area under the curve.
[a]Patients with brain metastases, squamous cell histology, on anticoagulants, or a recent history of thromboembolic events should *NOT* receive bevacizumab off of a clinical study

c. Inhibitors of angiogenesis. Inhibition of angiogenesis is based on the observations that neovascularization occurs in tumor tissues and rarely in other physiologic processes except wound healing. Theoretical advantages for targeting angiogenesis include the fact that endothelial cells are diploid, nonmutated cells and therefore less likely to be able to develop resistance to drugs. Vascular endothelial growth factor (VEGF) is a potent stimulator for formation of new blood vessels. Through binding to its receptor (vascular endothelial growth factor receptor [VEGFR]) on endothelial cells, VEGF initiates biologic pathways leading to different events including endothelial cell proliferation and migration, remodeling of extracellular matrix, and tumor vascularization. Although many antiangiogenesis agents are under investigation, such as VEGFR tyrosine kinase inhibitors, the drug that has been shown to have survival benefit in NSCLC is the anti-VEGF monoclonal antibody bevacizumab (Avastin).

Bevacizumab has been evaluated in a randomized ECOG trial in combination with standard cytotoxic chemotherapy for advanced NSCLC. In this recently reported trial, 878 chemonaive patients with advanced NSCLC were randomized to receive carboplatin and paclitaxel with or without bevacizumab (15 mg/kg) every 3 weeks for six cycles. Bevacizumab was continued for up to 1 year in patients with nonprogressing disease. Patients with squamous cell histology, brain metastases, history of bleeding or hemorrhagic disorders, and individuals on anticoagulation were excluded on the basis of phase II data showing increased hemorrhagic events as a complication with bevacizumab therapy. The study demonstrated an improvement in median survival (12.5 vs. 10.2 months; $p = 0.007$), overall response rates (27.2% vs. 10.0%) and progression-free survival (6.4 vs. 4.5 months), favoring the bevacizumab arm.

d. Duration of therapy. Four randomized studies failed to show a survival difference with "prolonged" (more than six) cycles of chemotherapy compared with a fewer (four to six) number of cycles. Therefore, continuing chemotherapy until progression cannot be routinely recommended.

e. "Doublets" versus "triplets". Most randomized trials have failed to demonstrate a survival advantage of three drugs over two, and have been at the expense of enhanced toxicity. Therefore, three-drug regimens cannot be routinely recommended outside of a clinical trial.

f. Non–platin-based regimens. Given the toxicities associated with cisplatin, there is considerable interest in combining two nonplatin drugs. Most recent randomized trials have failed to show a significant difference in survival with platin regimens compared with non–platin-based regimens, although the toxicity profile is different.

g. Isolated brain metastases. In patients with controlled disease outside of the brain who have an isolated cerebral metastasis in a resectable area, resection followed by whole-brain radiotherapy is superior to whole-brain radiotherapy alone.

4. **Second-line chemotherapy.** Docetaxel, pemetrexed, and erlotinib are currently approved by the U.S. Food and Drug Administration (FDA) for second-line monotherapy for patients with metastatic NSCLC.

a. **Docetaxel.** There have been two randomized trials evaluating second-line docetaxel versus best supportive care in patients who have failed first-line therapy. Docetaxel at a dose of 75 mg/m^2 every 3 weeks prolongs survival significantly in comparison with best supportive care and, in comparison with either vinorelbine or ifosfamide, improves time to progression and 1-year survival. Moreover, it also improves quality of life. It was noted that previous paclitaxel exposure did not affect patients' response to docetaxel, suggesting no cross-resistance between the two taxane agents.

b. **Pemetrexed.** Pemetrexed, a multitargeted antifolate, has similar antitumor activity as docetaxel in the second-line setting, with less toxicity. In a randomized trial, patients were treated with pemetrexed 500 mg/m^2 or docetaxel 75 mg/m^2 every 3 weeks and the overall response rates were similar (9.1% vs. 8.8% for pemetrexed and docetaxel, respectively) with no differences in median survival (8.3 vs. 7.9 months for pemetrexed and docetaxel, respectively). Docetaxel was associated with higher rates of neutropenia, neutropenic fever, and hospitalization due to neutropenic events or other drug-related adverse events as compared with pemetrexed.

c. **EGFR tyrosine kinase inhibitors.**

(1) **Gefitinib.** Monotherapy with gefitinib has been investigated in two phase II multicenter trials: one conducted in the United States and the other primarily in Japan and Europe. Both studies included advanced NSCLC patients who failed at least one chemotherapeutic regimen. In the European/Japanese study, 210 patients who had primarily one prior chemotherapy were randomly assigned to receive 250 or 500 mg of gefitinib orally daily. The overall response rate was 18.7%, with no difference between the two doses. In the U.S. study involving patients with two prior chemotherapeutic regimens, including docetaxel, the response rate was 11%. On the basis of these favorable results, gefitinib was subsequently approved in the United States in 2003 as third-line treatment of patients with NSCLC who have progressed either during or after therapy with platinum and docetaxel. However, the data of a large randomized trial of gefitinib 250 mg daily versus best supportive care have recently been published with negative results. In this trial of 1,692 patients with locally advanced or metastatic NSCLC who had received one or two prior chemotherapeutic regimens,

no survival benefit was seen with gefitinib treatment in the overall population (medial survival of 5.6 vs. 5.1 months for gefitinib and best supportive care, respectively). However, subgroup analysis showed significant benefit for patients of Asian origin and in nonsmokers (median survival 8.9 vs. 6.1 months; $p = 0.012$). Until 2005, the FDA has limited the use of gefitinib in patients with NSCLC who have previously taken gefitinib and who are or have benefited from its use.

(2) Erlotinib. Erlotinib is a similar orally available tyrosine kinase inhibitor of EGFR. Single-agent treatment with erlotinib in the second- and third-line setting for metastatic NSCLC has been evaluated in a recently published randomized trial, BR21, from Canada. This study randomized 731 patients with stage IIIB or IV NSCLC who had failed one or two prior treatment regimens in a 2:1 ratio to receive erlotinib versus placebo. The overall response rate for erlotinib was 9% versus <1% for placebo ($p < 0.001$). Stable disease was observed in 35% of patients on the erlotinib arm as compared with 27% of patients on placebo. In contrast to the results with gefitinib, there was a significant improvement in progression-free survival (2.2 vs. 1.8 months; $p < 0.001$) and overall survival (6.7 vs. 4.7 months; $p < 0.001$), in favor of erlotinib. The reason for the different outcomes with erlotinib as compared to those with gefitinib is unclear. Possible explanations include differences in drug disease, patient demographics and/or intrinsic differences in drug activity.

Clinical parameters that appear to predict response to these drugs include never-smoking history, East Asian ethnicity, adenocarcinoma, and female gender. However, in BR21, all patient subtypes derived a survival benefit, although the hazard ratio of 0.4 for never-smokers was significantly different statistically than the hazard ratio of 0.9 for smokers. ($p \leq 0.001$). Mutations of the EGFR appear to predict dramatic response, while mutations and overexpression by fluorescent *in situ* hybridization (FISH) and immunohistochemistry also appear to predict for survival.

Both gefitinib and erlotinib have been studied in the first-line setting in combination with cytotoxic chemotherapy. Randomized trials have demonstrated no benefit of adding either erlotinib or gefitinib to standard platinum-based doublet chemotherapy. Interestingly, in one of the studies, in a prospectively designed subset analysis, a subgroup of never-smokers treated with combined chemotherapy and erlotinib did significantly better as compared with treatment with chemotherapy alone.

V. Small cell carcinoma. SCLC differs from NSCLC in a number of important ways. First, it has a more rapid clinical course and natural history, with the rapid development of metastases, symptoms, and death. Untreated, the median survival time for patients with local disease is typically 12 to 15 weeks and for those with advanced disease, it is 6 to 9 weeks. Second, it exhibits features of neuroendocrine differentiation in many patients (which may be distinguishable histopathologically) and is associated with paraneoplastic syndromes. Third, unlike NSCLC, SCLC is exquisitely sensitive to both chemotherapy and radiotherapy, although resistant disease often develops. Because of the rapid development of distant disease and its extreme sensitivity to the cytotoxic effects of chemotherapy, this mode of therapy forms the backbone of treatment for this disease, irrespective of stage.

A. Staging. Although SCLC has a propensity to metastasize quickly and micrometastatic disease is presumed to be present in all patients at the time of diagnosis, this disease is usually classified into either a local or an extensive stage. Local disease is typically defined as disease that can be encompassed within one radiation port, usually considered limited to the hemithorax and to regional nodes, including mediastinal and ipsilateral supraclavicular nodes. Extensive-stage disease is usually defined as disease that has spread outside these areas.

B. Pretreatment evaluation. Common sites of metastases for SCLC include the brain, liver, bone marrow, bone, and CNS. For this reason, a complete staging workup has traditionally consisted of a complete blood cell count; liver function tests; CT of the brain, chest, and abdomen; a bone scan; and bone marrow aspiration and biopsy. However, this complete staging workup need not be undertaken unless the patient is a candidate for combined-modality treatment with chest radiation and chemotherapy, the patient is being evaluated for a clinical study, or the information is helpful for prognostic reasons. If the patient is not a candidate for combined-modality treatment or a clinical study, stopping the staging at the first evidence of extensive-stage disease is usually appropriate. Given that isolated bone marrow metastases are rare, bone marrow biopsies and aspirates are not usually done.

C. Prognostic factors. As in NSCLC, the major pretreatment prognostic factors are stage, performance status, and bulky disease. Hepatic metastases also confer a poorer prognosis. If the patient's initial poor performance status is due to the underlying malignancy, these symptoms often disappear quickly with treatment, resulting in a net improvement in quality of life. However, major organ dysfunction from nonmalignant causes often results in an inability of the patient to tolerate chemotherapy.

D. Therapy. A number of combination chemotherapeutic regimens are available for SCLC (Table 7.6). No clear survival advantage has been consistently demonstrated for any one regimen over another. With these chemotherapeutic regimens, overall response rates of 75% to 90% and complete response rates of 50% for localized disease can be anticipated. For extensive-stage disease, overall response rates of approximately 75% and complete response rates of 25% are common. Despite these high response rates, however, the median survival time remains approximately 14 months for limited-stage disease and 7 to 9 months for extensive-stage disease. Less

Table 7.6. Chemotherapeutic regimens for small cell lung cancer

Cisplatin-based regimens

Etoposide	120 mg/m^2 IV on days 1–3 *or*
	120 mg/m^2 PO b.i.d. on days 1–3
Cisplatin	60 mg/m^2 IV on day 1
or	
Cisplatin	25 mg/m^2 IV on days 1–3
Etoposide	100 mg/m^2 IV on days 1–3
	Repeat cycle every 3 weeks

Carboplatin-based regimens

Carboplatin	300 mg/m^2 IV on day 1
Etoposide	100 mg/m^2 IV on days 1–3
or	
Carboplatin	100 mg/m^2 IV on days 1–3
Etoposide	120 mg/m^2 IV on days 1–3
	Repeat cycle every 4 weeks

Irinotecan plus cisplatin

Irinotecan	60 mg/m^2 IV on days 1, 8, and 15
Cisplatin	60 mg/m^2 IV on day 1
	Repeat cycle every 4 weeks

than 5% of patients with extensive-stage disease survive for more than 2 years.

At present, either cisplatin or carboplatin, together with etoposide, is the standard of care in North America for the treatment of SCLC. In a randomized phase III study from Japan published in 2002, four cycles of irinotecan/cisplatin were compared with four cycles of etoposide/cisplatin. The enrollment was stopped early because of an interim analysis showing a clear survival benefit in the investigational arm, with a median survival of 12.8 months for the irinotecan/cisplatin group versus 9.4 months for the etoposide/cisplatin group. The 1- and 2-year survival for the two groups were 58% and 19.5% versus 38% and 5%. A randomized trial from the United States has been conducted to confirm these results and the results have recently been reported. This study randomly assigned previously untreated patients with extensive-stage SCLC to etoposide/cisplatin or irinotecan/cisplatin and there was no difference in response rates, time to progression or median survival between the two treatment arms. Potential explanations as to why these results differed from the Japanese study include biologic differences in drug metabolism and activity between different study populations and/or dosing or scheduling of chemotherapy between the two studies.

1. Dose intensity. A dose intensity meta-analysis of chemotherapy in SCLC, which evaluated doses not requiring bone marrow transplantation support, showed no consistent correlation between dose intensity and outcome. There have been several phase I and II clinical trials evaluating the role of marrow-ablative doses of chemotherapy with subsequent progenitor cell replacement (e.g., autologous bone marrow transplantation) with disappointing survival results. In a randomized phase III study, when compared with conventional-dose chemotherapy, high-dose regimen with stem cell support prolonged relapse-free, but not overall survival.

2. Duration of therapy. Most randomized studies do not show a survival benefit for prolonged administration of chemotherapy. Several studies have demonstrated no survival benefit of prolonged first-line treatment over treatment on relapse. The optimal duration of treatment for SCLC is 4 to 6 months.

3. Second-line therapy. No curative regimens for patients with recurrent disease have been identified. The only drug approved for second-line therapy of SCLC is topotecan, which has a 20% to 40% response rate in patients with *sensitive* SCLC (those patients in whom disease relapsed 2 to 3 or more months after the first-line therapy), with a median survival of 22 to 27 weeks. For patients with *refractory* disease (progressed through or within 3 months of completion of first-line therapy), the response rate in phase II studies is only between 3% and 11%. Median survival is approximately 20 weeks. Other agents including oral etoposide and the combination of cyclophosphamide, doxorubicin, and vincristine have been used with low response rates.

E. Chemotherapy plus chest irradiation. Numerous studies have been done with chemotherapy and thoracic radiotherapy for patients with limited-stage SCLC. Conflicting results have been attributed to differences in chemotherapeutic regimens and different schedules integrating chemotherapy and thoracic radiation (concurrent, sequential, and "sandwich" approach). Two meta-analyses concluded that thoracic irradiation does result in a small but significant improvement in survival and major control of the disease in the chest, although no conclusions could be made regarding the optimal sequencing of chemotherapy and thoracic radiation. In one randomized study, twice-daily hyperfractionated radiation was compared with a once-daily schedule; both were given concurrently with four cycles of cisplatin and etoposide. Survival was significantly higher with the twice-daily regimen (median survival of 23 vs. 19 months, 5-year survival of 26% vs. 16%), albeit at the expense of more grade 3 esophagitis. In another randomized trial, early administration of thoracic irradiation in the combined-modality therapy of limited-stage SCLC was superior to late or consolidative thoracic irradiation. These data suggest that patients with good performance status and with limited disease should receive concurrent chemoradiation, preferably with twice-daily hyperfractionation.

F. Prophylactic cranial irradiation. Most randomized trials failed to show that prophylactic brain irradiation enhanced survival but did demonstrate a decrease in the risk of brain metastases without a decrease in mental function. However, in a meta-analysis of seven randomized trials, prophylactic cranial irradiation was shown to significantly increase 3-year survival with a net gain of 5.4%. It also increased disease-free survival and decreased the risk of developing brain metastasis.

VI. Palliation

A. Radiotherapy. Palliative radiotherapy is often helpful in controlling the pain due to bone metastases or neurologic function in patients with brain metastases. Chest radiotherapy may help control hemoptysis, superior vena cava syndrome, airway obstruction, laryngeal nerve compression, and other local complications.

B. Pleural effusions. Common sclerosing agents include doxycycline, talc, and bleomycin. The disadvantage of bleomycin is its cost; talc, although effective, had the disadvantage of requiring a thoracoscopy and general anesthesia for insufflation. Comparative randomized trials are under way.

C. Brachytherapy. For patients with bronchial obstruction who have received maximum external-beam radiotherapy, the use of high-dose endobronchial irradiation may be of temporary benefit.

D. Cachexia. Megestrol acetate 160 to 800 mg daily may improve the appetite of some patients.

E. Chemotherapy. In randomized trials involving both NSCLC and SCLC patients, chemotherapy has been shown to reduce the incidence of cancer-related symptoms such as pain, cough, hemoptysis, and shortness of breath.

F. Colony-stimulating factors. Filgrastim (granulocyte colony-stimulating factor) decreases the incidence of neutropenic fevers, the median duration of neutropenia, days of hospitalization, and days of antibiotic treatment in patients. However, the clinical benefit of maintaining a dose-intense approach in the treatment of patients with lung cancer has not been established. In addition, caution must be exercised when using colony-stimulating factors in patients receiving combined-modality treatment with both chemotherapy and thoracic irradiation. A randomized study by the SWOG found that patients receiving sargramostim (granulocyte–macrophage colony-stimulating factor) and chemotherapy with concurrent thoracic irradiation had a significant increase in thrombocytopenia over patients receiving concurrent chemotherapy and radiation therapy without growth factor.

G. Fatigue. Stimulants such methylphenidate (Ritalin) may be helpful in improving fatigue.

SUGGESTED READINGS

Cappuzzo F, Hirsch FR, Rossi E, et al. Epidermal growth factor receptor gene and protein and gefitinib sensitivity in non-small-cell lung cancer. *J Natl Cancer Inst* 2005;97:643–655.

Dillman RO, Herndon J, Seagren SL, et al. Improved survival in stage III non–small cell lung cancer: seven-year follow-up of CALGB 8433. *J Natl Cancer Inst* 1996;88:1210–1215.

Eddy DM. Screening for lung cancer. *Ann Intern Med* 1989;111:232–237.

Fukuoka M, Yano S, Giaccone G, et al. Multi-institutional randomized phase II trial of gefitinib for previously treated patients with advanced non-small-cell lung cancer (the IDEAL Trial). *J Clin Oncol* 2003;21:2237–2246.

Furuse K, Fukuoka M, Kawahara M, et al. Phase III study of concurrent versus sequential thoracic radiotherapy in combination with mitomycin, vindesine, and cisplatin in unresectable stage III non–small cell lung cancer. *J Clin Oncol* 1999;17:2692–2699.

Giaccone G, Dalesio O, McVie GJ, et al. Maintenance chemotherapy in small cell lung cancer: long-term results of a randomized trial. *J Clin Oncol* 1993;11:1230–1240.

Hanna N, Shepherd FA, Fossella FV, et al. Randomized phase III trial of pemetrexed versus docetaxel in patients with non-small-cell lung cancer previously treated with chemotherapy. *J Clin Oncol* 2004;22:1589–1597.

Herbst RS, Giaccone G, Schiller JH, et al. Gefitinib in combination with paclitaxel and carboplatin in advanced non-small-cell lung cancer: a phase III trial- INTACT 2. *J Clin Oncol* 2004;22:785–794.

Herbst RS, Prager D, Hermann R, et al. TRIBUTE: a phase III trial of erlotinib hydrochloride (OSI-774) combined with carboplatin and paclitaxel chemotherapy in advanced non-small-cell lung cancer. *J Clin Oncol* 2004;23:5892–5899.

The International Adjuvant Lung Cancer Trial Collaborative Group. Cisplatin-based adjuvant chemotherapy in patients with completely resected non-small-cell lung cancer. *N Engl J Med* 2004;350:351–360.

Klasa R, Murray N, Coldman A. Dose-intensity meta-analysis of chemotherapy regimens in small-cell carcinoma of the lung. *J Clin Oncol* 1991;9:499–508.

Kris MG, Natale RB, Herbst RS, et al. Efficacy of gefitinib, an inhibitor of epidermal growth factor receptor tyrosine kinase, in symptomatic patients with non-small cell lung cancer: a randomized trial. *JAMA* 2003;290:2149–2158.

Lynch TJ, Bell DW, Sordella R, et al. Activating mutations in the epidermal growth factor receptor underlying responsiveness of non-small-cell lung cancer to gefitinib. *N Engl J Med* 2004;350:2129–2139.

Mountain CF. Revisions in the international system for staging lung cancer. *Chest* 1997;111:1710–1717.

Murray N, Coy P, Pater J, et al. Importance of timing for thoracic irradiation in the combined modality treatment of limited-stage small-cell lung cancer. *J Clin Oncol* 1993;11:336–344.

Neal CR, Amdur RJ, Mendenhall WM, et al. Pancoast tumor: radiation therapy alone vs. preoperative radiation and surgery. *Int J Radiat Oncol Biol Phys* 1991;21:651–660.

Noda K, Nishiwaki Y, Kawahara M, et al. Irinotecan plus cisplatin compared with etoposide plus cisplatin for extensive small cell lung cancer. *N Engl J Med* 2002;346:85–91.

Non–Small Cell Lung Cancer Collaborative Group. Chemotherapy in non–small cell lung cancer: a meta-analysis using updated data on individual patients from 52 randomized clinical trials. *Br Med J* 1995;311:899–909.

Pignon JP, Arriagada R, Ihde DC, et al. A meta-analysis of thoracic radiotherapy for small-cell lung cancer. *N Engl J Med* 1992;327:1618–1624.

Rosell R, Gomez-Codina J, Camps C, et al. A randomized trial comparing preoperative chemotherapy plus surgery with surgery alone in patients with non–small-cell lung cancer. *N Engl J Med* 1994;330:153–158.

Sause W, Scott C, Taylor S, et al., for the Radiation Therapy Oncology Group (RTOG) 88–08 and ECOG 3488. Preliminary results of a phase III trial in regionally advanced, unresectable non–small cell lung cancer. *J Natl Cancer Inst* 1995;87:198–205.

Schiller JH, Harrington D, Belani C, et al. Comparison of four chemotherapy regimens for advanced non–small cell lung cancer. *N Engl J Med* 2002;346:92–98.

Shepherd FA, Pereira JR, Ciuleanu T, et al. Erlotinib in previously treated non-small-cell lung cancer. *N Engl J Med* 2005;353:123–132.

Tsao MS, Sakurada A, Cutz JC, et al. Erlotinib in lung cancer—molecular and clinical predictors of outcome. *N Engl J Med* 2005;353:133–144.

Thatcher N, Chang A, Parikh P, et al. Gefitinib plus best supportive care in previously treated patients with refractory advanced non-small cell lung cancer: results from a randomized, placebo-controlled multicentre study (Iressa survival evaluation in lung cancer). *Lancet* 2005;366:1527–1537.

Turrisi AT, Kim K, Blum R, et al. Twice-daily compared with once-daily thoracic radiotherapy in limited small-cell lung cancer treated concurrently with cisplatin and etoposide. *N Engl J Med* 1999;340:265–271.

Von Pawel J, Schiller JH, Shepherd FA, et al. Topotecan versus cyclophosphamide, doxorubicin, and vincristine for the treatment of recurrent small-cell lung cancer. *J Clin Oncol* 1999;2:658–667.

Warde P, Payne D. Does thoracic irradiation improve survival and local control in limited-stage small-cell carcinoma of the lung? A meta-analysis. *J Clin Oncol* 1992;10:890.

Winton T, Livingston R, Johnson D, et al. Vinorelbine plus cisplatin vs. observation in resected non-small-cell lung cancer. *N Engl J Med* 2005;352:2589–2597.

CHAPTER 8

Carcinomas of the Gastrointestinal Tract

Al B. Benson, III

Cancers of the gastrointestinal (GI) tract (esophagus, stomach, small and large intestines, and anus) account for approximately 14% of all cases of cancer in the United States and for approximately 15% of cancer deaths. Colon cancer is by far the most common of these malignancies, with cancer of the rectum, stomach, esophagus, small intestine, and anus occurring with decreasing frequency. Surgery continues to be the principal curative modality, but irradiation and chemotherapy have increasingly important roles and, in certain adjuvant situations, improve the cure rate produced by surgery. Select patients with isolated, resectable metastatic colorectal cancer lesions also may be cured with surgical resection. Chemotherapy alone is not curative in patients with overt metastatic disease. Recent combination drug regimens have produced objective responses in up to 60% of patients, with increasing numbers of individuals obtaining stabilization of their disease. There is little question that meaningful palliation and an increase in survival can be achieved in patients who respond to chemotherapy or achieve disease stabilization. Controlled clinical trials, often by cooperative groups, have been useful in defining the natural history and therapeutic benefit of various treatment modalities. Participation in such clinical trials should be encouraged.

I. **Carcinoma of the esophagus**
   A. **General considerations and aims of therapy**
      1. **Epidemiology.** Cancer of the esophagus has been predominantly of squamous cell (epidermoid) histology and represents approximately 1% of the cases of cancers in the United States. Risk factors include heavy tobacco and alcohol use. It is more common in men than in women and occurs more often in blacks than in whites. The average patient is in his or her sixties at presentation. In certain parts of China, epidermoid esophageal cancer is the most common kind of cancer, which is thought to be related to dietary habits of the region and perhaps a consequence of fungal contamination of pickled vegetables. Other predisposing factors for esophageal cancer include achalasia, a history of lye burns of the esophagus, and prior epidermoid carcinomas of the aerodigestive tract.
      In recent years, the incidence of adenocarcinoma of the esophagus (along with adenocarcinoma of the proximal stomach) has increased greatly. By the mid-1980s, it accounted for approximately one third of all esophageal cancer cases among white men and in some institutions, it is approaching 60% of newly diagnosed cancers of the esophagus. Adenocarcinoma is predominantly a disease of

middle-aged white men, is less strongly linked with alcohol and tobacco use, and is frequently associated with Barrett's esophagus (epithelial metaplasia of the lower esophagus), which is sometimes seen with reflux esophagitis. The rate of increase of adenocarcinomas of the esophagus and gastric cardia during the 1970s and 1980s exceeded that of any other cancer, including lung cancer, non–Hodgkin's lymphoma, and melanoma. The cause of this impressive increase is not known, although recent epidemiologic studies have implicated obesity, which has been increasing in the U.S. population during the last few decades. This may in turn be associated with epithelial metaplasia in the esophagus (Barrett's esophagus). Adenocarcinomas of the esophagus tend to involve the lower third of that organ, whereas the middle third is the most common site for the epidermoid subtype. Optimal chemotherapy for the two histologic types of esophageal cancer is not known to be different, with little or no difference in response rate in most series. It has been suggested, however, that a lower expression of thymidylate synthase in squamous cell carcinoma than in adenocarcinoma may make the former more sensitive to fluorouracil-based chemotherapy. Other predictive molecular markers or laboratory correlates are under investigation. For example, investigators have recently genotyped patients with resectable squamous cell or adenocarcinoma of the esophagus or gastroesophageal junction that has resulted in a correlation of genetic markers with efficacy, including pathologic response and survival.

2. Clinical manifestations and pretreatment evaluation. Carcinoma of the esophagus is usually associated with progressive and persistent dysphagia. Pain, hoarseness, weight loss, and chronic cough are unfavorable manifestations that indicate spread to regional structures (e.g., mediastinal nodes), recurrent laryngeal nerve, or fistula formation between the esophagus and the airway. The most common sites of metastasis are regional lymph nodes (which may include cervical, supraclavicular, intrathoracic, diaphragmatic, celiac axis, or periaortic), the liver, and the lungs.

Diagnosis is usually made by barium swallow, endoscopy, and biopsy or lavage cytology. Staging should be based on chest radiographic appearance, computed tomography (CT) scan of the abdomen and chest, and careful physical examination of the cervical and supraclavicular nodes. Endoscopic esophageal ultrasound may be useful in assessing the depth of tumor invasion. The preoperative staging of esophageal cancer is still inadequate, owing to the inability to evaluate lymph nodes accurately. Bronchoscopy should be done for upper and middle third tumors, and a bone scan is useful in patients with bone pain or tenderness. Recent studies investigating positron emission tomography scanning suggest improved nodal evaluation as compared with endoscopic esophageal ultrasound and CT. In addition, a Cancer and Leukemia Group B (CALGB) trial

**Table 8.1.   TNM stages for carcinoma
of the esophagus**

Primary tumor	
Tis	Carcinoma *in situ*
T1	Invades lamina propria or submucosa
T2	Invades muscularis propria
T3	Invades adventitia
T4	Invades adjacent structures
Regional lymph nodes	
N0	No nodal metastasis
N1	Regional node metastasis
Distant metastasis	
M0	None
M1	Present
Stage grouping	
0	Tis, N0, M0
I	T1, N0, M0
IIA	T2 or T3, N0, M0
IIB	T1 or T2, N1, M0
III	T3, N1, M0
	T4, any N, M0
IV	Any T, any N, M1

Modified from American Joint Committee on Cancer. *AJCC staging manual,*
6th ed. New York: Springer-Verlag, 2002.

demonstrated that thoracoscopy and laparoscopy also may refine staging accuracy. Survival is related to pathologic stage, which can be defined only surgically (Table 8.1).

3. Treatment and prognosis. The primary treatment of stage I and II carcinoma of the esophagus is surgical resection. Approximately half of esophageal cancers are operable, and half of these are resectable. Complete surgical resection (R0 resection) results in a median survival of approximately 18 months with 15% to 20% of patients surviving 5 years. Patients with more advanced disease (stage III) are best treated, at least initially, with nonsurgical means, usually a combination of radiation therapy and chemotherapy. In patients who respond to such treatment, the carcinoma may subsequently be operable, whereas patients with metastatic disease to the liver, lung, or bone are best treated with systemic therapy. Palliative feeding procedures such as with a jejunostomy or gastrostomy tube may be useful if subsequent surgical resection is not to be done. The overall median survival time is less than 1 year, and the overall 5-year survival rate is 5% to 10%. The prognosis is related to the size of the lesion, the depth of penetration of the esophagus, and nodal involvement. Current controlled clinical trials help evaluate the relative roles of chemotherapy, radiation, and surgery in all stages of the two predominant histologic types. Most emphasis has been on preoperative ("neoadjuvant") combined-modality treatment, with few supporting data available for postoperative treatment, although the concept is being evaluated as more patients survive initial combined-modality therapy. This is important because many patients who achieve good local control have disease recurrence in distant sites subsequent to surgery. Recent randomized clinical trials, however, have produced conflicting results with respect to the long-term survival benefits of neoadjuvant therapy.

B. Combined-modality treatment for potentially curable patients. The poor results with immediate surgery, due in part to inadequate staging techniques, have focused attention for some years on preoperative combined-modality treatment with radiation therapy, chemotherapy, or both, followed by surgery (or, in some instances, not followed by surgery). This approach is controversial because of uncertainty of staging and conflicting results from randomized clinical trials. When this approach is used, aggressive staging including endoscopic ultrasound, CT scanning, and laparoscopy is needed and is often combined with jejunostomy feeding tube placement for nutritional support. Despite conflicting results from randomized trials, patients with stage II and III disease are often treated in this manner.

1. Preoperative chemotherapy. The National Cancer Institute Gastrointestinal Intergroup has reported a randomized trial of 440 patients with either adenocarcinoma or epidermoid cancer of the esophagus, which compared preoperative chemotherapy (cisplatin and fluorouracil for three cycles) versus surgery alone. After a median follow-up of 55.4 months, there were no median, 1-year, or 2-year survival differences between the two groups. These results differ when compared with recent data from the Medical Research Council Clinical Trials Unit in the United Kingdom, which included 802 patients randomized to receive either two cycles of preoperative cisplatin and fluorouracil followed by surgery or surgery alone. Approximately 66% of patients had adenocarcinoma. In this study, the median survival was 16.8 months for the preoperative chemotherapy patients as compared with 13.3 months for the patients treated with surgery alone, a statistically significant difference. The 2-year survival rates were 43% and 34%, respectively. Different proportions of the two different histologies contribute to the difficulties in interpretation of these trials.

2. Radiation therapy with surgery, chemotherapy, or both. Radiation therapy, as either a preoperative or a postoperative adjunct to surgery, has not improved overall survival in most series. Radiation therapy alone has 5-year survival rates ranging from 0% to 10%. Combined-modality treatment of radiotherapy with chemotherapy has been superior. In a randomized trial comparing radiotherapy alone with radiotherapy plus chemotherapy in 121 patients, 88% of whom had squamous cell cancer, the Radiation Therapy Oncology Group reported a 5-year survival rate of 27% for the combined-modality group and 0% for the radiation therapy alone group. Median survival times were 14.1 and 9.3 months, respectively. Most patients had stage T2 disease and were node negative by CT scanning. The Eastern Cooperative Oncology Group (ECOG) performed a similar trial of 135 patients with stage I or II squamous cell cancer of the esophagus. Patients were randomized to receive 40 Gy of radiation alone or radiation with a 96-hour continuous infusion of fluorouracil plus mitomycin. Median survival was improved for patients treated with chemoradiation (14.8 months) as compared with those receiving radiation therapy alone (9.2 months). A recent German study of 172 patients with locally advanced squamous cell carcinoma of the esophagus evaluated induction chemotherapy (fluorouracil, leucovorin, etoposide, and cisplatin) followed by chemoradiotherapy (40 Gy, cisplatin, etoposide) followed by surgery versus induction chemotherapy followed by chemoradiotherapy (at least 65 Gy) without surgery. The surgical group of patients demonstrated superior 2-year progression-free survival (64.3% vs. 40.7%, $p = 0.003$); however, treatment-related mortality was increased in the surgery group (12.8% vs. 3.5%, $p = 0.03$). There was no difference in survival. A recently reported meta-analysis of randomized controlled trials comparing neoadjuvant chemoradiation and surgery alone included nine randomized trials with 1,116 patients. The meta-analysis demonstrated that neoadjuvant chemoradiation and surgery improved the 3-year survival and reduced local-regional cancer recurrence ($p = 0.038$). There was also a higher rate of complete resection, although there was a nonsignificant trend toward increased treatment mortality with neoadjuvant chemoradiation. In addition, concurrent use of chemotherapy and radiotherapy was superior to sequentially administered treatment. More recent phase II trials have explored radiation with alternative chemotherapy combinations, including oxaliplatin, irinotecan, docitaxel, and paclitaxel alone and with molecular targeted agents. Combined chemotherapy and radiotherapy is therefore a reasonable approach for patients who refuse surgery or whose disease is unresectable for anatomic or physiologic reasons, particularly those with epidermoid carcinoma.

  a. Radiation therapy + fluorouracil + cisplatin

    (1) Radiation therapy of 180 to 200 cGy/day for 3 weeks, 5 days weekly, and then additional radiation for 2 weeks to the boost field for a total of 5,040 cGy, *and*

    (2) Fluorouracil 1,000 mg/m²/day by continuous infusion for 4 days on weeks 1, 5, 8, and 11, with cisplatin 75 mg/m² IV at 1 mg/minute on the first day of each course. Reduce fluorouracil for severe diarrhea or stomatitis and cisplatin for severe neutropenia or thrombocytopenia.

    (3) Surgery, when it can be done, is probably appropriate because most patients treated with chemotherapy and radiotherapy still have residual tumor. Even though a high proportion of patients, 25% in many

series, have complete pathologic responses at surgery, the preoperative identification of these patients is not accurate.

A randomized trial from Ireland of 113 patients with adenocarcinoma of the esophagus has shown a 3-year survival rate of 32% for patients treated with preoperative chemotherapy with fluorouracil and cisplatin (CF) and with radiotherapy followed by surgery as compared with 6% for patients treated with surgery alone. Similarly, a study from the University of Michigan of 100 patients (68% adenocarcinoma) has shown a 3-year survival rate of 30% for combined-modality treatment as compared with 16% for surgery alone, with a reduction in local recurrence in the combined group (42% vs. 19%). At a median follow-up of 8.2 years, there was no difference in survival between the two groups (17.6 and 16.9 months, respectively). Optimal results may involve all three major treatment modalities, with at least some of the chemotherapy being given concurrently with radiation therapy. Alternative preoperative treatments are being defined in phase II trials, incorporating such agents as paclitaxel and irinotecan, and postoperative chemotherapy is also being evaluated. The following regimens have been used in potentially resectable patients:

b. Cisplatin + fluorouracil + radiotherapy (Dublin regimen)

   (1) Fluorouracil 15 mg/kg (555 mg/m^2) IV over 16 hours daily, days 1 to 5, *and*

   (2) Cisplatin 75 mg/m^2 IV infused over 8 hours on day 7 after 1 full day of hydration. Repeat both drugs at 6 weeks.

   (3) Radiotherapy of 40 Gy in 15 fractions over 3 weeks, beginning on the first day of chemotherapy.

   (4) Surgery is done 8 weeks after beginning treatment, blood counts permitting.

c. Fluorouracil + cisplatin + vinblastine + radiotherapy (Michigan regimen)

   (1) Vinblastine 1 mg/m^2 IV on days 1 to 4 and 17 to 20 of radiotherapy, *and*

   (2) Cisplatin 20 mg/m^2/day by continuous IV infusion on days 1 to 5 and 17 to 21 of radiotherapy, *and*

   (3) Fluorouracil 300 mg/m^2/day by continuous IV infusion on days 1 to 21 of radiotherapy, *and*

   (4) Radiotherapy 45 Gy in 15 fractions (300 cGy b.i.d.) for 3 weeks

   (5) Surgery done at 6 weeks.

C. Treatment of advanced (metastatic) disease. Various agents with modest activity when used alone are available. These include cisplatin, carboplatin, fluorouracil, bleomycin, paclitaxel, docetaxel, irinotecan, gemcitabine, methotrexate, mitomycin, vinorelbine, and doxorubicin. Response rates range from 15% to 30% and are usually brief. Most data are for epidermoid carcinoma, the exception being paclitaxel, which appears equally effective in both histologic types. The most active drugs appear to be cisplatin, paclitaxel, and fluorouracil. Patients with no history of prior chemotherapy are more likely to respond than those who have had previous treatment. Single agents are less helpful than combination chemotherapy because of their lower response rates and brief duration of response. Cisplatin-based regimens have been most extensively tested. Among the most active are the following (for adenocarcinoma of the distal esophagus and gastroesophageal junction also see Section II, in this chapter):

1. **Cisplatin + fluorouracil**
   a. Cisplatin 75 to 100 mg/m^2 IV on day 1.
   b. Fluorouracil 1,000 mg/m^2/day as a continuous IV infusion on days 1 to 5. Repeat every 28 days.
2. **Paclitaxel + cisplatin**
   a. Paclitaxel 175 mg/m^2 IV.
   b. Cisplatin 75 mg/m^2 IV. Repeat every 21 days.
3. **Carboplatin + paclitaxel**
   a. Carboplatin area under the curve (AUC) 5 IV.
   b. Paclitaxel 150 mg/m^2 IV. Repeat every 21 days.
4. **Paclitaxel + cisplatin + fluorouracil**
   a. Paclitaxel 175 mg/m^2 IV over 3 hours on day 1.
   b. Cisplatin 20 mg/m^2/day IV on days 1 to 5.
   c. Fluorouracil (fluorouracil) 750 mg/m^2/day continuous IV on days 1 to 5. Repeat every 28 days.
5. **Cisplatin + irinotecan**
   a. Irinotecan 65 mg/m^2 IV days 1, 8.
   b. Cisplatin 30 mg/m^2 IV days 1, 8.
   The regimen is repeated every 21 days.
6. **Second-line therapy.** May be chosen from the list of alternative combination therapies or the single agents, including methotrexate 40 mg/m^2 IV weekly; bleomycin 15 U/m^2 IV twice weekly; vinorelbine 25 mg/m^2 IV weekly; or mitomycin 20 mg/m^2 IV every 4 to 6 weeks.

D. Supportive care. Esophagitis during a combined-modality treatment program is nearly universal, and nutritional support frequently is required, preferably using alimentation by feeding tube placed by enterostomy. Peripheral alimentation is difficult with the continuous chemotherapy administration. Gastrostomy tubes are to be avoided because of the usual requirement for a gastric pull-up after resection of the esophageal tumor.

E. Follow-up studies. For asymptomatic patients with potentially curative therapy, history and physical examination may be done every 4 months for 1 year, then every 6 months for 2 years. Chest radiographs, CT scans, endoscopy, chemistries, and complete blood count should be evaluated as clinically indicated.

II. **Gastric carcinoma**
   A. **General considerations and aims of therapy**
      1. **Epidemiology.** The incidence of stomach cancer has decreased dramatically in the United States since the beginning of the century, although it has stabilized in the last 20 years. The leading cause of cancer death in 1930, it now ranks eighth; however, worldwide it is the second most lethal cancer. No improvement has been seen, however, in 5-year survival rates, which range from 90% (T1, N0) to 30% to 50% (T3, N0) and from 30% to 40% (stage II) to less than 10% (stage IIIB). A recent large randomized

U.S. clinical trial, however, has shown improved survival for individuals treated with surgery followed by combined radiation and chemotherapy. The man-to-woman ratio is approximately two to one. Stomach cancer is still the leading cause of cancer deaths among men in Japan and is also common in China, Finland, Poland, Peru, and Chile. A high rate of chronic gastritis and intestinal metaplasia of the stomach is associated with a high incidence of gastric cancer. *Helicobacter pylori* has been implicated in such changes and in gastric cancer, particularly the more distal "intestinal" type, as well as in peptic ulcer. Although the incidence in the United States has decreased, the location of gastric cancers has migrated proximally. Nearly half the stomach cancers occurring in white men are located proximally (gastroesophageal [GE] junction, cardia and proximal lesser curvature).

2. Clinical manifestations and evaluation. The most common symptoms are weight loss, abdominal pain, nausea, vomiting, changes in bowel habits, fatigue, anorexia, and dysphagia. The diagnosis generally is made by endoscopy and biopsy, although barium swallow is frequently helpful. Endoscopic ultrasonography is increasingly used; it is more accurate in gauging the depth of the cancer in the gastric wall than in determining nodal involvement. Laparoscopy is also helpful in improving clinical staging since it can more accurately identify peritoneal metastases and further evaluate the liver. Metastases are to the liver, pancreas, omentum, esophagus, and bile ducts by direct extension and to regional and distant lymph nodes such as those in the left supraclavicular area. Pulmonary and bone metastases are a late finding. Staging of suspected gastric cancer should initially include CT scans of the chest, abdomen, and pelvis. Tumor markers such as carcinoembryonic antigen (CEA), CA 19-9, and CA 72-4 may be useful for subsequent assessment of the response to therapy. Prognosis is reflected by accurate staging (Table 8.2). The revised staging method classifies patients according to the number of pathologically involved regional lymph nodes. The groupings are 1 to 6 (N1), 7 to 15 (N2), and more than 15 involved lymph nodes (N3).

3. Treatment and prognosis. Most stomach cancers are adenocarcinomas. Important prognostic factors include tumor grade and gross appearance. Diffusely infiltrating lesions are less likely to be cured than sharply circumscribed, nonulcerating lesions. The presence of regional lymph node involvement or involvement of contiguous organs in the surgical specimen indicates an increased likelihood of recurrence, as does the presence of dysphagia at the time of diagnosis. Patients with proximal lesions or lesions requiring total, rather than distal subtotal, gastrectomy are also at greater risk.

There has been controversy as to the contribution of extensive lymphadenectomy (D1 vs. D2 dissection) to survival benefit. Japanese surgeons have widely promoted the D2 dissection; however, randomized clinical trials including the Dutch Gastric Cancer Group and the Medical Research

Table 8.2. TNM stages for carcinoma of the stomach

Primary tumor

Tis	Carcinoma *in situ*
T1	Invades lamina propria or submucosa
T2	Invades muscularis propria or subserosa
T3	Penetrates serosa (visceral peritoneum)
T4	Invades adjacent structures

Regional lymph nodes

N0	No nodal metastasis
N1	Metastasis in 1–6 regional lymph nodes
N2	Metastasis in 7–15 regional lymph nodes
N3	Metastasis in >15 regional lymph nodes

Distant metastasis

M0	None
M1	Present

Stage grouping

0	Tis, N0, M0
IA	T1, N0, M0
IB	T1, N1, M0
	T2, N0, M0
II	T1, N2, M0
	T2, N1, M0
	T3, N0, M0
IIIA	T2, N2, M0
	T3, N1, M0
	T4, N0, M0
IIIB	T3, N2, M0
IV	T4, N1, M0
	T1, N3, M0
	T2, N3, M0
	T3, N3, M0
	T4, N2, M0
	T4, N3, M0
	Any T, any N, M1

Modified from American Joint Committee on Cancer. *AJCC staging manual,* 6th ed. New York: Springer-Verlag, 2002.

Council trials did not show a survival benefit of D2 over D1 lymphadenectomy. However, there was increased morbidity and mortality for those patients who underwent the D2 dissection.

B. Treatment of advanced (metastatic, locally unresectable, or recurrent) disease

1. Single agents with activity include epirubicin, mitomycin, doxorubicin, cisplatin, etoposide, fluorouracil, irinotecan, hydroxyurea, the taxanes, and the nitrosoureas. Single agents have low response rates (15%–30%), brief durations of response, and few complete responses, and they have little impact on survival.

2. Combinations of drugs are more widely used than single agents, largely because of higher response rates, more frequent complete responses, and the theoretical potential of longer survival. A controlled trial (1985) of fluorouracil alone versus fluorouracil plus doxorubicin (Adriamycin) (FA) versus fluorouracil, doxorubicin, and mitomycin (FAM), however, failed to show a survival benefit for the combinations, which were more costly and toxic. Response rates, which were measurable in only approximately half the patients, were higher with the combinations. An European study compared methotrexate, fluorouracil, and doxorubicin (FAMTX) with etoposide, leucovorin, and fluorouracil (ELF) and with CF, showing no significant difference among the combinations. Another European trial compared epirubicin, cisplatin, and fluorouracil (ECF) to FAMTX, which favored ECF with improved response rate (45% vs. 20%) and a 2-month improvement in median survival. More recently, a large international advanced gastric cancer trial of 457 patients compared docetaxel, cisplatin, and fluorouracil (DCF) versus CF. The DCF regimen demonstrated significant toxicity including fatigue; however, it showed improved response rate (36% vs. 26%), improved time to tumor progression (5.6 vs. 3.7 months), and improved one- and 2-year survival (40.2% vs. 31.8%; 18.4% vs. 8.8%, respectively). DCF as a treatment for advanced disease, therefore, represents an important proof of principle; however, the toxicity is of significant concern. Recent clinical trials are exploring other docetaxel-containing combination regimens (e.g., oxaliplatin) in an effort to maintain efficacy but to reduce toxicity.

a. DCF (docetaxel, cisplatin, and fluorouracil). Dexamethosone 8 mg PO b.i.d. 1 day before chemotherapy, on the day of treatment, and the day after.

(1) Docetaxel 75 mg/m^2 as a 1-hour IV infusion.

(2) Cisplatin 75 mg/m^2 as a 2-hour IV infusion.

(3) Fluorouracil 750 mg/m^2 daily as a continuous intravenous infusion days 1 to 5.

The regimen is repeated every 21 days.

b. ECF (epirubicin, cisplatin, and fluorouracil)

(1) Epirubicin 50 mg/m^2 IV bolus on day one followed by

(2) Cisplatin 60 mg/m^2 IV over 2 hours on day one

(3) Fluorouracil 200 mg/m^2 daily as a continuous intravenous infusion days 1 to 21.

The regimen is repeated every 21 days.

c. CF (cisplatin, fluorouracil)

(1) Cisplatin 100 mg/m^2 IV over 2 hours on day 1.

(2) Fluorouracil 1,000 mg/m^2 daily as a continuous IV infusion on days 1 to 5.

The regimen is repeated every 28 days.

d. Irinotecan and cisplatin
   (1) Irinotecan 65 mg/m^2 over 30 minutes IV on days 1 and 8.
   (2) Cisplatin 30 mg/m^2 IV over 1 hour, days 1, 8.
   The regimen is repeated every 21 days.

e. Irinotecan + cisplatin
   (1) Irinotecan 70 mg/m^2 IV over 30 minutes on days 1 and 15.
   (2) Cisplatin 80 mg/m^2 IV over 2 hours on day 1.
   The cycle is repeated every 28 days.

f. FAMTX. Before methotrexate administration, hydrate with 1 L of isotonic sodium bicarbonate (1.4% bicarbonate; urine pH must be higher than 7.0). Infuse 2 L of an identical solution over 24 hours after methotrexate is given. The regimen is as follows:
   (1) Methotrexate 1.5 g/m^2 by IV bolus infusion after the hydration and urine alkalinization on day 1, *and*
   (2) Fluorouracil 1.5 g/m^2 by IV bolus infusion starting 1 hour after the end of the methotrexate infusion, *and*
   (3) Leucovorin 15 mg/m^2 orally starting 24 hours later on day 2, given every 6 hours for 3 days or until the methotrexate level is less than $2 \times 10^{-8}M$. If the methotrexate level is more than $2.5 \times 10^{-6}M$ at 24 hours, increase leucovorin dose to 30 mg/m^2 every 6 hours for 96 hours.
   (4) Doxorubicin 30 mg/m^2 IV on day 15 if the white blood cell count is more than 3,000/μL or the absolute neutrophil count is more than 1,500/μL and the platelet count is more than 70,000/μL.
The cycle is repeated every 4 weeks. Renal function must be normal and blood levels of methotrexate should be monitored with this regimen.

g. ELF. The ELF (leucovorin, etoposide, and fluorouracil) regimen was designed to be less toxic as compared to adriamycin- and cisplatin-containing regimens. The regimen is as follows:
   (1) Leucovorin 300 mg/m^2 as a 10-minute IV infusion, *followed by*
   (2) Etoposide 120 mg/m^2 as a 50-minute IV infusion, *followed by*
   (3) Fluorouracil 500 mg/m^2 IV as a 10-minute infusion.
All agents are given on days 1, 2, and 3. The course is repeated in 21 to 28 days.

h. Hydroxyurea + leucovorin + fluorouracil + cisplatin. A large phase II study of this regimen in France has reported a response rate of 62% and median survival time of 11 months. The regimen is as follows:
   (1) Hydroxyurea 1.5 to 2 g PO on days 0, 1, and 2, *and*
   (2) Leucovorin 200 mg/m^2 IV as a 2-hour infusion on days 1 and 2, *before*
   (3) Fluorouracil 400 mg/m^2 IV bolus and 600 mg/m^2 by 22-hour infusion on days 1 and 2, *then*

(4) Cisplatin 80 mg/m^2 IV on day 3 every other cycle.

The cycle is repeated every 14 days.

C. Adjuvant chemotherapy. Although no single randomized phase III adjuvant gastric chemotherapy trial has demonstrated a survival benefit, a meta-analysis published in 2001 of over 3,658 clinical trial patients (21 comparisons) who were randomized to receive adjuvant chemotherapy versus surgery alone showed a small survival benefit for those who received adjuvant therapy (18% reduced risk of death, HR = 0.82, $p < 0.001$).

Most recently, the European MAGIC Medical Research Council Adjuvant Gastric Infusional Chemotherapy trial included 503 patients with gastric cancer to receive surgery alone versus three preoperative and three postoperative cycles of the DCF regimen. The patients who received chemotherapy demonstrated significant downstaging of their tumors with improved progression-free survival (19 vs. 13 months, $p = 0.0001$), median survival (24 vs. 20 months, $p = 0.02$), and 5-year survival (36% vs. 23%, $p = 0.009$). Since only 55% of patients were able to begin postoperative therapy, it is postulated that the preoperative chemotherapy provided the most significant benefit. Other neoadjuvant regimens, including combinations with radiation, are under study.

D. Combined-modality therapy. The U.S. Gastrointestinal Intergroup has reported the results of a 556-patient randomized trial comparing surgery with or without postoperative chemotherapy (fluorouracil and leucovorin) and combined chemotherapy and radiation followed by two additional cycles of chemotherapy. Patients had resected stages IB through stage IV M0 adenocarcinoma of the stomach or gastroesophageal junction. Postoperative combined therapy produced a statistically significant median survival benefit (36 vs. 27 months, respectively; $p = 0.005$). Although the study did not show any significant difference in relapse-free or overall survival according to the extent of lymph node dissection, 54% of patients had a D0 lymphadenectomy (surgery that did not remove all of the N1 nodes), 36% had a D1 dissection, and only 10% underwent a D2 dissection (includes perigastric, celiac, splenic, hepatic artery, and cardial lymph nodes). Major toxic effects (grade 3 or higher) in the chemoradiotherapy group were predominantly hematologic (54%) and gastrointestinal (GI) (33%).

E. Recommended postoperative adjuvant combined-modality regimen

   1. **Preradiation chemotherapy** (cycle 1)
       a. Leucovorin 20 mg/m^2 IV bolus on days 1 to 5
       b. Fluorouracil 425 mg/m^2 IV bolus on days 1 to 5
   2. **Radiotherapy and Chemotherapy**
       a. Radiation therapy. 45 Gy at 180 cGy/day to the tumor (or tumor bed) and nodal chains daily for 5 days weekly × 5 weeks (begin 28 days after initial chemotherapy).
       b. Chemotherapy. Started on the first day of radiotherapy and repeated during the last 3 days of radiation.

(1) Leucovorin 20 mg/m^2 IV bolus on days 1 to 4
(2) Fluorouracil 400 mg/m^2 IV bolus on days 1 to 4, each dose given after the leucovorin

3. Postradiation chemotherapy. One month after completing chemoradiation, begin two 5-day cycles of leucovorin and fluorouracil as given during cycle 1.

F. Follow-up studies. Reasonable follow-up studies for patients in remission after surgery consist of history and physical examination every 4 to 6 months for 3 years, and then annually. Complete blood cell count, chemistries, endoscopy, and radiologic imaging should be evaluated as clinically indicated. Vitamin B$_{12}$ supplementation is recommended for patients who have had proximal resections or total gastrectomy.

G. Complications. Hematologic and GI toxicities from the chemotherapy may be accentuated by concurrent radiotherapy. If the complications are sufficiently severe, chemotherapy, radiotherapy, or both should be withheld until improvement. Consideration is given to treating at reduced doses. Hematopoietic growth factors may be of benefit in preventing severe infections secondary to neutropenia, but their use has not yet resulted in improved survival.

H. Treatment of refractory disease. If the patient's disease recurs or progresses with the recommended regimens, it is reasonable to consider combinations containing drugs not previously administered or any of the single agents mentioned in Section II.B.1.

III. Cancer of the small intestine

A. Carcinoid tumors. Carcinoid tumors are the most common tumors of the appendix and ileum. They may develop in other parts of the GI tract but much less frequently. The usual histologic criteria of malignancy are not always applicable. Invasion and evidence of distant spread are more useful prognostic features. In one series, the 60% of patients with intestinal carcinoids that were still confined to the wall of the gut had a 5-year survival rate of 85%, whereas those with tumors invading the serosa or beyond had a 5% survival rate at 5 years. Patients in the latter group were nearly always symptomatic, whereas patients in the former group were not. (Their tumors were discovered at surgery for appendicitis or other causes.) Tumors of the appendix are usually benign by these criteria, whereas those of the ileum are more often invasive. Surgical resection is the definitive therapy. Currently, with approximately 2,500 new cases of malignant carcinoid per year, it is expected that at least 50% of patients will survive 5 years.

1. Carcinoid syndrome. Approximately 10% of patients with carcinoid tumors have the carcinoid syndrome, which includes diarrhea, abdominal cramps, malabsorption, flushing, bronchoconstriction, and cardiac valvular disease (late sequela). With tumors of intestinal origin, liver metastases are nearly always present. Serotonin is thought to be responsible for the abdominal symptoms. Its metabolite, 5-hydroxyindoleacetic acid (5-HIAA), is excreted in large quantities in the urine and is a useful marker of disease activity. Other markers may be elevated, including chromogranin A, which is the most frequently elevated carinoid marker. The symptoms may respond to simple antidiarrheal therapy. The flushing caused by the syndrome has been attributed to bradykinin, formed by the interaction of kallikrein (produced by the tumor) with a plasma protein. If simple symptomatic measures do not suffice, the best treatment is the synthetic long-acting somatostatin analog octreotide acetate (Sandostatin). This agent, injected at a usual initial dose of 150μg SC every 8 hours or as the long-acting formulation (octreotide LAR depot) 20 to 30 mg IM every month, effectively decreases the secretion of serotonin and other gastroenteropancreatic peptides such as insulin or gastrin. It has been helpful in ameliorating the symptoms of carcinoid tumors (e.g., flushing and diarrhea). There are even modest objective antitumor effects, and improvement in survival is suggested in limited reports. The excretion of 5-HIAA is reduced by octreotide.

2. **Treatment of advanced carcinoid tumors**

   a. **Effective agents.** The chemotherapy agents doxorubicin, fluorouracil, dacarbazine, and streptozocin have been shown to have limited activity in this disease. Response rates for combinations including fluorouracil and streptozocin, for example, are 25% to 35%, with response durations usually less than 9 months; the overall response rate for patients with tumors of intestinal origin is 41%. A median duration of response of 7 months may be expected, and patients with a good performance status have the greatest likelihood of response. Tumor response correlates well with reduction of 5-HIAA excretion. Some reports have indicated responses with interferon-α, including responses in combination with octreotide and in some patients previously treated with chemotherapy. When the disease is confined to the liver, it is sometimes possible to achieve good palliation with hepatic artery embolization, chemoembolization, or most recently, yttrium 90 microspheres. Of note, poorly differentiated neuroendocrine tumors or small cell/atypical lung carcinoids are managed with a small cell lung cancer regimen.

   b. **Recommended regimens**

      (1) Octreotide LAR 20 to 30 mg IM q14 to 28 days.
      (2) Interferon-α 3 to 6 × 10⁶ U/day or 10 × 10⁶ U three times per week.

   c. **Precautions.** Treatment of carcinoid tumors may precipitate or exacerbate the carcinoid syndrome during the first days of treatment, and the serotonin antagonists cyproheptadine and methysergide as well as octreotide should be available.

B. **Adenocarcinomas.** Adenocarcinomas of the small intestine are so uncommon that there is no large chemotherapy experience to report. Survival of patients with small intestinal cancer is a function of stage (Table 8.3). Radiation and infusional fluorouracil may be considered for patients with local recurrence or unresectable disease. The chemotherapy regimens employed for advanced colorectal cancer (e.g.,

Table 8.3.   TNM stages for carcinoma of the small intestine

Primary tumor

Tis	Carcinoma *in situ*
T1	Invades lamina propria or submucosa
T2	Invades muscularis propria
T3	Invades through the muscularis propria into subserosa or into nonperitonealized perimuscular tissue with extension of ≤ 2 cm
T4	Perforates visceral peritoneum or directly invades other organs or structures

Regional lymph nodes

N0	No nodal metastasis
N1	Regional node metastasis

Distant metastasis

M0	None
M1	Present

Stage grouping

0	Tis, N0, M0
I	T1 or T2, N0, M0
II	T3 or T4, N0, M0
III	Any T, N1, M0
IV	Any T, any N, M1

Modified from American Joint Committee on Cancer. *AJCC staging manual,* 6th ed. New York: Springer-Verlag, 2002.

oxaliplatin, irinotecan, fluorouracil, and leucovorin) also are generally used to treat patients with small intestine adenocarcinoma.

IV. Cancer of the large intestine

   A. General considerations and aims of therapy. Taken together, cancers of the colon and rectum are by far the most frequent malignancies of the GI tract, and account for the most deaths. Approximately half of patients found to have large bowel cancers are cured by surgery, which remains the only curative modality. Local recurrence is much more common for rectal cancer (40%–50% in nonirradiated patients). Approximately half of large bowel cancer recurrences are in the liver.

   1. Staging. In the past, a commonly used staging system was the Dukes' staging system, including the Astler–Coller modifications. TNM staging for colorectal cancer (Table 8.4) is currently the recommended system. The sixth edition of the American Joint Committee on Cancer (AJCC) Staging Manual has expanded the subsets of patients with stage II (IIA—T3, N0; IIB—T4, N0) and stage III (IIIA—T1–2, N1; IIIB—T3–4, N1; IIIC—any T, N2) disease, which more accurately reflects the wide variations in survival. Recent models utilizing the staging subsets have incorporated T stage, lymph node status and grade of tumor.

Table 8.4.   TNM stages for carcinoma of the colon and rectum

Primary tumor

Tis	Carcinoma *in situ* and intramucosal (within lamina propria)
T1	Invades through muscularis mucosa into submucosa
T2	Invades muscularis propria
T3	Invades through muscularis propria into subserosa or nonperitonealized pericolic or perirectal tissues
T4	Invades adjacent organs or structures or perforates visceral peritoneum

Regional lymph nodes

N0	No nodal metastasis
N1	Metastasis in 1–3 regional nodes
N2	Metastasis in <4 regional nodes

Distant metastasis

M0	None
M1	Present

Stage grouping

0	Tis, N0, M0
I	T1 or T2, N0, M0
IIA	T3, N0, M0
IIB	T4, N0, M0
IIIA	T1–2, N1, M0
IIIB	T3–4, N1, M0
IIIC	Any T, N2, M0
IV	Any T, any N, M1

Modified from American Joint Committee on Cancer. *AJCC staging manual,* 6th ed. New York: Springer-Verlag, 2002.

For example, a stage IIA patient with a low-grade tumor, has a predicted 5-year disease-free survival after surgery of approximately 74%; however, the survivorship of a IIB patient declines to 63%. Stage IIIA patients actually have a better chance of survival as compared to stage IIB patients even without adjuvant therapy (approximately 71% with a low-grade tumor). The worse prognosis is for a stage IIIC patient who has a projected 5-year disease-free survival of less than 25%, even with fluorouracil chemotherapy. This pathologic staging method is helpful for selecting patients who are at sufficiently high risk to justify adjuvant therapy such as chemotherapy or irradiation (rectal cancer). Staging is most accurately performed at the time of surgery. Abdominal, chest, and pelvic CT are helpful for preoperative assessment of extrabowel involvement, but the findings may be falsely negative when small peritoneal implants are present. Bone scans are seldom needed, except for assessment of bone pain, because bone metastases occur rather late in the course of the disease. Positron emission tomography scanning is considered to determine the presence of metastatic disease.

2. Serum CEA. CEA level may parallel disease activity, although it is not increased in all patients with colon cancer. It is worth measuring it preoperatively and, if elevated, postoperatively because failure of an elevated value to return to normal may signify incomplete removal of the tumor. Likewise, a serial rise in CEA values after an initial fall to normal indicates recurrence. CEA values may also be an indicator of response during chemotherapy treatment. Patients who have a normal serum CEA level preoperatively may still demonstrate an elevated CEA value at the time of recurrence. A rising CEA level is an indication for careful re-evaluation with CT, positron emission tomography, and possibly laparoscopy because some patients may have isolated, resectable, and thus potentially curable metastases, particularly involving the liver.

B. Treatment of advanced disease

1. Effective agents and combinations. For more than 40 years, fluorouracil has been the standard agent in the treatment of advanced colorectal disease not amenable to surgical or radiotherapeutic control. Response rates have varied widely, but a generally agreed-on figure is 10% to 15%. Recent chemotherapy combinations with fluorouracil, including leucovorin, irinotecan and oxaliplatin, have demonstrated improved response rates and survival. The addition of the antivascular endothelial growth factor (anti-VEGF) monoclonal antibody bevacizumab to chemotherapy has further improved response rates and survival.

Second-line treatment for metastatic colorectal cancer is of particular interest because of the benefits of single-agent irinotecan in this setting. Trials have demonstrated response rates of greater than 20%, with greater than 50% of patients achieving stable disease and with median survivals of approximately 12 months. In addition, an European study, which randomized metastatic colorectal cancer patients who had progressed within 6 months of treatment with fluorouracil to receive irinotecan versus supportive care, demonstrated a significant 1-year survival advantage (36.2% vs. 13.8%; $p = 0.0001$) for those patients receiving irinotecan, including an improved pain-free survival.

More recent second-line clinical trials have demonstrated the superiority of FOLFOX4 *(See the regimens associated with the acronyms in Section IV.B.3.)* as compared to the LV5FU2 regimen for patients who received previous IFL chemotherapy (time to tumor progression 5.6 vs. 2.6 months, $p < 0.0001$). Oxaliplatin as a single agent has been shown to be inactive. ECOG demonstrated that FOLFOX plus bevacizumab was superior to FOLFOX for previously treated patients (response rate 21.08% vs. 9.2%; progression-free survival 7.2 vs. 4.8 months, $p < 0.0001$; overall survival 12.9 vs. 10.8 months, $p = 0.0018$). Cetuximab given as a second- or third-line agent produces a response rate of approximately 10%, while cetuximab and irinotecan have a response rate of approximately 23% for patients who have progressed on a previous irinotecan regimen.

First-line irinotecan trials for previously untreated patients with advanced colorectal cancer also have demonstrated response and survival benefits as compared with fluorouracil and leucovorin. For example, a U.S. trial comparing weekly IFL (bolus fluorouracil) with fluorouracil and leucovorin and with irinotecan alone revealed an overall response rate favoring the three-drug combination (39% vs. 21% vs. 18%, respectively) and a median survival advantage (14.8 vs. 12.6 vs. 12 months, respectively; $p = 0.04$). An European trial evaluating infusional fluorouracil regimens with or without irinotecan also confirmed a response advantage for the three drugs (49% vs. 31%) and improved median survival (17.5% vs. 14.1%; $p = 0.03$).

More recent first-line clinical trials have demonstrated the superiority of FOLFOX versus IFL (response rate 45% vs. 31%, $p = 0.002$; time to progression 8.7 months vs. 6.9 months, $p = 0.0014$; and overall survival 19.5 months vs. 14.8 months, $p = 0.0001$). In addition, IFL plus bevacizumab has enhanced efficacy as compared to IFL (median survival 20.3 vs. 15.6 months, $p < 0.001$; progression-free survival 10.6 vs. 6.4 months, $p < 0.001$; overall response 45% vs. 35%, $p < 0.01$). Fluorouracil/leucovorin and bevacizumab also has activity with a median overall survival of 18.3 months and progression-free survival of 8.8 months.

Capecitabine is the only oral fluoropyrimidine available for use in colorectal cancer in the United States. Two trials have demonstrated a better response with capecitabine than with fluorouracil and leucovorin with similar median time to disease progression, median time to treatment failure, and median overall survival (approximately 13.3 months for fluorouracil/leucovorin and 12.5 months for fluorouracil/leucovorin in a U.S. study). Capecitabine is therefore available for first-line colorectal cancer patients, particularly those who may not be optimal candidates for an irinotecan or oxaliplatin combination.

The current principle of treatment strategy for patients with advanced colorectal cancer encompasses a new paradigm. **Treatment now represents a continuum whereby patients who are exposed to all active agents, including fluorouracil, irinotecan, oxaliplatin, and bevacizumab, over the course of their illness, will achieve the maximum survival advantage, now estimated as a median survival of more than 2 years.**
2. Liver metastasis. A 2-week continuous infusion with floxuridine with or without leucovorin plus dexamethasone given every 28 days and administered by an implantable or portable infusion pump produces one of the highest responses for metastatic colorectal cancer to the liver. The impact on survival, however, remains controversial, with no definitive survival benefit shown by the hepatic artery infusion. More recently, investigators have included systemic therapy alternating with the hepatic artery infusion.

3. **Recommended regimens**
   a. **mFOLFOX6**

- Oxaliplatin 85 mg/m^2 as a 2-hour IV infusion in 500 mL of D5W on day 1 **only,** *and*
- Leucovorin 400 mg/m^2 as a 2-hour IV infusion followed by
- Fluorouracil 400 mg/m^2 IV bolus on day 1 **only**, then followed by
- Fluorouracil 2.4 to 3.0 g/m^2 as a continuous IV infusion over 46 hours, repeated every 2 weeks.

The cycle is repeated every 14 days. Day 1 leucovorin may be given during the same 2-hour period as the oxaliplatin, but because of the incompatibility of oxaliplatin with saline, both drugs must be given in D5W.

b. **FOLFOX4**

- Oxaliplatin 85 mg/m^2 as a 2-hour IV infusion in 250 to 500 mL of D5W on day 1 **only** simultaneously with leucovorin,
- Leucovorin 200 mg/m^2 as a 2-hour IV infusion, days 1 and 2, followed by
- Fluorouracil 400 mg/m^2 IV bolus on day 1 then fluorouracil 600 mg/m^2 as a 22-hour infusion given on days 1 and 2 every 14 days.

c. **FOLFIRI**

- Irinotecan 180 mg/m^2
- Fluorouracil 400 mg/m^2 IV bolus, and
- Leucovorin 400 mg/m^2, all on day 1 followed by fluorouracil 2.4 to 3.0 g/m^2 as a continuous infusion over 24 hours

Repeat every 2 weeks.

d. **Irinotecan + infusional fluorouracil + leucovorin**

- Irinotecan 80 mg/m^2 plus
- Leucovorin 500 mg/m^2 with
- Fluorouracil 2,300 mg/m^2 by 24-hour infusion are administered weekly for 6 weeks with a 1-week break.

e. **Irinotecan + fluorouracil + leucovorin**

- Irinotecan 180 mg/m^2 on day 1
- Leucovorin 200 mg/m^2 days 1 and 2,
- Fluorouracil 400 mg/m^2 IV bolus days 1 and 2, and
- Fluorouracil 600 mg/m^2 as a continuous infusion over 24 hours on days 1 and 2, repeated every 2 weeks.

f. **Irinotecan + fluorouracil + leucovorin (IFL)**

- Irinotecan 125 mg/m^2 as a 90-minute IV infusion with
- Fluorouracil 500 mg/m^2 and
- Leucovorin 20 mg/m^2

administered weekly for 4 weeks with a 2-week rest. Recent toxicity data are such that many oncologists have begun using irinotecan 100 mg/m^2 and fluorouracil 400 mg/m^2 with leucovorin 20 mg/m^2. Dose escalation to full dose is an option for patients with minimal toxicity. **Note: This is an inferior regimen when given** alone, and is only to be given with bevacizumab. Toxicity concerns limit the usefulness of this combination, however, and recent data suggest that FOLFIRI and bevicizumab is a superior regimen.

g. Irinotecan. Irinotecan 125 mg/m^2 as a 90-minute IV infusion is given weekly for 4 weeks with a 2-week rest **or** 180 mg/m^2 every 2 weeks **or** 300 to 350 mg/m^2 every 3 weeks.

h. Fluorouracil + high-dose leucovorin (weekly)

- Leucovorin 500 mg/m^2 IV is given over 2 hour
- Fluorouracil 500 mg/m^2 IV bolus injected 1 hour after beginning the leucovorin infusion.

The combination is administered weekly for 6 weeks followed by a 2-week rest. This regimen is now widely favored as the preferred bolus fluorouracil + leucovorin combination.

i. Fluorouracil + leucovorin (5-day)

- Leucovorin 20 mg/m^2 IV is followed by
- Fluorouracil 425 mg/m^2 IV. The combination is given daily for 5 days. Courses are repeated every 4 weeks.

Significant numbers of patients require dose reductions, and therefore, the weekly regimen is now favored (Section IV.B.3.h) over this 5-day regimen.

j. Fluorouracil by 24-hour continuous infusion. Fluorouracil 2,600 mg/m^2 is given by 24-hour continuous IV infusion weekly.

k. Fluorouracil by protracted venous infusion. Fluorouracil 250 to 300 mg/m^2 over 24 hours is given continuously until toxicity (e.g., erythrodysesthesia, mucositis, or diarrhea) or for 4 weeks continuously followed by a 1-week break.

l. LV5FU2

- Leucovorin 400 mg/m^2 as a 120-minute IV infusion, followed by
- Fluorouracil 400 mg/m^2 IV bolus on day 1 **only**, then followed by
- Fluorouracil 2.4 to 3.0 g/m^2 as a continuous IV infusion over 46 hours

Repeated every 2 weeks.

m. Bevacizumab. Bevacizumab 5 mg/kg IV over 90 minutes (first cycle), 60 minutes (second cycle), and then over 30 minutes for each subsequent cycle every other week given with FOLFOX, FOLFIRI, IFL (not recommended) or LV5FU2.

n. Cetuximab. 400 mg/m^2 IV first infusion given over 2 hours, then 250 mg/m^2 weekly with or without irinotecan.

o. Capecitabine. Capecitabine 1,250 mg/m^2 administered twice daily orally on days 1 to 14 every 3 weeks (2,500 mg/m^2/day). Many oncologists have begun patients on a lower dose of 1,000 mg/m^2 PO b.i.d. on days 1 to 14 every 3 weeks because of toxicity including erythrodysesthesia and mucositis in particular.

The following regimens are used less commonly:
p. Capox

- Oxaliplatin 130 mg/m^2 IV day one with
- Capecitabine 850 mg/m^2 PO b.i.d. for 14 days every 21 days.

q. Fluorouracil + methotrexate + leucovorin

- Methotrexate 200 mg/m^2 IV is given over 30 minutes after hydration with 1,500 mL of 5% dextrose in 0.5N saline, followed at 24 hours by
- Fluorouracil 600 mg/m^2 IV bolus, followed by
- Leucovorin 10 mg/m^2 (to the nearest 5 mg) PO every 6 hours × six doses. The regimen is repeated every 2 weeks.

r. Hepatic artery infusion. Most patients are managed by an implantable pump. A preferred regimen includes floxuridine 0.25 mg/kg/day in heparinized saline (50,000 U of heparin) plus 20 mg of dexamethasone administered for 2 weeks, alternating with 2 weeks of heparinized saline without floxuridine. Some patients will need a dose reduction of floxuridine to 0.15 to 0.2 mg/kg. The dexamethasone has helped prevent biliary sclerosis that sometimes accompanies such treatment. If leucovorin is added, the recommended dose of floxuridine is 0.18 mg/kg.

C. Adjuvant chemotherapy

1. Colon cancer. For patients with node-positive (stage III) resectable colon cancer, the combination of fluorouracil plus leucovorin given either by the 5-day or the weekly schedule for 6 months improves the disease-free as well as the overall survival of patients. The recent MOSAIC (Multicenter International Study of Oxaliplatin/5-fluorouracil/ Leucovorin in the Adjuvant Treatment of Colon Cancer) trial, which evaluated FOLFOX4 versus LV5FU2 in patients with stage II/III colon cancer, has confirmed a 4-year disease-free survival advantage favoring FOLFOX, with a difference between the two arms of 6.6% ($p < 0.001$). The greatest percent difference between both arms was seen for stage III patients with N$_2$ disease (11.5%). Overall survival data are not yet available. In addition, the NSABP (National Surgical Adjuvant Breast and Bowel Project) trial evaluating a bolus regimen of fluorouracil and oxaliplatin (FLOX) compared to weekly fluorouracil and leucovorin produced comparable 3-year disease-free survival statistics as seen with MOSAIC for stage II and III patients, favoring the FLOX regimen. Three recent adjuvant trials for patients with stage III colon cancer comparing irinotecan with either infusional fluorouracil or bolus fluorouracil versus fluorouracil and leucovorin failed to show a disease-free survival advantage for the combination; therefore, **irinotecan cannot be recommended as an adjuvant therapy strategy** at this time. Additional trials comparing capecitabine versus fluorouracil/leucovorin and infusional fluorouracil versus bolus fluorouracil and leucovorin have demonstrated that each of these approaches produce comparable results. For patients who are candidates for combination therapy, the FOLFOX regimen has become a standard for patients with stage III colon cancer.

Most randomized clinical trials have not demonstrated a survival advantage for stage II patients who have been treated with adjuvant chemotherapy, and the current standard is observation. Current guidelines from The American Society of Clinical Oncology (ASCO) suggest detailed discussion between the oncologist and patient as to the risk versus benefit of receiving adjuvant chemotherapy for stage II disease. There are high-risk stage II patients (e.g., stage IIB) where adjuvant therapy is a consideration based upon risk. A current Gastrointestinal Intergroup trial will define risk for stage II patients on the basis of molecular markers including 18q allele deletion and microsatellite instability.

Although historical data support the use of postoperative radiotherapy for locally advanced colon cancer (Dukes B3 or C3 or any T4 lesion), a small intergroup trial did not confirm its efficacy. Combination chemotherapy should probably be incorporated into the regimen and used for a total of 6 months after radiation therapy.

The recommended colon cancer adjuvant regimens for node-positive patients (stage III) are as follows:

   a. Fluorouracil + high-dose leucovorin (weekly) as in Section IVB.3.h.. Many physicians now favor this weekly regimen because of the toxicity noted with the 5-day schedule in Section IV.C.1.B.

   b. Fluorouracil + leucovorin (5-day).

- Leucovorin 20 mg/m^2 IV daily × 5 and
- Fluorouracil 425 mg/m^2 IV daily × 5 on weeks 1, 5, 9, 14, 19, and 24.

   c. LV5FU2. (See Section IV.B.3.l.)

   d. Capecitabine. (See Section IV.B.3.o.) Eight cycles are administered.

   e. mFOLFOX6. (See Section IV.B.3.a.)

   f. FOLFOX4. (See Section IV.B.3.b.)

   g. FLOX

- Oxaliplatin 85 mg/m^2 as a 120-minute IV infusion on weeks 1, 3, and 5 of each 8-week cycle.
- Fluorouracil 500 mg/m^2 IV bolus weekly for 6 weeks.
- Leucovorin 500 mg/m^2 IV bolus weekly for 6 weeks.

   There are three 8-week cycles administered.

   2. Resected hepatic metastases. Past data have demonstrated that patients with resected hepatic metastases secondary to colorectal cancer have a survival of at least 25%. Two recent clinical trials evaluating hepatic artery infusion with floxuridine compared to surgery have demonstrated significant reduction in recurrence of hepatic metastases with a trend toward improved survival for the patients receiving the hepatic artery infusion. Recent retrospective clinical trial analyses suggest that neoadjuvant chemotherapy (FOLFOX or FOLFIRI with or without bevacizumab) may improve the hepatic resection rate. Ongoing clinical trials should provide confirmatory data.

3. **Rectal cancer**
   a. **Preoperative irradiation.** Several studies have shown that preoperative irradiation benefits patients with rectal cancer, although there are disadvantages in terms of accuracy of staging, delay before surgery, incomplete knowledge of the extent of tumor for treatment planning, and inappropriate administration of radiation to patients with early (stage I) disease or most patients with advanced (stage IV) disease. Possible advantages include downstaging of tumor, improved sphincter preservation, improved resectability, and earlier initiation of systemic therapy. Better preoperative staging includes the use of magnetic resonance imaging and endorectal ultrasound. Ongoing clinical trials are exploring combinations of neoadjuvant therapy incorporating capecitabine, bevacizumab, and oxaliplatin as attempts to improve the pathologic complete response rate for patients with clinical stage II and III rectal cancer. Currently, preoperative chemoradiation employing fluorouracil 225 mg/m^2 daily as a continuous infusion during the course of the radiation therapy has become a U.S. and European standard. Capecitabine 825 mg/m^2 PO twice daily on the days of radiation is an alternative to the continuous infusion of fluorouracil that is used by some oncologists, but has not been compared for efficacy.
   b. **Postoperative irradiation, with and without chemotherapy.** Several controlled clinical trials have shown convincingly that radiation therapy alone reduces local recurrence but has little or no effect on overall survival. Fluorouracil-based chemotherapy added to radiation therapy is superior to either modality alone in terms of both local control and distant disease, thus improving overall survival. The optimal administration of fluorouracil during radiation therapy appears to be by protracted venous infusion, requiring a port and ambulatory pump, or by bolus with leucovorin. New adjuvant chemotherapy trials (for patients who receive preoperative chemoradiation) are investigating the use of FOLFOX with or without bevacizumab.
   The recommended postoperative adjuvant regimen for stage II or III rectal cancers is as follows:
      (1) Fluorouracil 500 mg/m^2 IV bolus daily on days 1 to 5 and days 36 to 40.
      (2) Radiation therapy 4,500 cGy in 180-cGy fractions over 5 weeks, with tumor boost of 540 to 900 cGy, beginning on day 64.
      (3) Fluorouracil 225 mg/m^2/day by protracted venous infusion throughout the period of radiation therapy, days 64 to 105.
      (4) Fluorouracil 500 mg/m^2 IV bolus daily, on days 134 to 138 and days 169 to 173.
      If leucovorin is added to the fluorouracil schedule (without radiation), the dose of leucovorin is 20 mg/m^2 and the dose of fluorouracil is 425 mg/m^2/day for 5 days before radiation. After radiation, fluorouracil

should be reduced to 380 mg/m^2/day with the leucovorin.

As with the preoperative chemoradiation, capecitabine 825 mg/m^2 PO twice daily on the days of radiation is an alternative to the continuous infusion of fluorouracil that is used by some oncologists, but has not been compared for efficacy. If capecitabine is used before and after radiation, the starting dose should be 1,000 to 1,250 mg/m^2 PO twice daily for 14 days of each 21-day cycle.

D. Follow-up. A recent pooled analysis of clinical trials suggests that 80% of colorectal cancer recurrences will occur within 3 years. In the asymptomatic patient, follow-up after treatment includes history, physical examination, and CEA every 3 months for 2 years, then every 6 months for 3 years. Colonoscopy is often performed 1 year after surgery and then every 3 years if no polyps are found. CT scans may be considered yearly for 3 years for patients at high risk for recurrence.

E. Complications of therapy or disease. The complications of chemotherapy are those attributable to the individual drugs. Myelosuppression, nausea, vomiting, and diarrhea are common and may require dose modification and symptomatic treatment. Radiation complications are similar and also include dysuria, tenesmus, and rectal discharge of blood or mucus. Phenazopyridine (Pyridium) is useful in treating dysuria, and loperamide (Imodium) or diphenoxylate (Lomotil) is recommended for diarrhea. If toxicity is substantial (grade 3 or 4) during radiotherapy, a treatment delay of at least 1 week is warranted. During chemotherapy with fluorouracil-based regimens, mild diarrhea (grade 1) may be treated symptomatically. Moderate diarrhea (grade 2 or 3) is an indication for dose reduction by 50%, and severe diarrhea (grade 3 or 4) is an indication for stopping chemotherapy for 1 week or longer. Dehydration is a real risk with grade 3 or 4 diarrhea, and IV hydration may be necessary. Tincture of opium or octreotide 150μ g t.i.d. may help to alleviate severe diarrhea.

Recent recommendations for management of irinotecan toxicity include evaluation for a GI syndrome, which can encompass diarrhea, nausea, vomiting, anorexia, abdominal cramping, dehydration, neutropenia, fever, and electrolyte abnormalities. There is also a vascular syndrome, which can include myocardial infarction, pulmonary embolus, or cerebral vascular accident. Patients receiving irinotecan should undergo weekly assessment, at least during the first cycle, looking for concurrent toxicities. In addition to treating the diarrhea with loperamide, tincture of opium, or octreotide, oral fluoroquinolone should be initiated in any patient experiencing neutropenia even in the absence of fever or diarrhea or in any patient experiencing fever and diarrhea even in the absence of neutropenia. Antibiotics should be initiated in any hospitalized patient with prolonged diarrhea regardless of granulocyte count and should be continued until resolution of diarrhea. Any patient who experiences significant treatment-related diarrhea should not receive irinotecan until he or she is diarrhea-free or at baseline bowel function for at least 24 hours without the use of antidiarrheal agents or antibiotics. In addition, abdominal cramping should be considered equivalent to diarrhea.

Oral mucositis can often be prevented on subsequent courses without dose reduction by holding ice in the mouth for 20 minutes before, during, and after the IV bolus of fluorouracil. Nausea is usually not severe with fluorouracil regimens and usually responds to prochlorperazine or dexamethasone. Hematopoietic growth factors are seldom warranted for the mild neutropenia that is observed with bolus fluorouracil therapy.

Oxaliplatin causes an acute cold sensitivity associated with distal dysesthesia/paresthesias and a chronic sensory neuropathy. Potential bevacizumab toxicities include hypertension, bleeding, delayed wound healing, arterial thrombosis, proteinuria, and GI perforation. Cetuximab is associated with acneiform rash, hypersensitivity, interstitial lung disease, and infusion reactions.

V. Cancer of the anal canal. These cancers, constituting only 1% to 3% of all cases of large bowel cancer, were historically treated by abdominoperineal resection with approximately a 50% cure rate. They have been seen more commonly in women. However, in recent years, there is an increase of these cancers in men, particularly homosexuals. The human papillomavirus has been implicated in some patients, and anal warts are sometimes seen as well. Patients infected with the human immunodeficiency virus also have an increased incidence of anal cancer.

A. Local disease. It has been found that combined-modality treatment with chemotherapy and irradiation is curative in 75% to 80% of patients and therefore allows avoidance of abdominoperineal resection with retention of anal function. The following regimen is recommended:

1. Radiotherapy 4,500 cGy in 25 fractions (5 weeks), *and concurrently*

2. Fluorouracil 1,000 mg/m^2 by continuous IV infusion daily × 4 days (days 1 to 4 and 29 to 32), *and*

3. Mitomycin 10 mg/m^2 IV on days 1 and 29.

A biopsy should be done 8 weeks after radiation therapy only for a suspicious residual area of abnormality. If negative, no further treatment is needed. If positive, consider an additional 900 cGy (five fractions) and a 4-day course of fluorouracil 1,000 mg/m^2 by continuous IV infusion on days 1 to 4 and cisplatin 100 mg/m^2 IV on day 2. If the biopsy is persistently positive, an abdominoperineal resection is appropriate.

A large U.S. Gastrointestinal Intergroup trial compared the standard regimen of mitomycin and fluorouracil versus preradiation chemotherapy followed by chemoradiotherapy using

- Cisplatin 75 mg/m^2 IV on days 1, 29, 57, and 85 and
- Fluorouracil 1,000 mg/m^2 by continuous IV infusion on days 1 to 4, 29 to 32, 57 to 60, and 85 to 88 plus
- Radiation 45 to 59 Gy, starting day 57.

Overall survival was not statistically different (5-year: 69%) nor was time to local-regional/distal relapse. The colostomy

rate, however, favored the standard regimen of mitomycin and fluorouracil (5-year: 10% vs. 20%, $p = 0.12$).
B. Metastatic disease. For metastatic disease, the following regimen may be considered:

1. Mitomycin 10 mg/m^2 IV every 4 weeks × 2, then every 10 weeks, *and*
2. Doxorubicin 30 mg/m^2 IV every 4 weeks × 2, then every 5 weeks, *and*
3. Cisplatin 60 mg/m^2 IV, every 4 weeks × 2, then every 5 weeks.

SUGGESTED READINGS

American Joint Committee on Cancer. *AJCC staging manual*, 6th ed. New York: Springer-Verlag, 2002:89–125.
National Comprehensive Cancer Network. *Clinical Practice Guidelines in Oncology.* http://www.nccn.org, 2007.

Esophagus

Berger AC, Farma J, Scott WJ, et al. Complete response to neoadjuvant chemoradiotherapy in esophageal carcinoma is associated with significantly improved survival. *J Clin Oncol* 2005;23:4330–4337.
Lightdale CJ, Kulkarni KG. Role of endoscopic ultrasonography in the staging and follow-up of esophageal cancer. *J Clin Oncol* 2005;23:4483–4489.
Smith TJ, Ryan LM, Douglass HO, et al. Combined chemoradiotherapy vs. radiotherapy alone for early stage squamous cell carcinoma of the esophagus: a study of the Eastern Cooperative Oncology Group. *Int J Radiat Oncol Biol Phys* 1998;42:269–276.
Stahl M, Stuschke M, Lehmann N, et al. Chemoradiation with or without surgery in patients with locally advanced squamous cell carcinoma of the esophagus. *J Clin Oncol* 2005;23:2310–2317.

Stomach

Cunningham D, Allum WH, Stenning SP, et al. Perioperative chemotherapy versus surgery alone for resectable gastroesophageal cancer. *N Engl J Med* 2006;355:11–20.
Jansen EPM, Boot H, Berheij M, et al. Optimal locoregional treatment in gastric cancer. *J Clin Oncol* 2005;23:4509–4517.
Lee W-J. No therapeutic effect of extended lymph node dissection for gastric cancer. *J Clin Oncol* 2005;23:1592–1593.
Macdonald JS, Smalley SR, Benedetti J, et al. Chemoradiotherapy after surgery compared with surgery alone for adenocarcinoma of the stomach or gastroesophageal junction. *N Engl J Med* 2001;345:725–730.
Moiseyenko VM, Ajani JA, Tjulandin SA, et al. Final results of a randomized controlled phase III trial (TAX 325) comparing docetaxel (T) combined with cisplatin (C) and fluorouracil (F) to CF in patients (pts) with metastatic gastric adeno carcinoma (MGC). *Proc Am Soc Clin Oncol* 2005;23(Suppl 16):A4002.
Smith DD, Schwartz RR, Schwartz RE. Impact of total lymph node count on staging and survival after gastrectomy for gastric cancer: data from a large US-population database. *J Clin Oncol* 2005;23:7114–7124.

Waters JS, Norman A, Cunningham D, et al. Long-term survival after epirubicin, cisplatin and fluorouracil for gastric cancer: results of a randomized trial. *Br J Cancer* 1999;80:269–272.

Small Intestine

Gupta S, Johnson MM, Murthy R, et al. Hepatic arterial emboliza- tion and chemoembolization for the treatment of patients with metastatic neuroendocrine tumors: variables affecting response rates and survival. *Cancer* 2005;104:1590–1602.

Panzuto F, Di Fondo M, Iannicelli E, et al. Long-term clinical outcome of somatostatin analogues for treatment of progressive, metastatic, well-differentiated entero-pancreatic endocrine carcinoma. *Ann Oncol* 2006;17:461–466.

Large Intestine

Andre T, Boni C, Mounedji-Boudiaf L, et al. Multicenter interna- tional study of oxaliplatin/5-fluououracil/leucovorin in the adjuvant treatment of colon cancer (MOSAIC) investigators: oxaliplatin, flu- orouracil, and leucovorin as adjuvant treatment for colon cancer. *N Engl J Med* 2004;350:2343–2351.

Benson AB III, Schrag D, Somerfield MR, et al. American Society of Clinical Oncology recommendations on adjuvant chemotherapy for stage II colon cancer. *J Clin Oncol* 2004;22:3408–3419.

Cunningham D, Humblet Y, Siena S, et al. Cetuximab monotherapy and cetuximab plus irinotecan in irinotecan-refractory metastatic colorectal cancer. *N Engl J Med* 2004;351:337–345.

Desch CE, Benson AB III, Somerfield MR, et al. Colorectal can- cer surveillance: 2005 update of an American Society of Clinical Oncology practice guideline. *J Clin Oncol* 2005;33:8512–8519.

Folprecht G, Grothey A, Alberts S, et al. Neoadjuvant treatment of unresectable colorectal liver metastases: correlation between tumour response and resection rates. *Ann Oncol* 2005;16:1311– 1319.

Gill S, Loprinzi CL, Sargent DJ, et al. Pooled analysis of fluorouracil- based adjuvant therapy for stage II and III colon cancer: who benefits and by how much? *J Clin Oncol* 2004;22:1797–1806.

Goldberg RM, Sargent DJ, Morton RF, et al. A randomized controlled trial of fluorouracil plus leucovorin, irinotecan, and oxaliplatin combinations in patients with previously untreated metastatic colorectal cancer. *J Clin Oncol* 2004;22:23–30.

Grothey A, Sargent D. Overall survival in patients with advanced colorectal cancer correlates with availability of fluorouracil, irinote- can, and oxaliplatin regardless of whether doublet or single-agent therapy is used first-line. *J Clin Oncol* 2005;23:9441–9442. [letter to the editor].

Gunderson LL, Sargent DJ, Tepper JF, et al. Impact of T and N stage and treatment on survival and relapse in adjuvant rectal cancer: a pooled analysis. *J Clin Oncol* 2004;22:1785–1796.

Hoff PM, Ansari R, Batist G, et al. Comparison of oral capecitabine versus IV fluorouracil plus leucovorin as first-line treatment in 605 patients with metastatic colorectal cancer: results of a randomized phase III study. *J Clin Oncol* 2001;19:2282–2292.

Hurwitz H, Fehrenbacher L, Novotny W, et al. Bevacizumab plus irinotecan, fluorouracil, and leucovorin for metastatic colorectal cancer. *N Engl J Med* 2004;350:2335–2342.

Le Voyer TE, Sigurdson ER, Hanlon AL, et al. Colon cancer survival is associated with increasing number of lymph nodes analyzed: a secondary survey of intergroup trial INT-0089. *J Clin Oncol* 2003;21:2912–2919.

Pfister DG, Benson AB III, Somerfield MR. Clinical practice. Surveillance strategies after curative treatment of colorectal cancer. *N Engl J Med* 2004;350:2375–2382.

Poston GJ, Adam R, Alberts S, et al. OncoSurge: a strategy for improving resectability with curative intent in metastatic colorectal cancer. *J Clin Oncol* 2005;23:7125–7134.

Saltz LB, Lenz H, Hochster H, et al. Randomized phase II trial of cetuximab/bevacizumab/irinotecan (CBI) versus cetuximab/bevacizumab (CB) in irinotecan-refractory colorectal cancer. *Proc Am Soc Clin Oncol* 2005;23(16S):3508. Abstract.

Sargent DJ, Wieand HS, Haller DG, et al. Disease-free survival versus overall survival as a primary end point for adjuvant colon cancer studies: individual patient data from 20,898 patients on 18 randomized trials. *J Clin Oncol* 2005;23:8664–8670.

Smalley SR, Benedetti J, Williamson S, et al. Intergroup 0144 - phase III trial of Fluorouracil based chemotherapy regimens plus radiotherapy (XRT) in postoperative adjuvant rectal cancer. Bolus Fluorouracil vs prolonged venous infusion (PVI) before and after XRT + PVI vs bolus Fluorouracil + leucovorin (LV) + levamisole (LEV) before and after XRT + bolus Fluorouracil + LV. *Proc Am Soc Clin Oncol*. 2003;21:1006.

Twelves C, Wong A, Nowacki MP, et al. Capecitabine as adjuvant treatment for stage III colon. *N Engl J Med* 2005;352:2696–2704.

Walsh TN, Noonan N, Hollywood D, et al. A comparison of multimodal therapy and surgery for esophageal adeno-carcinoma. *N Engl J Med* 1996;335:462–467.

Watanabe T, Tsung-Teh W, Catalano PJ, et al. Molecular predictors of survival after adjuvant chemotherapy for colon cancer. *N Engl J Med* 2001;344:1196–1206.

Wolmark N, Wieand HS, Hyams DM, et al. Randomized trial of postoperative adjuvant chemotherapy with or without radiotherapy for carcinoma of the rectum: National Surgical Adjuvant Breast and Bowel Project protocol R-02. *J Natl Cancer Inst* 2000;92:388–396.

Wolmark N, Wieand HS, Kuebler JP, et al. A phase III trial comparing FULV to FULV + oxaliplatin in stage II or III carcinoma of the colon: results of NSABP protocol C-07. *Proc Am Soc Clin Oncol* 2005;23:3500. Abstract.

Anus

Ajani JA, Winter KA, Gunderson LL, et al. Intergroup RTOG 98-11: a phase III randomized study of fluorouracil (Fluorouracil), mitomycin, and radiotherapy versus fluorouracil, cisplatin and radiotherapy in carcinoma of the anal canal. *Proc Am Soc Clin Oncol* 2006;24(18S):4009. Abstract.

CHAPTER 9

Carcinomas of the Pancreas, Liver, Gallbladder, and Bile Ducts

Rekha T. Chaudhary

Carcinomas of the pancreas, liver, and biliary passages account for approximately 2% of all cases of cancer and for 5% of all cancer-related deaths in the United States. Virtually all patients with these cancers die from this disease.

I. **Adenocarcinoma of the pancreas**
    A. **Epidemiology and etiology.** There were approximately 32,000 cases of pancreatic cancer in 2005 and almost all patients died from the disease. Pancreatic cancer is currently the fifth leading cause of cancer-related deaths in the United States in women and the fourth leading cause of death in men. Risk factors for pancreatic cancer include age, sex, and race. Blacks, men, and patients older than the age of 50 have a higher risk of developing pancreatic cancer. It is rare before 30 years of age, and the incidence rises throughout life, with peak occurrence during the seventh decade. Smokers have 1.6 to 3.9 times the risk of developing pancreatic cancer as compared with nonsmokers. Chronic pancreatitis is commonly associated with carcinoma of the pancreas in pathologic specimens. It is not certain whether this association is causal. Patients with familial pancreatitis appear to have a greater risk. Hereditary pancreatic cancer has been observed in rare families with an autosomal site-specific pattern, in families with *BRCA2* mutations, and in families with hereditary nonpolyposis colorectal cancer. Likewise, families with *p*16 germline mutations may be at a higher risk of developing pancreatic cancer. More than 80% of resected pancreatic cancers harbor either activating point mutations in *K-ras* or inactivating mutations of the tumor suppressor genes *p*16, *p*53, and *DPC4*.
    B. **Presenting signs and symptoms.** Pain is the most common presenting symptom. It occurs in three fourths of patients with carcinoma of the head of the pancreas and in virtually all patients with carcinoma of the body or tail. Usually, the pain is a dull ache in the epigastrium that radiates to the right upper quadrant when the tumor is in the head of the pancreas or to the left upper quadrant when the tumor is in the body or tail or it may be located in the lumbar region of the back. As many as one fifth of patients also present with nonspecific symptoms including weight loss, anorexia, nausea, vomiting, and constipation. The nonspecific, vague nature of these complaints may delay diagnosis for several months. Seventy percent of patients with carcinoma of the head of the pancreas have jaundice, whereas fewer than 15% of patients with carcinoma of the pancreatic body have jaundice. Physical

findings are generally associated with advanced carcinomas and include weight loss, hepatomegaly, and an abdominal mass. A palpable gallbladder in the absence of cholecystitis or cholangitis suggests malignant obstruction of the common bile duct (Courvoisier's sign), and it is present in approximately 25% of all patients with pancreatic cancer. Other physical findings, which can be indicative of distant metastases, include Trousseau's syndrome (migratory superficial phlebitis), ascites, palpable left supraclavicular node (Virchow's node), a periumbilical mass (Sister Mary Joseph's node), or a palpable pelvic shelf on rectal examination (Blumer's shelf).

C. Diagnostic evaluation. Abdominal ultrasonography and computed tomography (CT) demonstrate masses in the pancreas or dilation of the pancreatic duct or the common bile duct. Sensitivity and specificity of CT are approximately 90%, whereas sensitivity and specificity of ultrasonography are somewhat less. Both tests detect relatively large mass lesions of the pancreas and usually miss 1- to 2-cm carcinomas. Endoscopic retrograde cholangiopancreatography (ERCP) demonstrates subtle ductal abnormalities; sensitivity and specificity are in excess of 90%, with biopsies detecting tumors smaller than 1 to 2 cm in diameter. Endoscopic ultrasound (EUS) may be useful for staging (i.e., nodal status), determination of major vessel invasion and at times for fine needle aspiration (FNA) for pathologic determination of tumor. To determine vascular invasion there are three options: helical CT, magnetic resonance arteriography or EUS. Percutaneous FNA of suspicious abnormalities identified on CT scan can confirm the diagnosis of pancreatic cancer, with 80% to 90% sensitivity and 100% specificity. A common histologic hallmark of pancreatic adenocarcinoma is an associated desmoplastic reaction that, in a given tumor mass, can vastly overestimate the malignant cell mass. Furthermore, pancreatic cancer may be associated with varying degrees of acute or chronic pancreatitis or cyst formation, which may make it difficult to make a diagnosis with needle aspiration and may lead to false-negative results.

D. Laboratory tests. CA 19-9 is a cell surface glycoprotein associated with pancreatic cancer. Rising serum levels may be a useful early indicator of recurrent or progressive disease once a diagnosis has been established but because of low specificity it is not used as screening method. However, there is data to support the need to obtain a CA19-9 level in all patients in whom pancreatic cancer is suspected.

E. Staging and preoperative evaluation

  1. Staging. The primary tumor, regional lymph nodes, and potential sites of metastatic disease must be carefully assessed (Table 9.1). The staging system has been modified to better account for "resectability" of disease. Resectable disease is loosely defined as disease confined to the pancreas without involvement of the celiac axis or major vessels. A surgeon experienced in pancreatic surgery should evaluate each case individually when determining resectability as there are numerous clinical caveats.

  2. Preoperative evaluation. Preoperative evaluation should be performed stepwise from least invasive to most invasive as indicated by the clinical situation. Preoperative

Table 9.1. TNM staging for pancreatic cancer

Stage	Definition
IA	T1 (tumor ≤2 cm, confined to pancreas), N0, M0
IB	T2 (tumor >2 cm, confined to pancreas), N0, M0
IIA	T3 (extrapancreatic extension but no celiac axis or major vessel involvement), N0, M0
IIB	T1–3, N1, M0
III	T4 (involvement of celiac axis or superior mesenteric artery), N0–1, M0
IV	T1–4, N0–1, M1

N1, any nodal metastases; M1, any distant metastases.
From American Joint Committee on Cancer. *AJCC staging manual,* 6th ed.
New York: Springer-Verlag, 2002.

evaluation can be stopped when metastatic disease or definite evidence for unresectable locoregional spread is identified. All patients should undergo abdominal CT scanning. More recently, helical CT has emerged as a preferred technique for increasing the accuracy of detecting pancreatic carcinoma in general and vessel encasement, in particular. If no major blood vessel involvement is identified, then laparoscopy can be used to identify small metastases in the liver or peritoneum. Laparoscopy can be used to identify metastatic disease in patients with pancreatic cancer in whom equivocal results have been obtained from the tests mentioned in the preceding text or in whom, despite negative tests, the clinician still has a high suspicion for extrapancreatic disease. The use of positron emission tomography (PET) with 2-[^{18}F]fluoro-2-deoxy-D-glucose in the preoperative evaluation of patients with pancreatic cancer is expanding but is still controversial.

F. Primary therapy

1. **Surgery.** Three fourths of patients with pancreatic cancer are operative candidates, but only 15% to 20% have resectable tumors. Patients without evident metastatic cancer or major blood vessel involvement, whose performance status permits operative intervention, are candidates for curative surgery. Eight percent to 11% of the patients resected for cure survive 5 years. Surgical bypass procedures may also palliate obstructive jaundice and gastric outlet obstruction. ERCP stent placement may palliate obstructive jaundice.

2. **Radiation therapy.** External-beam radiation therapy can palliate unresectable carcinomas. It may also be used as a surgical adjuvant in combination with chemotherapy. Great care and expertise must be exercised to plan the radiation fields. These fields must encompass known disease without excessive involvement of adjacent normal tissue. Surgical clips placed at laparotomy or laparoscopy can guide treatment. Intraoperative external-beam radiotherapy has been successful in placing a high dose on the local tumor

while protecting the surrounding normal tissues but has not increased the cure rate of pancreas cancer in most hands.

3. **Combined-modality therapy**

   a. **Resected carcinomas.** Local and distant failures are common problems after resection of pancreatic cancer. A prospective randomized study by the Gastrointestinal Tumor Study Group (GITSG) compared observation to postoperative radiochemotherapy. The study showed an overall survival benefit (median survival: 20 vs. 11 months, $p = 0.03$) and a 2-year survival benefit (42% vs. 15%) for the radiochemotherapy arm, but this study is criticized for small patient numbers, low radiation doses, long accrual time, and early termination. The European Organization for Research and Treatment of Cancer did a similar trial that showed a trend toward being positive in the treatment group (median survival: 17.1 vs. 12.6 months $p = 0.099$). This study is also criticized for low radiation doses and underpowering of the study. A complicated trial in a 2×2 design was completed by the European Group for Pancreatic Cancer (ESPAC-1) that is difficult to interpret and has some trial design concerns including selection bias and treatment variability. An intriguing outcome of the analysis is that the chemotherapy group seemed to have a survival benefit; however, the chemoradiotherapy group seemed to do worse than the controls. The toxicity from the combination of chemotherapy and radiation may blur the survival advantage of the chemoradiotherapy arm. Finally, a recent Radiation Therapy Oncology Group (RTOG) trial 97-04 has the benefit of modern radiation doses and the addition of gemcitabine to the chemotherapy regimen. There is no standard of care for adjuvant treatment of pancreas cancer as there is no trial yet to confirm the results of the GITSG trial. All the trials agree, however, that in the acceptable candidate, chemotherapy is useful; however, the addition of radiotherapy is still controversial.

   b. Alternative adjuvant chemotherapy regimens (with or without radiotherapy) include the following:

   (1) Fluorouracil 225 mg/m^2 by continuous IV infusion throughout radiation therapy followed by four to six courses of bolus fluorouracil weekly, or gemcitabine (1,000 mg/m^2 on days 1, 8, 15 with 1-week break) *or*

   (2) Fluorouracil 425 mg/m^2 by IV push 1 hour after leucovorin, 20 mg/m^2 by IV push daily for 4 days during the first week of radiation therapy and for 3 days during the fifth week of radiation therapy followed by four to six courses of bolus fluorouracil weekly or gemcitabine (1,000 mg/m^2 on days 1, 8, 15 with 1-week break) *or*

   (3) Gemcitabine alone (1,000 mg/m^2 on days 1, 8, 15 with 1-week break) *or*

   (4) Capecitabine 1,500 mg/m^2 daily in divided doses with radiation therapy followed by four to six courses of bolus fluorouracil weekly or gemcitabine (1,000 mg/m^2 on days 1, 8, 15 with 1-week break).

Capecitabine can be used in the chemotherapy only part of regimen as well but there is no phase III data to confirm capecitabine in this setting.

c. Localized unresectable carcinoma. A series of randomized trials conducted by the GITSG demonstrated superior survival of patients with localized but unresectable pancreatic cancer when treated with combined-modality therapy as compared with patients treated with radiation therapy or chemotherapy alone. These clinical trials also used split-course radiation therapy. Current clinical trials do not support a specific combined-modality treatment program; however, doses of chemotherapy as discussed in Section I.F.3.b are used. A dose of 60 Gy of radiation should be delivered in a single course of external-beam radiation to gross tumor and 40 to 50 Gy to microscopic cancer. Paclitaxel is also being used at 50 mg/m^2 in a 3-hour infusion along with radiotherapy of approximately 50 Gy with similar benefits and tolerability as historical controls. Neoadjuvant chemotherapy and chemoradiotherapy are being studied to improve the number of patients eligible for resection but only approximately 10% patients were deemed resectable after various chemotherapy and chemoradiotherapy regimens.

G. Chemotherapy of metastatic disease. Patients with pancreatic cancer are often poor candidates for chemotherapy because of severe weight loss, poor performance status, severe pain, lack of measurable or evaluable disease, and presence of jaundice or hepatic involvement, which may interfere with clearance of therapeutic agents. However, two recent randomized clinical trials demonstrated survival and quality-of-life benefits from chemotherapy in selected patients with advanced pancreatic cancer.

1. Single agents. A number of single agents have demonstrated activity although no agent has demonstrated consistent complete and partial response rates of 20% or greater using CT to measure response. Gemcitabine has been accepted as first-line therapy for metastatic pancreatic cancer in patients with adequate performance status on the basis of a phase III trial that compared bolus fluorouracil and gemcitabine, with the primary endpoint being "clinical benefit score." Clinical benefit was defined as sustained (>4 weeks) improvement of one of the following parameters without worsening of any of the others: performance status, composite pain measurement (average pain intensity and narcotic analgesic use), and weight. The improvement in clinical benefit score in the gemcitabine and fluorouracil arms were 25% and 5%, respectively. In addition, there was a significant improvement in survival and in response rates, 16% versus 0%, respectively.

2. Combination chemotherapy. Combination chemotherapy has been investigated. The most commonly used regimens are fluorouracil + doxorubicin + mitomycin (FAM) and streptozocin + mitomycin + fluorouracil (SMF), with response rates reported between 13% and 43%. Other popular combinations using newer agents that have been recently attempted are (1) docetaxel and gemcitabine, (2) gemcitabine, docetaxel, and capecitabine (GTX), (3) gemcitabine/platinum combinations (i.e., gemcitabine and oxaliplatin [GemOx] or gemcitabine and cisplatin), and (4) Capecitabine and gemcitabine. GemOx was compared to gemcitabine alone in a phase III trial. GemOx had a superior response rate (26.8% vs. 17.3%; $p = 0.03$) but did not have a significantly superior overall and median survival. Capecitabine and gemcitabine were compared in a randomized controlled manner to gemcitabine alone but no differences were seen except in a subgroup with Karnofsky performance status of greater than 90. Although gemcitabine doublets did not show a benefit in randomized trials, a significant improvement has been observed in the subgroup of patients with good performance status.

3. Novel agents. Targeted agents such as bevacizumab, cetuximab, and erlotinib in combination with chemotherapy and alone are being investigated for all stages of pancreatic cancer. Erlotinib in particular has shown some promise in a randomized phase III trial of erlotinib versus chemotherapy alone. Initial reports show no increases in response rates but a modest yet statistically significant increase in 1-year survival (24% vs. 17%). This led to the approval of this medication in combination with gemcitabine for the treatment of metastatic pancreatic cancer.

4. Current recommendations

a. Single-agent therapy with gemcitabine 1,000 mg/m^2 IV of 4-week cycles of three weekly doses followed by 1-week rest is recommended for patients with metastatic pancreatic cancer and with an Eastern Cooperative Oncology Group performance status of 0 to 2, who are not eligible for clinical trials.

b. Patients with a very good performance status can use a doublet such as GemOx, with gemcitabine 1,000 mg/m^2 on days 1 and 8 plus oxaliplatin 130 mg/m^2 over 2 hours on day 8 every 3 weeks *or*

c. Capecitabine and gemcitabine (CapGem), with capecitabine at 1,500 mg/m^2 daily in twice-daily divided doses on days 1 to 14 and gemcitabine 1,000 mg/m^2 on days 1 and 8 every 3 weeks *or*

d. Capecitabine and oxaliplatin (CapOx), with capecitabine at 1,500 mg/m^2 daily in twice-daily divided doses on days 1 to 14 plus oxaliplatin 130 mg/m^2 on day 1 every 3 weeks.

e. Erlotinib 100 mg PO daily plus gemcitabine 1,000 mg/m^2 weekly for 3 weeks with a 1-week break.

II. Malignant islet cell carcinomas

A. Epidemiology and natural history. Islet cell neoplasms occur in approximately 1 in 100,000 people per year. These tumors cover a spectrum of neoplasms, many, but not all, of which originate from the pancreatic islets of Langerhans. Eighty percent of these tumors secrete one or more hormones excessively: most commonly insulin or gastrin, less commonly glucagon, serotonin, or adrenocorticotropic hormone, and rarely vasoactive intestinal peptides (VIPs), growth hormone–releasing hormone, or somatostatin. Twenty percent are nonfunctional. Islet cell tumors may occur with the multiple endocrine neoplasia type 1 (MEN-1) syndrome. In families with this autosomal dominant syndrome, 80% of affected members develop islet cell tumors, most commonly gastrinoma (54%), insulinoma (21%), glucagonoma (3%), or VIPoma (1%). The gene for MEN-1 has been localized to the long arm of chromosome 11 and was recently identified and named *MENIN*. Approximately one fourth of gastrinomas are associated with MEN-1. Eighty percent to 90% of gastrinomas occur in the head of the pancreas. Insulinomas are equally common in the head, body, and tail. Gastrinomas tend to be multiple small tumors, whereas insulinomas tend to be single tumors and glucagonomas and VIPomas are single large tumors. The median age of patients is in the sixth decade. Islet cell tumors generally present with symptoms caused by hormone hypersecretion, most commonly fasting hypoglycemia. VIPomas are associated with episodic severe secretory diarrhea with hypokalemia, hypochlorhydria, and metabolic acidosis. Classically, glucagonomas are associated with necrolytic migratory erythema, mild diabetes, severe muscle wasting, and marked hyperaminoaciduria.

Sixty percent of gastrinomas are malignant. Histologic appearance and tumor size do not predict malignancy; only the presence of metastatic disease confirms malignancy. Ninety percent of malignant gastrinomas have liver metastases. Other sites of spread include abdominal nodes, peritoneum, bone, and lung. Median survival from time of diagnosis of metastatic disease is approximately 2.5 years. Only 10% of insulinomas are malignant. They are usually larger than 2.5 cm, whereas benign insulinomas are generally smaller than 2.5 cm. Most glucagonomas and VIPomas are malignant (60%–80%).

B. Treatment of advanced disease

1. Endocrine syndromes. The first goal of treatment must be to control endocrine syndromes.

> **a. Gastric acid suppression.** The H^+, K^+-adenosine triphosphatase inhibitors omeprazole and lansoprazole successfully control gastric acid secretion in patients with gastrinoma. Optimal doses must be individualized and periodically re-evaluated. Gastric acid secretion in the hour preceding the next dose of omeprazole or lansoprazole should be less than 10 mEq in patients who have had no previous gastric surgery and less than 5 mEq in those who have had an acid-reducing procedure. The starting dose is 60 mg/day with both agents. Doses greater than 80 mg/day should be divided. Similar, newer agents in the same class of proton pump inhibitors are equally efficacious.

> **b. Insulin suppression.** Diazoxide, an insulin release inhibitor, when given at 3 to 8 mg/kg/day PO divided in three doses (e.g., 50 to 150 mg PO t.i.d.), is the therapy of choice for hypoglycemia associated with insulinoma when dietary measures fail. A diuretic should be given with diazoxide to prevent water retention.

> **c. Octreotide acetate (Sandostatin).** Octreotide acetate is a somatostatin analog that inhibits gut hormone secretion. It is generally useful for carcinoid and

VIPoma syndromes and is possibly useful for controlling symptoms in patients with glucagonomas, gonadotrophic hormone–releasing hormone tumors, and gastrinomas. In patients with unresectable insulinoma, it can reduce insulin secretion by 50% and return blood glucose levels to normal. However, it must be initiated cautiously in patients in the hospital because profound hypoglycemia may occur. The usual starting dose of octreotide is 50 μg SC b.i.d.; thereafter, the dose and frequency of injections can be increased to 100 μg t.i.d. More recently, a long-acting preparation (Octreotide LAR) has become available. The dose should be 20 to 30 mg IM monthly, depending on the dose of the short-acting preparation that the patient was requiring. It is designed to provide the convenience of once-a-month or twice-a-month injections once a stable dose of the shorter-acting preparation is established.

2. Chemotherapy for advanced islet cell tumors. Streptozocin is the most active single agent, with a 50% response rate. Doxorubicin is also an active agent. The combination of streptozocin and doxorubicin was demonstrated to have a superior response rate (69%), time to tumor progression (20 months), and survival time (2.2 years) than the combination of streptozocin and fluorouracil or single-agent chlorozotocin in a North Central Cancer Treatment Group study. Current recommendations for treatment are as follows:

a. Streptozocin 500 mg/m^2 IV on days 1 to 5 and doxorubicin 50 mg/m^2 IV, on days 1 and 22. Repeat every 6 weeks. Renal impairment occurs in approximately 30% of patients receiving a streptozocin-based regimen; approximately one third of those with renal insufficiency have creatinine levels higher than 2 mg/dL. Nausea and vomiting occur in approximately 60% of patients. Leukopenia occurs in approximately 75%, but only 10% have a white blood cell count of less than 1,000/μL. Stomatitis is uncommon. Liver function test abnormalities may also occur. Deaths caused by treatment are rare.

b. Interferon-α may diminish excess hormone secretion and induce shrinkage of tumors; some trials have reported 50% response rates.

c. Newer approaches include bevacizumab, sunitinib, and metaiodobenzylguanidine (MIBG) radiotherapy. MIBG ([^{131}I]metaiodobenzylguanidine) is a radiolabelled substance similar to norepinephrine that in retrospective studies has been found to produce symptomatic and objective responses in patients with metastatic carcinoid.

III. Ampullary carcinomas. In up to 80% of people, the common bile duct and main pancreatic duct empty into a common channel, the ampulla of Vater. Periampullary carcinomas can be classified according to their site of origin. Type 1 tumors originate in the ampulla of Vater or the duodenal portion of the common bile duct. Type 2 carcinomas are duodenal tumors involving the ampulla of Vater. Type 3 tumors are mixed ampullary–periampullary carcinomas, and type 4 tumors are pancreatic head carcinomas involving the ampulla. Type 4 tumors carry a much worse prognosis and should be distinguished from the ampullary or periampullary carcinomas. Types 1 to 3 periampullary and ampullary carcinomas generally can be extirpated surgically. Large tumors require a Whipple resection, whereas local excision may be curative for small tumors. The overall 5-year survival rate is 40% to 50% for patients with types 1 to 3 carcinomas. The roles of irradiation and chemotherapy are uncertain. Tumors larger than 2 cm in diameter should be treated as adenocarcinoma of the pancreas.

IV. Carcinoma of the bile ducts (cholangiocarcinoma)

    A. Epidemiology and natural history. The incidence of primary biliary tree carcinoma is approximately 2 per 100,000 population. Men are affected more commonly than women. Tumors occur most often in late-middle-aged and elderly patients. They are associated with cholelithiasis, ulcerative colitis, obesity, liver flukes, exposure to thorium oxide (Thorotrast), primary sclerosing cholangitis, and congenital anomalies of the pancreaticobiliary tree. Patients present with obstructive jaundice, except for the occasional patient with a carcinoma identified at laparotomy for cholelithiasis. Approximately half the number of bile duct tumors are located proximally. Ten percent have multicentric involvement of the bile ducts. Local invasion is common. Liver involvement occurs in nearly half of these patients. Surgical cure is uncommon. Bypass procedures or intubation of the biliary tree may offer palliation to patients whose tumors cannot be resected. Radiation therapy may relieve proximal obstruction without intubation or a bypass procedure. Combined-modality therapy with radiation and fluorouracil should be considered in patients with an unresectable but localized cancer.

    B. Chemotherapy for advanced disease. Few reports are available for this unusual tumor with low response rates and median survival of approaching 6 months. Fluorouracil has response rates of approximately 10%. Newer agents and combinations have been tried including gemcitabine alone, gemcitabine and fluorouracil, gemcitabine and oxaliplatin, capecitabine and oxaliplatin, and capecitabine and gemcitabine. Outside the context of a clinical trial in patients with an acceptable performance status, one of the following regimens is recommended:

    1. Fluorouracil 500 mg/m^2 IV push on days 1 to 5 every 4 weeks or 500 mg/m^2 IV weekly

    2. Fluorouracil 400 mg/m^2 IV on days 1 to 5 and streptozocin 500 mg/m^2 IV on days 1 to 5

    3. Patients with a very good performance status can use a doublet such as GemOx with gemcitabine 1,000 mg/m^2 on day 1 and 8 plus oxaliplatin 130 mg/m^2 over 2 hours on day 8 every 3 weeks *or*

    4. Gemcitabine 1,000 mg/m^2, fluorouracil 600 mg/m^2, leucovorin 20 mg/m^2 IV days 1, 8, and 15 every 4 weeks

    5. Capecitabine 1,500 mg/m^2 daily in twice-daily divided doses on days 1 to 14 and gemcitabine 1,000 mg/m^2 on days 1 and 8 every 3 weeks *or*

6. Capecitabine 1,500 mg/m² daily in twice-daily divided doses on days 1 to 14 plus oxaliplatin 130 mg/m² on day 1 every 3 weeks.

V. **Carcinoma of the gallbladder**

A. **Epidemiology and natural history.** Carcinomas of the gallbladder are seen predominantly in late-middle-aged and elderly women, with the highest incidence in native Americans and the populations of Central and Eastern Europe and Israel. The areas of high frequency also report a high incidence of cholelithiasis. Patients with "porcelain" or calcified gallbladders identified on radiographs have a 12% to 62% risk of cancer. Carcinoma of the gallbladder most commonly presents with pain, nausea and vomiting, and weight loss. Jaundice occurs in only one third of patients. Anorexia, abdominal distention, pruritus, and melena occur in some patients. One percent of patients undergoing cholecystectomy are found to have carcinoma of the gallbladder. Overall survival is poor; less than 5% of patients who undergo resection survive 5 years. When the tumor is histologically confined to the mucosa or submucosa, survival rates of 64% at 5 years and 44% at 10 years have been reported. Gallbladder carcinomas may invade locally into the bile ducts, liver, pancreas, stomach, or duodenum. They may also spread to regional lymph nodes and distantly to liver. There is no definitive data for adjuvant therapy but usually disease that is locally advanced is treated with a combination of radiation and chemotherapy (usually fluorouracil-based).

B. **Chemotherapy for advanced disease.** Although there is no data that indicates that chemotherapy treatment in advanced disease is better than the best supportive care alone, chemotherapy is often used for symptom palliation. Combinations are similar to those mentioned in the preceding text for cholangiocarcinomas. Gemcitabine alone or in combination with capecitabine or leucovorin are the commonly used regimens.

VI. **Primary carcinoma of the liver**

A. **Epidemiology.** Primary carcinoma of the liver is rare in the United States. There are fewer than 10,000 new patients annually, accounting for less than 2% of all malignancies. However, it is the leading cause of cancer death in parts of Africa and Asia. Ninety percent of primary cancers of the liver are hepatocellular carcinomas or hepatoma; the remaining cancers include cholangiocarcinomas (~7%), hepatoblastomas, angiosarcomas, and other sarcomas. Histologic subsets of hepatocellular carcinoma have been recognized. Fibrolamellar carcinomas occur in young patients and are more likely to be resectable and cured. Hepatocellular carcinomas are more common in men than in women. The peak occurrence is during the sixth decade, with the highest incidence during the ninth decade. There appear to be three major factors associated with hepatocellular carcinoma: viral hepatitis B and C, alcohol abuse, and aflatoxin exposure. Seventy-five percent of patients with hepatocellular carcinoma have concomitant cirrhosis, and 4% to 20% of patients with cirrhosis have hepatocellular carcinoma at autopsy, depending on the population studied. Among the patients with hepatocellular carcinoma, 15% to 80% have hepatitis B surface antigenemia. In China, the incidence of hepatocellular carcinoma parallels the incidence of hepatitis B infection. The introduction of an effective hepatitis B vaccine may reduce the risk of hepatocellular carcinoma in these areas. In Africa, the increased risk appears to be related to exposure to aflatoxin, which is produced by the fungi *Aspergillus flavus* and *Aspergillus parasiticus* during improper food storage. Three percent to 27% of patients with long-standing hemochromatosis develop hepatocellular carcinoma. Anabolic steroids have also been associated with hepatocellular carcinoma. Tumors induced by anabolic steroids may retain hormone dependence and regress after withdrawal of the steroid.

B.   Presentation. Patients with primary carcinoma of the liver commonly complain of right upper quadrant pain, abdominal distention, or weight loss. The pain is usually dull or aching but may be acute and radiate to the right shoulder. Fatigue, loss of appetite, and unexplained fever may occur. Patients with underlying cirrhosis may present with hepatic decompensation: new ascites, variceal bleeding, jaundice, or encephalopathy. Rarely, patients present with paraneoplastic syndromes: erythrocytosis is the most common; hypercalcemia, hyperthyroidism, and carcinoid syndrome have also been described. Physical findings include nodular hepatomegaly with an arterial bruit and hepatic rub. Extrahepatic spread occurs in approximately 50% of patients during the course of the illness. Twenty percent of patients have lung metastases.

C.   Diagnostic evaluation and screening. α-Fetoprotein levels are elevated in 70% of patients and are associated with a poor prognosis. Ultrasonography and CT have a high sensitivity when lesions are larger than 2 cm; however, small lesions are frequently missed. Magnetic resonance imaging is generally equivalent to CT but at a greater cost. FNA with cytology or biopsy usually confirms the diagnosis. Screening is controversial because although some studies have shown a survival benefit with screening, there are concerns about lead-time bias. Serial α-fetoprotein measurements and liver ultrasonography every 4 to 6 months should be considered in high-risk patients with hepatitis B antigenemia and with hepatitis C and cirrhosis (Child-Pugh class A and/or patients who are suitable for hepatectomy).

D.   Staging. Staging procedures should include a chest radiograph, CT of the abdomen, complete blood cell count, blood chemistry profile, and α-fetoprotein measurement (Table 9.2). If these do not disclose unresectable cancer or sites of metastatic cancer, then CT of the chest and arteriogram (upper abdominal and hepatic) should be performed to guide surgical intervention and further screening for extrahepatic involvement.

E.   Primary therapy. At presentation, 25% of patients with hepatocellular carcinoma have potentially resectable lesions. Liver transplantation may permit resection of small tumors in patients with advanced cirrhosis, and survival is similar to or better than that seen after resection without transplantation Patients with hepatocellular carcinoma who meet the Milan criteria for transplantation are those patients with one nodule less than 5 cm or two to three nodules less than 3 cm and have low recurrence rates after transplantation with 5-year

Table 9.2.   TNM staging for hepatocellular cancer

Stage	Definition
I	T1 (solitary tumor, any size without vascular invasion), N0, M0
II	T2 (solitary tumor, any size with vascular invasion; or multiple tumors, none >5 cm), N0, M0
IIIA	T3 (multiple tumors 75 cm or tumor involving a major branch of the portal or hepatic vein[s]), N0, M0
IIIB	T4 (direct invasion of adjacent organs other than gall bladder or with perforation of visceral peritoneum)
IIIC	Any T, N1, M0
IVB	Any T, any N, M1

Modified from American Joint Committee on Cancer. *AJCC staging manual,* 6th ed. New York: Springer-Verlag, 2002.

survival rates of 75%. The main problem with transplantation is timely organ availability. Resection is an option for patients with good liver function and resectable lesions. Patients who are not candidates for either therapy can be considered for ablative therapies. Radiofrequency ablation is superior to percutaneous ethanol injection. Chemoembolization can be used in patients who have liver-only disease but are not candidates for transplant, resection or ablative treatment for palliation of symptoms.

F. Therapy of advanced hepatocellular carcinoma
   1. Single agents. Numerous single agents have been tested in primary hepatocellular carcinoma: alkylating agents, antimetabolites, plant alkaloids, and cisplatin have been ineffective. Doxorubicin 60 mg/m^2 IV every 21 days is recommended. This regimen results in a partial response rate of approximately 2%. There is really no effective chemotherapy in this situation and patients should be considered for clinical trials.

SUGGESTED READINGS

Burris HA, Moore MJ, Andersen J, et al. Improvements in survival and clinical benefit with gemcitabine as first-line therapy for patients with advanced pancreas cancer: a randomized trial. *J Clin Oncol* 1997;15:2403–2413.

Collier J, Sherman M. Screening for hepatocellular carcinoma. *Hepatology* 1998;27:273–278.

Gastrointestinal Tumor Study Group. Further evidence of effective adjuvant combined radiation and chemotherapy following curative resection of pancreatic cancer. *Cancer* 1987;59:2006–2010.

Glimelius B, Hoffman K, Sjoden PO, et al. Chemotherapy improves survival and quality of life in advanced pancreatic and biliary cancer. *Ann Oncol* 1996;7:593–600.

Jensen RT, Fraker DL. Zollinger–Ellison syndrome: advances in treatment of gastric hypersecretion and the gastrinoma. *JAMA* 1994;271:1429–1435.

Kalser MH, Ellenberg SS. Pancreatic cancer: adjuvant combined radiation and chemotherapy following curative resection. *Arch Surg* 1985;120:899–903.

Katz MH, Savides TJ, Moossa AR, et al. An evidence-based approach to the diagnosis and staging of pancreatic cancer. *Pancreatology* 2005;5:576–590.

Klinkenbijl JH, Jeekel J, Shamoud T, et al. Adjuvant radiotherapy and 5-fluorouracil after curative resection of cancer of the pancreas and periampullary region: phase III trial of the EORTC gastrointestinal tract cancer cooperative group. *Ann Surg* 1999;230(6): 776–782.

Louvet C, Labianca R, Hammel P, et al. Gemcitabine in combination with oxaliplatin compared with gemcitabine alone in locally advanced or metastatic pancreatic cancer: results of a GERCOR and GISCAD phase III trial. *J Clin Oncol* 2005;23(15):3509–3516.

Moertel CG, Hahn RG, O'Connell MS. Therapy of locally unresectable pancreatic carcinoma: a randomized comparison of high dose (6000 rads) radiation alone, moderate dose radiation (4000 rads–5-fluorouracil), and high dose radiation–5-fluorouracil. Gastrointestinal Tumor Study Group. *Cancer* 1981;48:1705–1710.

Moertel CG, Lefkopoulo M, Lipsitz S, et al. Streptozocin–doxorubicin, streptozocin–fluorouracil, or chlorozotocin in the treatment of advanced islet-cell carcinoma. *N Engl J Med* 1992;326:519–523.

Neoptolemos JP, Dunn JA, Stocken DD, et al. Adjuvant chemoradiotherapy and chemotherapy in resectable pancreatic cancer: a randomised controlled trial. *Lancet* 2001;358(9293):1576–1585.

Rao S, Cunningham D, Hawkins RE, et al. Phase III study of fluorouracil, etoposide and leucovorin (FELV) compared to epirubicin, cisplatin and fluorouracil (ECF) in previously untreated patients with advanced biliary cancer. *Br J Cancer* 2005;92(9):1650–1654.

Rich T, Harris J, Abrams R, et al. Phase II study of external irradiation and weekly paclitaxel for nonmetastatic, unresectable pancreatic cancer: RTOG-98-12. *Am J Clin Oncol* 2004;27(1):51–56.

Safford SD, Coleman RE, Gockerman JP, et al. Iodine-131 metaiodo benzylguanidine treatment for metastatic carcinoid. Results in 98 patients. *Cancer* 2004;101(9):1987–1993.

Tsukuma H, Hiyama T, Tanaka S, et al. Risk factors for hepatocellular carcinoma among patients with chronic liver disease. *N Engl J Med* 1993;328:1797–1801.

CHAPTER 10

Carcinoma of the Breast

Iman Mohamed

I. **Natural history, evaluation, and modes of treatment**
   A. **Epidemiology and risk factors.** Carcinoma of the breast gave way to carcinoma of the lung as the most common cause of cancer deaths among women in the United States in 1986. Nonetheless, in 2005, more than 250,000 new cases of breast cancer were diagnosed, and there were approximately 40,000 women who died from this cancer. More women survive because of earlier diagnosis and better therapy. The disease-specific mortality from breast cancer is reported to have decreased by 2.2% per year since 1990.

   The incidence of breast cancer varies widely among different populations. Women in Western Europe and the United States have a higher incidence than women in most other parts of the world, possibly in part because of the high intake of animal protein and fat. White women in the United States are more likely to develop breast cancer as compared with African American women. Mortality from breast cancer, however, is higher in African American women than in other ethnic or racial groups. Although discrete causes of breast cancer cannot be identified in individual women, many factors increase a woman's risk of developing the disease. Among the strongest of the risk factors is family history, particularly if more than one family member has developed breast cancer at an early age. Genetic linkage analysis has led to the discovery of dominant germ-line mutations in two tumor suppressor genes, *BRCA1* and *BRCA2*, localized to chromosomes 17 and 13, respectively, which are associated with a high risk of female breast cancer as well as ovarian cancer (*BRCA1* and *BRCA2*), male breast cancer (*BRCA2*), and other cancers. Although these mutations account for less than 10% of all cases of breast cancer, together they may account for over 70% of inherited cases in high-risk populations. It is important to note that most patients with a family history of breast cancer do not have a defined inherited mutation. However, if a woman with breast cancer is under the age of 50 and has any relative who developed breast cancer before she was 50, her chance of having a mutation in *BRCA1* or *BRCA2* rises to 25%. Other factors that increase the probability of a mutation include any relative with ovarian cancer or a personal history of bilateral breast cancer or ovarian cancer. Carriers of these mutations have up to a 70% lifetime risk of breast cancer, depending on familial history, perhaps the specific mutation, and other cellular genes that may modify penetrance. The 5-year survival rate of patients with either of the *BRCA* mutations is not significantly less than for other patients with breast cancer. Other less common or less well-defined genetic mutations may be present in other familial breast cancers. Additional factors that increase breast cancer risk are early menarche, late age at birth of first child, and prior benign breast disease (particularly if there is a high degree of benign epithelial atypia). Present use of birth control pills appears to have a small effect on the risk of developing breast cancer (relative risk, 1.24); risk from prior use diminishes over time. Although breast cancer may occur among men, such cases represent fewer than 1% of all breast cancers and are infrequently seen in most hospitals. Male carriers of *BRCA2* mutations have a 6% lifetime risk of breast cancer, significantly increasing their risk in comparison to the general population.

Hormone replacement therapy can possibly increase the risk of breast cancer. In the Women Health Initiative study, researchers found an increased breast cancer risk of approximately 10% for every 5 years of use. There was a greater risk with combined estrogen and progesterone products than with estrogen therapy alone.

B. Prevention. Until recently, it was unknown whether any preventive measures would be effective in reducing the incidence of breast cancer. Two trials using selective estrogen receptor modulators (SERMs) have demonstrated that 3 to 5 years of preventive treatment with these agents reduces the rate of cancer development over a short term. Women at increased risk because of family history, age, and other risk factors, who are treated with tamoxifen, 20 mg/day, were found to have a 45% reduction in the rate of occurrence of invasive breast cancer as compared with women treated with placebo. Noninvasive disease and preneoplastic breast lesions are also decreased. Raloxifene, 60 or 120 mg/day, also appears to reduce the risk of breast cancer in postmenopausal women (who had osteoporosis and a standard or reduced risk of breast cancer), with a relative risk of 0.26. Raloxifene appears to have a lower risk for the development of endometrial cancer than tamoxifen that has been associated with an increased risk for endometrial cancer of 1.5 to 2 times that in untreated women. Effects on survival, when used in breast cancer prevention, have not yet been demonstrated for either agent. The results of the STAR trial (Study of Tamoxifen against Raloxifene) have recently been published. Raloxifene was found not to decrease the incidence of preinvasive carcinomas despite a seemingly better outcome than tamoxifen for prevention of invasive cancers. This makes the initial enthusiasm about this drug (which is currently primarily used for treatment of osteoporosis) difficult to sustain. Clearly, decisions regarding prevention are complex and require consideration of cost, benefit, and potential side effects of drugs.

The approach to management of women at very high risk because of family history or known suppressor gene mutations is evolving. Increased surveillance, such as increasing the frequency of mammography to once in every 6 months, has been suggested as a reasonable conservative approach. In mutation carriers who are at risk for both breast and ovarian cancers, bilateral oophorectomy after child-bearing age has been recommended because of the inadequacy of screening tests for ovarian cancer. Some women may prefer prophylactic mastectomy. In a recent study from Mayo Clinic, bilateral simple mastectomy in mutation carriers was found to reduce the risk of breast cancer by 90%. A small risk of breast cancer in residual breast glandular tissue persists, and the irreversible loss of nipple sensation may be distressing to some women. Bilateral oophorectomy in the premenopausal woman who has completed her family reduces the risk of breast cancer by approximately 50% and avoids the psychological trauma of bilateral mastectomy.

The role of SERMs in patients with these *BRCA1* and *BRCA2* mutations is evolving as well. Analysis of blood samples of women who participated in the prevention trial with tamoxifen showed that mutation carriers also had a 47% lower risk of breast cancer, suggesting a useful role for this group of drugs in mutation carriers. Another approach to managing high-risk patients is increased surveillance. This involves clinical examination and imaging of suspicious palpable findings in a timely manner. As discussed in the following text, the use of magnetic resonance imaging (MRI) is currently approved for screening high-risk populations in addition to regular mammography.

C. Detection, diagnosis, and pretreatment evaluation

   1. Screening. Because more lives can be saved if breast cancer is diagnosed at an early stage, many screening programs have been designed to detect small, early cancers. Monthly breast self-examination for all women after puberty and yearly breast examinations by a physician or other trained professional after a woman is 20 years of age are recommended. Notwithstanding some skepticism in the literature, most breast cancer specialists and statistical analyses have concluded that mammography, when done on a regular basis, can reduce mortality due to breast cancer by 25% to 30% in women older than 50 years. The benefit for women aged 40 to 50 years has been more difficult to demonstrate. Mammography is recommended at age 40 as a baseline, once every 1 to 2 years between the ages of 40 and 50 (depending on risk factors and the recommending organization), and yearly after 50 years of age. An upper age of effectiveness is not established. For high-risk women and in family members of mutation-positive patients, annual mammography should be initiated 5 years earlier than the age of the youngest diagnosed relative. Patients with Hodgkin's disease (regardless of a history of mantle field irradiation) should have a baseline mammogram by age 25. In mutation *BRCA1* or *BRCA2* carriers, MRI of the breast has recently been approved for screening in addition to annual mammography. Although each method for early detection can be of some help in finding early lesions that can be successfully removed before metastasis has occurred, mammography is capable of detecting the smallest and therefore the most curable lesions. Therefore, despite the high cost of screening mammography ($75 to $140 in many areas of the United States), it is highly recommended that the guidelines mentioned in the preceding text be followed. Mammography has clearly led to the discovery of many earlier cancers and sharply increased the discovery of preinvasive cancers (ductal carcinoma *in situ* [DCIS]). Screening breast ultrasound is commonly used in Europe. Its role in the United States remains limited to evaluation of palpable lesions, especially in premenopausal women where mammography has a high false-negative rate due to higher breast radiographic density.

2. Presenting signs and symptoms. Although an increasing number of nonpalpable cancers are found by mammography, invasive breast cancer is still most often discovered by a woman herself as an isolated, painless lump in the breast. If the mass has gone unnoticed, ignored, or neglected for a time, there may be fixation to the skin or underlying chest wall, ulceration, pain, or inflammation. Some early lesions present with discharge or bleeding from the nipple. At times, the primary lesion is not discovered, and the woman presents with symptoms of metastatic disease, such as pleural effusion, nodal disease, or bony metastases. Approximately half of all lesions are in the upper outer quadrant of the breast (where most of the glandular tissue of the breast is), approximately 20% are central masses, and 10% are in each of the other quadrants. Up to one fourth of all women with breast cancer have axillary node metastasis at the time of diagnosis, although this is less common when the primary tumor has been detected by screening mammography or other screening methods.

3. Staging. Carcinoma of the breast is staged according to the size and characteristics of the primary tumor (T), the involvement of regional lymph nodes (N), and the presence of metastatic disease (M). An abridged version of the commonly used TNM classification of breast cancer is shown in Table 10.1, and the stage grouping is outlined in Table 10.2. As of January 2003, the revised American Joint Commission on Cancer (AJCC) staging system for breast cancer has been officially adopted for use in tumor registries. Although preliminary staging is commonly done before surgery, definitive staging that can be used for prognostic and further treatment planning purposes usually must await postsurgical pathologic evaluation when the primary tumor size and the histologic involvement of the lymph nodes are established. In up to 30% of patients with palpable breast masses (not found by mammography), but without clinical evidence of axillary lymph node involvement, the histologic evaluation of the nodes reveals cancer. In patients with negative nodes on routine histologic evaluation, serial sectioning may reveal microscopic cancer deposits in additional patients. The principal changes in the new staging system take into consideration the widespread use of immunohistochemical (IHC) and molecular biologic techniques that afford pathologists the ability to detect microscopic metastatic lesions down to isolated tumor cell level. It is less certain whether there is prognostic value if cancer cells in nodes are detected by molecular markers (reverse transcriptase-polymerase chain reaction [RT-PCR]). The current staging system designates nodes to be pathologically negative if cells are identified by polymerase chain reaction (PCR) and not by haematoxylin and eosin stain (H&E) or by IHC but a designator mol+ or mol− is added. Pathologists agree that the size of the metastatic deposit is of utmost significance as opposed to how the deposit was

Table 10.1. Abridged TNM classification of breast cancer

Primary tumor

TX Primary tumor cannot be assessed

T0 No evidence of primary tumor

Tis Carcinoma *in situ*: intraductal carcinoma, lobular carcinoma *in situ*, or Paget's disease of the nipple with no tumor

T1 Tumor ≤2 cm

  T1mic ≤0.1 cm

  T1a >0.1–0.5 cm

  T1b >0.5–1 cm

  T1c >1–2 cm

T2 Tumor >2 to 5 cm

T3 Tumor >5 cm

T4 Any size with extension to chest wall or skin (chest wall includes ribs, intercostal muscles, and serratus anterior muscle, but not pectoral muscles)

T4a Extension to chest wall

  T4b Edema, skin ulceration, or satellite skin nodules confined to same breast

  T4c Both (T4a and T4b) criteria

  T4d Inflammatory carcinoma

Regional lymph nodes (N)—*clinical*

NX Regional lymph nodes cannot be assessed (e.g., previously removed)

N0 No regional lymph node metastasis

N1 Metastasis to movable ipsilateral lymph node(s)

N2 Metastasis in ipsilateral axillary lymph nodes, fixed or matted, or in clinically apparent ipsilateral internal mammary nodes in the absence of clinically evident axillary lymph node metastasis

N2a Metastasis in ipsilateral axillary lymph nodes fixed to one another (matted) or to other structures

N2b Metastasis only in clinically apparent ipsilateral internal mammary nodes in the absence of clinically evident axillary lymph node metastasis.

N3 Metastasis in ipsilateral infraclavicular lymph node(s), with or without axillary lymph node involvement, or in clinically apparent ipsilateral internal mammary lymph nodes in the presence of clinically evident axillary lymph node metastasis; or metastasis in ipsilateral supraclavicular lymph node(s), with or without axillary or internal mammary lymph node involvement.

N3a Metastasis in ipsilateral infraclavicular lymph node(s)

N3b Metastasis in ipsilateral internal mammary lymph nodes in the presence of clinically evident axillary lymph node metastasis

N3c Metastasis in ipsilateral supraclavicular lymph node(s), with or without axillary or internal mammary node involvement

Distant metastasis (M)

MX Distant metastasis cannot be assessed

M0 No distant metastasis

M1 Metastases present, including to ipsilateral supraclavicular lymph nodes

Table 10.2.   Stage grouping of breast cancer[a]

Stage	Description
0	Tis, N0, M0
I	T1, N0, M0
IIA	T0–1, N1, M0
	T2, N0, M0
IIB	T2, N1, M0
	T3, N0, M0
IIIA	T0–2, N2, M0
	T3, N1–2, M0
IIIB	T4, any N, M0
IIIC	Any T, N3, M0
IV	Any T, any N, M1

New classification for nodal metastasis to infraclavicular, internal mammary, and supraclavicular nodes.
[a]Patients are staged in the highest group possible for their composite TNM. For example, a patient with T1a, N2, M0 would have stage IIIA disease because of the N2 status. Modified from American Joint Committee on Cancer. Breast. *AJCC staging manual*, 6th ed. New York:Springer-Verlag, 2002:171–180.

detected. The AJCC Staging manual (6th edition) reviews the basis for these changes in the discussion section of breast cancer staging.

4. **Diagnostic evaluation**

a. **Before biopsy,** the woman should have a careful **history**, during which attention should be paid to risk factors, and a **physical examination**, with a focus not only on the involved breast but also on the opposite breast, all regional lymph node areas, the lungs, bone, and liver. This examination should be followed by bilateral mammography to help assess the extent of involvement and to look for additional ipsilateral or contralateral disease.

b. **Excisional or core needle biopsy of the primary lesion** is performed, and the specimen is given intact (not in formalin) to the pathologist, who can divide the specimen for histologic examination, hormone receptor assays, overexpression of genes such as *HER2*, flow cytometric measurements of ploidy and the percentage of cells in the S phase, and other specialized tests.

c. **After confirmation of the histology,** the patient is evaluated for possible metastatic disease.

(1) **Mandatory studies** include a chest radiograph, complete blood count, blood chemistry profile, and estrogen and progesterone receptor assays and HER2 assessment on the primary breast carcinoma and grossly cancerous nodal tissues.

(2) **Other studies,** including radionuclide scan of the bones, skeletal survey (usually obtained only if the radionuclide scan is positive), and computed

tomography scan of the liver (abdomen) are optional unless the history, physical examination, or blood studies suggest a poor prognosis or point to specific organ involvement.

(3) Histology. Approximately 75% to 80% of all breast cancers are infiltrating ductal carcinomas, and 10% are infiltrating lobular carcinomas; these two types have similar biologic behavior. The remainder of the histologic types of invasive breast carcinoma may have a somewhat better prognosis but are usually managed more according to the stage than to the histologic type. With the recent development of microarray technology breast cancer is now thought of as a disease with distinct subtypes. One subtype (the basal epithelial subtype) is commonly referred to as *triple negative or basaloid breast cancer*. It constitutes approximately 15% of all invasive breast cancers and is distinctly different from tumors arising from inner milk-secreting luminal cells (luminal breast cancer) that constitute most breast cancers in the United States and Northern Europe. Basaloid breast cancer lacks hormone receptor expression and the cells do not overexpress her2-neu. Triple negative tumors are seen in association with *BRCA1* mutations and in women of African ancestry. This type is associated with a poor prognosis.

D. Approach to therapy

1. Consultation with a surgeon, radiotherapist, and medical oncologist is critical once the diagnosis of carcinoma is highly suspected or histologically confirmed. Multimodal therapy has had a more beneficial impact on carcinoma of the breast than on any other common cancer affecting adults. It is important to have all these oncology specialists see the patient before final decisions regarding therapy are made, so the primary physician and the patient can have opinions from several perspectives about optimal management. This is best achieved during **multidisciplinary** treatment planning conferences where opportunities arise to discuss treatment, identify patients who require psychosocial support, identify patients who may benefit from genetic testing, and those eligible for clinical trials. It is also critical to have the patient (and her family if she desires) share in the therapy decisions after hearing the options, the relative advantages and disadvantages of each option, and the recommendations of the consultants. The patient should be given an opportunity to hear why the recommended treatment is thought by the physicians to be best and to decide whether that is acceptable to her.

2. Goals of therapy differ depending on the stage of disease being treated.

a. For early disease, the goal of therapy is to eradicate micrometastases to render the patient free of disease and prevent recurrence. If eradication of cancer cells cannot be achieved, long-term suppression is desirable. This may be accomplished by tamoxifen and other SERMs (hormonal manipulation). Coincident with therapy is the goal of avoiding unnecessarily excessive drug-induced toxicity, both short and long term. Of particular concern is the increased incidence of second cancers (myelodysplasia and leukemias in particular) arising years after the completion of chemotherapy. Therefore, a goal of investigational studies has been to try to determine the minimum therapy that is effective for preventing the maximum number of recurrences in any given clinical situation.

b. For locally advanced disease, defined as patients with stage IIIA or T3–4 disease, including inflammatory breast cancer and patients with positive ipsilateral supraclavicular or infraclavicular nodes, the goal of therapy (commonly referred to as ***neoadjuvant*** *therapy*) is to reduce the size of an initially unresectable tumor, improve local control and decrease the spread of metastatic disease. Such preoperative administration of chemotherapy allows the opportunity to test therapeutic efficacy of drugs as well as test novel therapies and biomarkers.

c. For advanced disease, the goal is usually to reduce the tumor burden and the resultant disability in order to alleviate the patient's symptoms, improve performance, and prolong meaningful survival (palliation). Whereas long-term toxicity is not usually of great importance, short-term toxicity is a major area of concern for both physician and patient because the aim of therapy is to improve how the patient feels (quality of life) as well as to prolong survival time.

3. Surgery has been and remains the most frequently used mode of primary therapy for most women with carcinoma of the breast. The role of surgery in the primary management of carcinoma of the breast has been evolving with a **trend to lesser surgery (lumpectomy)** together with axillary node dissection. Surgical margins should be free (3–4 mm). Complete axillary node dissection may become unnecessary when the reliability of **sentinel node identification,** removal, and histologic assessment is established with greater certainty. This technique may spare many women the additional surgical procedure of axillary node dissection and its attendant risk of lymphedema. At this point, full axillary dissection remains the standard of care if the sentinel node(s) was found to be positive for breast cancer cells. **Lumpectomy and axillary node evaluation are followed by radiotherapy** to control the microscopic cancer remaining in the breast. Depending on the stage of the cancer, additional radiotherapy may be used to treat upper internal mammary nodes. For most women, this therapy yields therapeutic results that are as good as with **modified radical mastectomy** without the need for amputating the breast and its attendant physical deformity and psychological trauma. Many surgeons believe that in the modern management of breast cancer, and unless requested by the patient herself, a mastectomy is only indicated in cases of inability to completely excise the primary tumor, if the patient has multicentric disease or if she has a contraindication to radiation therapy.

Although many women and their physicians are opting for lesser surgery, some version of the modified radical mastectomy is still more commonly performed in many areas of the United States; in this operation, the breast, pectoralis fascia (with or without the pectoralis minor muscle), and lymph nodes are removed. There are wide geographic variations in the use of breast-conserving surgery throughout the United States. For most women, surgeries more extensive than the modified radical mastectomy are probably of no benefit, and lesser surgeries that are not combined with radiotherapy are insufficient in terms of providing important prognostic information regarding the status of the axillary lymph nodes and controlling the local disease (40% of women treated with excisional biopsy alone have recurrence in the ipsilateral breast).

For patients who have had mastectomy, reconstruction is being done with increasing frequency. It may be done at the time of mastectomy or delayed for a period (usually 1 to 2 years). Options include insertion of a silicone or saline implant or transposition of a muscle flap. Neither procedure has resulted in worsening of the prognosis from the breast cancer or a significant increase in the difficulty in detecting local recurrences.

4. Radiation therapy. The role of radiation therapy in the management of carcinoma of the breast has been expanded since the early 1970s. Radiotherapy is now commonly used in conjunction with lumpectomy as part of the primary therapy. In this circumstance, radiotherapy is commonly delivered using external-beam therapy to the entire breast with a boost of therapy to the tumor bed using either external-beam therapy or implantation of radioactive substances. Radiotherapy may also be given after mastectomy in women who have a high likelihood of local recurrence, and it is highly effective in preventing the reappearance of disease in the treated fields. In some circumstances it may also improve survival. Postmastectomy radiation is indicated if the primary is larger than 5 cm or if four or more positive lymph nodes were found in the axilla. Radiation may be omitted in patients older than 70 years with estrogen receptor–positive tumors smaller than 2 cm if they were treated with antiestrogen therapy. Radiation therapy is usually started after completion of cytotoxic therapy. Many trials (e.g., MammoSite) are currently defining the role of brachytherapy in the management of patients with early breast cancer. Such therapy is given over a short period of time (typically 5 days) and delivers a higher dose of radiation through a catheter or balloon placed in the lumpectomy cavity. Patients are treated twice a day. This allows patients to complete their radiation therapy before initiating systemic therapy if indicated. Radiation therapy is also helpful as adjunct therapy for advanced disease. Local recurrences and distant metastases also are frequently treated successfully with radiotherapy. This mode of treatment is particularly critical to the management of painful bony lesions or sites of impending pathologic fracture.

5. Chemotherapy and endocrine therapy (systemic therapy) are used to reduce the likelihood of recurrence in early disease and to treat more advanced disease with or without distant metastasis. The Early Breast Cancer Trialists' Collaborative Group (EBCTCG) analysis of adjuvant therapy demonstrated a **clear benefit of postoperative chemotherapy or hormonal therapy** (including ovarian ablation in premenopausal women). Such therapy will on average reduce the risk of recurrence by 20% to 35%. Similarly the odds of death were also reduced by 15% to 30%. The same **proportional risk reduction** was seen in node-positive as well as node-negative patients. Patients with node-negative disease benefit from adjuvant therapy with a percentage decrease in mortality similar to that for node-positive women but the lower baseline mortality for node-negative women results in less absolute benefit per 100 women treated. Current clinical trials use tumor size, hormone receptor status, DNA synthesis rate (percentage of cells in S phase), and other factors to aid in identifying the patients, among those with negative nodes, who are most likely to relapse and thereby most likely to benefit from adjuvant therapy. Commercially available tests that map out a gene profile for node-negative cancers (see Section I.E. in the following text) may also help in treatment decisions in this population and thereby help clinicians avoid unnecessary treatment. The physiologic age of the patient and comorbid conditions will become important considerations in adjuvant therapy decisions.

Endocrine therapy may result from surgical, radiotherapeutic, or chemotherapeutic ablation or inhibition of the ovaries or adrenal glands; or it may consist of additive therapy with antiestrogens, aromatase inhibitors (AIs), progestins, androgens, or luteinizing hormone–releasing hormone (LHRH) agonists. Endocrine therapy is generally ineffective (as sole therapy) for the treatment of metastatic disease in patients with low levels of estrogen and progesterone receptors in the cancer cells and is increasingly effective as the level of receptors rises. The best responses can be expected in women in whom the estrogen receptor level is high and progesterone receptors are present.

E. Prognosis. There is a broad spectrum in the biologic behavior of breast carcinoma from aggressive, rapidly fatal, inflammatory carcinoma to relatively indolent disease with late-appearing metastasis and survival time of 10 to 15 years. The likelihood of relapse and survival are influenced by a number of factors:

1. Stage. Axillary node involvement and the size of the primary tumor are major determinants of the likelihood of survival.

    a. Nodes. In one large National Surgical Adjuvant Breast Project (NSABP) study, before the use of modern adjuvant therapy, 65% of all patients who underwent radical mastectomy survived 5 years and 45% survived 10 years. When no axillary nodes were positive, the 5-year survival rate was approximately 80% and the 10-year survival rate was 65%. If any axillary nodes were positive, the 5-year survival rate was less than 50% and the 10-year survival rate was 25%. If four or more nodes were positive, the 5-year survival rate was 30% and the 10-year survival rate less than 15%. Since that time (1975), there has been improvement, with 5-year survival rates of 87% for stage I, 75% for stage II, 45% for stage III, and 13% for stage IV breast cancer. Lymph node involvement remains the single most important prognostic factor in making survival predictions and treatment decisions.

b. Primary tumor. Patients with large primary tumors do not do as well as patients with small tumors, irrespective of the nodal status, although patients with large primary tumors are more likely to have node involvement. Tumors that are fixed to the skin or to the chest wall do worse than those that are not. Patients with inflammatory carcinomas have a particularly poor prognosis, with a median survival time of less than 2 years and a 5-year survival rate of less than 10% in some series. Aggressive initial (neoadjuvant) chemotherapy has improved the outcome of many of these patients.

2. Estrogen and progesterone receptors. Patients without estrogen or progesterone receptors (or with very low levels) are twice as likely to relapse during the first 2 years after diagnosis as those who are receptor positive. This observation is true for both premenopausal and postmenopausal patients within each major node group (0, 1 to 3, and 4 or more).

3. *Her-2/neu* amplification is associated with impaired survival in early-stage breast cancer. This is a proto-oncogene that codes for a transmembrane receptor of the epidermal growth factor receptor family. Amplification (as is seen in 25%–30% of early breast cancer) results in worse prognosis with earlier appearance of metastatic disease.

4. Gene profiling. As of January 2004, the U.S. Food and Drug Administration (FDA) approved the use of a 21-gene PCR assay, the Oncotype Dx (Genomic Health, Inc., Redwood City, California) breast cancer assay, for use in patients who are hormone-receptor positive with negative nodes. These patients tend to be overtreated (~50% of the time). This technology is based on gene expression studies on tumors in paraffin-embedded tissues. After a detailed selection process of candidate genes, a panel of 16 cancer genes and 5 reference genes was selected. The gene expression levels were formulated in an algorithm that allows computation of a recurrence score (RS) for each tumor. The test demonstrated the ability (in randomized clinical trials) to quantify the risk of recurrence as well as predict benefit from chemotherapy for this group of hormone-dependent tumors. A report is sent out on each patient, with a number representing their RS (a continuum from 0–100).

Patients with a RS less than 18 (~50% of patients in most series) are considered low risk and will probably not benefit from the addition of cytotoxic therapy to their hormonal manipulation. Patients with an RS of greater than 30 have a high risk of systemic disease and will obtain the maximum benefit from chemotherapy. Patients with intermediate score (18–30) currently represent a decision-making dilemma and trials are underway to better define the approach to therapy in this patient population.

5. Other prognostic factors are still under study as to whether they can provide information as independent prognostic factors, particularly for node-negative cancers. These include the percentage of cells in DNA synthesis (low percentage in S phase better than high percentage) and the ploidy of the breast cancer cells (diploid better than aneuploid). Additional tumor markers that may have predictive value include cathepsin D, *c-myc* oncogene amplification, and *p*53 suppressor gene expression.

II. Systemic therapy of breast cancer

A. Cytotoxic therapy. As with other cancers, the basis for the effectiveness of cytotoxic drugs in the treatment of carcinoma of the breast is not completely understood. It is clear, however, that combinations of drugs are considerably more effective in the adjuvant setting than single agents (although how many is enough is not as certain). Nearly all treatment programs use the drugs in various combinations, at least during initial therapy. In addition to their cytotoxic effects, chemotherapeutic agents may induce menopause in premenopausal women, thereby affecting estrogen production as well as killing cells directly. Recent studies suggest a trend toward a lower recurrence rate in women who develop chemotherapy-induced amenorrhea.

1. Response to therapy. In the adjuvant setting, it is impossible to determine whether individual patients have responded to treatment for micrometastatic disease unless they relapse, because there are no parameters to measure. New testing modalities for chemotherapy responsiveness are being evaluated. Currently, they are used more commonly in the metastatic setting but we anticipate widespread use in the next few years. The effectiveness of adjuvant therapy must therefore depend on population studies. Because breast cancer may have a long natural history, and the disease may recur even beyond 10 years, it is critical to defer final conclusions regarding any study until at least 5 years and preferably 10 years have passed.

Chemotherapy improves both disease-free survival (DFS) and overall survival (OS) by approximately 25% in all groups of patients. Although the proportional reduction in death rate is similar for both high- and low-risk patients (e.g., node-positive and node-negative), the absolute benefit is greater for those at higher risk of recurrence and death (e.g., younger patients with positive nodes).

2. Treatment of early disease (adjuvant therapy). Standard treatment of early disease depends on primary tumor size, nodal status, menopausal status of the patient, hormone receptor status of the tumor, and other tumor characteristics. Because there is no optimal therapy yet for any subset of women with breast cancer, the patient and her physician should be encouraged to participate in clinical trials. If none is available or the patient declines, Table 10.3

Table 10.3. Prognostic factors for assessing risk of recurrence of breast cancer

Value	Parameter
Nodal status	Risk increases with presence of metastasis and numbers of nodes involved
Tumor size	Risk increases with tumor size independent of nodal status
Estrogen and progesterone receptors	Positive receptors confer better prognosis
Age	Complex factor (biology chronology): women aged 45 to 49 years have best prognosis, with increasing likelihood of deaths from their breast cancer in older and younger age groups
Morphology	Higher nuclear grade, higher histologic grade, tumor necrosis, peritumoral lymphatic vessel invasion, and increased microvessel density tumors have worse prognosis
DNA content and proliferative capacity	Tumors that are diploid and have low S-phase fraction do better than those that are aneuploid or have a high S-phase fraction (by flow cytometry)
HER2/neu (c-erbB-2)	Amplification has association with earlier relapse and shorter survival. HER2/neu (c-erbB-2) testing by either **FISH** (fluorescent in situ hybridization) expressed as molecules/gene copy ratio (2.0 or more copies) or by **IHC** staining expressed as 0–3+ where 3+ correlates best with FISH positivity
BRCA1 and BRCA2 mutations	Seem to have little effect on prognosis

can be used as a guide for assessing risk. Table 10.4 may be used as a guide to select the type of therapy, depending on stage of disease, menopausal state, age, receptor status, and other risk factors. Cytotoxic therapy is recommended for all premenopausal and most postmenopausal women with positive nodes, irrespective of hormone receptor status. It should also be used in higher-risk premenopausal and postmenopausal women with negative nodes, particularly if they have negative hormone receptors. The goal of adjuvant chemotherapy is to decrease the risk of systemic

Table 10.4. Systemic adjuvant therapy for breast cancer—suggested guidelines

Tumor Category	Premenopausal Women	Postmenopausal Women[a] ≤70 yr	Postmenopausal Women[a] >70 yr
Node positive			
ER and/or PR positive	CT with TAM or oophorectomy	AI with or without CT	AI
ER and PR negative	CT	CT	None or CT
Node negative			
ER and PR indeterminate because tumor too small	TAM	? AI	None
ER and/or PR positive			
≤2 cm			
Low risk[b]	TAM	AI	AI or none
High risk	CT plus TAM	AI ± CT	AI
>2 cm	CT plus TAM	CT + AI	AI
ER and PR negative	CT	CT	None

ER, estrogen receptor; PR, progesterone receptor; CT, chemotherapy; AC (doxorubicin [Adriamycin] plus cyclophosphamide) for four cycles; CAF (cyclophosphamide, doxorubicin, fluorouracil); CMF (cyclophosphamide, methotrexate, fluorouracil); CMFP (cyclophosphamide, methotrexate, fluorouracil, prednisone) for six cycles; other chemotherapy may be of equal or better efficacy (such as AC followed by paclitaxel); TAM, tamoxifen (for 5 years, alone or after completion of chemotherapy). AI, aromatase inhibitor.

[a]Comorbid conditions may modify decision to treat and choice of therapy.

[b]Based on factors such as size <1 cm, low histologic grade, or a low percentage (<6%–10%) of cells in S phase (see Table 10.3).

disease. We are less inclined to use cytotoxic therapy in the adjuvant treatment of older women (over 70 years of age with comorbid conditions, over 80 years of age without comorbid conditions), particularly if they are hormone receptor positive and are at lower risk. How much, if any, cytotoxic therapy adds to antiestrogen (tamoxifen) therapy in lower-risk, node-negative, hormone receptor–positive patients is not established.

Many practicing oncologists use AC (doxorubicin [Adriamycin] and cyclophosphamide) more commonly in women with a higher risk of recurrence, and CMF (cyclophosphamide, methotrexate, and fluorouracil) more in those who have lesser risks (e.g., are node negative), who have comorbid conditions, or in whom cardiac risk of doxorubicin is deemed important. Anthracyclines, however, remain the minimum standard of care in healthy node-positive patients. In 1998, the International Consensus Panel on the Treatment of Breast Cancer in St. Gallen, Switzerland agreed that anthracycline-based therapy is superior to CMF. The Oxford overview and the EBCTCG update showed a 3% absolute survival and recurrence benefit with anthracycline-based regimens as compared with CMF at 5 years and 4% benefit at 10 years. Retrospective analysis suggests that the superiority of anthracyclines may be limited to *her-2-neu–* positive disease. We highly recommend reviewing the EBCTCG update *Lancet* 2005 paper (included in our list of *Suggested Readings*) for a better understanding of the evolution of breast cancer therapy.

a. **Use of taxanes in node-positive disease.** Three phase III trials have evaluated the addition of taxanes (paclitaxel or docetaxel) in node-positive patients. These patients have a higher risk for relapse. Both the pivotal Cancer and Leukemia Group B (CALGB) protocol 9934 and the NSABP B28 trial supported the use of paclitaxel after AC for node-positive breast cancer regardless of the receptor status, tamoxifen use, age of the patient, or the number of positive lymph nodes. Although all patients benefit, hormone receptor–negative patients benefit to a greater extent. Both trials were positive for DFS. There was a 14% improved OS in the CALGB trial. A slightly differently designed trial (BCIRG 001) addressed the same question. In this trial, six cycles of TAC (docetaxel, doxorubicin, and cyclophosphamide) were compared to six cycles of FAC (fluorouracil, doxorubicin and cyclophosphamide) as adjuvant therapy for node-positive patients. The study showed superiority of TAC in all patient groups. Long-term follow-up (at 55 months) showed a reduction of relapse by 28% and an improvement of 30% in OS. This improvement was independent of all variables. There were more episodes of febrile neutropenia in the TAC arm but no septic deaths. Similar findings were noted when epirubicin was used instead of doxorubicin. Three cycles of FEC followed by three cycles of docetaxel were found to be superior to six cycles of FEC in node-positive patients by the French Adjuvant Study Group.

b. Dose-dense therapy. A superior DFS (albeit with a very small difference [2%] for OS) was seen when chemotherapy was administered on a 2-weekly basis (AC-T) in the CALGB 9741 landmark trial. All patients had early breast cancer with positive nodes. Such regimen requires growth factor support. Longer follow-up is needed before the oncology community switches to every 2 weeks therapy. It was apparent, however, that it is feasible to administer chemotherapy with an absolute neutrophil count of 1,000 cells/μL.

c. Trastuzumab in the adjuvant setting. Her-2-neu–positive breast cancer accounts for 20% of all cases of breast cancer. Such patients have a higher risk of recurrence and a more aggressive course in the adjuvant setting. Trastuzumab has been used for the past 7 years in combination with chemotherapy as standard therapy for metastatic her-2-neu–positive disease. Results from large adjuvant trials have now established the role of trastuzumab in the adjuvant setting as well. The detailed description of these trials is beyond the scope of this book. At this point, the use of trastuzumab along with chemotherapy (a taxane was included in four of these trials) in high-risk node-negative as well as node-positive patients was associated with a 39% to 52% reduction in the risk of recurrence. We have also learned from these trials that earlier use of the monoclonal antibody is associated with survival benefit (as opposed to using trastuzumab when patients recur). We still do not understand the mechanism of trastuzumab resistance. Trastuzumab does not cross the blood–brain barrier (BBB). Newer small molecules (e.g., lapatinib) are awaiting FDA approval after their promising role in this subset of patients when combined with capecitabine if resistance to trastuzumab develops. Smaller molecules also cross the BBB and provide potential for reducing brain metastasis in this patient population.

d. High-dose chemotherapy. Moderate escalation of the doses of the standard chemotherapy regimens does not appear to be of benefit in improving survival and may increase the risk for treatment-related myelodysplasia and leukemia. Very high-dose chemotherapy with autologous bone marrow or peripheral blood progenitor cell reinfusion has not fulfilled the promise of improving the survival of women at very high risk of recurrence. After analysis of recently completed clinical trials, it has become clear that no single group of patients with advanced breast cancer, regardless of tumor factors or clinical features demonstrated benefits from high-dose chemotherapy. The potential benefit for women with a large number of positive lymph nodes remains investigational.

e. Some commonly used regimens. (Please refer to discussion in the preceding text about choice of regimen based on nodal status.)

- **CAF**

  Cyclophosphamide 100 mg/m^2 PO on days 1 to 14
  Doxorubicin 30 mg/m^2 IV on days 1 and 8
  Fluorouracil 500 mg/m^2 IV on days 1 and 8.
  Repeat the cycle every 4 weeks.

- **AC**

  Doxorubicin 60 mg/m^2 IV push through a rapidly running IV
  Cyclophosphamide 600 mg/m^2 IV.
  Repeat every 3 weeks.

- **CMFP**

  Cyclophosphamide 100 mg/m^2 PO on days 1 to 14
  Methotrexate 40 mg/m^2 IV on days 1 and 8
  Fluorouracil 600 mg/m^2 IV on days 1 and 8
  Prednisone 40 mg/m^2 PO on days 1 to 14, during the first three cycles only.
  Repeat the cycle every 4 weeks.

- **Doxorubicin plus paclitaxel** with or without filgrastim (Neupogen)

  Doxorubicin 50 to 60 mg/m^2 IV, *followed in 4 hours by*
  Paclitaxel 150 mg/m^2 IV over 3 to 24 hours
  Filgrastim 300μg/day SC starting 24 hours after the end of chemotherapy, for 10 days.
  Repeat every three weeks.

- **FEC**

  Fluorouracil 500 mg/m^2 IV on day 1
  Epirubicin 100 mg/m^2 IV on day 1
  Cyclophosphamide 500 mg/m^2 IV on day 1.
  Repeat cycle every 21 days.

- **TAC**

  Taxotere (docetaxel) 75 mg/m^2 on day 1
  Adriamycin (doxorubicin) 50 mg/m^2 on day 1
  Cyclophosphamide 500 mg/m^2 on day 1.
  Repeat cycle every 21 days.

- Trastuzumab may be added to paclitaxel after completion of four cycles of AC

  Paclitaxel 80 mg/m^2 weekly × 12 given concurrently with trastuzumab 4 mg/m^2 as an initial loading dose, followed by 2 mg/m^2 weekly, which is continued for 52 weeks.

  Tips:

  (1) Limit the number of cycles of doxorubicin in any combination regimen to six (300 to 360 mg/m^2) to reduce enhanced cardiotoxicity from the combination.

  (2) No safety data for trastuzumab (Herceptin) in combination with anthracyclines in the adjuvant setting, so administer sequentially.

  (3) Monitor for peripheral neuropathy especially in patients with diabetes and older patients with paclitaxel.

3. **Cytotoxic therapy of advanced (metastatic) disease.** Among the cytotoxic drugs, the most commonly used agents include doxorubicin, cyclophosphamide, methotrexate, fluorouracil, paclitaxel, docetaxel, gemcitabine, capecitabine, vinorelbine, mitoxantrone, thiotepa, and vincristine. Each of these agents has a response rate of 20% to 40% when used as a single agent. Because combinations are so much more effective (60%–80% response rate) than single agents, these drugs are rarely used alone as initial therapy. With very few exceptions, the data have not supported a survival advantage in the metastatic setting with combination chemotherapy. The choice of single agent therapy versus a combination regimen should be made on the basis of the tempo of the metastatic process, the patient's age, performance status, and access to care.

Cytotoxic combination chemotherapy is used as first-line treatment for advanced disease, in hormone receptor–negative patients, and at times in patients with several organs involved because the responses are more rapid and the rate of response is greater when drugs are used in combination than when endocrine therapy is used alone. For patients over 65 years of age, however, initiation of hormone therapy alone may be justified, with cytotoxic therapy being reserved for patients who have failed one or more hormonal treatments.

Cytotoxic chemotherapy produces responses in 60% to 80% of patients regardless of their estrogen receptor status. The responses to therapy are at times durable, but the median duration in most studies is less than 1 year. Clearly, improved survival is desirable. This is not achievable with most current regimens with the exception of regimens that include trastuzumab. The benefits of trastuzumab (Herceptin) are limited to patients who are *HER2* 3+ by immunohistochemistry or those who are FISH positive. Carboplatin in combination with paclitaxel and trastuzumab (TCH) is being tested in various schedules with the hope of finding an active regimen without the cardiotoxicity of the doxorubicin–trastuzumab combination. Other forms of taxanes are a new addition to the drugs active in the metastatic setting. **Nanoparticle albumin-bound (nab) paclitaxel (Abraxane)** is the first in a novel class of compounds combining human albumin with paclitaxel in the nanoparticle state. A phase III trial showed superiority of the drug given in this form to paclitaxel given every 3 weeks. There were fewer associated hypersensitivity reactions, a shorter infusion time, and a more reversible peripheral neuropathy.

Second-line therapy depends on what treatment the patient has initially received. If the patient relapses while on treatment or within 6 months of finishing treatment for micrometastatic disease (adjuvant therapy), it is not likely that these drugs used in combination can be helpful in achieving a second remission. Because doxorubicin is among the most effective agents against breast carcinoma, it should be used in any combination in this situation, provided it has not been given adjuvantly as discussed in the preceding text. One of the regimens listed previously may be used. **Additional choices include the following:**

- **Paclitaxel** 150 to 175 mg/m² IV over 3 hours every 3 weeks, *or* 80 mg/m² over 1 hour weekly.
- **Docetaxel,** 60 to 100 mg/m² IV over 1 hour every 3 weeks (premedication with oral corticosteroids such as dexamethasone, 8 mg b.i.d., for 3 days starting 1 day before starting docetaxel is necessary to reduce the severity of fluid retention and hypersensitivity reactions), *or*
- **Vinorelbine,** 30 mg/m² IV over 6 to 10 minutes weekly.
- **Capecitabine/docetaxel**

  Capecitabine 1,250 mg/m² orally twice daily on days 1 to 14 followed by 1-week rest, *plus*
  Docetaxel 75 mg/m² IV over 1 hour on day 1
  Repeat cycle every 3 weeks.

- **Gemcitabine/paclitaxel**

  Gemcitabine 1,250 mg/m² IV on days 1 and 8 followed by a week's rest, *plus*
  Paclitaxel 175 mg/m² IV on day 1
  Repeat every 3 weeks.

- **Weekly trastuzumab and paclitaxel**

  Trastuzumab 4 mg/m² IV as an initial loading dose, followed by 2 mg/m² weekly *and*
  Paclitaxel 200 mg/m² IV every 3 weeks.

- **Lapatinib plus Capecitabine (after failure on anthracyclline, taxane, and trastuzumab)**

  Lapatinib 1250 mg PO daily and
  Capecitabine 2000 mg/m² in two divided doses daily on days 1 through 14 of a 21-day cycle.

- **Abraxane** 260 mg/m² IV over 30 minutes given every 3 weeks.
- **TCH(Taxotere [docetaxel]/carboplatin/ Herceptin[trastuzumab])**

  Carboplatin at an area under the curve (AUC) of 6 IV day 1
  Docetaxel 75 mg/m² IV day 1
  Trastuzumab (see dose mentioned earlier).

Note: This is by no means an all-inclusive list. Regimens listed are what the author commonly uses.

4. **Dose modifications** are outlined in Table 10.5.

B. **Endocrine (hormonal) therapy of advanced disease** is presumed to be effective because the breast cancer tissue retains some of the endocrine sensitivity of the normal breast tissue. In premenopausal women, if the breast cancer growth is supported by estrogen production from the ovary, antiestrogen therapy, removal of endogenous estrogen by oophorectomy, or suppression of estrogen production using an LHRH agonist logically results in regression of the cancer—at least those tumor cells that are dependent on the estrogen. (The dependent cells seem to be those that have the estrogen receptors.) Other

Table 10.5.   Dose modification for chemotherapy of breast carcinoma

Dysfunction			Percentage of full dose
Hematologic Toxicity ANC (WBC)/μL on Day of Scheduled Treatment		Platelets/μL on Day of Scheduled Treatment	Dose as Percentage of Immediately Preceding Cycle
=1,800 (=3,500)	and	>100,000	100
1,500–1,800 (3,000–3,500)	or	75,000–100,000	75[a]
1,000–1,500 (2,500–3,000)	or	50,000–75,000	50
<1,000 (<2,500)	or	<50,000	0 (delay 1 wk)

[a]Absolute neutrophil count (ANC) is the preferred parameter if available. Some use 100% dosing for ANC 1,500–1,800. If counts are rising at the end of a treatment cycle, an alternative is to delay by a few days to a week and then treat at a higher dose according to the count on the day of actual treatment. If the nadir ANC is <1,000/μL and is associated with fever >38.3°C (101°F) or the nadir platelet count is <40,000/μL, decrease dose by 25% in subsequent cycles. If the nadir white blood cell (WBC) count is >3,500/μL and the platelet count is >125,000/μL, increase the dose by 25%.

mechanisms of action of the antiestrogen tamoxifen include inhibition of the epithelial growth factor, transforming growth factor-α (TGF-α), and stimulation of the epithelial inhibitory factor TGF-β. Complicating the anticipated interactions of SERMs further is the presence of different classes of estrogen receptors, different ligands, many receptor-interacting proteins, a host of transcription-activating factors, and several response elements.

1. Treatment of early disease (adjuvant therapy). Among the antihormonal drugs, the most commonly used agent is tamoxifen (the other SERMs toremifene and raloxifene are not as widely used). The AIs (anastrozole, letrozole, and exemestane) block estrogen production at the cellular level by inhibiting reversibly or irreversibly the aromatase enzyme (responsible for conversion of male hormones to estrogen in postmenopausal patients). Current data support that in postmenopausal women, AIs offer additional benefit to what was observed with 5 years of tamoxifen including a survival advantage in node-positive receptor-positive patients. Both the ATAC (Arimidex or Tamoxifen Alone or in Combination) trial and the Breast International Group (BIG) 1–98 trials demonstrated an advantage to upfront use of an AI (Arimidex and letrozole, respectively). Results of the Intergroup Exemestane Study (IES) study demonstrated a superior DFS with sequential therapy using exemestane following 2 to 3 years of tamoxifen as compared to 5 years of tamoxifen alone. Fewer side effects are seen in this population with the use of AIs in comparison to that of tamoxifen. Of the most clinical relevance is the lower incidence of venous thromboembolic events and endometrial carcinoma with AIs. These drugs, however, are associated with a higher incidence of osteoporosis and musculoskeletal complaints.

Tamoxifen, 20 mg daily, is recommended in hormone receptor–positive women with positive nodes. It should be continued for 5 years. Longer durations do not improve survival. It is also beneficial in hormone receptor–positive premenopausal women with negative nodes who are not determined to be at low risk of recurrence (*see discussion in the preceding text about gene profiling*). In patients who are receptor positive and who receive cytotoxic chemotherapy, tamoxifen appears to have an added benefit. It has a relatively low risk in the adjuvant setting, and our current recommendations generally include tamoxifen where it is indicated in addition to chemotherapy in Table 10.4.

Tamoxifen (and probably other SERMs) improves DFS and OS in most estrogen receptor–positive patients. Although the proportional reduction (~25%) in death rate is similar for both high- and low-risk patients (e.g., node-positive and node-negative), the absolute benefit is greater for those at higher risk of recurrence and death. The improvement in DFS is superior with all AIs and there is an associated more significant reduction in contralateral breast cancer with these drugs in comparison to tamoxifen.

2. Treatment of advanced (metastatic) disease. Hormonal therapy is indicated in women who have had a positive test for estrogen or progesterone receptors in their tumor tissue. It is not generally recommended as the sole therapy for women who have low receptor levels or have previously been shown to be unresponsive to hormonal manipulation. It is also not the appropriate therapy for women with brain metastasis, lymphangitic pulmonary metastasis, or other dire visceral disease, such as extensive liver metastasis, in which a slow response could jeopardize survival. For **premenopausal women**, oophorectomy may still be the treatment of choice. The LHRH analogs goserelin and leuprolide can achieve the equivalent of a medical oophorectomy. This treatment may then be combined with an AI. **For postmenopausal women**, an AI should be used as the initial hormonal therapy. Adrenal suppression with aminoglutethimide is less commonly used because of greater side effects but is still effective. Responses to endocrine therapy tend to last longer than responses to cytotoxic chemotherapy, frequently lasting for 12 to 24 months. Second-line hormonal manipulation, for example, using a SERD (selective estrogen receptor downregulator), is a reasonable option if the tempo of disease progression allows it. This approach is usually helpful in patients who present with skeletal metastases. We also use IV bisphosphonates in this patient population because of their role in reduction of skeletal events.

a. Doses of commonly used drugs:

- Tamoxifen, 20 mg PO daily
- Anastrozole, 1 mg PO daily (alternative letrozole, 2.5 mg PO daily, or exemestane, 25 mg PO daily)
- Fulvestrant, 250 mg IM (into buttock) monthly as either a single 5-mL or two 2.5-mL injections
- Megestrol acetate, 40 mg PO q.i.d.

- Aminoglutethimide, 250 mg PO q.i.d.; hydrocortisone, 100 mg PO in divided doses daily for the first 2 weeks, then 40 mg PO in divided doses daily. Fludrocortisone, 0.05 to 0.1 mg PO may be given daily or every other day if there is evidence of salt wasting.
- **IV bisphosphonates**

  Zoledronic acid 4 mg over 15 minutes
  Pamidronate 60 to 90 mg over 1 to 2 hours.

3. Complications of therapy. Acute toxicities are primarily hematologic and gastrointestinal. Subacute toxicities include alopecia, hemorrhagic cystitis, hypertension, edema, and psychoneurologic abnormalities. Chronic or long-term toxicities may be cardiac, neoplastic, or psychoneurologic. Dose modifications for the more common problems are given in Table 10.5. These guidelines are de signed to be helpful in selecting a course of therapy that will be effective with the least risk of life-threatening toxicity. Because of individual differences, toxicities that are worse than expected may occur, and the responsible physician must always be alert to special circumstances that dictate further attenuation of the drug doses. The drug data listed in Chapter 4 should be consulted for the individual toxicities, precautions, and toxicity-prevention measures for each drug.

Adjuvant tamoxifen therapy also has consequences. These include a twofold to fourfold increase in endometrial cancer, an increase in cataracts, and an increase in thromboembolic disease. Hot flashes are common but can be ameliorated in some women with venlafaxine, 25 to 50 mg daily. While there is also reduction in the hot flashes from using a progestin, such as megestrol, 20 mg b.i.d., the effect of the progestin on the risk of recurrence is not known. Adverse effects on vaginal mucosa may be ameliorated with minimal systemic estrogen effect by the estradiol vaginal ring. Whereas fractures related to osteoporosis decrease with tamoxifen, there does not appear to be any reduction in cardiovascular events. AIs, on the other hand, may worsen osteoporosis despite an absence of increased fracture incidence in many trials. Caution and possibly anticoagulation should be exercised in treating women with Factor V Leiden who begin treatment with tamoxifen, AIs or other SERMs in the prevention or adjuvant setting.

SUGGESTED READINGS

Albain K, Nag S, Calderillo-Ruiz G, et al. Global phase III study of gemcitabine plus paclitaxel vs. paclitaxel as frontline therapy for metastatic breast cancer: first report of overall survival. *Proc Am Soc Clin Oncol* 2004;23:5. Abstract 510.

American Joint Committee on Cancer. Breast. *AJCC staging manual,* 6th ed. New York:Springer-Verlag, 2002:221–240.

Auquier A, Rutqvist LE, Host H, et al. Post-mastectomy megavoltage radiotherapy: the Oslo and Stockholm trials. *Eur J Cancer* 1992;28(2–3):433–437.

Bonadonna G, Valagussa P. Adjuvant systemic therapy for resectable breast cancer. *J Clin Oncol* 1985;3:259–275.

The Breast International Group (BIG) 1–98 Collaborative Group. A comparison of letrozole and tamoxifen in post-menopausal women with early breast cancer. *N Engl J Med* 2005;353:2747–2757.

Collaborative Group on Hormonal Factors in Breast Cancer. Breast cancer and hormonal contraceptives: collaborative reanalysis of individual data on 53,297 women with breast cancer and 100,239 women without breast cancer from 54 epidemiological studies. *Lancet* 1996;347(9017):1713–1727.

Coombes RC, Hall E, Gibson LJ, et al. The Intergroup Exemestane Study: a randomized trial of exemestane after 2–3 years of tamoxifen therapy in postmenopausal women with primary breast cancer. *N Engl J Med* 2004;350:1081–1092.

Early Breast Cancer Trialists' Collaborative Group. Ovarian ablation in early breast cancer: overview of the randomised trials. *Lancet* 1996;348:1189–1196.

Early Breast Cancer Trialists'Collaborative Group. Effects of chemotherapy and hormonal therapy for early breast cancer on recurrence and a 15-year survival :an overview of the randomized trials. *Lancet* 2005;365:1687–1717.

Fisher B, Costantino JP, Wickerham DL, et al. Surgical adjuvant breast and bowel project P–1 Study. *J Natl Cancer Inst* 1998; 90:1371–1388.

Fisher B, Dignam J, Mamounas EP, et al. Sequential methotrexate and fluorouracil for the treatment of node-negative breast cancer patients with estrogen receptor-negative tumors: eight-year results from National Surgical Adjuvant Breast and Bowel Project (NSABP) B-13 and first report of findings from NSABP B-19 comparing methotrexate and fluorouracil with conventional cyclophosphamide, methotrexate, and fluorouracil. *J Clin Oncol* 1996;14(7):1982–1992.

Fowble BL, Solin LJ, Schultz DJ, et al. Ten year results of conservative surgery and irradiation for stage I and II breast cancer. *Int J Radiat Oncol Biol Phys* 1991;21:269–277.

Goldhirsch A, Glick JH, Gelber RD, et al. Meeting highlights: International Consensus Panel on the Treatment of Primary Breast Cancer. Seventh international conference on adjuvant therapy of primary breast cancer. *J Clin Oncol* 2001;19:3817–3827.

Henderson IC, Berry D, Demetri G, et al. Improved disease-free and overall survival from the addition of sequential paclitaxel but not from the escalation of doxorubicin dose level in the adjuvant chemotherapy of patients with node-positive breast cancer. *Proc Am Soc Clin Oncol* 1998;17:101a.

Howell A, Cuzick J, Baum M, et al. Results, of the ATAC (Arimidex, Tamoxifen Alone or in Combination) trial after completion of 5 years of adjuvant treatment for breast cancer. *Lancet* 2005; 365:60–62.

Ingle JN, Krook JE, Green SJ, et al. Randomized trial of bilateral oophorectomy versus tamoxifen in premenopausal women with metastatic breast cancer. *J Clin Oncol* 1986;4:178–185.

Mouridsen H, Gershanovich M, Sun Y, et al. Superior efficacy of letrozole (Femara) versus tamoxifen as first-line therapy for post-menopausal women with advanced breast cancer: results of a phase III study of the International Letrozole Breast Cancer Group. *J Clin Oncol* 2001;19:2596–2606.

Paik S, Shak S, Tang G, et al. A multigene assay to predict recurrence in tamoxifen-treated, node negative breast cancer. *N Engl J Med* 2004;351:2817–2826.

Phillips K-A, Andrulis IL, Goodwin PH. Breast Carcinomas arising in carriers of mutations in *BRCA1* or *BRCA2*: are they prognostically different? *J Clin Oncol* 1999;17:3653–3663.

Pickle LW, Johnson KA. Estimating the long-term probability of developing breast cancer. *J Natl Cancer Inst* 1989;81:1854–1855.

Pritchard KI, Paterson AH, Paul NA, et al. Increased thromboembolic complications with concurrent tamoxifen and chemotherapy in a randomized trial of adjuvant therapy for women with breast cancer. *J Clin Oncol* 1996;14(10):2731–2737.

Rivkin SE, Green S, Metch B, et al. Adjuvant CMFVP vs tamoxifen vs concurrent CMFVP and tamoxifen for postmenopausal, node-positive, and estrogen receptor-positive breast cancer patients: a Southwest Oncology Group study. *J Clin Oncol* 1994;12:2078–2085.

Ross RK, Paganini-Hill A, Wan PC, et al. Effect of hormone replacement therapy on breast cancer risk: estrogen versus estrogen plus progestin. *J Natl Cancer Inst* 2000;92:328–332.

Singeltary SE, Allred C, Ashley P, et al. Revision of the American Joint Committee on Cancer staging system for breast cancer. *J Clin Oncol* 2002;20:3628–3636.

Slamon DJ, Leyland-Jones B, Shak S, et al. Use of chemotherapy plus a monoclonal antibody against HER2 for metastatic breast cancer that overexpresses HER2. *N Engl J Med* 2001;344:783–792.

Smith IE, Ross Gm. Breast radiotherapy after lumpectomy-no longer always necessary. *N Engl J Med* 2004;351:1021–1023.

Taylor SG, Gelman RSFalkson G, et al. IV Combination chemotherapy compared to tamoxifen as initial therapy for stage IV breast cancer in elderly women. *Ann Intern Med* 1986;104:455–461.

Van Dam FSAM, Schagen SB, Muller MJ, et al. Impairment of cognitive function in women receiving adjuvant treatment for high-risk breast cancer: high-dose versus standard-dose chemotherapy. *J Natl Cancer Inst* 1998;90:210–218.

CHAPTER 11

Gynecologic Cancer

Stephen Andrews

In 2006, there were an estimated 77,250 new female genital tract cancers in the United States and more than 28,000 deaths. The history of gynecologic cancer treatment in the United States has witnessed many successes such as the widespread acceptance of routine screening for cervical cancer with the Papanicolaou (Pap) smear. The Pap smear is credited with dramatic reduction in both the incidence rate and the death rate of cervical cancer over the past 40 years. More recent success includes the use of combined chemoradiotherapy to increase survival in the treatment of advanced cervical cancer and the increased survival realized with combined use of both intraperitoneal and intravenous chemotherapy for advanced ovarian cancer. The elucidation of the human papilloma virus (HPV) as the causative agent for cervical cancer worldwide has opened new techniques for cervical cancer screening. The use of HPV DNA detection on a cervical cytology specimen can identify those women who are at increased risk for developing cervical dysplasia and cervical cancer. The research on HPV has allowed the introduction of an HPV vaccine that will hopefully decrease further, if not eliminate, cervical cancer. In addition, there is now evidence that the involvement of a gynecologic oncologist in the treatment of a woman with a gynecologic cancer will enhance the outcome of treatment.

Despite many advances, there are still challenges ahead. Ovarian cancer is responsible for the overwhelming majority of deaths from gynecologic cancers because of the advanced stage at time of diagnosis and the lack of an effective screening test for this dreaded disease. Although the Pap smear is an effective screening test for cervical cancer, most women who develop invasive cervical cancer come from an unscreened or an under-screened population. Quality of life (QOL), the ramifications of sexual dysfunction after treatment for a gynecologic cancer, and fertility preservation for younger women with a gynecologic malignancy are all important issues that are now moved to the forefront of clinical research.

Women diagnosed with a gynecologic malignancy are best treated with a team approach. Review of all pertinent data at a prospective, multidisciplinary tumor board is recommended for optimal care. The oncologist should discuss treatment options based upon evidence-based research with the patient in a quiet, supportive setting with adequate time to address all her concerns. An open dialogue combined with an empathetic clinical support staff who understand and are committed to the care of women with gynecologic cancers will optimize the patient's treatment and QOL.

I. Carcinoma of the cervix. In 2006, there were approximately 9,710 new cases of invasive cervical cancer and 3,700 deaths from the disease in the United States. In developed countries with cervical cancer screening programs by Pap smears the incidence and death rate of invasive cervical cancer have decreased dramatically. However, cervical cancer is the second most common malignancy the world over, especially in nondeveloped countries that lack Pap smear screening programs. The relation between HPV infection and invasive cervical cancer is well established, especially HPV types 16 and 18 that account for 70% of all cervical cancers worldwide. Other risk factors for cervical cancer include early onset of coitus, multiple sex partners, high parity, tobacco use, human immunodeficiency virus and the "high-risk" male. This is a man who has had multiple sex partners, has frequented prostitutes or is positive for high-risk HPV types.

A. **Pathology and patterns of spread**
   1. **Histology.** Approximately 80% of cervical cancers are squamous cell carcinomas, both keratinizing and nonkeratinizing. The other 20% are adenocarcinomas. Squamous cell carcinomas typically arise from the squamo–columnar junction, an active zone of squamous metaplasia on the ectocervix. Adenocarcinomas arise from the endocervical canal. Both are associated with HPV, although squamous cells are more likely to be HPV-16 positive and adenocarcinomas HPV-18 positive. Adenosquamous carcinomas and adenoid cystic carcinomas, both of which have a worse prognosis stage for stage, are less commonly seen. A particularly virulent, and fortunately rare, type is small cell carcinoma of neuroendocrine origin. The most common metastatic lesions to the cervix are from other gynecologic cancers, especially endometrial.
   2. **The continuum of neoplasia.** The dramatic decrease in the incidence of invasive cervical cancer in the United States is due to the detection of cervical dysplasia through Pap smear screening. This allows preclinical disease to be diagnosed and treated. In 1988, the Bethesda system for reporting Pap smears was established and has undergone three revisions. The most recent American Cancer Society (ACS) guidelines for Pap smear screening recommends initiation of Pap smears 3 years after the onset of vaginal coitus, or by the age of 21. Dysplasias are divided into high-grade squamous intraepithelial lesions (HGSILs) and low-grade squamous intraepithelial lesions (LGSILs). The goal of Pap smear screening is to identify HGSIL (moderate dysplasia, severe dysplasia, and carcinoma *in situ*). Since most (91% over 36 months) of LGSILs (mild dysplasia and HPV changes) resolve spontaneously, observation alone is warranted and recommended. Biopsy-proved HGSIL changes can be treated conservatively with loop electrosurgical excision, cryotherapy, or CO_2 laser ablation.

   Glandular dysplasias are more difficult to detect and diagnose. Any glandular abnormality of a Pap smear requires immediate evaluation with colposcopy, directed biopsies, endocervical curettings, and possibly endometrial sampling. A cervical biopsy showing glandular dysplasia requires further sampling with cervical conization. There does not appear to be a spectrum of dysplastic changes in glandular epithelium akin to cervical epithelium. In addition, the histologic boundary within the cervical stroma makes delineation of margins more difficult for the pathologist. Therefore, after a diagnosis of adenocarcinoma *in situ*, even with clear margins, simple hysterectomy is recommended if the patient's childbearing is complete.

3. Spread patterns. The most common spread pattern is by direct extension through the cervical stroma and into the parametrial tissues (cardinal ligaments) and/or directly onto the vaginal wall. Pelvic spread is typically lateral rather than anterior or posterior into the bladder or rectum due to the investing fascia of the cardinal ligaments. Lymphatic metastasis is not uncommon because of the rich lymphatic drainage of the cervix with a typical orderly spread pattern from the pelvic nodes (obturator, internal iliac, external iliac, and common iliac) to the para-aortic nodes. Hematogenous metastasis is found in approximately 10% of patients, with the most common site being lung or bone.

B. Diagnosis and staging

1. Clinical manifestations. The classic symptom of cervical cancer is abnormal vaginal bleeding, typically postcoital bleeding, although intramenstrual bleeding and sudden vaginal hemorrhage are not uncommon. An abnormal vaginal discharge is also common. Pain, typically sciatic, lumbosacral, or flank pain is usually a sign of locally advanced disease.

2. Diagnosis. Biopsy of a cervical lesion is the only way to diagnose cervical cancer. Any suspicious or gross lesion of the cervix should be biopsied. A Pap smear should only be performed on a clinically normal cervix.

3. Staging (Table 11.1). Cervical cancer is staged clinically on the basis of international standards. Procedures allowed include examination under anesthesia, cystoscopy, proctoscopy, chest x-ray and an intravenous pyelogram (IVP). However, in the United States, there is a tendency to perform a computed tomography (CT) of the abdomen or pelvis to evaluate the retroperitoneum for lymphadenopathy. Positron emission tomography (PET) imaging has also been used to evaluate cervical cancer spread. Although CT and PET may be used in treatment planning, they cannot be used to change the clinical stage. Surgical staging with either laparoscopic or retroperitoneal lymphadenectomy (LND) has been promoted by some; however, the sensitivity of PET scanning may allow for nonsurgical staging.

C. Treatment

1. Early clinical disease

a. Microinvasive. The definition of a microinvasive cervical cancer adopted by the Society of Gynecologic Oncologists (SGO) states that invasion must be less than or equal to 3 mm below the basement membrane, with absence of lymphatic or vascular invasion and negative margins on a conization specimen. The SGO definition closely corresponds to International Federation of Gynecology and Obstetrics (FIGO) stage IA1 and represents a lesion with essentially a zero chance of lymph node metastasis. This stage of disease can be treated with

Table 11.1.   1995 International Federation of Gynecology and Obstetrics Staging (Montreal) for carcinoma of the cervix uteri

Stage Grouping	Definition
I	The carcinoma is strictly confined to the cervix (extension to the corpus should be disregarded)
IA	Invasive cancer identified only microscopically. All gross lesions even with superficial invasion are stage IB cancers. Invasion is limited to measured stromal invasion with maximum depth of 5 mm and no wider than 7 mm
IA-1	Measured invasion of stroma no greater than 3 mm in depth and no wider than 7 mm
IA-2	Measured invasion of stroma >3 mm, no greater than 5 mm, and no wider than 7 mm. The depth of invasion should not be more than 5 mm, taken from the base of the epithelium, either surface or glandular, from which it originates. Preformed space involvement (vascular or lymphatic) should not alter the staging but should be specifically recorded to determine whether it should affect treatment decisions in the future
IB	Clinical lesions confined to the cervix or preclinical lesions greater than those of stage IA
IB-1	Clinical lesions no greater than 4 cm in size
IB-2	Clinical lesions >4 cm in size
II	The carcinoma extends beyond the cervix but has not extended to the pelvic wall. The carcinoma involves the vagina but does not extend as far as the lower third
IIA	No obvious parametrial involvement
IIB	Obvious parametrial involvement
III	The carcinoma has extended to the pelvic wall. On rectal examination, there is no cancer-free space between the tumor and the pelvic wall. The tumor involves the lower third of the vagina. All cases with hydronephrosis or nonfunctioning kidney are included unless they are known to be due to other causes
IIIA	No extension to the pelvic wall
IIIB	Extension to the pelvic wall and/or hydronephrosis or nonfunctioning kidney
IV	The carcinoma has extended beyond the true pelvis or has clinically involved the mucosa of the bladder or rectum. (Bullous edema does not permit a case to be allotted to stage IV)
IVA	Spread of the growth to adjacent organs
IVB	Spread to distant organs

simple hysterectomy, or if the patient desires further childbearing, conization alone.

b. Stage IA2, IB1. Patients with a gross lesion on the cervix less than or equal to 4.0 cm or a microinvasive lesion with greater than 3 mm of invasion require more aggressive therapy. The incidence of pelvic lymph node metastasis with microinvasion between 3.1 and 5.0 mm is reported at 7%.

- Patients in this category require radical hysterectomy with pelvic LND. For patients thought to be poor surgical candidates the use of radiation therapy (RT) offers similar cure rates. However, surgical therapy offers the advantages of ovarian preservation, less long-term morbidity and better posttreatment sexual function. Risk stratification for recurrence after surgical treatment is based upon clinicopathologic criteria.

Patients at the highest risk for recurrence include those with positive pelvic lymph nodes, positive margins, or disease in the parametrial tissue. Patients with one or more of these poor prognostic factors do better with chemotherapy plus radiation versus RT alone as shown by 4-year disease-free (80% vs. 63%) and overall survival (81% vs. 71%). Recommended treatment is

- 4,930 cGy external beam pelvic RT and
- Cisplatin 70 mg/m^2 IV and a 96-hour continuous infusion of fluoruracil, 1,000 mg/m^2/day × 4 days, given every 3 weeks for a total of 4 cycles.
- The first two cycles are administered concurrently with RT.

Patients with intermediate-risk factors based upon tumor size, depth of invasion and presence of lymph-vascular space involvements appear to benefit from postoperative pelvic RT although at the cost of increased morbidity.

c. Stage IB2 (bulky). The optimal treatment of bulky stage I tumors (>4.0 cm) is controversial. Survival rates for these bulky cancers are substantially worse than those for smaller IB cancers.

- RT with cisplatin at 40 mg/m^2 IV weekly × 6 (maximum dose 70 mg) has been shown in a Gynecologic Oncology Group (GOG) study to offer a survival advantage over RT alone.

The role of the postradiation hysterectomy is debated as it most likely only benefits those with residual cancer in the cervix postchemoradiotherapy.

2. Advanced disease
   a. Stage IIA. Very early–stage IIA disease with only minimal involvement of the upper vagina (classically seen in the postmenopausal women because of atrophy of the cervix) can be adequately treated with radical hysterectomy with upper vaginectomy and pelvic LND. However, bulky stage IIA is best treated with RT and radiosensitizing chemotherapy as detailed in the preceding text.

b. Stage IIB to IVA. These locally advanced cancers are best treated with RT, teletherapy and brachytherapy, along with radiosensitizing chemotherapy.

- RT doses usually include 5,000 cGy to the whole pelvis initially to shrink the tumor, followed by 3,000 cGy delivered by high-dose rate brachytherapy.
- Cisplatin 40 mg/m^2 (maximum 70 mg) infused IV at a rate of 1 mg/minute is given weekly for 6 weeks as radiosensitizing drug. On the day of infusion, chemotherapy should precede the RT fraction.

c. Stage IVB. These patients should have the treatment individualized as they are not considered curable. RT to alleviate bleeding and chemotherapy (see Section 2.d.(3) below) in the palliative setting is acceptable.

d. Recurrent disease

    (1) Surgical therapy. The only accepted role for surgical excision in recurrent cervical cancer is in the patient who presents with a central pelvic recurrence. These patients can be offered pelvic exenteration with an expected 5-year survival of 50% to 60%. The use of continent urinary diversion, low rectal reanastomosis and neovaginal reconstruction allows for a better QOL for these women.

    (2) Chemotherapy. Patients with recurrent or persistent (failed radiochemotherapy) cervical cancers represent the largest group referred for systemic chemotherapy. Unfortunately, these women who are not exenteration candidates are not considered curable. The response rates to chemotherapy are significantly lower for patients with disease in a previously irradiated area or those who have received prior chemotherapy. Responses are generally short lived and do not affect progression-free and overall survival to a great extent.

    (3) Chemotherapy options. The standard treatment for recurrent or metastatic disease for the past 25 years is single-agent cisplatin—50 mg/m^2 IV every 3 weeks.

    This has an expected overall response rate of 38%. Subsequent studies have reported on cisplatin combined with several other agents, such as ifosfamide, dibromodulcitol, mitomycin C, bleomycin, and paclitaxel. Most of these studies showed increased response rate with multiagent chemotherapy (up to 69% with bleomycin, ifosfamide and cisplatin) but with no significant change in overall survival versus single agent cisplatin, and at the cost of increased toxicity. The exception is a combination of

- Cisplatin 50 mg/m^2 on day 1 *plus*
- Topotecan 0.75 mg/m^2 IV on days 1 to 3.
- Repeat every 21 days.

    This regimen has shown a significant increased survival advantage of 2.9 months as compared to patients treated with cisplatin alone. In addition, the QOL scores were similar between these two regimens. Interestingly, those patients who had received cisplatin as a radiosensitizing agent had poorer response rates overall. In addition, the time to recurrence was a powerful prognostic predictor of response, similar to the platinum-free interval in epithelial ovarian cancer (EOC).

Other active single agents include paclitaxel, ifosfamide, vinorelbine, fluorouracil, and mitomycin.

(4) Future developments. For patients with recurrent disease, combinations of cytotoxic agents (e.g., cisplatin combined with paclitaxel, gemcitabine, vinorelbine or topotecan) and molecularly targeted agents should offer further insight into the optimal treatment of these patients.

II. Endometrial cancer. Endometrial cancer is the most common of gynecologic malignancies. In 2006, it is estimated there were approximately 41,200 new cases and 7,350 deaths from endometrial cancer in the United States. Risk factor for developing endometrial cancer include advancing age, nulliparity, chronic anovulation, obesity, and unopposed estrogen and tamoxifen use. Of these, obesity carries the highest relative risk, especially for those women who are more than 100 pounds overweight. These patients typically present with postmenopausal bleeding, or dysfunctional uterine bleeding for those not yet postmenopausal. The diagnosis can often be made in the office with an endometrial biopsy or by a dilatation and curettage (D & C) in the operating room. A transvaginal sonogram of the uterus for the endometrial stripe can be performed on those women who may be difficult to biopsy because of a stenotic cervix. A stripe greater than 5 mm in a postmenopausal woman is considered abnormal and would require surgical sampling to rule out endometrial cancer.

A. Pathology and patterns of spread

1. Histology. The classic endometrial cancer is an endometrioid adenocarcinoma, accounting for approximately 90% of all uterine cancers. Grading is a function of the amount of solid areas in the tumor specimen. The presence of squamous metaplasia, adenocanthoma, does not harbor a worse prognosis. However, the presence of malignant squamous elements, adenosquamous carcinoma, typically portends a poorer prognosis, as they are usually poorly differentiated tumors. Approximately 5% of uterine cancers will be adenocarcinoma subtypes such as papillary serous or clear carcinoma, both of which are poor-prognosis cell types. The remaining 5% of uterine cancers will be the uterine sarcomas, comprising carcinosarcoma (mixed mullerian tumors [MMTs]), leiomyosarcoma (LMS) and endometrial stromal sarcomas (ESSs).

2. Patterns of spread. Endometrioid adenocarcinoma begins in the endometrial lining and then invades into the underlying myometrium where it can then invade lymph and vascular spaces. The pelvic and para-aortic lymph nodes are the most common sites of lymphatic metastasis. Spread to the vagina or cervix is not uncommon. Another pattern of spread can be into the abdominal cavity, either by direct extension through the uterine serosa or by exfoliation through the fallopian tubes. Distant spread to the liver, lungs, and brain are usually late events. However, extrauterine spread into the abdominal cavity is not uncommon with the uterine sarcomas and the papillary serous and clear cell adenocarcinomas.

B. Pretreatment evaluation

1. Diagnostic tests. In clinically early endometrial cancer, extensive imaging and testing are not necessary. A complete physical examination looking for evidence of vaginal or lymphatic spread is performed. A chest radiograph is obtained to rule out pulmonary metastasis. If the clinical examination or history suggests advanced disease, then CT imaging, cystoscopy, or proctoscopy may be useful. If intraabdominal spread is suspected, a preoperative CA125 level may be useful as a tumor marker.

2. Staging. By international convention, endometrial cancer is staged surgically (Table 11.2) requiring hysterectomy, bilateral salpingo-oophorectomy (BSO), peritoneal washings, and pelvic and para-aortic lymph node sampling. In addition, any suspected intra-abdominal metastasis should be biopsied and resected. Owing to early symptoms, most endometrial cancers (80%) are found in stage I.

C. Management

1. Surgery. The classic therapy for endometrial cancer or uterine sarcoma is surgical with extrafascial hysterectomy and BSO. To complete the surgical staging, pelvic and para-aortic lymph node sampling and peritoneal washings should be obtained. In addition to staging, selective pelvic

Table 11.2. International Federation of Gynecology and Obstetrics Staging for carcinoma of the corpus uteri

Stage	Definition
I	Tumor confined to the uterine fundus
IA	Tumor limited to the endometrium
IB	Invasion to less than one-half of the myometrium
IC	Invasion to more than one-half of the myometrium
II	Tumor extends to the cervix
IIA	Endocervical glandular involvement only
IIB	Cervical stromal invasion
III	Regional tumor spread
IIIA	Tumor invades the serosa and/or adnexa and/or has positive peritoneal cytology
IIIB	Vaginal metastases
IIIC	Metastases to pelvic and/or periaortic lymph nodes
IV	Bulky pelvic disease or distant spread
IVA	Tumor invasion of the bladder and/or bowel mucosa
IVB	Distant metastases, including intra-abdominal and/or inguinal lymph nodes

and para-aortic lymph node sampling may also have a therapeutic effect. Patients undergoing lymph node sampling seem to have a survival advantage across all risk groups. In the event of intra-abdominal spread, complete surgical excision is beneficial.

2. Special cases. Patients who present with gross cervical involvement that is not deemed surgically resectable may be offered preoperative radiation therapy to shrink the tumor. This may then allow a postradiation hysterectomy. For patients who are poor surgical candidates, radiation therapy (both teletherapy and brachytherapy) is the best option; however, the cure rate is inferior to surgical therapy. Rarely, endometrial cancer will develop in a young woman who still desires fertility. This usually occurs in a woman with long-standing anovulatory cycles (polycystic ovarian disease). There are reports of these young women being treated successfully with uterine curettage followed by high-dose progestins. After reversal of the cancer, documented by repeat uterine curettage, ovulation induction is often necessary for conception.

3. Postoperative management

a. Risk stratification. After surgical staging, patients can generally be placed in one of three categories: (1) those with a low incidence of recurrence (low risk); (2) those who have an increased rate of recurrence who may or may not benefit from additional therapy (intermediate risk); and (3) those at high risk for recurrence without some type of additional therapy (high risk). Risk factors for recurrence in stage I disease (confined to the uterine corpus) include increasing grade, increasing depth of invasion (especially invasion of the outer third), lymph-vascular space invasion, older age, and depth of myometrial invasion.

b. Adjuvant treatment. Patients in the low-risk group are those with stage IA or IB disease with grade 1 or 2 tumors. These patients are adequately treated with surgery alone. Adjuvant therapy for the intermediate-risk group is not well established. This group includes patients with deep myometrial invasion of any grade (IC), patients with grade 3 tumors, and those with cervical involvement (IIA and IIB). Studies in both staged and unstaged patients have shown adjuvant pelvic RT to decrease the risk of locoregional recurrence, but without a significant increase in survival. A study of unstaged patients showed a locoregional relapse rate of 14% in the observation group versus 4% in those treated with pelvic RT. A randomized study in staged patients showed a 2-year recurrence rate of 12% in the observation arm versus 3% in the pelvic RT arm. The role of vaginal brachytherapy alone in the adjuvant setting for this group is also not clear. Those at high risk for recurrence include patients with disease outside of the uterus such as adnexal involvement, nodal disease, intraperitoneal spread, or distant metastasis (stage III and IV). These patients require additional therapy after surgical staging.

c. Advanced disease treatment

(1) **Radiotherapy (RT).** Patients with evidence of retroperitoneal (nodal) disease only (stage IIIC) are typically treated with tailored RT. Those who are found to have intra-abdominal disease can be offered systemic chemotherapy or whole abdominal radiotherapy (WART). However, a recent randomized phase III trial in more than 400 women with stage III and IV disease receiving WART with a pelvic boost versus eight cycles of doxorubicin 60 mg/m^2 and cisplatin 50 mg/m^2 every 3 weeks showed a significant improvement in both progression-free and overall survival in the chemotherapy arm. WART appears to be most effective in patients with maximally resected disease. A study of 180 evaluable patients with stage III and IV disease showed survival rates of 35% with WART, although no patient with gross residual disease after surgical staging survived. The trend in those patients with intraperitoneal disease is for systemic treatment with chemotherapy.

(2) **Systemic therapy.** Patients with intra-abdominal spread are candidates for chemotherapy after maximal surgical reduction. Active agents include cisplatin, the anthracyclines, and the taxanes:

- TAP, a three-drug regimen of
  — Cisplatin (**P**latinol) 50 mg/m^2 IV *and*
  — Doxorubicin (**A**driamycin) 45 mg/m^2 IV day 1 followed by
  — Paclitaxel (**T**axol)160 mg/m^2 day 2 with filgrastim support
  repeated every 21 days, improves response rate (57% vs. 34%), progression-free survival (median, 8.3 vs. 5.3 months) and overall survival (median, 15.3 vs. 12.3 months), compared with cisplatin and doxorubicin alone, but with increased toxicity, especially neuropathy.
- The doublet of carboplatin an area under the curve (AUC) of 6 and paclitaxel at 175 mg/m^2 every 3 weeks has also been reported with 60% to 70% response rates in phase II trials.

(3) **Recurrent disease.** Patients who present with isolated vaginal cuff recurrences who have not been irradiated represent the only clinical situation where cure rates of 50% to 60% are reported. Surgical restaging with possible upper vaginectomy may be considered to help rule out intra-abdominal spread and to completely resect the tumor. Patients who present with distant metastasis present difficult clinical situations. These patients are often elderly, obese and harbor other medical comorbidities that complicate aggressive chemotherapy. In the chemonaive patient, treatment with TAP or carboplatin and taxol may be considered. Patients who have failed primary therapy have few good options. Liposomal doxorubicin, topotecan, ifosfamide and etoposide all have response

rates in the range of 15% to 30%. The use of systemic progestins is best reserved with patients with late, asymptomatic recurrences that are well-differentiated tumors. The response rate of progestins varies inversely with the grade of the tumor. However, for tumors with positive progesterone receptors, a response rate of 37% was reported by the GOG. Risks of progestins include weight gain and thrombosis. Drugs include megestrol acetate at 160 mg/day or medroxyprogesterone acetate at 200 mg/day.

4. Special cases. A variety of less common uterine neoplasms can occur. These need to be treated according to the unique biology.

    a. Uterine papillary serous carcinoma (UPSC) and clear cell carcinoma. These histologies have a predilection for early intra-abdominal spread and distant recurrences. At the time of presentation, approximately 70% of patients with UPSC will have disease outside of the uterus. Patients diagnosed with UPSC or clear cell endometrial cancer should be referred to a gynecologic oncologist for complete surgical staging to include total abdominal hysterectomy (TAH/BSO), pelvic and para-aortic lymph node sampling, peritoneal washings, omentectomy and careful assessment of the entire peritoneal cavity. Overall, patients with stage I disease have recurrence rates of 40% to 50%. Recommendations for adjuvant therapy for stage I UPSC and clear cell carcinomas have varied considerably and a clear consensus is lacking.

- Stage IA patients with no residual disease in the hysterectomy specimen can be observed.
- Patients with stage I disease with residual disease in the hysterectomy specimen should be treated with adjuvant chemotherapy with carboplatin AUC 5 and paclitaxel 175 mg/m^2 every 3 weeks and vaginal cuff brachytherapy.
- Patients with advanced-stage UPSC and clear cell carcinoma require platinum-based chemotherapy after maximal tumor reduction.

    b. Uterine sarcomas. Approximately 5% of uterine neoplasms will be sarcomas. The carcinosarcoma or MMT is the most common of the uterine sarcomas. As with most sarcomas, early systemic spread with distant recurrence is common. Unlike endometrial adenocarcinomas, patients with stage I uterine sarcomas have 5-year survival rates of 40% to 60%. Recurrences are approximately evenly divided between local (pelvic) and distant sites.

- For stage I uterine sarcomas, adjuvant pelvic RT has been shown to decrease the local recurrence rate, but not change overall survival, principally because of distant disease. However, adjuvant chemotherapy does not appear to be of benefit.
- Patients with advanced or recurrent MMT are best treated with ifosfamide 1.2 to 1.5 g/m^2/day IV on days

1 to 4 with mesna protection along with cisplatin 20 mg/m^2/day IV for 4 days.

Several phase II trials have also shown carboplatin with an AUC of 5 to 6 and paclitaxel 135 to 175 mg/m^2 to be effective.

The second most common uterine sarcoma is the LMS. These patients tend to be younger than those with MMT and the disease is rarely diagnosed preoperatively. Adjuvant RT to the pelvis for stage I and II disease will decrease local recurrence rate but not affect overall survival. The role of adjuvant chemotherapy is unclear. Patients with advanced-stage or recurrent LMS are best treated with an adriamycin-based regimen such as adriamycin and cisplatin. Recently, the combination gemcitabine 900 mg/m^2 IV on days 1 and 8 with docetaxel 100 mg/m^2 on day 8 with filgrastim support showed a 53% overall response rate. Single-agent etoposide also has activity with LMS.

Patients with advanced-stage low-grade ESSs are best treated with progestins as they are typically rich in progesterone receptors.

III. Fallopian tube cancer. Fallopian tube cancer is rarely suspected preoperatively and accounts for less than 1% of all gynecologic malignancies. Patients usually undergo surgery for a complex pelvic mass or may present in a manner similar to advanced ovarian cancer with ascites and evidence of intra-abdominal spread. Preoperative symptoms that are unique to fallopian tube cancer include a watery vaginal discharge associated with a colicky pelvic pain. Rarely, a Pap smear showing serous adenocarcinoma or psammoma bodies lead to the diagnosis. Fallopian tube cancer is staged and managed surgically in a manner identical to ovarian cancer.

IV. Ovarian cancer. Ovarian cancer is the leading killer among gynecologic malignancies accounting for more deaths than all the other gynecologic cancers combined. In 2006, there were approximately 20,180 new cases and 15,310 deaths. The ovary is formed from three embryologic tissues; germ cells, stroma, and epithelium. Each of these groups gives rise to a distinct neoplasm that is biologically diverse and is treated differently.

A. Histologic types and treatment of germ cell and stromal tumors

1. Germ cell ovarian cancers. Germ cell tumors (GCTs) of the ovary account for approximately 5% of all ovarian malignancies. They are found in a young age group and are curable. GCTs are typically fast-growing neoplasms and often present with the sudden onset of abdominal or pelvic pain. Surgical therapy for GCT is conservative with removal of the affected ovary and comprehensive staging. Even in the event of advanced disease, preservation of the contralateral ovary and uterus is recommended because of the sensitivity of GCT to chemotherapy. For chemotherapy purposes, GCTs are usually divided into dysgerminomas and nondysgerminomas.

All nondysgerminoma GCTs, except for stage IA grade 1 immature teratoma, will require chemotherapy. Patients with completely resected nondysgerminoma GCT require

Table 11.3.   Multiagent chemotherapy in germ cell cancers of the ovary

BEP: Bleomycin 20 units/m^2 IV (maximum 30 units) weekly
  Etoposide 100 mg/m^2 IV daily × 5 days q3 week
  Cisplatin 20 mg/m^2 IV daily × 5 days q3 week
VAC: Vincristine 1.5 mg/m^2 IV (maximum 2 mg) q2 week
  Actinomycin-D 350 μg/m^2 IV daily × 5 days q4 week
  Cyclophosphamide 150 mg/m^2 IV daily × 5 days q4 week

three courses of adjuvant bleomycin, etoposide, and cisplatin (BEP, Table 11.3). With adjuvant therapy, relapse rates should be less than 5%, but without adjuvant BEP, the rates are 40% to 80%. Those with incompletely resected nondysgerminoma GCT require four courses.

Patients with a completely staged IA dysgerminoma do not require chemotherapy and may be observed. The recurrence rate in this group will be approximately 20%; however, they can be successfully treated with BEP. All other stages of dysgerminoma require BEP similar to nondysgerminomas. Most patients with a dysgerminoma will not be completely staged. Few of these patients are managed surgically by a gynecologic oncologist and the diagnosis is most often made postoperatively. Careful surveillance is recommended in this group of patients to allow early detection of recurrence and chemotherapy with BEP.

Patients with GCT who relapse or cannot receive BEP as primary therapy, should receive a combination of vincristine, actinomycin-D, and cyclophosphamide (VAC) (Table 11.3).

2. Stromal tumors. Stromal tumors represent the least common of the ovarian neoplasms. They are derived from the sex cords and the ovarian stroma of the ovary and are usually divided into those tumors that represent the female cells (granulosa and theca cells) and the male cells (Sertoli and Leydig cells). Occasionally, they are characterized by their hormonal production, especially in the rare juvenile granulosa cell tumor where estrogen production will cause precocious pseudopuberty. Stromal tumors of the ovary are usually found at stage I and allow for conservative surgery consisting of a unilateral salpingo-oophorectomy in those patients who still desire childbearing. Typically, they are slow-growing, indolent neoplasms that are managed surgically. Chemotherapy is reserved for advanced stage or for recurrent disease. Options for chemotherapy include BEP (see Table 11.3) or a platinum and a taxane, as with EOC.

3. Epithelial ovarian cancer (EOC). The overwhelming majority of ovarian malignancies belong to the epithelial group (e.g., serous, mucinous, endometrioid, clear cell). In contrast to GCT, EOC generally occurs after menopause, is advanced at the time of diagnosis, and is rarely curable. The remainder of this section deals with the diagnosis and management of this common variety of ovarian cancer.

B. **Diagnosis and screening of EOC**
  1. Diagnosis. The diagnosis of early-staged EOC is difficult because of the lack of early signs or symptoms. In the
  United States, 70% to 80% of ovarian cancers are diagnosed
  at an advanced stage when cure is difficult. Rarely, an
  asymptomatic pelvic mass will be felt on pelvic examination. Symptoms of early EOC are often pelvic or lower abdominal pressure, pain or discomfort. Imaging studies, such
  as a pelvic CT or ultrasound (USD) will reveal a pelvic mass.
  Radiologic characteristics of an ovarian malignancy include
  the presence of solid areas within the mass ("complex"), ascites, bilaterality, and irregularity in the shape of the mass.
  Most benign pelvic or ovarian masses will be completely
  cystic and rounded on imaging studies. As the age of the patient increases, the chance of a pelvic mass being malignant
  increases as well. Patients with advanced EOC will often
  have as a presenting symptom a sudden increase in abdominal girth due to ascites. These women will often have vague
  abdominal complaints such as pelvic or abdominal full-
  ness, urinary frequency, early satiety, or pelvic discomfort
  for several months preceding the diagnosis. Imaging studies will often reveal widespread ascites, omental caking,
  peritoneal implants, and pleural effusions. Preoperative
  diagnostic tests such as needle biopsies and paracenteses
  are generally meddlesome, carry the risk of disseminating
  disease, and do not alter the ultimate need for surgery. The
  diagnosis will be made by surgical exploration, preferably
  by a fellowship-trained gynecologic oncologist. In the case
  of early-staged EOC, a frozen section should be obtained
  during surgical exploration to make the diagnosis and allow
  for complete surgical staging in the case of malignancy.
  2. Screening. The overall 5-year survival for stage I or II
  EOC is 80% to 90%; however, the overall 5-year survival
  for stage III or IV EOC is 30% to 35%. The potential
  value for earlier diagnosis is unequivocal, but neither
  the use of transvaginal ultrasound (TVS) with or without Doppler flow studies nor serum screening for CA125
  has the necessary sensitivity and specificity to accurately
  predict early-stage EOC, and these are therefore not good
  screening tools in the average risk woman.
    This is in distinction to the observation that two classes of
  serum tumor markers, monoclonal antibodies (e.g., CA125
  with EOCs) and peptide markers (e.g., α-fetoprotein with
  endodermal sinus tumors, müllerian-inhibiting factor, and
  inhibin with granulosa cell tumors) have proved **useful in
  monitoring the treatment** of ovarian cancer. Additionally, preoperative evaluation of tumor markers and pelvic
  USD may be useful in estimating risk of malignancy and
  aid in appropriate preoperative patient triage.
    Overall lifetime risk of developing EOC is 1 in 70 or ap-
  proximately 1.4%. The strongest risk factor for developing
  EOC is a positive family history. Unfortunately, only 10%
  of new patients with EOC will have a suggestive family
  history. Factors that decrease a woman's risk include pregnancy, lactation, oral contraceptive use, tubal ligation, and
  hysterectomy. Women with a family history suggestive of

familial ovarian cancer or any woman of Ashkenazi Jewish descent who develops breast or ovarian cancer should be referred for genetic counseling and possible genetic studies for the *BRCA1* and *BRCA2* gene mutations. The breast and ovarian cancer syndrome, associated with germline *BRCA1* and *BRCA2* mutations that function as tumor suppressor genes, is inherited in an autosomal dominant manner. Female carriers of a mutation in the *BRCA1* or *BRCA2* gene have a 15% to 60% risk of developing EOC by the age of 70, with the risk being lower for *BRCA2* than for *BRCA1*. Approximately 5% to 10% of ovarian cancer cases are likely attributable to such mutations. Women at high risk for developing EOC and those who harbor a *BRCA1* or *BRCA2* germline mutation should consider prophylactic oophorectomy after childbearing. This procedure will decrease dramatically the patient's chance of developing an ovarian cancer and also decrease her risk of developing a breast cancer. Women in this high-risk group who decide to retain their ovaries should consider surveillance with TVS twice yearly. Increased surveillance in the form of CA125 levels can also be valuable, especially in the postmenopausal setting. An increased risk of ovarian cancer is also associated with hereditary nonpolyposis colon cancer (HNPCC), with mutations documented in the mismatch repair genes *MSH2, MLH1, PMS1*, and *PMS2*.

C. **Management**

1. **Surgery.** Ovarian cancer is staged surgically (Table 11.4). Any woman with a suspicious ovarian or pelvic mass requires surgical exploration. Surgery allows for accurate diagnosis, thorough staging of disease, and, in advanced disease, valuable tumor debulking.

a. **Early disease and surgical staging.** At surgical exploration, the ovarian mass is resected intact if possible (i.e., without rupture), and diagnosis is established on the basis of frozen-section evaluation. During surgery, 20% of EOCs appear visually or grossly confined to the ovary (i.e., stage I), but 30% to 50% of these patients will have extraovarian microscopic disease. A thorough surgical staging will identify those patients with more advanced-stage disease and allow for selection of appropriate chemotherapy.

b. **Advanced disease.** Eighty percent of women have advanced disease (stage III or IV) at diagnosis. Most of the women have disease disseminating throughout the abdominal cavity with ascites. The finding of advanced EOC often portrays a seemingly insurmountable picture of unresectable peritoneal and bulky pelvic and abdominal tumor. Fortunately, with the proper surgical approach, maximal tumor resection is possible in 80% of patients. The benefit of optimal debulking has been recognized in several retrospective reviews. A recent meta-analysis of patients with advanced ovarian cancer treated postoperatively with platinum-based chemotherapy showed that each 10% increase in maximal cytoreduction was associated with a 5.5% increase

Table 11.4. **International Federation of Gynecology and Obstetrics staging system for ovarian cancer**

Stage	Definition
I	Growth limited to the ovaries
IA	Growth limited to one ovary; no ascites; no tumor on the external surfaces; capsule intact
IB	Growth limited to both ovaries; no ascites; no tumor on the external surfaces; capsule intact
IC	Tumor either stage IA or IB but with tumor on the surface of one or both ovaries; or with capsule ruptured; or with ascites present containing malignant cells or with positive peritoneal washings
II	Growth involving one or both ovaries with pelvic extension
IIA	Extension and/or metastases to the uterus and/or tubes
IIB	Extension to other pelvic tissues
IIC	Tumor either stage IIA or IIB but with tumor on the surface of one or both ovaries; or with capsule ruptured; or with ascites present containing malignant cells or with positive peritoneal washings
III	Tumor involving one or both ovaries with peritoneal implants outside the pelvis and/or positive retroperitoneal or inguinal nodes; surface liver metastasis equals stage III; tumor is limited to the true pelvis but with histologically verified malignant extension to small bowel, large bowel, or omentum
IIIA	Tumor grossly limited to the true pelvis with negative nodes but with histologically confirmed microscopic seeding of abdominal peritoneal surfaces
IIIB	Tumor of one or both ovaries; histologically confirmed implants of abdominal peritoneal surfaces, none exceeding 2 cm in diameter; nodes negative
IIIC	Abdominal implants >2 cm in diameter and/or positive retroperitoneal or inguinal nodes
IV	Growth involving one or both ovaries with distant metastases; if pleural effusion is present, there must be positive cytologic test results to allot a case to stage IV; parenchymal liver metastases equals stage IV

in median survival time. Another multi-institutional review reported a median survival of 38.4 months in those patients optimally debulked versus only 10.3 months in the nonoptimally debulked patients. Therefore, initial therapy for advanced EOC is optimal surgical debulking. The value of a focused expertise in managing EOC has been directly recognized by the National Cancer Institute (NCI) in their recommendation that where the potential for such cases exists, they be managed by fellowship-trained gynecologic oncologists.

2. Systemic chemotherapy. The need and route of administration for postsurgery chemotherapy is determined in the context of histology, grade, stage, and amount of residual tumor. Patients with ovarian tumors of low malignant potential (or borderline ovarian tumors) are treated with surgical resection alone and do not require chemotherapy.

a. Early stage, low risk. Patients with a thoroughly staged IA or IB, grade 1 or 2 EOC are considered at low risk for recurrence, have an expected 5-year survival rate of greater than 90%, and do not require chemotherapy.

b. Early stage, high risk. Patients with early-stage EOC who are considered at high risk for relapse include all patients with stage IA/IB with grade 3 or clear cell histologies, stage IC and stage II disease. Adjuvant platinum-based chemotherapy has proved to prolong disease-free survival and possibly survival itself. The standard treatment for patients with high-risk, stage I or II EOC is three courses of carboplatin and paclitaxel.

- Carboplatin AUC of 7.5 IV *and*
- Paclitaxel 175 mg/m^2 IV every 21 days.

c. Stage III and IV, advanced disease. Patients with more advanced disease are currently treated with a platin and paclitaxel regimen after debulking surgery. For patients with optimally debulked stage III EOC, a combination of IP and IV chemotherapy has been shown to be superior to standard IV chemotherapy (see Section IV.C.3). For patients with suboptimally debulked EOC, appropriate intravenous regimens include the following:

1. Carboplatin AUC of 5 to 7.5 IV *plus* paclitaxel 175 mg/m^2 IV over 3 hours *or*
2. Cisplatin 50 mg/m^2 IV *plus* paclitaxel 135 mg/m^2 IV over 24 hours (high neurotoxicity otherwise) *or*
3. Carboplatin AUC of 5 to 7.5 IV *plus* docetaxel 60 to 80 mg/m^2 IV.

Each of these regimens is repeated every 21 days for a total of 6 to 8 courses.

Recent data suggest that docetaxel, when substituted for paclitaxel in combination with carboplatin, has a similar overall efficacy for initial treatment of EOC with a more favorable neurotoxicity profile. Therefore, this regimen is an alternative for patients at high risk for, or with preexisting neuropathy. Several prospective, randomized studies have shown carboplatin to be similar in efficacy to cisplatin with a toxicity profile favoring carboplatin. This, in addition to the ease of administration in an outpatient setting, favors carboplatin over cisplatin.

Overall, the response rate to paclitaxel and carboplatin as first-line treatment of EOC (complete response plus partial response) is 70% to 80%, of which 50% are complete clinical responses and 30% complete pathologic responses. Patients are carefully monitored during chemotherapy to determine treatment efficacy. Before receiving each cycle, they should undergo physical examination, CA125 determination, and other studies as indicated to assess disease response.

If any parameter suggests treatment failure (i.e., progression of disease), the regimen is immediately curtailed, and strategic options that remain are presented to the patient. Patients who progress during initial platinum-based chemotherapy generally do not respond well to second-line agents. Patients opting for second-line treatment, on or off protocol, should do so realistically and with a great concern for maintaining the best possible QOL under difficult circumstances.

3. Intraperitoneal (IP) chemotherapy. A recent prospective study on patients with stage III optimally debulked EOC or primary peritoneal cancer, defined as no residual mass greater than 1.0 cm, was reported. This showed that when IP was added to IV therapy, there was an increase in the median duration of progression-free survival to 23.8 months in the IP/IV arm versus 18.3 months in the IV arm. The median duration of overall survival was 65.6 months in the IP/IV arm and 49.7 months in the IV arm. The regimen recommended is

- Paclitaxel 135 mg/m^2 IV over 24 hours followed by
- Cisplatin 100 mg/m^2 IP on day 2 and
- Paclitaxel 60 mg/m^2 IP on day 8. The cycle is repeated every 21 days for 6 courses.

Only 42% of the patients in the IP/IV arm completed all six courses. A QOL index was significantly worse in the IP/IV group before cycle four and 3 to 6 weeks after treatment, but was not different 1 year after treatment. Although the IP mode of therapy is more difficult for the patient to tolerate, a clear survival advantage was seen and changed the standard of care for patients with optimally debulked stage III EOC and primary peritoneal cancer.

4. Maintenance therapy. As noted earlier, even with advanced EOC, it is expected that approximately 60% to 70% of patients will achieve a clinical remission after initial platinum-based chemotherapy. However, most of these women are destined to recur with eventual death from their disease. Therefore, the concept of maintenance chemotherapy to extend survival is attractive. Studies have shown that extending combined carboplatin and paclitaxel beyond six courses does not prolong survival. A recent trial looking at four additional courses of topotecan after initial platinum-based therapy also showed no survival advantage. However, one trial studied women with advanced EOC who achieved a complete clinical remission after carboplatin and taxol. They were then randomized to an additional 3 or 12 cycles of paclitaxel alone at 175 mg/m^2 every 28 days. A statistically significant progression-free survival of 28 versus 21 months in the arm with 12 additional courses of paclitaxel was seen. To date, this has been the only trial showing an advantage with extended or maintenance chemotherapy.

5. Second-look laparotomy. Once a part of standard ovarian cancer treatment, second-look laparotomy is rarely performed currently. Recent data has not shown any survival advantage to routine second-look surgery at the end of primary treatment and should not be offered outside of an approved clinical trial. Even after a pathologically negative second-look laparotomy, more than 50% of patients will eventually have a recurrence and die of their disease.

D. Follow-up. After six courses of a platinum-based chemotherapy, patients in complete clinical remission can be offered entry into a clinical trial of consolidation or maintenance therapy, maintenance therapy with an additional 12 courses of paclitaxel on a monthly basis, or close observation with reinitiating chemotherapy for documented recurrence. Observation usually entails monitoring of the CA125 level, physical examination, and directed radiologic studies such as CT or PET scan on a scheduled basis.

E. Recurrent and persistent disease. Patients with recurrent EOC are generally grouped based upon their duration of response from initial platinum-based therapy. Patients who have a recurrence within 6 months of their last dose of platinum-based therapy are termed *platinum resistant* and are best treated with a non–cross-resistant drug or placed on a research protocol. Patients who have a disease-free interval of greater than 6 months are termed *platinum sensitive*. The length of this disease-free interval directly corresponds to the anticipated response rate of retreatment with platinum. Patients who have a long disease-free interval from their initial platinum regimen (12 or more months) are probably best retreated with their initial regimen of a platinum drug and a taxane.

Many patients will demonstrate marker-only relapse (elevated CA125) without symptoms and without evidence of recurrence by examination or CT scan. The decision to treat on the basis of tumor marker elevation only is often difficult for the patient and for the physician. These women may be enjoying a good QOL, and introduction of chemotherapy for an asymptomatic disease will reduce this quality. A frank and honest discussion with the patient is warranted. The patient may be a good candidate for observation or enrollment in a clinical trial. However, most gynecologic oncologists, as well as most patients, elect to treat with chemotherapy on the basis of the belief that retreatment with low tumor volume may enhance the possibility of a second remission. Once the decision to utilize chemotherapy is made, the choice of agent is based upon the patient's platinum-free interval, as discussed in the preceding text.

Several agents are available for those who are platinum resistant. The selection of a drug is based upon balancing anticipated toxicities with scheduling, as second-line chemotherapy regimens have yielded similar responses. Generally, single-agent therapy is used, unless the patient is on protocol. Taxanes (paclitaxel and docetaxel) can be given if they are not used up front or if the patient has received a taxane up front but is not considered taxane resistant. Various schedules of taxanes and other agents with reported activity include the following (used as single agents, not in combinations):

- Paclitaxel 135 to 175 mg/m^2 IV over 3 hours every 21 days
- Paclitaxel 50 to 80 mg/m^2 IV over 1 hour on days 1, 8, and 15 every 28 days

- Docetaxel 60 to 80 mg/m² IV every 21 days
- Docetaxel 25 to 35 mg/m² IV days on 1, 8, and 15 every 28 days
- Liposomal doxorubicin (Doxil) 40 to 50 mg/m² IV every 3 weeks
- Topotecan 1.0 to 1.5 mg/m² IV on days 1 to 5 every 3 weeks *or* Topotecan 3 to 4 mg/m² days 1, 8 and 15 every 28 days
- Oral etoposide 50 mg/m² (30 mg/m² for prior RT) on days 1 to 21 every 28 days
- Gemcitabine 800 to 1,000 mg/m² IV on days 1, 8, and 15 every 28 days
- Vinorelbine 30 mg/m² IV on days 1, 8, and 15 every 28 days
- Tamoxifen 20 mg PO b.i.d.
- Oral altretamine (hexamethylmelamine, Hexalen) 260 mg/m²

Responses with second-line treatment range from 20% to 40%. Most are short, but responses can occasionally exceed 1 to 2 years, justifying the concept of second-line chemotherapy for the informed patient who still wishes to try. High-dose therapy including peripheral blood stem cell transplant has not been found to improve survival in EOC. In the setting of a relapse, patients should be encouraged to participate in clinical trials.

The addition of gemcitabine to cisplatin has been shown *in vitro* in an ovarian cancer cell line to demonstrate synergetic activity. In an attempt to reverse platin resistance, a trial in platin- and paclitaxel-resistant patients using gemcitabine 750 mg/m² IV over 30 minutes followed by cisplatin 30 mg/m² on days 1 and 8 every 21 days was reported. An overall response rate of 43% with a median response duration of 11 months was seen in this refractory group of patients.

The use of targeted therapeutics has been reported in recurrent disease. A monoclonal antibody directed against vascular endothelial growth factor (VEGF), bevacizumab, was used in combination with oral cytoxan in a group of heavily pretreated patients with recurrent, refractory EOC, and primary peritoneal cancer. Patients were treated with bevacizumab 10 mg/kg IV on days 1, 8 and 15, then every 2 weeks along with oral cyclophosphamide 50 mg PO daily until the disease progresses. Toxicities were minimal and this combination showed a 21% partial response, 59% stable disease, and a progression-free survival of 5.8 months.

V. Gestational trophoblastic neoplasm (GTN). GTN comprises a spectrum of neoplastic growth ranging from hydatidiform mole (HM), invasive molar disease, choriocarcinoma and the rare placental site trophoblastic tumor (PSTT). All of these represent abnormal proliferation of trophoblastic tissue. The terminology and classification systems used for these disorders can be confusing. GTN is now considered the more appropriate term to encompass the variety of clinical situations encountered. The evaluation and management of GTN has been standardized to make it one of the most curable gynecologic malignancies. Reasons for the high cure rate include the presence of a sensitive tumor marker, β-human chorionic gonadotropin (β-hCG), that is directly related to the extent of disease, the extreme sensitivity of GTN to a variety of chemotherapeutic agents, the identification of high-risk factors to allow for individualization of treatment, and the aggressive use of multiagent chemotherapy combined with other modalities such as surgery and radiation for recalcitrant cases.

A. Hydatidiform mole (HM). The most common form of GTN is the HM, with the complete HM being found more frequently than the partial HM. A complete HM is the result of fertilization of an anucleate ovum by a sperm. Cytogenetic studies have shown that all genetic material in a complete HM is paternal. They are always diploid (> 90% 46 XX) and are devoid of any fetal tissue. The partial HM, in contrast, is associated with triploidy (usually 69 XXY) and fetal tissue. Risk factors for developing an HM include being at the extremes of the reproductive age, prior history of GTN, and being of Asian descent. The most common symptom is first trimester vaginal bleeding or the passage of vesicular tissue from the vagina. Although a high β-hCG is often associated with GTN, there is no single level that is diagnostic of GTN. The development of pre-eclampsia before the 20th week of gestation is pathognomonic of GTN. Diagnosis is made by an USD of the uterus, showing the classic "snowstorm" appearance with multiple small vesicles in the case of a complete GTN, and of a large hydropic placenta with a fetus in the event of a partial HM.

1. Management. Once the diagnosis of an HM is made by USD, the patient should be scheduled for uterine evacuation in the operating room expeditiously. Preoperative evaluation includes a baseline β-hCG, complete blood count (CBC), chest x-ray, and a careful physical examination to rule out evidence of genital metastasis (especially vaginal) and for any signs of hyperthyroidism or pre-eclampsia. Liver and thyroid function tests may be considered, based on the physical findings. If the USD shows evidence of theca luetin cysts (they can be quite large) they should be followed expectantly, as they will resolve after evacuation of the HM. The optimal method of evacuation for a complete HM is by suction curettage. Prostaglandin induction should not be performed. In the event of an extremely large uterus, larger than 16 weeks size, intraoperative USD guidance to avoid uterine perforation and insure complete evacuation of all molar tissue is recommended. Evacuation of an incomplete HM usually involves a combination of prostaglandin induction and suction curettage.

2. Monitoring. After evacuation of an HM, serum β-hCG levels are monitored weekly until three consecutive normal values (<5 mIU/mL) are obtained. Monthly titers are then drawn for 6 months. An effective form of contraception should be used to avoid pregnancy. Approximately 15% to 20% of complete HM and 3% to 5% of partial HM will recur. Risk factors for persistence or metastasis include patients with paraneoplastic disorders such as hyperthyroidism or pre-eclampsia, uterus being greater than 16-weeks size at diagnosis, extremely high baseline β-hCG levels, and the presence of theca luetin cysts. During the follow-up, if there is a plateau or a rise in the β-hCG level, than prompt evaluation and staging are imperative. Referral of these women to a trophoblastic disease center or to a gynecologic oncologist is highly recommended to optimize outcome.

B. Persistent GTN. During follow-up for an HM, a plateau or a rise in the β-hCG level mandates prompt staging and treatment. At the minimum, a complete physical and pelvic examination, chest x-ray, liver function tests, and CBC are necessary. If residual disease is suspected in the uterus, a pelvic sonography can be performed. The only indication for repeat curettage is in the setting of residual disease in the uterus. If any evidence of metastatic disease is found on these preliminary studies or suspected on physical examination, then a CT of the abdomen and pelvis and head is necessary. There are several staging systems for GTN. The most clinically relevant is the American College of Obstetricians and Gynecologists (ACOG) staging (Table 11.5). The FIGO staging system and the World Health Organization (WHO) classification are also used but are more cumbersome (Table 11.6). All patients with persistent GTN require treatment with chemotherapy. The key treatment monitor for persistent GTN is the serum β-hCG level. Using the ACOG classification system, patients can be divided into three separate groups based upon the presence of absence of metastatic disease.

1. Nonmetastatic GTN. By definition, patients with nonmetastatic GTN are 100% curable since all the disease is still contained in the uterus. Treatment involves single-agent chemotherapy with either methotrexate (MTX) or dactinomycin (Actinomycin-D, Act-D). Cure rates are similar between the two drugs. Recommended dosages and schedule for Act-D include 10 to 13μg/m² IV daily for 5 days every 14 days. However, Act-D 1.25 mg/m² IV every 2 weeks is often preferred as it is logistically easier for the patient. Schedules acceptable for MTX include 0.5 mg/kg IM daily for 5 days every 2 weeks; 1 mg/kg on days 1, 3, 5, and 7 followed by leucovorin 0.1 mg/kg on days 2, 4, 6, and 8 every 15 to 18 days; and MTX 30 to 50 mg/m² IM weekly. The latter regimen has increased in popularity because of its ease of administration. Treatment is continued until the β-hCG level normalizes. Fortunately, few patients with nonmetastatic GTN fail primary therapy. Those who do can be switched to the alternative single-agent therapy. In the event of resistance to both Act-D and MTX, patients should be switched to multiagent therapy with EMA-CO or EMA-EP (see Table 11.7). Patients with nonmetastatic GTN who

Table 11.5. International Federation of Gynecology and Obstetrics staging for gestational trophoblastic neoplasia

Stage	Definition
I	Strictly confined to uterine corpus
II	Extends outside uterus but limited to genital structures
III	Extends to lungs with or without genital tract involvement
IV	All other metastatic sites

Greene FL, Page DL, Fleming ID, et al. *AJCC cancer staging handbook*, 6th ed. Springer-Verlag, 2002.

Table 11.6.   Modified American College of Obstetricians and Gynecologists classification of gestational trophoblastic neoplasm

1. Nonmalignant GTN
   a. Hydatidiform mole
      1. Complete
      2. Incomplete
2. Malignant GTN
   a. Nonmetastatic GTN: no evidence of disease outside of uterus, not assigned to prognostic category
   b. Metastatic GTN: any metastases
      1. Good-prognosis metastatic GTN
         Short duration (<4 months)
         Low β-hCG level (<40,000 mIU/mL serum β-hCG)
         No metastases to brain or liver
         No antecedent term pregnancy
         No prior chemotherapy
      2. Poor-prognosis metastatic GTN: any high-risk factor
         Long duration (>4 months since last pregnancy)
         High pretreatment β-hCG level (> 40,000 mIU/mL serum β-hCG)
         Brain or liver metastases
         Antecedent term pregnancy
         Prior chemotherapy

GTN, gestational trophoblastic neoplasm; β-hCG, β-human chorionic gonadotropin.

no longer desire fertility can be considered for hysterectomy as primary therapy. The use of hysterectomy will decrease the number of cycles of chemotherapy necessary for remission. Additionally, patients with refractory nonmetastatic disease can also be considered for hysterectomy in the salvage setting. If a nodule of GTN deep in the myometrium is present on imaging studies, successful remission with resection of the lesion or intrapelvic chemotherapy infusion and preservation of the uterus has been reported.

2. Low-risk metastatic GTN. Patients in this group are treated in a manner similar to those with nonmetastatic GTN with single agent ACT-D or MTX. Therapy is continued for at least one course past a normal β-hCG titer. Patients who fail single-agent therapy are candidates for multiagent chemotherapy with EMA-CO.

3. High-risk metastatic GTN. This group of patients represents a significant challenge to the clinician. They have often developed drug resistance, as well as toxicity, and depleted bone marrow reserves from prior therapy. The current treatment of choice is the use of multiagent chemotherapy with EMA-CO every 2 weeks (see Table 11.7) with expected cure rates of 70% to 90%. Treatment is continued until three consecutive weekly normal β-hCG levels have been obtained and at least two to four cycles of therapy have been delivered after normalization of the β-hCG.

Table 11.7. Multiagent chemotherapy regimens for gestational trophoblastic disease

Regimen	Schedule and Doses	Regimen	Repeated
EMA-CO	Etoposide	100 mg/m^2 IV day 1–2	Every 2 week
	Actinomycin	0.5 mg IV push day 1–2	
	Methotrexate	100 mg/m^2 IV push, then	
		200 mg/m^2 IV over 12 h day 1	
	Leucovorin	15 mg IM or PO q12 h × 4	
		24 h after MTX	
	Vincristine	1 mg/m^2 IV push day 8	
	Cyclophosphamide	600 mg/m^2 IV push day 8	
EMA-EP	Etoposide[a]	100 mg/m^2 IV push day 8	
	Cisplatin[a]	80 mg/m^2 IV day 8	

[a]Same as EMA-CO, except substitute etoposide/cisplatin for vincristine cyclophosphamide.

Patients who fail EMA-CO have been salvaged with replacement of the cyclophosphamide and vincristine on day 8 with etoposide 100 mg/m^2 IV and cisplatin 80 mg/m^2 IV (EMA-EP). Alternative regimens for the refractory patient, although less effective than EMA-EP include platinum, vinblastine and bleomycin (PVB), and bleomycin, etoposide, and cisplatin (BEP), or single-agent paclitaxel, topotecan, gemcitabine, irinotecan, and oxaliplatin.

4. Special situations. Owing to the usually young age of these patients and of the potential for salvage, aggressive multimodality therapy and aggressive support should be considered for those patients with resistant or refractory disease. Patients with refractory disease should undergo investigation for solitary lesions that may be surgically resectable such as an isolated pulmonary, hepatic or cerebral metastasis. Additionally, intrathecal chemotherapy with MTX or whole brain irradiation may be considered for central nervous system (CNS) disease. Patients with hepatic lesions may be candidates for whole-liver radiation in conjunction with chemotherapy to help reduce the risk of hepatic hemorrhage.

5. Placental site trophoblastic tumors (PSTT). Treatment guidelines for patients with PSTT are less well established owing to their rarity. These rare tumors arise from the intermediate trophoblastic cell and are usually slow-growing, indolent neoplasms. Diagnosis of PSTT several years after pregnancy is not unusual. They produce low levels of β-hCG, and human placental lactogen has been used as a reliable tumor marker. Hysterectomy is considered the treatment of choice. For patients with metastatic or recurrent disease, treatment with EMA-CO or EMA-EP is recommended. However, owing to their low growth fraction, chemotherapy is rarely successful.

VI. Vulvar cancer. Primary malignancy of the vulva is rare, accounting for 4% to 5% of all gynecologic malignancies. This is usually a disease of elderly women with most cases diagnosed in the seventh or eighth decade of life. Recently there has been an increased incidence of invasive vulvar cancer in younger women. These younger women will very often have a long history of HPV infection, multifocal vulvar dysplasia and tobacco abuse. Symptoms of vulvar cancer include vulvar pruritus, vulvar pain, vulvar bleeding, or a noticeable lump or mass.

A. Pathology. Squamous cell cancers represent 90% of all vulvar cancers followed in decreasing frequency by melanoma, adenocarcinoma (usually of the Bartholin's gland), and sarcomas.

B. Diagnosis and evaluation. Diagnosis is by biopsy of the lesion. Vulvar cancers can spread by lymphatic dissemination first to the groin/inguinal lymph nodes, then to pelvic and para-aortic nodes, or by direct spread to the vagina, urethra, or anus. Evaluation of a woman with invasive vulvar cancer includes chest x-ray, routine laboratory studies, and careful physical examination of the vulvar and inguinal area to assess the clinical extent of the disease. CT imaging of the pelvis and abdomen may be considered if suspicious adenopathy is found in the inguinal nodes to rule out spread to the pelvic or para-aortic nodes.

C. Treatment

1. Surgery. Vulvar cancer is treated primarily with surgery. In select cases preoperative chemotherapy (Section VI.C.3) and radiation is warranted. Surgical treatment involves a radical wide local resection of the primary lesion with a 1-cm gross margin combined with an inguinal lymph node dissection. An ipsilateral inguinal node dissection can be performed through a separate incision. Bilateral inguinal node dissection should be performed if the ipsilateral inguinal nodes are positive or if the primary lesion involves midline structures (clitoris, urethra, vagina, perineum or anus). A lesion less than 2 cm in diameter with less than 1 mm of invasion (stage IA) can be safely treated with wide resection alone. All lesions with more than 1.0 mm of invasion require an inguinal node dissection. The use of lymphatic mapping and sentinel lymph node biopsy is still considered investigational. Often, for large vulvar lesions, reconstruction with a skin or myocutaneous flap may be necessary.

2. Staging, risk stratification (Table 11.8). Vulvar cancer is surgically staged on the basis of the size of the primary lesion, direct extension to the vagina, anus or urethra, and by the pathologic status of the inguinal lymph

Table 11.8.   1995 International Federation of Gynecology and Obstetrics staging for carcinoma of the vulva

Stage	Definition
0	Carcinoma *in situ*; intraepithelial carcinoma (Tis)
I	Tumor confined to the vulva and/or perineum, ≤ 2 cm in greatest dimension; nodes are negative (T1, N0, M0)
IA	Lesions ≤ 2 cm in size confined to the vulva or perineum with stromal invasion no greater than 1 mm No nodal metastases. The depth of invasion is defined as the measurement of the tumor from the epithelial–stromal junction of the adjacent most superficial derma papilla to the deepest point of invasion
IB	Lesions ≤ 2 cm in size confined to the vulva or perineum with stromal invasion >1 mm; no nodal metastases
II	Tumor confined to the vulva and/or perineum, >2 cm in greatest dimension; nodes are negative (T2, N0, M0)
III	Tumor of any size with (a) adjacent spread to the lower urethra and/or the vagina or to the anus; and/or (b) unilateral regional lymph node metastasis (T3, N0, M0; T3, N1, M0; T1, N1, M0; T2, N1, M0)
IVA	Tumor invades any of the following: upper urethra, bladder mucosa, rectal mucosa, pelvic bone; and/or bilateral regional node metastasis (T1, N2, M0; T2, N2, M0; T3, N2, M0; T4, any N, M0)
IVB	Any distant metastasis, including pelvic lymph nodes (any T, any N, M1)

TNM classification

Primary tumor

Tis	Preinvasive carcinoma (carcinoma *in situ*)
T1	Tumor confined to the vulva and/or perineum <2 cm in greatest dimension
T2	Tumor confined to the vulva and/or perineum >2 cm in greatest dimension
T3	Tumor of any size with adjacent spread to the urethra and/or vagina and/or to the anus
T4	Tumor of any size infiltrating the bladder mucosa and/or the rectal mucosa, including the upper part of the urethral mucosa and/or fixed to the bone

Regional lymph nodes

N0	No lymph node metastasis
N1	Unilateral regional lymph node metastasis
N2	Bilateral regional lymph node metastasis

Distant metastasis

M0	No clinical metastasis
M1	Distant metastasis (including pelvic lymph node metastasis)

nodes. Clinical staging is often used to direct primary therapy. However, clinical evaluation of normal inguinal lymph nodes is historically inaccurate with disease in up to 20% of patients with palpably normal inguinal nodes. The impact of spread to the inguinal lymph nodes is prognostically significant. A patient with a T1 lesion and negative inguinal lymph nodes (stage IB) will have a 5-year survival of more than 90%. Pathologic spread to the inguinal nodes with the same size of primary lesion (stage III) will portend a 5-year survival of approximately 60%. After surgical staging, patients with negative inguinal lymph nodes and negative surgical margins are in a low-risk group and are generally observed. Patients with evidence of pathologic spread to the inguinal nodes are offered adjuvant RT to the affected groin and pelvis.

3. Candidates for chemotherapy. Patients with distant disease are candidates for chemotherapy. Clinical data on the optimal choice of chemotherapy for these patients are lacking owing to the rarity of the disease. Most agents that are effective against squamous cell cancers occurring at other sites are deemed effective in the treatment of distant metastasis from vulvar cancer. Cisplatin, bleomycin, topotecan, flurouracil, methotrexate, mitomycin, and doxorubicin all have reported activity. However, response of distant disease to chemotherapy is usually brief.

Patients who initially present with locally advanced disease (T3 or T4) that would require exenterative type radical resection are also candidates for combined chemotherapy and RT. This includes patients presenting with fixed or ulcerative (N3 or N4) inguinal nodes. A prospective clinical trial treated 73 patients with locally advanced disease with local irradiation and concurrent chemotherapy; cisplatin 50 mg/m^2 IV on day 1 plus flurouracil 1,000 mg/m^2 as a continuous IV infusion on days 1 to 4 every 3 weeks during radiation gave a 46% complete response rate and only three patients required interruption of the gastrointestinal or genitourinary system. Chemoradiation appears to be the treatment of choice for those patients who present with locally advanced vulvar or inguinal disease. However, a recent trial involved 14 patients with locally advanced vulvar cancer involving the anal sphincter and/or urethra who were treated with neoadjuvant chemotherapy alone consisting of cisplatin and flurouracil followed by radical vulvectomy. A response rate of 100% with preservation of the urethra and anal sphincter in all patients was observed.

SUGGESTED READINGS

General

Carney ME, Lancaster JM, Ford C, et al. A population-based study of patterns of care for ovarian cancer: who is seen by a gynecologic oncologist and who is not? *Gynecol Oncol* 2002;84:36–42.

Earle CC, Schrag D, Neville BA, et al. Effect of surgeon specialty on processes of care and outcomes for ovarian cancer patients. *J Natl Cancer Inst* 2006;98:172–180.

Carcinoma of the Cervix

Keys HM, Bundy BN, Stehman FB, et al. Cisplatin, radiation, and adjuvant hysterectomy compared with radiation and adjuvant hysterectomy for bulky stage Ib cervical carcinoma. *N Engl J Med* 1999;340:1154–1161.

Long HJ III, Bundy BN, Grendys, ED Jr, et al. Randomized phase III trial of cisplatin with or without topotecan in carcinoma of the uterine cervix: a gynecologic oncology group study. *J Clin Oncol* 2005;23:4626–4633.

Moore DH, Blessing JA, McQuellon RP, et al. Phase II study of cisplatin with or without paclitaxel in stage IVB, recurrent, or persistent squamous cell carcinoma of the cervix; a Gynecologic Oncology Group study. *J Clin Oncol* 2004;22:3113–3119.

Moore DH, Blessing JA, McQuellon RP, et al. Phase III study of cisplatin with or without paclitaxel in stage IVB, recurrent or persistent squamous cell carcinoma of the cervix; a Gynecologic Oncology Group study. *J Clin Oncol* 2004;22:3223–3219.

Morris M, Eifel PJ, Lu J, et al. Pelvic radiation with concurrent chemotherapy compared with pelvic and para-aortic radiation for high-risk cervical cancer. *N Engl J Med* 1999;340:1137–1143.

Peters WA III, Liu PY, Barrett RJII, et al. Concurrent chemotherapy and pelvic radiation therapy compared with pelvic radiation therapy alone as adjuvant therapy after radical surgery in high-risk early-stage cancer of the cervix. *J Clin Oncol* 2000;18:1606–1613.

Rose PG, Blessing JA, Gershenson DM, et al. Paclitaxel and cisplatin as first-line therapy in recurrent or advanced squamous cell carcinoma of the cervix: a Gynecologic Oncology Group study. *J Clin Oncol* 1999;17:2676–2680.

Rose PG, Bundy BN, Watkins EB, et al. Concurrent cisplatin-based radiotherapy and chemotherapy for locally advanced cervical cancer. *N Engl J Med* 1999;340:1144–1153.

Thigpen T, Shingleton H, Homesley H, et al. Cis-platinum in treatment of advanced or recurrent squamous cell carcinoma of the cervix; a phase II study of the Gynecologic Oncology Group. *Cancer* 1981;48:899–903.

Whitney CW, Sause W, Bundy BN, et al. Randomized comparison of fluorouracil plus cisplatin versus hydroxyurea as an adjunct to radiation therapy in stage IIb–IVa carcinoma of the cervix with negative para-aortic lymph nodes: a Gynecologic Oncology Group and Southwest Oncology Group Study. *J Clin Oncol* 1999;17:1339–1348.

Endometrial Carcinoma

Ball HG, Blessing JA, Lentz SS, et al. A phase II trial of paclitaxel in advanced and recurrent adenocarcinoma of the endometrium: a Gynecologic Oncology Group study. *Gynecol Oncol* 1995;56:120.

Creutzberg CL, van Putten WL, Koper PC, et al. Surgery and postoperative radiotherapy versus surgery alone for patients with stage I endometrial carcinoma: multicentre randomised trial. *Lancet* 2000;355:1404–1411.

Fleming GF, Brunetto VL, Cella D, et al. Phase III trial of doxorubicin plus cisplatin with or without paclitaxel plus filgrastim in advanced endometrial carcinoma: a Gynecologic Oncology Group study. *J Clin Oncol* 2004;22:2159–2166.

Hensley ML, Maki R, Venkatraman E, et al. Gemcitabine and docetaxel in patients with unresectable leiomyosarcoma: results of a phase II trial. *J Clin Oncol* 2002;20:2824–2831.

Keys HM, Roberts JA, Brunetto VL, et al. A phase III trail of surgery with or without adjunctive external pelvic radiation therapy in intermediate risk endometrial adenocarcinoma: a Gynecologic Oncology Group study. *Gynecol Oncol* 2004;92:744–751.

Kilgore LC, Partridge EE, Alvarez RD, et al. Adenocarcinoma of the endometrium: survival comparisons of patients with and without pelvic node sampling. *Gynecol Oncol* 1995;56:29–33.

Lee SW, Russell AH, Kinney WK. Whole abdomen radiotherapy for patients with peritoneal dissemination of endometrial adenocarcinoma. *Int J Radiat Oncol Biol Phys* 2003;56:788–792.

Mariani A, Webb MJ, Galli L, et al. Potential therapeutic role of para-aortic lymphadenectomy in node-positive endometrial cancer. *Gynecol Oncol* 2000;76:348–356.

Morrow CP, Bundy BN, Kurman RJ, et al. Relationship between surgical-pathological risk factors and outcome in clinical stage I and II carcinoma of the endometrium: a Gynecologic Oncology Group study. *Gynecol Oncol* 1991;40:55–65.

Randall ME, Filiaci VL, Muss H, et al. Randomized phase III trail of whole-abdominal irradiation versus doxorubicin and cisplatin chemotherapy in advanced endometrial carcinoma: a Gynecologic Oncology Group study. *J Clin Oncol* 2006;24:36–44.

Small WS Jr, Lurain JR. Current management of endometrial cancer: surgical staging and postoperative radiotherapy. *Am J Oncol Rev* 2006;5:165–166.

Sutton G, Axelrod JH, Bundy BN, et al. Whole abdominal radiotherapy in the adjuvant treatment of patients with stage III and IV endometrial cancer: a Gynecologic Oncology Group study. *Gynecol Oncol* 2005;97:755–763.

Carcinoma of the Ovary

Armstrong DK, Bundy B, Wenzel L, et al. Intraperitoneal cisplatin and paclitaxel in ovarian cancer. *N Engl J Med* 2006;354:34–43.

Bristow RE, Tomacruz RS, Armstrong DK, et al. Survival effect of maximal cytoreductive surgery for advanced ovarian carcinoma during the platinum era: a meta-analysis. *J Clin Oncol* 2002;20:1248–1259.

Burger RA, Sill M, Monk BJ, et al. Phase II trial of bevacizumab in persistent or recurrent epithelial ovarian cancer (EOC) or primary peritoneal cancer (PPC): a Gynecologic Oncology Group (GOG) study. *Presented at the 41st Annual Meeting of the American Society of Clinical Oncology in Orlando*, Florida: ASCO Oral #5010. Available at http://www.asco.org/ac/1.1003. 12-002511-00 18-0034-00 19–003624.00.asp, May 13–17, 2005.

Garcia AA, Oza AM, Hirte H, et al. Interim report of a phase II clinical trial of bevacizumab and low dose metronomic oral cyclophosphamide in recurrent ovarian cancer: a trial conducted by the California, Princess Margaret Hospital and University of Chicago Phase II Consortia. *Presented at the American Society of Clinical Oncology in Orlando*, Florida: ASCO Oral #5000. Available at http://www.asco.org/ac/1.1003. 12-002511-00 18-0034-00 19–003449.00.asp, May 13–17, 2005.

Markman M, Markman J, Webster K, et al. Duration of response to second-line, platinum-based chemotherapy for ovarian cancer:

implications for patient management and clinical trial design. *J Clin Oncol* 2004;22:3120–3125.

Markman M, Walker JL. Intraperitoneal chemotherapy of ovarian cancer: a review, with a focus on practical aspects of treatment. *J Clin Oncol* 2006;24:1–6.

Michener CM, Belinson JL. Modern management of recurrent ovarian carcinoma. *Oncology* 2005;19:1277–1285.

NIH Consensus Conference. Ovarian cancer screening, treatment and follow-up. *JAMA* 1995;273:491.

Ozols RF, Bundy BN, Greer BE, et al. Phase III trial of carboplatin and paclitaxel compared with cisplatin and paclitaxel in patients with optimally resected stage III ovarian cancer: a Gynecologic Oncology Group study. *J Clin Oncol* 2003;21:3194–3200.

Parmar MK, Ledermann JA, Colombo N, et al. Paclitaxel plus platinum-based chemotherapy versus conventional platinum-based chemotherapy in women with relapsed ovarian cancer. The ICON4/AGO-OVAR-2.2 trial. *Lancet* 2003;361:2099–2106.

Rose PG, Blessing JA, Mayer AR, et al. Prolonged oral etoposide as second-line therapy for platinum-resistant and platinum-sensitive ovarian carcinoma: a Gynecologic Oncology Group study. *J Clin Oncol* 1998;16:405–410.

Rose PG, Mossbruger K, Fusco N, et al. Gemcitabine reverses cisplatin resistance: demonstration of activity in platinum- and multidrug-resistant ovarian and peritoneal carcinoma. *Gynecol Oncol* 2002;88:17–21.

Schrag D, Kuntz KM, Garber JE, et al. Decision analysis—effects of prophylactic mastectomy and oophorectomy on life expectancy among women with BRCA1 or BRCA2 mutations. *N Engl J Med* 1997;336:1465–1471.

Gestational Trophoblastic Disease

Newlands ES, Bower M, Holden L, et al. Management of resistant gestational trophoblastic tumors. *J Reprod Med* 1998;43:111–118.

Petrilli ES, Twiggs LB, Blessing JA, et al. Single-dose actinomycin-D treatment for nonmetastatic gestational trophoblastic disease. *Cancer* 1987;60:2173–2176.

Carcinoma of the Vulva

Burke TW, Levenback C, Coleman RL, et al. Surgical therapy of t1 and t2 vulvar carcinoma: further experience with radical wide excision and selective inguinal lymphadenectomy. *Gynecol Oncol* 1995;57:215–220.

Geisler JP, Manahan KJ, Buller RE. Neoadjuvant chemotherapy in vulvar cancer: avoiding primary exenteration. *Gynecol Oncol* 2006;100:53–57.

Han SC, Kim DH, Higgins SA, et al. Chemoradiation as primary or adjuvant treatment for locally advanced carcinoma of the vulva. *Int J Radiat Oncol Biol Phys* 2000;47:1235–1244.

Montana G, Thomas GM, Moore DH, et al. Preoperative chemoradiation for carcinoma of the vulva with N2/N3 nodes: a Gynecologic Oncology Group study. *Int J Radiat Oncol Biol Phys* 2000;48:1007–1013.

CHAPTER 12

Urologic and Male Genital Cancers

Joseph S. Chan, Scott B. Saxman, and Craig R. Nichols

I. **Bladder cancer**
   A. **General considerations and staging.** Cancer arising in the bladder is usually transitional cell carcinoma (TCC), although occasionally squamous cell carcinoma, neuroendocrine carcinoma, and adenocarcinoma are seen. TCC falls into two major groups: superficial and invasive. The biology and natural history of these two groups differ markedly. When planning treatment for bladder cancer, one must take into account the stage of the tumor (0 to IV), histologic grade (1–3), and location of the tumor within the bladder (related to surgical considerations of partial vs. total cystectomy).

   The standard evaluation of a patient with invasive bladder cancer should include a computed tomography (CT) scan of the abdomen and pelvis, chest radiograph, complete blood cell count, and serum chemistry profile. In certain circumstances, urine cytology, chest CT, magnetic resonance imaging (MRI), and bone scan may also be helpful. The TNM staging system is summarized in Table 12.1.

   B. **General approach to therapy**
      1. **Superficial-stage, low-grade tumors.** Patients with stage 0 or I tumors are usually treated by transurethral resection (TUR) and fulguration, which may provide local control. However, most patients will have recurrence at other sites of the bladder. The risk of recurrence may be reduced by administration of intravesical therapy. Diffuse carcinoma *in situ* may also be treated with intravesicular therapy.
      2. **Deep-stage, high-grade tumors.** Patients with larger stage II lesions or with stage III disease are usually managed by radical cystectomy. Partial cystectomy may be used in highly select patients with small and ideally located focal disease. The responsiveness of TCC to cisplatin-based combination chemotherapy suggests its potential in the neoadjuvant and adjuvant setting. With a significant rate of recurrence after surgery, the addition of chemotherapy to radical cystectomy, especially in a clinical trial, may be considered in patients with muscle-invasive bladder cancer. The addition of chemotherapy and radiation to local resection in bladder-sparing protocols is also under active investigation.
      3. **Advanced and metastatic tumors.** Patients with locally advanced disease or local recurrences can be considered for radiation therapy. Patients with advanced or metastatic disease are candidates for systemic chemotherapy. There is evidence that chemotherapy can prolong

Table 12.1.   TNM staging of bladder cancer

TX: Primary tumor cannot be assessed

T0: No evidence of primary tumor

Ta: Noninvasive papillary carcinoma

Tis: Carcinoma *in situ*

T1: Tumor invades subepithelial connective tissue

T2: Tumor invades muscle

T2a: Superficial (inner half)

T2b: Deep (outer half)

T3: Tumor invades perivesical fat

T3a: Microscopically

T3b: Macroscopically (extravesical mass)

T4: Tumor invades any of the following: prostate, uterus, vagina, pelvic wall, or abdominal wall

T4a: Tumor invades the prostate, uterus, or vagina

T4b: Tumor invades the pelvic wall or abdominal wall

Stage groupings

Stage 0: Ta or Tis, N0, M0

Stage I: T1, N0, M0

Stage II: T2, N0, M0

Stage III: T3 or T4a, N0, M0

Stage IV: T4b, N0, M0; any T, N1–3, M0–1

---

survival and that combination chemotherapy is superior to single agents.

C. **Treatment regimens and evaluation of response**

1. **Intravesical chemotherapy**

a. **Method of administration and follow-up.** Intravesical therapy is usually administered in a volume of 40 to 60 mL through a Foley catheter. The catheter is then clamped and the agent retained for 2 hours. This procedure delivers a high local concentration to the tumor area while usually avoiding systemic effects. Patients with superficial bladder cancers require lifelong surveillance with periodic cystoscopy (initially every 3 months, then every 6 months, then annually) because even with intravesical therapy, an increased risk of new primary tumors persists. Patients being treated for diffuse carcinoma *in situ* should have biopsy confirmation of the return of normal mucosa after the instillation of therapy has been completed. These patients also require lifelong cystoscopic surveillance.

b. **Selection of patients for intravesical therapy.** Only patients with superficial or small, minimally invasive tumors (T1) should be treated. The grade of the tumor is also a significant predictor of progression. Patients with lesions at high risk for progression, especially those that persist or recur after initial intravesical therapy may be considered for cystectomy. Possible objectives for intravesical therapy are as follows:

(1) Prevention of relapse in patients with high-grade Ta and stage I lesions treated with TUR.

(2) Prevention of new bladder tumors. Patients with two or more previously resected bladder tumors may be treated in an effort to prevent development of de novo malignancies.

(3) Treatment of carcinoma *in situ*, which may involve the bladder diffusely and therefore not be amenable to TUR. A course of instillation therapy is usually given, followed by repeat biopsies. Persistence of carcinoma *in situ* is an indication for more aggressive local management such as cystectomy.

c. Specific intravesical therapeutic regimens

Bacillus Calmette-Guerin (BCG) 120 mg weekly for 6 to 8 weeks, *or*

Thiotepa 30 to 60 mg weekly for 4 to 6 weeks, *or*

Mitomycin 20 to 40 mg weekly for 6 to 8 weeks, *or*

Doxorubicin 50 to 60 mg weekly for 6 to 8 weeks

d. Selection of therapy. Two separate studies have shown BCG to be superior to thiotepa and doxorubicin in preventing recurrence. Two published meta-analyses suggest significantly less tumor recurrence with BCG as compared to mitomycin. In addition, BCG demonstrates higher rates of response in treatment of carcinoma *in situ*. Therefore, BCG should be considered the agent of choice for intravesical therapy. The benefit of maintenance BCG therapy is controversial.

e. Response to therapy. In patients with Ta or T1 disease, intravesical BCG decreases tumor recurrence by approximately 50%. The complete response rate with BCG in carcinoma *in situ* is approximately 70% to 80%. However, the benefit of intravesical therapy in preventing progression to invasive or metastatic bladder cancer is still unclear.

f. Complications of therapy. All of the agents mentioned can cause symptoms of bladder irritation (pain, urgency, and hematuria) and allergic reactions. Thiotepa is systemically absorbed and can occasionally cause myelosuppression. This is rare with mitomycin and doxorubicin. Patients receiving thiotepa should have their blood cell counts monitored closely. Mitomycin can cause dermatitis in the perineal area and hands. BCG is occasionally associated with systemic symptoms including fever, chills, malaise, arthralgias, and skin rash. Septic reactions and disseminated BCG infections are rare.

2. Adjuvant chemotherapy. With the encouraging response rates of cisplatin-based chemotherapy in advanced bladder cancer, there has been enthusiasm for using this therapy in the neoadjuvant and adjuvant setting. However, there are only a few select studies suggesting a survival benefit. The US Intergroup trial, which randomized patients to neoadjuvant MVAC (methotrexate, vinblastine, doxorubicin, and cisplatin) or radical cystectomy alone, suggested a survival benefit for neoadjuvant chemotherapy. Two other meta-analyses also suggest a small improvement in overall survival with neoadjuvant cisplatin-based combination chemotherapy. There is also strong enthusiasm for using adjuvant chemotherapy as it does not delay possible curative surgery. However, studies of adjuvant therapy are flawed and its use is still controversial.

3. **Bladder-sparing therapy.** Reports of success with combination chemotherapy and radiotherapy as definitive treatment for muscle-invasive bladder cancer is compelling especially for patients who wish to keep their native bladder. However, there is no randomized trial directly comparing bladder preservation therapy with radical cystectomy. Bladder-sparing therapy does not avoid the possibility of new bladder tumors nor the distinct toxicities of chemotherapy and radiotherapy. Patients with favorable tumors and those who are unfit for radical cystectomy because comorbidities may be the best candidates for bladder-sparing protocols.

4. **Systemic chemotherapy for advanced disease**
   a. **Specific chemotherapy drugs and regimens.** Drugs active against bladder cancer include cisplatin, doxorubicin, vinblastine, methotrexate, cyclophosphamide, gemcitabine, carboplatin, paclitaxel, and docetaxel. Of these, cisplatin is probably the most active drug as a single agent. The MVAC combination is the most standard therapy because of its significant survival advantage over single-agent cisplatin. However, the use of GC (gemcitabine and cisplatin) is increasing substantially due to similar response rates and survival data with fewer side effects. Specific regimens are shown in Table 12.2.

   b. **Response to therapy.** MVAC may be expected to produce a complete response in approximately 15% of patients and a partial response in 35%, for an overall response rate of approximately 50% in patients with metastatic disease. The median survival time is approximately 14 months. The toxicity of the regimen is substantial and patient selection in regards to medical comorbidities and performance status is important. Response to any chemotherapy is monitored by periodic measurement of tumor masses with the expectation that most patients who will respond will do so within the first one to two cycles of treatment.

   A trial comparing MVAC with GC demonstrated similar response rates and overall survival. An update of the trial's results demonstrated that these survival outcomes were maintained after long-term follow-up. However, the study was not powered statistically to prove equivalence of the two regimens. Despite this statistical argument, the GC regimen has entered common usage as first-line therapy in patients with advanced TCC.

   Patients who will not tolerate cisplatin-based chemotherapy because of poor performance status or renal insufficiency may be considered for carboplatin or nonplatin-based therapy. Combinations containing

Table 12.2. Combination chemotherapy and active single agents for cancer of the bladder

Regimen or Single Agent	Doses and Schedules
MVAC	Methotrexate 30 mg/m^2 IV on day 1
	Vinblastine 3 mg/m^2 IV on day 2
	Doxorubicin 30 mg/m^2 IV on day 2
	Cisplatin 70 mg/m^2 IV on day 2 (with adequate pre- and postchemotherapy hydration)
	Repeat methotrexate and vinblastine on days 15 and 22 if white blood cell count >2, 000/μL and platelet count >50, 000/μL. Cycles should be repeated every 28 days
GC	Gemcitabine 1,000 mg/m^2 day 1
	Cisplatin 70 mg/m^2 on day 2
	Repeat gemcitabine on days 8 and 15 if white blood cell count >2, 000/μL and platelet count >50, 000/μL. Cycles should be repeated every 28 days
Carboplatin/gemcitabine	Carboplatin AUC 5 day 1
	Gemcitabine 1,000 mg/m^2 days 1 and 8
	Cycles repeated every 21 days
Carboplatin/paclitaxel	Carboplatin AUC 6
	Paclitaxel 225 mg/m^2
	Cycles repeated every 21 days
Paclitaxel	250 mg/m^2 IV over 24 h every 21 days

AUC, area under the curve.

carboplatin, gemcitabine, docetaxel, or paclitaxel have all shown activity.

Management of the non-TCC histologies arising from the bladder is difficult. Local therapies should be identical to TCC, but the role of chemotherapy is limited. Non-TCC histologies respond poorly to chemotherapy. Neuroendocrine tumors of the bladder are usually treated in a manner similar to small cell lung cancer with cisplatin/etoposide-based regimens and local radiation for those with disease confined to the bladder. **c. Complications of systemic therapy.** The major dose-limiting toxicity of MVAC is myelosuppression, which often precludes the administration of chemotherapy on days 15 and 22. GC produces significantly less neutropenia and mucositis but more thrombocytopenia. Cisplatin can cause renal damage, but this can usually be prevented by vigorous hydration and saline diuresis. Nausea, vomiting and malaise are also commonly seen.

d. Follow-up. Patients with advanced disease can be followed up every few months for symptomatic progression. Serial x-ray studies or bone scans are costly and are of minimal value.

II. Prostate cancer

A. Background. Carcinoma of the prostate is the most common cancer in the United States, with the exception of nonmelanoma skin cancer. Largely because of aggressive screening using prostate-specific antigen (PSA), the estimated number of new cases increased to more than 230,000 in 2006. However, the median survival of patients with early prostate cancer may be over 10 years. The benefit of aggressive surgical or radiotherapeutic management of these patients is largely dependant on individual patient comorbidities and the biology of the tumor.

B. Staging. Staging is usually done using a combination of clinical and pathologic indicators. Pathologic staging is necessary for a completely accurate staging of low-stage disease but it is often not needed, once the disease has become metastatic to the bones or visceral organs. Accurate determination of extension beyond the prostate capsule and into the lymph nodes may be difficult. Full assessment of stage may not be possible until after surgery and pathologic evaluation. Nomograms such as the ones published by Memorial Sloan Kettering Cancer Center are often helpful in predicting pathologic stage, determining patient outcome, and guiding treatment. These nomograms utilize the degree of elevation in PSA value and differentiation of the tumor using the Gleason score in determining prognostic information.

Full staging of prostate cancer may also include abdominal and pelvic CT scans, chest radiographs, bone scans, liver function tests, and acid phosphatase measurements. The most common staging system is the TNM system shown in Table 12.3. The modified Whitmore-Jewett or American Urologic Association system is also used. In the American Urologic Association system, stages A, B, C, and D correspond closely to stages I, II, III, and IV in the TNM system.

C. General considerations and goals of therapy. Selection of therapy for prostate cancer is complex and is based on the extent of disease as well as on the age and general medical condition of the patient. Although many biases exist, there are no good randomized trials comparing treatment modalities in patients with organ-confined disease.

With the possible exception of young patients less than 60 years of age, T1a prostate cancer may be followed up without further therapy as few patients will have disease progression. For other patients with organ-confined disease (T1b, T1c, T2), several treatment options exist. Radical prostatectomy and external beam radiation therapy are probably equivalent treatment modalities when PSA and Gleason score are taken into account. Observation or active surveillance should also be considered for patients with low-grade, organ-confined tumors. However, there is no good direct comparison between these treatments and the choice of these options must take into account the patient's performance status and the toxicities of each modality. Toxicities of radical prostatectomy

Table 12.3.   TNM staging of prostate cancer

T-stage

TX: Primary tumor cannot be assessed

T0: No evidence of primary tumor

T1: Clinically inapparent tumor not palpable or visible by imaging

T1a: Tumor incidental histologic finding in 5% or less of tissue resected

T1b: Tumor incidental histologic finding in more than 5% of tissue resected

T1c: Tumor identified by needle biopsy (e.g., because of elevated PSA)

T2: Tumor confined within prostate

T3: Tumor extends through the prostatic capsule

T4: Tumor is fixed or invades adjacent structures other than seminal vesicles

Stage groupings

Stage I: T1a, N0, M0, G1

Stage II: T1a, N0, M0, G2–4

T1b, T1c, N0, M0, any G

T2, N0, M0, any G

Stage III: T3, N0, M0, any G

Stage IV: T4, N0, M0, any G

Any T, N1–3, M0, any G

Any T, any N, M1, any G

PSA, prostate-specific antigen.

include anesthesia, bleeding, urinary leakage, and erectile dysfunction. Diarrhea, tenesmus, and rectal bleeding are more common with radiation therapy. In general, younger men are more likely to receive radical prostatectomy whereas older men are more likely to receive radiation therapy. Lastly, brachytherapy and cryosurgery may also be alternatives for treating localized disease.

Patients with stage III tumors are often treated with radiation therapy. However, very elderly patients or patients in poor general health may be followed up with observation because the natural history of prostate cancer can be slow with progression over years rather than months. The addition of early hormonal therapy to radiation therapy may be considered in higher stage disease. Currently the addition of chemotherapy in high-risk, localized prostate cancer is being studied.

D. Treatment of metastatic disease. Patients with metastatic disease are usually treated initially with hormonal therapy. Radiation for symptomatic localized metastasis may also be considered.

    1. Hormonal therapy. Hormonal therapy results in subjective response in approximately 75% of patients treated, lasting an average of 18 months. Most of these patients also have objective response, measured either radiographically or by a decreasing PSA level. In general, either luteinizing hormone–releasing hormone (LHRH) analogs or orchiectomy is the primary initial treatment. There is little evidence to suggest that one treatment is better than the other, and patient preference, existing medical conditions, and cost often determine treatment choice. There are currently no good predictive markers for response in clinical practice.

a. Orchiectomy is still the standard modality of treatment for metastatic disease because it is relatively inexpensive and obviates the need for injections or daily medications. This procedure can often be done on an outpatient basis. However, most men choose a nonsurgical method of hormonal therapy.

b. Luteinizing hormone–releasing hormone (LHRH) analogs are synthetic peptides, which, when administered by parenteral injection, occupy the receptors for LHRH in the pituitary gland. Initially the release of luteinizing hormone (LH) is increased, causing a rise in the serum testosterone level. The continuous administration of therapeutic (super physiologic) doses of the LHRH analog blocks the physiologic pulsatile LH release from the pituitary, causing a fall in the serum testosterone to castrate levels. Currently used agents include the following:

- **Leuprolide** 7.5 mg IM depot monthly or 22.5 mg IM depot every 3 months or 30 mg IM depot every 4 months.
- **Goserelin** 3.6 mg SC depot monthly or 10.8 mg SC every 3 months

There is a potential for rapid worsening during the initial few weeks of therapy due to the paradoxical transient increase in testosterone production. This flare can usually be avoided by the concurrent use of antiandrogens. Another disadvantage is the potential for poor patient compliance and the high cost of treatment. The possible benefit of intermittent hormonal therapy is currently being studied.

c. LHRH analogs and antiandrogens (total androgen blockade) have been used in combination. Synthetic antiandrogens such as flutamide, bicalutamide, and nilutamide act by competing with testosterone at the level of the cellular receptor. However, a large randomized trial of flutamide given after orchiectomy did not show improvement in survival. Because of the lack of consistent evidence of benefit as well as added cost and toxicity, total androgen blockade is not considered standard initial treatment in patients with metastatic disease.

d. Estrogens. Diethylstilbestrol (DES) is effective but not frequently used because of concern about potential cardiotoxicity and thrombophlebitis. Historically 3 to 5 mg/day of DES has been given; however, 1 mg/day produces fewer side effects without shortening survival. Painful gynecomastia can be prevented by superficial radiation (5 Gy) to the breast tissue before the start of therapy.

e. **Second-line hormonal therapies** have low response rates (<20%) and are of brief duration. Initial hormone therapy should be continued to maintain castrate levels of testosterone. Second-line therapies include addition of antiandrogens, estrogens, ketoconazole, and progestins. Patients who were initially treated with combined-modality therapy occasionally respond to withdrawal of the antiandrogen. This should be considered before proceeding to more toxic therapies.

2. **Cytotoxic chemotherapy.** Patients who relapse from or fail to respond to hormonal therapies can be considered for cytotoxic chemotherapy. Previous trials of chemotherapy were disappointing and the role of chemotherapy in treatment of hormone-refractory prostate cancer was unclear.

a. **Mitoxantrone.** A study of mitoxantrone 12 mg/m^2 every three weeks and prednisone 5 mg b.i.d. demonstrated improved pain control and reduced need for analgesic medications as compared to patients treated with prednisone alone in a randomized trial with no improvement in overall survival. This regimen remains a possible treatment choice with a relatively low toxicity profile.

b. **Docetaxel.** Recently, two large randomized trials of docetaxel-based chemotherapy were the first to demonstrate a survival benefit over mitoxantrone and prednisone.

- **Docetaxel** 75 mg/m^2 every 3 weeks, and prednisone 5 mg b.i.d. *or*
- **Estramustine** 280 mg t.i.d. PO on days 1 to 5 and **docetaxel** 60 mg/m^2 IV on day 2 and **prednisone** 5 mg b.i.d. during 3-week cycles.

Owing to the survival benefit docetaxel-based chemotherapy is considered a standard treatment option for patients with hormone-refractory prostate cancer.

3. **Evaluation of response.** Evaluating the response is often difficult because many patients do not have measurable disease. However, the serum PSA is often elevated and can be serially measured as a marker for response. Bone scans are difficult to interpret because "hot spots" can reflect either the presence of disease or healing of bone in response to tumor regression.

4. **Complications of therapy.** All effective hormonal therapies will cause sexual dysfunction, including impotence and decreased libido. Orchiectomy can rarely be complicated by local infection or hematoma. LHRH analogs can cause an initial flare of the disease and are frequently associated with hot flashes. Antiandrogens can cause diarrhea and hepatic dysfunction. Estrogens are associated with thromboembolic disease, fluid retention, and cardiac disease. Side effects of chemotherapy include nausea and vomiting, mucositis, marrow suppression, and alopecia.

5. Follow-up. Patients treated with radical prostatectomy can be followed up with PSA measurements every 3 to 6 months. Patients with a rising PSA level, evidence of local recurrence, and no evidence of metastatic disease can be considered for salvage radiation therapy to the prostatic bed. Some patients can be considered for bisphosphonate therapy. Osteoporosis is a complication of androgen deprivation therapy and may benefit from treatment. Monthly IV bisphosphonate therapy with zoledronic acid may decrease the incidence of skeletal–related complications such as pathologic fractures in patients with hormone-refractory prostate cancer.

III. Testicular cancer (germ cell tumors [GCTs])

A. Overview. Although primary neoplasms of the testis can arise from Leydig or Sertoli cells, more than 95% of testicular cancers are of spermatogenic or germ cell origin. GCTs are rare, accounting for 1% of all malignancies in men. However, they are important malignancies because they represent the most common solid tumor in young men and because of their high degree of curability. With the advent of cisplatin-based chemotherapy, accurate tumor markers, and aggressive surgical approaches, overall cure rates for patients with disseminated disease approach 80%, and patients with early stage disease are nearly always cured. GCT is also one of the few solid tumors for which salvage chemotherapy can be curative.

B. Histology. GCTs are categorized as either seminomatous or nonseminomatous (which includes a variety of other histologies such as embryonal cell carcinoma, choriocarcinoma, and yolk sac tumors). Pure seminoma accounts for 40% of patients with GCTs. Although mild elevations of the β-subunit of human chorionic gonadotropin (hCG) may be seen, pure seminoma is never associated with an elevation of α-fetoprotein (AFP). Nonseminomatous GCT can cause elevations of hCG, AFP, or both.

C. Staging. Pretreatment staging should include serum tumor markers (AFP, hCG) and CT of the abdomen and chest. Other radiographic procedures should be undertaken only if symptoms or physical examination dictate.

Stage I: Tumor confined to the testis with or without involvement of the spermatic cord or epididymis

Stage II: Tumor with metastasis limited to retroperitoneal lymph nodes

Stage III: Tumor spread beyond retroperitoneal lymph nodes

D. Treatment strategies and management of specific situations. The therapeutic approach to the patient with testicular cancer depends on the histology of the tumor and the clinical or pathologic stage of the disease.

1. Seminoma. Most patients with seminoma present with early- stage disease and are nearly always cured with radiation therapy. Patients with stage I disease are treated with 2,500 cGy given to abdominal nodes in daily fractions over 3 to 4 weeks. Patients with lymph node involvement on lymphangiogram or CT scans receive a slightly higher dose of 3,000 to 3,500 cGy. The contralateral testis should be shielded to maintain fertility. Radiation to the mediastinum is contraindicated and can compromise subsequent chemotherapy. Surveillance for clinical stage I seminoma is a competitive option for motivated patients and physicians. Residual radiographic abnormalities are most often scar tissue or necrosis and do not need to be surgically resected. Patients with bulky retroperitoneal disease larger than 5 cm or stage III disease should be treated with chemotherapy (see Section III.D.2.d.).

2. **Nonseminoma**

   a. **Stage I disease.** Historically, these patients have been pathologically staged and treated with a retroperitoneal lymph node dissection (RPLND). Patients with pathologically confirmed stage I disease do not need any further therapy because only approximately 10% show relapse. In approximately 25% of patients, clinical stage I disease is found to be stage II pathologically at RPLND, and the treatment for these patients is discussed in the following section. The major complication of RPLND has been retrograde ejaculation with subsequent infertility, although its occurrence is rare in experienced centers using nerve-sparing procedures. The other option for selected patients is surveillance without RPLND. These patients should be chosen carefully and must be committed to careful lengthy follow-up. Because 30% of these patients eventually experience relapse, they must be followed up closely with monthly measurements of serum markers and chest radiographs for the first year and every other month the year after that. Abdominal CT scans should also be performed every 2 months the first year, every 4 months the second year, and every 6 months thereafter. If patients are selected and followed up appropriately, overall survival appears to be the same as for patients undergoing RPLND.

   b. **Stage II disease.** Patients with lymph nodes larger than 2 to 3 cm should be treated primarily with chemotherapy. If the lymph nodes measure less than 2 cm, an RPLND can be considered. Patients with pathologically confirmed and completely resected stage II disease have a relapse rate of approximately 30%. Patients with fully resected pathologic stage II disease can be either treated with two cycles of adjuvant chemotherapy after RPLND or followed up closely and treated with standard chemotherapy if they show relapse. Patients who choose to be under observation should receive monthly chest radiograph and serum marker evaluations and should be treated immediately if the disease recurs. Patients with stage II disease who have elevated markers after RPLND or whose disease is not completely resected should be treated in the same manner as patients with stage III disease.

   c. **Stage III disease.** Approximately 30% of patients present with stage III disease. The most common site of involvement is the lungs, but liver, bone, and brain can also be involved with metastatic disease. These patients are further categorized as good, intermediate, or poor risk on the basis of the primary site, level of marker elevation, and involvement of brain liver or bone. An international germ cell prognostic classification has been developed on the basis of a retrospective analysis of more than 5,000 patients with metastatic GCTs. Poor-risk (poor prognosis) patients according to the International Germ Cell Cancer Consensus Classification System include those with the following:

- Mediastinal primary site *or*
- Nonpulmonary visceral metastasis (e.g., liver, bone, and brain) *or*
- Elevation of AFP ($>10,000$ ng/mL), hCG ($>10,000$ ng/mL), or lactate dehydrogenase (LDH) $>10\times$ upper limit of normal (ULN);

Patients with nonseminoma without mediastinal primary or nonpulmonary visceral metastasis have the following:

- A good prognosis with the AFP <1,000 ng/mL, hCG <1,000 ng/mL, and LDH $<1.5\times$ ULN;
- An intermediate prognosis if any of the markers is in the intermediate range (AFP 1,000–10,000 ng/mL, hCG 1,000–10,000 ng/mL, and LDH $1.5–10\times$ (ULN).

d. Recommended therapy. All patients with stage II or III disease who require chemotherapy should receive cisplatin-based chemotherapy, **BEP,** as follows:

Cisplatin 20 mg/m^2 IV over 30 minutes on days 1 to 5, *and*

Etoposide 100 mg/m^2 IV on days 1 to 5, *and*

Bleomycin 30 U IV push weekly on days 1, 8, and 15

Repeat cycle every 21 days regardless of blood cell counts for two (adjuvant therapy), three (good-risk patients), or four (intermediate or poor risk patients) cycles.

If the patient has fever associated with granulocytopenia, we would give the next cycle at the same doses, followed by daily SC injections of granulocyte colony-stimulating factor (filgrastim or pegfilgrastim). Other chemotherapy regimens such as VIP (etoposide, ifosfamide, cisplatin) have not improved outcome and are more toxic. Substitution of carboplatin for cisplatin is inferior therapy and should not be used.

e. Surgery for residual disease. Patients who have a complete response with chemotherapy should be followed up and do not require any further treatment. Patients whose marker levels normalize but who have not achieved a radiographic complete response should undergo complete surgical resection of residual disease. If the resected material reveals only teratoma, necrosis, or fibrosis, then no further therapy is necessary, and the patient should be followed up. If there is carcinoma in the resected specimen, the patient should receive two more cycles of cisplatin-based chemotherapy (cisplatin and etoposide).

f. Follow-up. Most patients who experience relapse do so within the first 2 years, although late relapses do occur. In general, patients should be followed up with every 2-month physical examination, chest x-ray studies, and serum marker measurements during the first year and every 4 months during the second year. Patients should then be followed up every 6 months for the third and fourth years, and yearly thereafter. Because tumors can arise in the contralateral testis, patients should be taught to do testicular self-examination.

E. Salvage chemotherapy

1. Standard-dose therapy. Patients who respond to first-line chemotherapy and then relapse are still curable with salvage regimens such as VIP:

- Vinblastine 0.11 mg/kg (4.1 mg/m^2) IV push on days 1 and 2,
- Ifosfamide 1.2 g/m^2 IV over 30 minutes on days 1 to 5, *and*
- Cisplatin 20 mg/m^2 IV over 30 minutes on days 1 to 5.

Repeat every 21 days for four cycles. Any radiographic abnormalities that persist after salvage chemotherapy should be considered for surgical resection.

2. High-dose chemotherapy with autologous stem cell transplantation (ASCT). High-dose chemotherapy with carboplatin and etoposide with or without cyclophosphamide/ifosfamide followed by ASCT should be considered for patients requiring salvage chemotherapy. Overall, approximately 15% to 25% of these patients are long-term survivors. The role of ASCT in the initial salvage setting is still under evaluation. Patients with incomplete response, high markers, high disease volume, and late relapse may be best candidates for initial salvage ASCT.

F. Prognosis. With these strategies, the overall cure rate for patients with stage I disease is more than 98%, that for stage II disease more than 95%, and that for stage III disease more than 80%.

G. Complications of therapy. Because patients are cured, the short- and long-term toxicities are of considerable importance. The short-term toxicities of the chemotherapy regimens described include nausea and vomiting, myelosuppression, renal toxicity, and hemorrhagic cystitis. Major long-term morbidities include infertility, pulmonary fibrosis, and a small but definite risk of secondary leukemia.

H. Mediastinal and other midline GCTs. GCTs can arise in several midline structures including the retroperitoneum, mediastinum, and pineal gland. All patients with GCTs at these sites should have a testicular ultrasound examination to exclude an occult primary tumor. Mediastinal nonseminomatous GCTs are associated with Klinefelter's syndrome and with rare hematologic malignancies (particularly acute megakaryocytic leukemia). Small mediastinal seminomas can be treated with radiation therapy alone. Widespread tumors or nonseminomatous tumors should be treated with four cycles of BEP chemotherapy. Salvage chemotherapy (including autologous bone marrow transplantation [ABMT]) in patients with nonseminomatous mediastinal GCT is ineffective.

IV. Cancer of the penis

A. General considerations. Penile cancer is rare in North America but is a significant health problem in many developing countries. These tumors are nearly always of squamous cell origin and are associated with the presence of a foreskin and poor hygiene. Typically, these tumors present as a nonhealing ulcer or mass on the foreskin or glans. The most common treatment is wide surgical excision or penectomy, depending on the size and location of the lesion. Prophylactic inguinal lymph node dissection is indicated in certain subgroups of patients. Radiation therapy can also provide local control, especially with small tumors. However, local relapse may be up to 30% and surgery is still considered standard management, especially for larger tumors.

B. Chemotherapy for systemic disease. Active single agents include bleomycin, cisplatin, and methotrexate, with response rates of 20% to 50%. Combination chemotherapy results in high response rates, but whether survival is improved over that with single agents is unknown. A reasonable regimen is cisplatin 100 mg/m² on day 1, with fluorouracil 1,000 mg/m²/day given by continuous infusion on days 1 to 4. Cycles can be repeated every 21 days.

SUGGESTED READINGS

Testis

Bhatia S, Abonour R, Porcu P, et al. High-dose chemotherapy as initial salvage chemotherapy in patients with relapsed testicular cancer. *J Clin Oncol* 2000;18(19):3346–3351.

Bosl GJ, Motzer RJ. Testicular germ-cell cancer. *N Engl J Med* 1997;337:242–254.

International Germ Cell Cancer Collaborative Group. International germ cell consensus classification: a prognostic factor-based staging system for metastatic germ cell cancer. *J Clin Oncol* 1997;15: 594–603.

Loehrer PJ Sr, Gonin R, Nichols CR, et al. Vinblastine plus ifosfamide plus cisplatin as initial salvage therapy in recurrent germ cell tumor. *J Clin Oncol* 1998;16:2500–2504.

Saxman SB, Finch D, Gonin R, et al. Long-term follow-up of a phase III study of three versus four cycles of bleomycin, etoposide, and cisplatin in favorable-prognosis germ-cell tumors: the Indiana University experience. *J Clin Oncol* 1998;16(2):702–706.

Williams SD, Birch R, Einhorn LH, et al. Treatment of disseminated germ-cell tumors with cisplatin, bleomycin, and either vinblastine or etoposide. *N Engl J Med* 1987;316:1435–1440.

Bladder

Grossman HG, Natale RB, Tangen CM, et al. Neoadjuvant chemotherapy plus cystectomy compared with cystectomy alone for locally advanced bladder cancer. *N Engl J Med* 2003;349:859–866.

Herr HW, Schwalb DM, Zhang ZF, et al. Intravesical bacillus Calmette–Guérin therapy prevents tumor progression and death from superficial bladder cancer: ten-year follow-up of a prospective randomized trial. *J Clin Oncol* 1995;13:1404–1408.

Lamm DL, Blumenstein BA, Crawford ED, et al. A randomized trial of intravesical doxorubicin and immunotherapy with bacille

Calmette–Guérin for transitional-cell carcinoma of the bladder. *N Engl J Med* 1991;325:1205–1209.

Loehrer PJ Sr, Einhorn LH, Elson PJ, et al. A randomized comparison of cisplatin alone or in combination with methotrexate, vinblastine, and doxorubicin in patients with metastatic urothelial carcinoma: a Cooperative Group study. *J Clin Oncol* 1992;10:1066–1073.

von der Maase H, Hansen SW, Roberts JT, et al. Gemcitabine and cisplatin versus methotrexate, vinblastine, doxorubicin, and cisplatin in advanced or metastatic bladder cancer : results of a large, randomized, multinational, multicenter, phase III study. *J Clin Oncol* 2000;17:3068–3077.

Okeke AA, Probert JL, Gillatt DA, et al. Is intravesical chemotherapy for superficial bladder cancer still justified? *BJU Int* 2005;96:763–767.

Prostate

Bill-Axelson A, Holmberg L, Ruutu M, et al. Radical prostatectomy versus watchful waiting in early prostate cancer. *N Engl J Med* 2005;352:1977–1984.

Eisenberger MA, Blumenstein BA, Crawford ED, et al. Bilateral orchiectomy with or without flutamide for metastatic prostate cancer. *N Engl J Med* 1998;339(15):1036–1042.

Messing EM, Manola J, Sarosdy M, et al. Immediate hormonal therapy compared with observation after radical prostatectomy and pelvic lymphadenectomy in men with node-positive prostate cancer. *N Engl J Med* 1999;341:1781–1788.

Partin AW, Kattan MW, Subong ENP, et al. Combination of PSA clinical stage and Gleason score to predict pathology in men with localized prostate cancer: a multiinstitutional update. *JAMA* 1997;277:1445–1451.

Tannock IF, Osoba D, Stockler MR, et al. Chemotherapy with mitoxantrone plus prednisone or prednisone alone for symptomatic hormone-resistant prostate cancer: a Canadian randomized trial with palliative end points. *J Clin Oncol* 1996;14:1756–1764.

Tannock IF, de Wit R, Berry WR, et al. Docetaxel plus prednisone or mitoxantrone plus prednisone for advanced prostate cancer. *N Eng J Med* 2004;351:1502–1512.

Penile Cancer

Culkin DJ, Beer TM. Advanced penile carcinoma. *J Urol* 2003;170:359–365.

Kroon BK, Horenblas S, Nieweg O. Contemporary management of penile squamous cell carcinoma. *J Surg Oncol* 2005;89:43–50.

CHAPTER 13

Kidney Cancer

Walter D. Y. Quan, Jr. and Mikhail Vinogradov

Approximately 38,800 Americans were diagnosed with kidney cancer in 2006. Males accounted for approximately 24,600 of these new cases and for approximately 8,000 of the 12,800 deaths that occurred. The incidence of kidney cancer is increasing.

I. Carcinoma of the kidney

A. Cell types. Clear cell cancer of the kidney, which is an adenocarcinoma that arises from renal parenchyma, accounts for 85% of primary renal neoplasms. Papillary (or chromophilic) cancer is responsible for approximately 10%. Less common are oncocytomas (well-differentiated adenocarcinomas) and chromophobic types. Wilms' tumor (nephroblastoma) is seen predominantly in childhood. The term *hypernephroma* is a historic term for kidney cancer and is no longer commonly used.

B. Risk factors. In general, cigarette smoking is felt to roughly double the risk of kidney cancer. Approximately 30% of men and 25% of women with this cancer have a history of tobacco use. Industrial exposure to asbestos, cadmium, and the drug phenacetin have also been associated with higher risk. Lesser risk factors include acquired multicystic disease in patients undergoing hemodialysis for chronic renal failure, obesity, and hypertension. An important link has been established with the *von Hippel-Lindau* gene on chromosome 3 wherein its inactivation or deletion is associated both with enhanced production of vascular endothelial growth factor (VEGF) and a higher incidence of clear cell carcinoma of the kidney. VEGF is therefore felt to augment the growth of new blood vessels typically seen with clear cell kidney cancer and its metastases ("kidney cancer is a vascular cancer"). Clear cell kidney cancer is also associated with tuberous sclerosis.

C. Clinical characteristics. Common clinical symptoms/findings of kidney cancer include hematuria (56% of patients), flank pain (38%), abdominal mass (36%), weight loss (27%), and fever (11%). The classic triad of hematuria, flank pain, and abdominal mass occurs in less than 20% of patients. Because of its propensity to display paraneoplastic syndromes, kidney cancer is sometimes described as being "the internist's tumor." Up to 20% of patients without bone metastases may exhibit hypercalcemia thought to be possibly due to parathyroid hormone (PTH)-like peptide, osteoclast activating factor, or tumor necrosis factor. Excess erythropoietin production has been described in as many as 3% of patients. Other clinical manifestations may include hypertension, fever, anemia, and hyperglycemia. Up to 20% of patients may exhibit Stauffer syndrome, evidence of elevated alkaline phosphatase, activated partial thromboplastin time, liver function tests, and hepatomegaly without liver metastases. The etiology is unclear—biopsies show nonspecific

Table 13.1. Staging and prognosis of kidney cancer

Stage	Clinical Characteristic(s)	TNM	Five-Year Survival (%)
I	Tumor 7 cm or smaller confined to the kidney	T1, N0, M0	75
II	Tumor >7 cm confined to the kidney	T2, N0, M0	64
III	Tumor extending into major veins, adrenal gland, or perinephric tissues but not beyond Gerota's fascia or metastasis to single node	T3, N0, M0; or T1–3, N1, M0	32
IV	Tumor invading beyond Gerota's fascia or multiple lymph node metastases or distant metastatic disease	T4, any N, M0; any T, N2, M0; or any T, any N, M1	<10

hepatitis—but may be related to cytokine release, particularly, interleukin 6 (IL-6). This syndrome is reversible with therapy including nephrectomy.

Metastatic disease is present at initial presentation in approximately 25% to 30% of patients. The most common sites of metastases are lung, lymph node, liver, and bone. Brain metastases are often a late manifestation. Untreated patients with metastases or patients in whom treatment fails to halt disease progression may have a particularly dire prognosis with the median survival being approximately 6 months.

D. Staging. The TNM staging system together with expected 5-year survival by stage is listed in Table 13.1. Factors adversely affecting prognosis include hypercalcemia, serum lactate dehydrogenase (LDH) level more than 1.5 times the upper limit of normal, Karnofsky performance status less than 80%, comorbid medical conditions, anemia, or multiple sites of metastases. Newer methods of molecular, genomic, and proteomic profiling may further delineate prognostic factors in the future.

E. Treatment considerations. The treatment of choice for nonmetastatic kidney cancer is radical nephrectomy, including removal of the perinephric fat and regional lymph nodes. Partial nephrectomy is an option in patients with bilateral renal tumors or a solitary kidney to avoid the necessity of dialysis. Rarely, patients with solitary metastatic lesions can be cured by surgical removal of a metastasis at the time of nephrectomy. Kidney cancer is relatively radioresistant; thus, adjuvant radiation therapy does not improve survival. Radiation therapy can be useful for palliation of painful metastasis. It is reasonable to consider patients with inoperable metastatic disease for treatment with biologic agents, particularly IL-2, or molecular targeted therapy. Neither hormonal therapy nor chemotherapy has been shown to be beneficial.

A question of some controversy centers on whether nephrectomy should be done as an adjunct to systemic treatment in patients with metastases. Two randomized studies in metastatic disease have shown improved survival in the group treated with nephrectomy followed by interferon α versus interferon α alone. In contrast, a recent study with high-dose IL-2 showed no difference in response rate or survival between those undergoing nephrectomy initially and those who received IL-2 alone. Data show that approximately 35% of patients with distant metastases who undergo nephrectomy, are never able to receive any systemic treatment, usually because of disease progression.

F. Treatment regimens

1. Biologic response modifiers

a. Interleukin 2 (IL-2; Proleukin, aldesleukin) mediates its antitumor effects through activation of a patient's lymphocytes, particularly those that are CD56+, converting them into lymphokine-activated killer (LAK) cells. IL-2, alone or in combination with *ex vivo*-activated LAK, results in overall response rates of up to 18%. Complete responses, when obtained, tend to be long-lasting. There is a wide range of IL-2 doses and schedules, but recent randomized data suggest that high-dose therapy is more likely to lead to complete responses and a higher overall response rate than lower, subcutaneously administered outpatient therapy. It is most commonly used in a "high-dose" regimen of 600,000 IU/kg given in 15-minute IV infusions every 8 hours for up to 14 doses. This schedule produces responses in 15% to 22% of patients, many of long duration. Because this drug is associated with a capillary leak syndrome that can include hypotension, fluid retention, renal and hepatic hypoperfusion, and pulmonary edema, the dose and schedule mentioned in the preceding text require inpatient care. It should be used only by those experienced in its administration. Inpatient continuous infusion schedules (18 MIU/m² given over 24 hours for up to 5 consecutive days) may also be administered.

b. Sunitinib is a tyrosine kinase receptor inhibitor that interferes with tumor angiogenesis. Typical dosing is 50 mg orally per day for 4 weeks followed by a 2-week rest. Partial response rates of up to 40% with median time to disease progression of more than 8 months have been reported.

c. Sorafenib is another tyrosine kinase inhibitor, which, at doses of 400 mg orally twice per day, has been shown to improve progression-free survival versus placebo (24 vs. 12 weeks).

d. Temsirolimus (TEMSR) is a novel kinase inhibitor that is a derivative of the macrolide antibiotic and immunosuppressant sirolimus (rapamycin). After temsirolimus complexes with the immunophilin FKBP12, the complex inhibits mTOR (mammalian Target Of Rapamycin) kinase activity. mTOR, as a master regulator of cell physiology, is involved in regulation of cell growth and angiogenesis, and changes that are induced downstream from mTOR as a consequence of the temsirolimus inhibition lead to cell cycle arrest at the G_1 phase. In a randomized trial comparing interferon (IFN) with TEMSR in poor-risk patients with advanced renal cell carcinoma (RCC), overall survival was statistically better in the TEMSR arm (7.3 vs. 10.9 months).

e. IFN yields response rates of approximately 10%. Numerous treatment doses and schedules have been utilized. A representative one is 5 MIU/m^2 SC three times per week. The median response durations range between studies from 6 to 12 months. Response correlates with Karnofsky performance status equal to or more than 80% and prior nephrectomy.

f. Bevacizumab, an antibody to VEGF, has response rates of 10% with some patients having progression-free intervals as long as 5 years. Doses of up to 10 mg/kg IV every 2 weeks have been utilized.

g. Combination therapy. Combinations of IFN and IL-2 have been tested but have not been shown to be superior to IL-2 alone. Newer doublets including bevacizumab and erlotinib (another tyrosine kinase receptor inhibitor), sunitinib and IFN, and sorafenib plus IFN hold promise.

2. Cytotoxic chemotherapy/hormonal therapy. Of historic note, vinblastine, medroxyprogesterone acetate, and tamoxifen at best produce responses in fewer than 5% of patients and therefore cannot be recommended.

3. Adjuvant therapy. No adjuvant therapy has been proven to improve survival to date after resection of all known disease. A randomized study of high-dose bolus IL-2 versus placebo was stopped early. However, a trial comparing tyrosine kinase receptor inhibitors versus placebo has been initiated.

SUGGESTED READINGS

Atkins MB, Hidalgo M, Stadler WM, et al. Randomised Phase II study of multiple dose levels of CCI-779, a novel mammalian target of rapamycin kinase inhibitor, in patients with advanced refractory renal cell carcinoma. *J Clin Oncol* 2004;22:909–918.

Childs R, Chernoff A, Contentin N, et al. Regression of metastatic renal-cell carcinoma after nonmyeloablative allogeneic peripheral-blood stem-cell transplantation. *N Engl J Med* 2000;343:750–758.

Escudier B, Szczylik C, Eisen T, et al. Randomized phase III trial of the raf kinase and VEGF inhibitor sorafenib (BAy 43–9006) in patients with advanced renal cell carcinoma (RCC). *J Clin Oncol* 2005;23:380.

Figlin RA, Pierce WC, Kaboo R, et al. Treatment of metastatic renal cell carcinoma with nephrectomy, interleukin-2, and cytokine-primed or CD8(+) selected tumor infiltrating lymphocytes from primary tumor. *J Urol* 1997;158(3):740–745.

Fisher RI, Rosenberg SA, Fyfe G. Long-term survival update for high-dose recombinant interleukin-2 therapy in patients with renal cell carcinoma. *Cancer J Sci Am* 2000;6(Suppl 1):S55–S57.

Gollob J, Richmond T, Jones J, et al. Phase II trial of sorafenib plus interferon alpha 2b as first or second-line therapy in patients with metastatic renal cell cancer. *J Clin Oncol* 2006;24(Suppl 18S):226s.

Hainsworth JD, Sosman JA, Spigel DR, et al. Treatment of metastatic renal cell carcinoma with a combination of bevacizumab and erlotinib. *J Clin Oncol* 2005;23(31):7889–7896.

Hudes G, Carducci P, Tomczak J, et al. A phase 3, randomized, 3-arm study of Temsirolimus (TEMSR) or interferon-alpha (IFN) or the combination of TEMSR + IFN in the treatment of first-line, poor-risk patients with advanced renal cell carcinoma (adv RCC). *J Clin Oncol* 2006;24(18S):LBA4. ASCO Annual Meeting Proceedings Part I.

Mandell JS, McLaughlin JK, Schlehofer B, et al. International renal-cell study. IV. Occupation. *Int J Cancer* 1995;61:601–605.

McDermott DF, Regan MM, Clark JI, et al. Randomized phase III trial of high-dose interleukin-2 versus subcutaneous interleukin-2 and interferon in patients with metastatic renal cell carcinoma. *J Clin Oncol* 2005;23(1):133–141.

Motzer RJ, Mazumdar M, Bacik J, et al. Survival and prognostic stratification of 670 patients with advanced renal cell carcinoma. *J Clin Oncol* 1999;17(8):2530–2540.

Motzer RJ, Michaelson MD, Redman BG, et al. Activity of SU11248, a multitargeted inhibitor of vascular endothelial growth factor receptor and platelet-derived growth factor receptor, in patients with metastatic renal cell carcinoma. *J Clin Oncol* 2006;24:16–24.

Rini BI, Small EJ. Biology and clinical development of vascular endothelial growth factor- targeted therapy in renal cell carcinoma. *J Clin Oncol* 2005;23:1028–1043.

Rosenberg SA, Lotze MT, Muul LM, et al. A progress report on the treatment of 157 patients with advanced cancer using lymphokine-activated killer cells and interleukin-2 or high-dose interleukin-2 alone. *N Engl J Med* 1987;316:889–897.

Rosenberg SA, Lotze MT, Yang JC, et al. Prospective randomized trial of high-dose interleukin-2 alone or in conjunction with lymphokine-activated killer cells for the treatment of patients with advanced cancer. *J Natl Cancer Inst* 1993;85:622–632.

Rosenberg SA, Yang JC, Topalian SL, et al. Treatment of 283 consecutive patients with metastatic melanoma or renal cell cancer using high-dose bolus interleukin-2. *JAMA* 1994;271:907–913.

Ryan CW, Goldman BH, Lara PN Jr, et al. Sorafenib plus interferon-a2b as first-line therapy for advanced renal cell carcinoma: SWOG 0412. *J Clin Oncol* 2006;24 (Suppl 18S):223s.

Schwartzentruber D. Guidelines for the safe administration of high-dose interleukin-2. *J Immunother* 2001;24:287–292.

Thompson JA, Shulman KL, Benyunes MC, et al. Prolonged continuous intravenous infusion interleukin-2 and lymphokine-activated killer-cell therapy for metastatic renal cell carcinoma. *J Clin Oncol* 1992;10:960–968.

Yang JC. Bevacizumab for patients with metastatic renal cancer: an update. *Clin Cancer Res* 2004;10(18 Pt 2):6367S–6370S.

CHAPTER 14

Thyroid and Adrenal Carcinomas

Haitham S. Abu-Lebdeh and Samir N. Khleif

Endocrine cancers account for 1.5% of all cancers diagnosed and for 0.4% of cancer deaths. Thyroid cancer is the most common endocrine malignancy, accounting for 90% of endocrine cancers and for 60% to 70% of the deaths from this group of diseases. Although the role of cytotoxic chemotherapy is limited in endocrine cancer, it is beneficial in select patients. Pancreatic islet cell carcinomas and other pancreatic malignancies are discussed in Chapter 9. Here, thyroid and adrenal carcinomas are discussed. The pathology, presentation, and biologic behavior of thyroid and adrenal carcinomas are important determinants of therapy and are briefly considered.

I. Thyroid carcinoma
A. Background
1. **Incidence.** Approximately 17,000 new cases of thyroid carcinoma are diagnosed each year, with approximately 1,200 deaths due to this cancer. The incidence of thyroid carcinoma is 5.9 per 100,000 women and 2.2 per 100,000 men, and the peak incidence is at age 40 in women and age 60 in men. The prevalence at autopsy is 5 to 15 per 100,000 subjects. The incidence of thyroid cancer is increasing each year. Thyroid carcinoma usually affects people between the ages of 25 and 65 years.

2. **Etiology and prevention.** In most instances, the cause of thyroid carcinoma is unknown, although experimentally prolonged stimulation by thyroid-stimulating hormone (TSH) may lead to the development of thyroid carcinoma. Some cases appear to be related to a dose-dependent phenomenon involving radiation to the neck during childhood. Thyroid malignancy has been observed 20 to 25 years after radiation exposure in atomic bomb survivors and in children treated with radiation therapy for benign conditions of the head and neck. The frequency increases exponentially with doses up to 12 Gy and then decreases, so that with doses over 20 Gy, the risk of developing malignancy becomes relatively low because such high doses lead to the destruction of cells rather than non-lethal damage of the deoxyribonucleic acid (DNA). In cases of accidental nuclear exposure, it is thought that the use of potassium iodide to block the thyroid uptake of radioactive iodine (RAI) in children is helpful in reducing the incidence of subsequent thyroid cancer. This measure was used in Eastern Europe after the Chernobyl accident. Although ionizing radiation for benign conditions of the head and neck is no longer being used, thyroid carcinomas related to prior exposure to radiation are still being seen. Some

cases of thyroid carcinoma (usually medullary carcinoma) are familial, as seen in the multiple endocrine neoplasia (MEN) syndrome, associated with germline mutation of the *RET* proto-oncogene. Furthermore, mutations in the follicular thyroid cell signaling pathway are associated with tumor development. For example, *RET/PTC* gene rearrangements and Ras, BRAF and MEK-ERK pathway mutations are present in 70% of papillary thyroid cancer. Abnormalities in the p53-catenin pathway are associated with the development of anaplastic thyroid cancer. The least understood cancer is follicular carcinoma, but this is also associated with Ras and mutations on chromosome 3 (pax8-PPAR mutations).

3. **Histologic types.** The most common histologic types of thyroid carcinoma are as follows:

   a. **Differentiated thyroid cancer (DTC).** DTC includes papillary carcinoma (75%–80%) and follicular carcinoma (11%). DTCs are derived from thyroglobulin-producing follicular cells and are typically RAI responsive, especially in initial stages.

   b. **Anaplastic or undifferentiated carcinoma (2%)**

   c. **Medullary carcinoma (4%).** Medullary carcinomas are derived from thyroid parafollicular or C cells. These cells produce both immunoreactive calcitonin and carcinoembryonic antigen (CEA).

   d. **Hürthle cell carcinoma (3%).** Hürthle cell carcinoma used to be considered a variant of follicular carcinoma. It is now considered as a separate pathologic entity, and is characterized by relative RAI resistance.

   e. **Thyroid lymphoma (5%)**

4. **Prognosis**

   a. **Cell types.** Papillary and mixed papillary and follicular histologies are considered to have similar biologic and prognostic behaviors. Patients with these cancers have an excellent prognosis, with less than 15% mortality at 20 years. However, survival rates are significantly reduced if distant metastasis is detected. Patients with pure follicular carcinoma do not do as well as those with papillary elements, at least in part because there is a tendency for the follicular carcinoma to spread through the bloodstream, whereas the papillary carcinoma spreads more by lymphatic channels. The 10-year relative survival rates are 85% and 93%, respectively. Recent studies have shown that patients having follicular carcinoma with vascular invasion have a relatively bad prognosis, whereas patients with follicular carcinoma without vascular invasion do almost as well as those with papillary carcinoma. Approximately 25% of medullary carcinomas are familial, as part of three clinical syndromes (MEN 2A, MEN 2B, and familial non-MEN medullary thyroid carcinoma). Regional lymph node and distant metastases are common in patients with medullary carcinomas and occur in early stages of the disease. The 10-year survival rate after surgical resection is 40% to 60%. Patients with anaplastic thyroid carcinoma have an abysmal prognosis, with a median survival time of 4 months, although occasional patients may be cured with combined radiotherapy and chemotherapy.

b. Other factors. In addition to the cell type, the prognosis of thyroid carcinoma is shown to be worse if the following factors are present:

- A large tumor size, especially more than 4 cm.
- Patient age more than 40 years.
- Distant metastases. DTC tends to metastasize to the lung or bone. Patients with bone metastases have survival rates of 53%, 38%, and 30% at 5, 10, and 15 years, respectively.
- Abnormal DNA content in tumor cells in the papillary type; the more pronounced the aneuploidy, the more aggressively the cancer behaves.
- Male sex, which may be related to the fact that men tend to be older at the time of diagnosis and are more likely to have a worse histologic type.

In contrast to most other cancers, limited regional lymph node metastasis of DTC does not influence survival substantially, and radiation-induced thyroid carcinoma is not associated with a worse prognosis.

B. Diagnosis and staging. Any solitary thyroid nodule should be considered a possible malignant tumor until proved otherwise, especially in patients younger than 25 years and men older than 60 years. Although toxic nodular goiters are less likely to contain carcinoma, a nodule in the setting of hyperthyroidism does not automatically confer benignity. The overall incidence of cancer in a "cold" nodule is 5% to 10%. Because most thyroid tumors spread primarily by local extension and regional nodal metastasis, assessment of the extent of disease is concentrated on the neck. Presurgical studies include careful physical examination, thyroid function tests, thyroid ultrasound and cytology by fine needle aspiration (FNA). Unlike core needle biopsy, FNA biopsy yields an aspirate of cells and not a tissue fragment. FNA does not require local anesthesia and is considered safer and easier to perform. The accuracy of needle aspiration biopsy ranges between 50% and 97%, depending on the experience of the pathologist and the institution.

Other studies such as indirect laryngoscopy, radionuclide scanning, esophagogram, and computed tomography (CT) scan of the neck can be performed on a case-by-case basis. In a few instances, a core needle biopsy might be considered. If there is a strong clinical suspicion of thyroid lymphoma and FNA is not diagnostic, then a core needle biopsy should be considered as an alternative to a surgical biopsy that requires general anesthesia. Chest radiography should be performed before surgery to rule out pulmonary metastasis. If there is any clinical or laboratory suggestion of bone metastases, skeletal x-rays, CT scan, or a radionuclide bone scan should be performed. Patients with thyroid carcinoma are typically euthyroid. Thyroid carcinoma rarely destroys thyroid tissue to the point of frank hypothyroidism. However, elevated TSH levels with increased thyroid peroxidase antibodies may be

Table 14.1. Pathologic TNM staging system for thyroid cancer

Stage	Papillary or Follicular, Age <45	Papillary or Follicular, Age >45; Medullary, Any Age	Anaplastic, Any Age
I	M0	T1, N0, M0	—
II	M1	T2, N0, M0	—
III	—	T3, N0, M0	—
		T1–3, N1a, M0	
IV	—	T4, Any N, M0	Any T, N, or M
		T1–3, N1b, M0	
		Any T, Any N, M1	

T4 = Any tumor invading tissue beyond thyroid capsule.
N1a = Metastasis to central lymph node compartment.
N1b = Metastasis to other lymph nodes.
M0 = no evidence for metastasis.
M1 = distant metastasis is present.

seen with Hashimoto's thyroiditis, which may coexist in 20% of patients with thyroid lymphoma.

The most widely accepted staging system is the pathologic TNM (pTNM) classification, which assesses tumor size and extent (T1, <2 cm; T2, 2–4 cm; T3, >4 cm), lymph node metastasis, and distant metastasis (Table 14.1). With the use of pTNM staging, any anaplastic thyroid cancer is considered stage IV, and there are no stage III or IV patients with DTC who are younger than 45 years. This staging system does not provide all the information needed. Other staging or risk-group assignment systems are used for providing prognostic information.

C. Treatment. The therapeutic approach to patients with thyroid carcinoma depends considerably on the histologic type.

1. Differentiated thyroid carcinoma (DTC)

a. Surgery is the only definitive therapy. Although the surgical approach may differ among surgeons and institutions, many surgeons prefer a bilateral, near-total, or total thyroidectomy, taking into consideration that with DTC, the incidence of disease in the contralateral lobe is 20% to 87%. Limited lymph node involvement does not substantially influence the survival rate, but it is associated with an increase in local recurrence and therefore routine central compartment neck dissection should be considered. Total thyroidectomy with modified neck dissection is often preferred for those who have lateral cervical lymph node involvement. Mortality after thyroidectomy in DTC approaches 0%. Complications include permanent recurrent laryngeal nerve damage in 2% of patients and permanent hypoparathyroidism in 1% to 2%.

b. TSH suppression is an essential component in the treatment of DTC because there is good evidence that cells are usually responsive to TSH. TSH suppresses the growth of malignant as well as normal thyroid tissue, and therefore the recurrence rate is reduced; in a few patients, metastatic lesions are diminished markedly. This hormonal suppression can be achieved by the administration of exogenous thyroid hormone. Usually 125 to 200 μg of levothyroxine (T4) daily is used to keep the TSH level in the range of 0.1 to 0.4 mIU/L. Complete TSH suppression (0.01–0.1 mIU/L) should be reserved for high-risk patients to avoid long-term adverse effects on bone and heart. Side effects and dose-limiting factors include symptoms of thyrotoxicosis, angina, and cardiac arrhythmia.

c. Radiotherapy. Destruction of residual normal thyroid tissue after thyroidectomy with radioactive iodine (RAI-[131I]) is termed *radioactive remnant ablation* (RRA). RRA is different from "RAI therapy." In RAI therapy larger doses of RAI are used to destroy persistent cancer or distant metastasis. RRA is widely used in the United States. When ablation is carried out postoperatively, it is usually done 4 to 6 weeks after thyroidectomy. RRA allows for better subsequent imaging with RAI when looking for metastasis. It also improves the sensitivity for thyroglobulin measurements (since remnant thyroid tissue is destroyed) and may destroy microscopic cancer cells within the remnant. A dose of 30 mCi (1,110 MBq) to 150 mCi (5,550 MBq) of RAI is usually used. Most centers use the lower dose of 30 mCi, which is estimated to expose the whole body to approximately 6 mSv. For patients who are at low risk (tumor size <1 cm), ablation is controversial. Many physicians still ablate to allow for an easier follow-up. RRA is strongly recommended for patients who are at high risk of recurrence or metastasis (patients older than 45 years or with large lesions or multifocal disease). Once ablation is successful, patients are placed on suppressive therapy.

Treatment with RAI (131I) (RAI therapy) is usually recommended for patients with DTC and known postoperative residual disease, patients with distant metastases, and patients with locally invasive lesions. For patients with nodal metastases that are not large enough to excise, a dose of 100 to 175 mCi of RAI is given (3,700–6,475 MBq). Locally invasive cancer that is not completely resected is treated with 150 to 200 mCi of RAI (5,550–7,400 MBq). Patients with distant metastasis are treated with 200 mCi (7,400 MBq). The exception is lung metastasis; a dose of up to 80 mCi of RAI (2,960 MBq) whole body retention as determined by dosimetry at 48 hours is generally used to avoid radiation-induced fibrosis. Effective use of RAI treatment requires the following:

1. Tumor cells that are capable of receiving and concentrating iodide (i.e., DTC), *and*
2. Appropriate patient preparation by either withholding thyroid hormone administration for a short period

of time to provide the iodine-concentrating cells with the highest endogenous TSH stimulation or by using recombinant thyroid-stimulating hormone (rhTSH) to stimulate thyroid cell uptake of RAI.

T3 is cleared from the body much more rapidly than T4. The shorter period of withdrawal minimizes the period of hypothyroidism. Accordingly, patients are switched from suppression therapy with T4 to a corresponding dose of T3 for 4 weeks to allow metabolic disposal of the T4. This is followed by 2 weeks of T3 withdrawal. Ideally, TSH of at least 25 to 30 µm/mL is required for successful ablation or radiotherapy. Potential side effects expected after radioiodine therapy include temporary bone marrow depression, nausea, sialoadenitis with possible permanent cessation of salivary flow (radiation mumps), skin reaction over the tissue concentrating the radioiodine, and pulmonary fibrosis. The use of high doses (cumulative effect) may be associated with acute myelogenous leukemia, bladder and breast cancer, and transient bone marrow depression. Patients with lung metastases treated with RAI have a 20-year survival rate of 54%. Scintigraphy should be performed 4 to 10 days after therapy to detect any residual carcinoma. Most DTCs grow very slowly. The rate of recurrence is 0.5% to 1.6% per year. Therefore, lifelong annual serum thyroglobulin assays are recommended. Several centers also advocate the use of neck ultrasounds for follow-up. The role of external radiation therapy in DTC is limited. It is considered for residual cervical tumors that do not concentrate iodine. It is also used for localized painful bony metastasis, or metastatic lesions that are not amenable to surgery such as in the pelvis, vertebra or central nervous system (CNS).

2. Medullary thyroid carcinoma. With familial medullary carcinoma, the disease is almost always bilateral. Regional lymph node involvement is common in early stages. Therefore, total thyroidectomy, central lymph node dissection, and lateral ipsilateral modified radical neck dissection are required. The overall 10-year survival rate after surgical resection is 40% to 60%. Serum calcitonin levels should be measured 8 to 12 weeks postoperatively to assess disease burden and residual cancer. Search for germline and not somatic *RET* proto-oncogene mutations identifies most familial cases. For other family members with a positive *RET* proto-oncogene, surgery is recommended as early as at an age of 2 years. Postoperative annual evaluation is recommended by measuring levels of calcitonin and CEA, both of which are secreted by the medullary thyroid carcinoma cells, as a follow-up for residual disease or recurrence. Suppressive therapy is of no benefit because medullary cells do not have TSH receptors. RAI and cytotoxic chemotherapy are of little utility. Cisplatin, streptozocin, carmustine, methotrexate, and fluorouracil have shown little, if any, benefit. However, some studies have shown doxorubicin chemotherapy to produce occasional responses of metastatic disease (see Section I.C.4).

Local radiation therapy is useful in some patients as palliative therapy.

3. Anaplastic thyroid carcinoma. Most anaplastic tumors are unresectable at the time of presentation. A more complete thyroid resection is associated with longer survival than biopsy alone. Combination chemotherapy or chemotherapy plus radiation therapy has shown encouraging results for local control, and few partial and complete remissions have been seen.

4. Chemotherapy

a. Single-agent chemotherapy. The most widely applied cytotoxic agents are doxorubicin, bleomycin, cisplatin, and etoposide. Each of these medications has demonstrated some activity against anaplastic and medullary thyroid carcinomas. Improved survival may be achieved in patients who respond to sequential exposure to these agents. Doxorubicin has proved to be the best single chemotherapeutic agent with the highest response rate.

- **Doxorubicin** in a dosage of 60 to 75 mg/m^2 IV every 3 weeks has resulted in objective responses in 20% to 45% (median 34%) of patients with advanced refractory metastatic thyroid carcinoma. The response rate is probably highest for the medullary type and lowest for undifferentiated thyroid carcinoma. A high single dose of doxorubicin, which should be increased in patients with no response, appears to be essential for a therapeutic effect. Because of its apparently lower cardiotoxicity, epirubicin, although almost as effective as doxorubicin, may be given at higher doses and over longer periods and is therefore preferred by some investigators.

b. Combination chemotherapy. Combination chemotherapy usually includes doxorubicin.

- **Cisplatin** 40 mg/m^2 IV plus **doxorubicin** 60 mg/m^2 IV every 3 weeks has yielded a higher rate and quality of response than doxorubicin alone. These results included complete remission in 12% of patients, several of whom may be expected to survive for more than 2 years. Toxicity was no worse with the combination therapy. Other combination-chemotherapy regimens are doxorubicin, bleomycin, vincristine, and melphalan, with a response rate of 36%, and doxorubicin, bleomycin, and vincristine, with an improved 64% response rate.

- **Doxorubicin** 10 mg/m^2 IV has been used in combination with **external beam radiotherapy** 90 minutes before the first radiation treatment and weekly thereafter. In this combination, the radiotherapy was given at a dose of 1.6 Gy/treatment twice a day for 3 consecutive days weekly for 6 weeks. Patients with undifferentiated thyroid carcinoma treated in this manner showed an improvement in the median survival as compared with historical control subjects.

- **Carboplatin** 300 mg/m^2 IV infusion and **epirubicin** 75 mg/m^2 IV bolus every 4 to 6 weeks for 6 courses used in a small study in association with rhTSH or thyroxine dose adjustments to stimulate the biological activity of thyroid cancer cells showed improved prognosis over historical controls.

In general, the highest response is observed in patients with pulmonary metastasis. If anaplastic thyroid carcinoma responds to chemotherapy, a prolongation of the median survival time from 3 to 5 months to 15 to 20 months can be achieved. The benefit of chemotherapy is modest at best; therefore, novel therapies targeting specific tumor signaling pathway are under way. These include angiogenesis inhibitors targeting vascular endothelial growth factors, tyrosine kinase inhibitors which target *RET/PTC* oncogene signal, proteasome inhibitor (bortezomib), and DNA methylation inhibitor (decitabine). For a list of active trials visit www.clinicaltrials.gov.

5. **Non–Hodgkin's lymphoma.** Non–Hodgkin's lymphoma is more thoroughly addressed in Chapter 23. The discussion here briefly highlights its significance concerning thyroid malignancies. By definition, lymphoma of the thyroid is, at the time of diagnosis, confined to the gland or to the gland and regional lymph nodes. The major histologic type is non–Hodgkin's lymphoma. Autoimmune thyroiditis is a predisposing factor. Lymphoma of the thyroid usually presents with rapid enlargement of the gland within a few weeks and is bilateral in 25% of patients. If the tumor is confined to the thyroid, surgical excision alone yields a 5-year survival rate of 70% to 90%. Once the lymphoma extends beyond the thyroid gland, however, surgical therapy does not improve survival, and radiation therapy and chemotherapy are indicated.

II. Adrenal carcinoma

A. Adrenocortical carcinoma (ACC)

1. **Incidence and etiology.** ACC is a rare tumor, with fewer than 200 new cases occurring yearly in the United States. It accounts for 0.05% to 0.20% of all cancers and for 0.2% of cancer deaths. It has a prevalence of 2 per 1 million population worldwide. The peak incidence of ACC is during the fourth and fifth decades of life. The incidence in women in most reports is approximately 2.5 times higher than that in men, who tend to be older at diagnosis. Women have a tendency to develop a functional (hormone-secreting) carcinoma, whereas men usually develop a nonfunctional malignancy. There is no family predilection, and no etiologic factors have been established, although loss of genes on chromosome 17 and gene rearrangements on chromosome 11 are associated with ACC. Most cancers are monoclonal, suggesting that a genetic alteration in a progenitor cell contributes to tumorigenesis. Sometimes, it occurs in the context of tumor-predisposing syndromes such as Beckwith-Wiedemann syndrome or Li-Fraumeni syndrome, which is caused by an inactivating

mutation in the TP53 tumor suppressor gene on chromosome 17.

2. Clinical picture. Adrenal carcinoma may present in several modes.

a. Forty percent to 60% of patients present with **functioning tumor**, with endocrine signs and symptoms of Cushing's syndrome; virilization, or feminization maybe detected. Such manifestations are due to an increase in the production of a wide variety of steroid hormones. Ten percent of ACCs are associated with virilization and 12% with feminization. Adrenal carcinoma is the cause of 10% of all cases of Cushing's syndrome.

b. Other frequent presenting symptoms include upper abdominal pain, weight loss, palpable abdominal mass, anorexia, and malaise. Usually, these symptoms are associated with advanced disease.

c. An abdominal mass maybe detected incidentally by abdominal imaging for some other purpose.

3. Pathology and diagnosis. Most malignant adrenal masses represent carcinomatous metastatic lesions, primarily from the lung and breast. Whether the coincidental finding of an adrenal mass requires complete screening of the patient for a hidden primary adrenal tumor depends on the clinical situation. There may be some difficulty distinguishing adenoma from carcinoma (Table 14.2). CT scan and magnetic resonance imaging (MRI) are helpful in diagnosing ACC. A CT finding of a large unilateral adrenal mass

Table 14.2. Diagnosis of malignancy in adrenocortical neoplasms

Reliability	Clinical Criteria	Pathologic Criteria
Diagnostic of malignancy	Weight loss, feminization, nodal or distant metastases	Tumor weight >100 g, tumor necrosis, fibrous bands, vascular invasion, mitoses
Consistent with malignancy	Virilism, Cushing's syndrome and virilism, no hormone production	Nuclear pleomorphism
Suggestive of malignancy	Elevated urinary 17-ketosteroid levels	Capsular invasion
Unreliable	Hypercortisolism, hyperaldosteronism	Tumor giant cells, cytoplasmic size variations, ratio between compact and clear cells

Adapted from Page DL, DeLellis RA, Hough AJ. Tumors of the adrenal. *In:* Hartmann WH, Sobin LH, eds. *Atlas of tumor pathology.* Washington, DC: Armed Forces Institute of Pathology, 1986.

with irregular borders and a heterogeneous and hypervascular interior is almost always an indication of adrenal cancer. On MRI, adrenal cancer has intermediate to high signal intensity on T2-weighted images in contrast to benign lesions, which have low signal intensity. In addition, MRI is a helpful tool in delineating ACC before surgery. Iodocholesterol scanning is rarely indicated. It shows poor uptake in carcinomas as compared with adenomas. ACC can be further divided into two categories according to the pathologic patterns of cellular arrangement and the cellular pleomorphism:

> **a. Well-differentiated ACC,** which occurs more commonly in women and usually presents with a functioning tumor, *and*
>
> **b. Anaplastic ACC,** which is more common in men and is often associated with a lack of hormone production.

4. Staging and prognosis. Most patients (70%) present with stage III or IV disease. ACC is a highly malignant cancer with an overall 5-year mortality rate of 75% to 90%, depending on the stage and morphology of the disease. The most commonly used staging system (derived from the TNM classification system) for ACC is presented in Table 14.3.

Metastases of ACC most commonly occur in the lung (60%), lymph nodes (43%), liver (53%), and bone (10%). The median survival time of patients with well-differentiated carcinoma is 40 months, whereas patients with anaplastic carcinoma have a more dismal median survival time of 5 months. The median survival time of patients with stage I, II, or III disease is 24 to 28 months and for stage IV disease, it is 12 months. Intratumoral hemorrhage, number of mitotic figures per high-power field, and tumor size correlate with survival rates.

5. Treatment. Because of the extremely low incidence of this disease, few medical centers have sufficient experience treating it, and an effort should be made to refer these patients to centers that have clinical trials pertaining to this disease. This caveat notwithstanding, several guidelines regarding its treatment can be given.

Table 14.3. TNM staging system for adrenocortical cancer

Stage	Size (cm)	Nodes or Local Invasion	Metastasis
I	≤5	−	−
II	>5	−	−
III	Any	+	−
IV	Any	Either present or absent	+

−, absent; +, present.

a. Surgery. In up to half the number of patients, ACCs can be resected, although incompletely in some patients; however, the remainder of patients have either local invasion that is too extensive or metastases to the abdomen, liver, lung, or other locations. Of the patients whose tumors are resected for cure, 40% remain disease free. The remainder die, usually with extensive metastatic disease, within an average of less than 1 year. Patients who undergo complete resection should initially be followed up on a monthly basis (with measurements of steroid levels if they have a functioning tumor) to detect recurrence. Serial MRI may also be used to evaluate for recurrence.

b. Radiotherapy. Radiation therapy provides symptomatic relief from pain due to local or metastatic disease, especially bony metastases. It has also been used to prevent local recurrence after surgical resection (40–55 Gy over 4 weeks), but the benefit is uncertain, and there is no proof that it improves survival.

c. Chemotherapy. Indications for chemotherapy include recurrent, metastatic, and nonresectable ACC. Agents used are the following:

(1) Adrenocortical suppressants

(a) Mitotane (*o,p′*-DDD, Lysodren). An unconventional chemotherapeutic agent and a close chemical relative of the insecticide 1,1-bis (*p*-chlorophenyl)-2,2,2-trichloroethane (DDT), mitotane has been used to treat ACC since 1960. It inhibits steroid biosynthesis and with prolonged use destroys adrenal cells. The cytotoxic effect of mitotane has been considered transient and inconsistent. Included in its effects is the destruction of the adrenocortical cells. The part that is most affected by this action is the zona reticularis and the least affected is the zona glomerulosa. Forty percent of the medication is absorbed from the gastrointestinal tract. The drug is highly lipid soluble and is subsequently concentrated in both normal and malignant adrenocortical cells. Reports of its plasma half-life range from 18 to 159 days.

(i) Dosage and administration. Treatment with mitotane is started at 2 to 6 g/day PO in three divided doses, then gradually increased monthly by 1 g/day until 9 to 10 g/day is reached or until the maximum tolerated dose is achieved with no side effects. Blood levels of *o,p′*-DDD should be maintained at more than 14 μg/mL to demonstrate a therapeutic response. Mitotane serum level was shown in a retrospective study to be the only significant prognostic factor for tumor response. Levels of more than 20 μg/mL have a higher incidence of toxicity. Starting at a small dose and increasing it gradually may delay achieving adequate plasma levels;

frequently, starting at a higher dose of 6 to 9 g may be tolerated and may shorten the time required to achieve a therapeutic effect.

(ii) Response and follow-up. Objective tumor regression usually occurs within 6 weeks of the initiation of therapy and is seen in 70% of patients as a decrease in excessive hormone production. However, the reduction in hormone production is not regularly accompanied by an objective tumor response. In approximately 30% to 40% of patients, the tumor size is reduced significantly, but complete remission is unlikely. The median duration of response is 10.5 months. If no clinical benefit is demonstrated at the maximum tolerated dose after 3 months, the case may be considered a clinical failure. Postoperative adjuvant therapy with mitotane has resulted in no improvement in survival. The combination of mitotane and radiation therapy has not conferred any additional benefit over mitotane alone.

(iii) Side effects. Nausea and vomiting occur in 80% of patients. Severe neurotoxicity, which may occur during long-term treatment, presents as somnolence, depression, ataxia, and weakness in 40% of patients. Reversible diffuse electroencephalographic changes may also occur. Adrenal insufficiency occurs in 50% of patients (without replacement), and dermatitis develops in 20% of patients. Because the maximal dosage is often limited by the severity of, and the patient's tolerance to, the side effects, the total dose may range widely from patient to patient.

(iv) Glucocorticoid replacement. During mitotane treatment, it is necessary to prevent hypoadrenalism. Replacement can be achieved by administering cortisone acetate 25 mg PO in the morning and 12.5 mg PO in the evening or equivalent glucocorticoid plus fludrocortisone acetate 0.1 mg PO in the morning. Plasma cortisol should be used to monitor adrenal function during mitotane use. If severe trauma or shock develops, mitotane should be discontinued immediately and larger doses of corticosteroids (e.g., hydrocortisone 100 mg t.i.d.) should be administered.

(b) Non-responders to mitotane. These patients can be treated with other adrenocortical suppressants including **metyrapone** (750 mg PO every 4 hours), which reduces cortisol production by inhibiting 11β-hydroxylase. However, this results in accumulation of deoxycorticosterone and can induce hypertension and hypokalemic alkalosis.

Another agent is **aminoglutethimide** (250 mg PO every 6 hours initially, with a stepwise increase in dosage to a total of 2 g/day or until limiting side effects that resemble those of mitotane appear). The latter drug inhibits conversion of cholesterol to pregnenolone. Neither of these medications has antitumor effects, but they are effective in relieving the signs and symptoms of excessive hormonal secretion. Combining both in smaller doses might reduce the side effects seen in taking higher doses of either agent alone. Another medication that can be used is **ketoconazole** 600 mg/day. It is a potent adrenal inhibitor that produces clinical alleviation of the signs and symptoms within 4 to 6 weeks. In addition, it may cause regression of pulmonary and hepatic metastases, although the mechanism is not clear. Other drugs that might be of benefit in controlling symptoms include those that block the action of steroids in their target tissues, including antimineralocorticoid and antiandrogenic agents and, more recently, antiglucocorticoid agents such as mifepristone (RU 486). None of these medications has an effect on tumor regression.

(2) Cytotoxic chemotherapy. Cytotoxic drugs are usually used in patients who show no response to mitotane. Because of the small number of patients who require such therapy, the experience with this treatment is limited despite many clinical trials. No cytotoxic monotherapy has shown definite effectiveness in the treatment of ACC, although doxorubicin, cisplatin, and suramin have been reported to produce partial responses in patients with metastatic disease.

- **Cisplatin** 75 to 100 mg/m^2 was combined with **mitotane** 4 g PO daily.

  This resulted in a 30% objective response that lasted for 7.9 months. The survival duration in this study was 11.8 months. Few combination-chemotherapy regimens have been effective.

- **Etoposide** 100 mg/m2 IV on day 1 to 3 plus **cisplatin** 100 mg/m^2 IV given in cycles every 4 weeks plus mitotane led to partial remission in 33% of 18 patients with ACC.

The most used regimen is

- **Etoposide** 100 mg/m^2 on days 5 to 7, **doxorubicin** 20 mg/m^2 on days 1 and 8, **cisplatin** 40 mg/m^2 on days 1 and 9 every 4 weeks, combined with **mitotane** 4 g/day (EPD + M) for 3 to 8 months.

This was associated with approximately 50% response rate. Another frequently used regimen is a combination of streptozotocin 1 g/day for 5 days then 2 g every 3 weeks combined with mitotane 1 to 4 g daily. A third regimen is used as salvage therapy for patients failing the protocol mentioned in the preceding text; this includes vincristine 1.5 mg/m^2 on day 1, cisplatin 100 mg/m^2 on day 2, teniposide 150 mg/m^2 on day 4, and cyclophosphamide 600 mg/m^2 on day 1 (OPEC) every 4 weeks for 6 months. This salvage regimen improved survival rates as compared to historical controls. Other combinations of natural-product chemotherapy with mitotane are being tested; this may be pharmacologically advantageous because mitotane has been shown to be a multidrug resistance–blocking agent. The role of vascular endothelial growth factor inhibitors, thalidomide and tyrosine kinase inhibitors are being evaluated in treatment of ACC as well.

d. Arterial embolization. Another modality used for palliation of ACC is arterial embolization. It is used to decrease the bulk of the tumor, suppress tumor function, and relieve pain. Embolic agents used include polyvinyl alcohol foam and surgical gelatin.

B. Pheochromocytoma

1. Description and diagnosis. Pheochromocytoma is a tumor that arises from chromaffin cells mainly in the adrenal medulla (90% of cases), paraganglia, as well as in other sites (e.g., urinary bladder, heart, and organ of Zuckerkandl). It is an uncommon tumor, with an estimated 800 cases diagnosed in the United States every year. It is found in up to 0.3% of autopsy subjects and is responsible for less than 0.1% to 0.5% of all cases of hypertension. Pheochromocytoma can be hereditary, as part of the MEN syndrome (MEN 2A, MEN 2B), or familial with no other manifestation of the MEN syndrome; when part of the MEN syndrome, it is almost always benign. Also, it may be found as part of von Hippel-Lindau disease, tuberous sclerosis, Sturge-Weber syndrome and Carney's syndrome. The incidence of malignant pheochromocytoma is approximately 10% of all pheochromocytomas. The only definite proof of malignancy is the presence of tumor in secondary sites where chromaffin tissue is not normally present. The diagnosis of pheochromocytoma depends on a thorough history and physical examination, increased catecholamine levels in the plasma and the urine (including epinephrine, norepinephrine, dopamine, and total metanephrines), cross-sectional imaging such as CT or MRI, or [131I]metaiodobenzylguanidine ([131I]MIBG) scintigraphy. The overall 5-year survival rate for patients with malignant pheochromocytoma is 36% to 44%. Although pheochromocytoma is a rare tumor, early detection and treatment are crucial, owing to its high morbidity and potential mortality (stroke and myocardial infarction). Patients with pheochromocytoma can present with sustained or episodic hypertension. Hypertension does not usually correlate with the amount of catecholamine production, and its severity varies widely among patients.

2. Treatment

a. Surgery. Surgery is the only definitive therapy for pheochromocytoma, for localized and regional unilateral or bilateral disease. Surgery requires careful preoperative preparation to achieve control of the blood pressure, blood volume, and heart rate. Phenoxybenzamine, an α-adrenergic receptor blocker, is started 1 to 2 weeks before surgery in a dose of 10 to 20 mg PO three or four times daily. Some patients require the addition of β-blockers (e.g., propranolol 80 to 120 mg/day), which are indicated for persistent supraventricular tachycardia or the presence of angina. To prevent hypertensive crisis secondary to unopposed vasoconstriction, the β-blocker should never be given before the α-antagonist. Other α-adrenergic blockers are used for the same purpose, including prazosin, which is a selective α₁-antagonist that has also been used successfully for preoperative preparation of pheochromocytoma. Metyrosine 250 mg four times daily (maximum 4 g/day) can also be used, but is associated with frequent side effects. Intraoperatively, blood pressure can be controlled by titration with nitroprusside.

Catecholamine and metanephrine levels should be measured 1 week after surgery to confirm total removal of the tumor. Surgical mortality is estimated to be approximately 2% and usually correlates with the severity of hypertension. Patients whose localized disease is fully resected should have normal life expectancy. Close postoperative follow-up is mandatory because of the possibility of postoperative residual tumor and because 10% of patients have metastasis, and another 10% have multiple primary tumors at the time of diagnosis.

Follow-up should include a history, physical examination, and catecholamine and metanephrine measurements at 3 months, followed by a similar evaluation yearly for life. Redevelopment of any sign or symptom suggesting pheochromocytoma or a rising trend in catecholamine levels requires imaging, including [131I]MIBG scintigraphy. A few centers recommend that [131I]MIBG scintigraphy be done yearly, regardless of the catecholamine levels or the clinical picture; this is not frequently practiced in the United States. The recurrence rate of pheochromocytoma postoperatively is 5% per year. Contralateral adrenalectomy of a normal gland is generally not recommended in patients with a high incidence of bilateral disease (e.g., MEN 2), despite the high risk of subsequent involvement. In patients with metastatic disease, there is no evidence to support improved survival after local debulking.

b. Chemotherapy. This is reserved for locally invasive, metastatic, and inoperable lesions. Response to chemotherapy or radiotherapy is evaluated by regression of tumor size and a decrease in the catecholamine levels. Owing to the small number of patients with pheochromocytoma, limited data are available regarding the effect of chemotherapy. Because of the functional and biologic similarities between pheochromocytoma and neuroblastoma, the combination of cyclophosphamide and dacarbazine, which induces an 80% response in neuroblastoma, was used in two series to treat pheochromocytoma. The chemotherapy regimen consisted of **cyclophosphamide** 750 mg/m^2 IV plus **vincristine** 1.4 mg/m^2 IV on day 1 and **dacarbazine** 600 mg/m^2 IV on days 1 and 2; it was repeated in 21- to 28-day cycles.

Analysis of 23 patients showed objective tumor size regression in 61% of patients, and the urinary catecholamine levels decreased in 74% of patients. The median response time averaged 28 months. Improvement of blood pressure control and performance status occurred with minimal toxicity. Because streptozocin has yielded favorable results in the treatment of neuroendocrine tumor in the gastrointestinal tract, it was used as a single agent in a patient with malignant pheochromocytoma. Streptozocin showed promising results, with a 73% reduction in urinary vanillylmandelic acid level and significant tumor size regression.

c. Radiation therapy. [^{131}I]MIBG is actively taken up and concentrated by pheochromocytoma cells with high sensitivity and specificity. Consequently, a high dose of [^{131}I]MIBG is used to treat pheochromocytoma. This treatment has shown some evidence of response in terms of tumor size regression and decreased catecholamine levels. The uptake of [^{131}I] MIBG by pheochromocytoma requires the presence of an active neuronal pump mechanism, which limits the use of this agent to patients with pheochromocytoma who have the ability to concentrate [^{131}I]MIBG in the cells. Therefore, initial screening of the ability of the pheochromocytoma to concentrate small doses of [^{131}I]MIBG is necessary to determine the probable efficacy of the treatment. High doses such as 800 mCi (37 MBq) have been used in a small study, achieving complete response in three patients; two had prior evidence of skeletal and soft tissue metastasis. In addition, combination [^{131}I]MIBG and chemotherapy produced additive effects in reducing tumor burden. External radiation to doses of 4,000 to 5,000 cGy over 4 to 5 weeks may provide local control to an inoperable tumor and may be used to control local bone metastasis.

d. Supportive pharmacologic therapy. α-Blockers should be used to prevent severe hypertension-related morbidity and mortality, especially in untreated patients and those receiving chemotherapy. Another pharmacologic agent that can be used is α-methyl-L-tyrosine (metyrosine), which inhibits tyrosine hydroxylase, a rate-limiting step in catecholamine biosynthesis. Metyrosine allows the use of lower doses of α-blockers and has been shown to be effective in catecholamine-induced cardiomyopathy. Other medications include β-blockers, which are used to control arrhythmia, angiotensin-converting enzyme inhibitors, and calcium-channel blockers, which are also used for hypertension control as discussed previously.

SUGGESTED READINGS

Thyroid Carcinoma

AACE/AME Task Force on Thyroid Nodules. American Association of Clinical Endocrinologists and Associazione Medici Endocrinologi medical guidelines for clinical practice for the diagnosis and management of thyroid nodule. *Endocr Pract* 2006;12(1):63–102.

Abbosh PH, Nephew KP. Multiple signaling pathways converge on beta-catenin in thyroid cancer. *Thyroid* 2005;15(6):551–561.

Ain KB. Pathobiology of antineoplastic therapy in undifferentiated thyroid cancer. *Cancer Treat Res* 2004;122:357–367.

Brierley JD, Tsang RW. External-beam radiation therapy in the treatment of differentiated thyroid cancer. *Semin Surg Oncol* 1999;16(1):42–49.

Brierley J, Tsang R, Panzarella T, et al. Prognostic factors and the effect of treatment with radioactive iodine and external beam radiation on patients with differentiated thyroid cancer seen at a single institution over 40 years. *Clin Endocrinol (Oxf)* 2005;63(4):418–427.

Cooper DS, Doherty GM, Haugen BR, et al. The American Thyroid Association Guidelines Taskforce. Management guidelines for patients with thyroid nodules and differentiated thyroid cancer. *Thyroid* 2006;16(2):109–142.

Farid NR. Molecular pathogenesis of thyroid cancer: the significance of oncogenes, tumor suppressor genes, and genomic instability. *Exp Clin Endocrinol Diabetes* 1996;104(Suppl 4):1–12.

Galloway RJ, Smallridge RC. Imaging in thyroid cancer. *Endocrinol Metab Clin North Am* 1996;25:93–113.

Giuffrida D, Gharib H. Anaplastic thyroid carcinoma: current diagnosis and treatment. *Ann Oncol* 2000;11:1083–1089.

Machens A, Holzhausen HJ, Dralle H. The prognostic value of primary tumor size in papillary and follicular thyroid carcinoma. *Cancer* 2005;103(11):2269–2273.

Mazzaferri EL, Jhiang SM. Long-term impact of initial surgical and medical therapy on papillary and follicular thyroid cancer. *Am J Med* 1994;97(5):418–428.

Modigliani E, Franc B, Niccoli-Sire P. Diagnosis and treatment of medullary thyroid cancer. Best practice and research. *Clin Endocrinol Metab* 2000;14:631–649.

Noguchi M, Katev N, Miwa K. Therapeutic strategies and long-term results in differentiated thyroid cancer. *J Surg Oncol* 1998;67:52–59.

Robbins J. Prognostic factors in the management of thyroid cancer. *J Endocrinol Invest* 1995;18:159–160.

Santini F, Bottici V, Elisei R, et al. Cytotoxic effects of carboplatinum and epirubicin in the setting of an elevated serum thyrotropin for advanced poorly differentiated thyroid cancer. *J Clin Endocrinol Metab* 2002;87(9):4160–4165.

Sawka AM, Thephamongkhol K, Brouwers M, et al. Clinical review 170: a systematic review and metaanalysis of the effectiveness of radioactive iodine remnant ablation for well-differentiated thyroid cancer. *J Clin Endocrinol Metab* 2004;89(8)3668–3676.

Soh EY, Clark OH. Surgical considerations and approach to thyroid cancer. *Endocrinol Metab Clin North Am* 1996;25:115–139.

Thyroid Carcinoma Task Force. AACE/AAES medical/surgical guidelines for clinical practice: management of thyroid carcinoma. *Endocr Pract* 2001;7:203–220.

Yeh SD, La Quaglia W. ^{131}I therapy for pediatric thyroid cancer. *Semin Pediatr Surg* 1997;6:128–133.

Adrenocortical Carcinoma

Abraham J, Bakke S, Rutt A, et al. A phase II trial of combination chemotherapy and surgical resection for the treatment of metastatic adrenocortical carcinoma: continuous infusion doxorubicin, vincristine, and etoposide with daily mitotane as a P-glycoprotein antagonist. *Cancer* 2002;94(9):2333–2343.

Berruti A, Terzolo M, Pia A, et al. Mitotane associated with etoposide, doxorubicin, and cisplatin in the treatment of advanced adrenocortical carcinoma. Italian Group for the Study of Adrenal Cancer. *Cancer* 1998;83(10):2194–2200.

Berruti A, Terzolo M, Sperone P, et al. Etoposide, doxorubicin and cisplatin plus mitotane in the treatment of advanced adrenocortical carcinoma: a large prospective phase II trial. *Endocr Relat Cancer* 2005;12(3):657–666.

Bornstein SR, Stratakis CA, Chrousos GP. Adrenocortical tumors: recent advances in basic concepts and clinical management. *Ann Intern Med* 1999;130:759–771.

Cook DM. Adrenal mass. *Endocrinol Metab Clin North Am* 1997;26:829–852.

Dackiw AP, Lee JE, Gagel RF, et al. Adrenal cortical carcinoma. *World J Surg* 2001;25(7):914–926.

Kendrick ML, Lloyd R, Erickson L, et al. Adrenocortical carcinoma: surgical progress or status quo? *Arch Surg* 2001;136:543–549.

Khan TS, Imam H, Juhlin C, et al. Streptozocin and o,p'DDD in the treatment of adrenocortical cancer patients: long-term survival in its adjuvant use. *Ann Oncol* 2000;11(10):1281–1287.

Khan TS, Sundin A, Juhlin C, et al. Vincristine, cisplatin, teniposide, and cyclophosphamide combination in the treatment of recurrent or metastatic adrenocortical cancer. *Med Oncol* 2004;21(2):167–177.

Krause DS, Van Etten RA. Tyrosine kinases as targets for cancer therapy. *N Engl J Med* 2005;353(2):172–187.

Luton JP, Cerdas S, Billaud L, et al. Clinical features of adrenocortical carcinoma, prognostic factors, and the effect of mitotane therapy. *N Engl J Med* 1990;322:1195–1201.

McGrath PC, Sloan DA, Schwartz RW, et al. Current advances in the diagnosis and therapy of adrenal tumors. *Curr Opin Oncol* 1998;10:52–57.

Miller JA, Norton JA. Multiple endocrine neoplasia. *Cancer Treat Res* 1997;90:213–225.

Schteingart DE, Doherty GM, Gauger PG, et al. Management of patients with adrenal cancer: recommendations of an international consensus conference. *Endocr Relat Cancer* 2005;12(3):667–680.

Williamson SK, Lew D, Miller GJ, et al. Phase II evaluation of cisplatin and etoposide followed by mitotane at disease progression in patients with locally advanced or metastatic adrenocortical carcinoma: a Southwest Oncology Group Study. *Cancer* 2000;88(5):1159–1165.

Pheochromocytoma

Averbuch SD, Steakley CS, Young RC, et al. Malignant pheochromocytoma: effective treatment with a combination of cyclophosphamide, vincristine, and dacarbazine. *Ann Intern Med* 1988;109: 267–273.

Kebebew E, Duh QY. Benign and malignant pheochromocytoma: diagnosis, treatment, and follow-up. *Surg Oncol Clin N Am* 1998;7: 765–789.

Kopf D, Goretzki PE, Lehnert H. Clinical management of malignant adrenal tumors. *J Cancer Res Clin Oncol* 2001;127(3):143–155.

Kulke MH, Stuart K, Enzinger PC, et al. Phase II study of temozolomide and thalidomide in patients with metastatic neuroendocrine tumors. *J Clin Oncol* 2006;24(3):401–406.

Lenders JWM, Pacak W, McClellan M, et al. Biochemical diagnosis of pheochromocytoma: which test is best? *JAMA* 2002;287:1427–1434.

Mukherjee JJ, Kaltsas GA, Islam N, et al. Treatment of metastatic carcinoid tumours, phaeochromocytoma, paraganglioma and medullary carcinoma of the thyroid with (131)I-meta-iodobenzylguanidine [(131)I-mIBG]. *Clin Endocrinol (Oxf)* 2001;55(1):47–60.

Pacak K, Linehan WM, Eisenhofer G, et al. Recent advances in genetics, diagnosis, localization, and treatment of pheochromocytoma. *Ann Intern Med* 2001;134:315–329.

Rose B, Matthay KK, Price D, et al. High-dose 131I-metaiodobenzylguanidine therapy for 12 patients with malignant pheochromocytoma. *Cancer* 2003;98(2):239–248.

Sisson JC. Radiopharmaceutical treatment of pheochromocytomas. *Ann N Y Acad Sci* 2002;970:54–60.

CHAPTER 15

Melanomas and Other Skin Malignancies

Karen S. Milligan and Walter D. Y. Quan, Jr.

More than 1 million Americans were diagnosed with skin cancer in 2006. Melanoma accounted for approximately 62,190 cases and was responsible for approximately 7,910 deaths, far surpassing the total deaths due to all other skin malignancies combined. Melanoma is increasing in incidence at a higher rate than any other cancer (except for non−small cell lung cancer in women) in the United States. Less common tumors of the skin include Merkel cell cancer, Kaposi's sarcoma (see Chapter 26), and mycosis fungoides (MF).

I. Melanoma
A. Natural history
1. **Etiology and epidemiology.** Melanoma arises from pigment-producing melanocytes that migrate to the skin and eye during embryologic development. Approximately 5% of melanoma occurs in extradermal sites such as the eye and mucous membranes of the oropharynx, vagina, and anus. In approximately 5% of cases, patients present with either regional lymph node involvement or metastatic organ involvement without any obvious primary being identified. Melanoma occurs more commonly in men than in women and has a peak age at incidence of approximately 50 years. Owing to the young age of many melanoma patients, this disease takes a striking toll in terms of the average number of years of life lost per patient in this country. The incidence of the disease has increased rapidly in the United States to the point where melanoma is now the sixth most common cancer. The substantial increase in incidence is presumably due to increased exposure to sunlight (primarily ultraviolet radiation), with the greatest risk of melanoma felt to be in those who have intermittent intense sun exposure, particularly in fair-skinned, light-haired individuals. The cultural emphasis on suntanned skin as an indicator of physical health and beauty has played a major role in this increase. Depletion of the ozone layer may contribute as well. Sunny parts of the United States have the highest incidence of the disease, especially Southern California, Florida, and Texas. One particular melanoma subtype, lentigo malignant melanoma, may be more closely associated with long-term occupational sun exposure as is seen in farmers and fishermen, for instance. Patient education in prevention, including use of sun-protective clothing, performing outdoor activities at times other than the brightest sunlit hours of the day, use of topical sunscreens, refraining from use of suntan parlors, use of skin self-examination, and avoiding suntanning ("tanned

skin = damaged skin"), should be emphasized. Individuals with xeroderma pigmentosa, an autosomal recessive disorder, typically incur multiple basal and squamous skin cancers and melanoma because their skin lacks the ability to repair damage induced by ultraviolet radiation.

2. Precursor lesions, genetics, and familial melanoma. Melanoma may arise not only from dysplastic nevi but also from congenital and acquired nevi. Dysplastic nevi may be sporadic or familial. Individuals who have more than 100 benign nevi may also be at risk for melanoma. Ten percent of patients with melanoma have a family history of this cancer. Careful follow-up should be carried out in patients with these risk factors. Suspicious-appearing lesions or lesions that appear to have changed should be excised. The familial atypical multiple mole melanoma (FAMMM) syndrome is characterized by earlier mean age at diagnosis (34 years) and multiple lesions. The most common germline mutation seen in familial melanoma occurs in the tumor suppressor gene *CDKN2A*. *CDKN2A, PTEN, NRAS*, and *BRAF* mutations have been seen in nonfamilial melanoma. Multiple chromosomal abnormalities have been identified and associated with melanoma, including chromosomal regions 10q, 9p, 6q, 6p, 7, 1p, and 11.

3. Types and appearance of primary lesions. Clinical features ("ABCD") suspicious for melanoma are as follows:

- **A**symmetry of a lesion
- **B**orders that are irregular
- **C**olor that is multihued
- **D**iameter greater than 6 mm (i.e., "larger than the diameter of a pencil eraser")

Other characteristics of concern could include history of recent growth, change in pigmentation, ulceration, itching, or bleeding. Nonpigmented skin lesions that behave like melanoma should be examined with the immunochemical stains S-100 and HMB-45 as 1% to 2% of melanoma lesions are amelanotic.

There are four clinical types of primary cutaneous melanoma. **Superficial spreading melanoma** is the most common type, accounting for 70% of melanomas. It is commonly found on the trunks of men and lower extremities of women. **Nodular melanoma** comprises 10% to 15% of melanomas and has an early vertical growth phase. It is commonly found on the trunks of men. **Lentigo malignant melanoma** accounts for approximately 10% of cases. It is characterized by flat, large (1- to 5-cm) lesions located on the arms, hands, and face of the elderly (median age 70 years) in particular and is known for a relatively longer radial phase. **Acral lentiginous melanoma** is seen in approximately 3% to 5% of cases and occurs primarily on the palmar surfaces of the hands, plantar surfaces of the feet, and under nails on the digits. This melanoma subtype is most commonly seen in individuals with darker-pigmented skin.

In general, melanoma is felt to show two distinct growth phases: an initial radial phase during which the melanoma enlarges in a horizontal/superficial pattern above the basal lamina of the skin, followed eventually by a vertical growth phase characterized by the cancer "diving deep" toward subcutaneous fat. It is during the vertical growth phase that metastases are felt to be at highest risk.

4. Patterns of metastases. Although much attention is rightly attached to assessing lymph node status (see following text), melanoma has a proclivity for hematogenous spread as well. Common sites of metastases include lung, liver, bone, subcutaneous areas, and, primarily in late stages, brain. However, melanoma can spread to virtually any site. Following diagnosis, approximately 25% of patients will develop visceral (non–lymph node) metastases. As many as an additional 15% may develop disease limited to lymph nodes alone. Patients who present with lymph node or metastatic involvement without any obvious primary site may have undergone spontaneous remission of the primary, a phenomenon that may be attributable to some degree of immune system involvement. Patients with "cancer of unknown primary" should have their biopsy material stained with the immunohistochemical stains S-100 and HMB-45 in consideration of the possibility of melanoma.

5. Ocular melanoma. Ocular melanoma is the most common malignancy of the eye in adults. It may occur in any eye structure that contains melanocytes, although uveal tract sites predominate, with choroid, ciliary body, and iris in decreasing frequency. Standard therapy may consist of either enucleation (often utilizing a "no touch" technique) or brachytherapy with radioisotopes such as iodine 125 (^{125}I). This tumor metastasizes most frequently to the liver and appears to be less sensitive to both biologic agents and chemotherapy than cutaneous melanoma.

B. Staging. Melanoma is staged according to the updated American Joint Committee on Cancer staging system (see Tables 15.1 to 15.3). All patients should have a careful history and physical examination with special attention to the skin including scalp, mucous membranes, and regional lymph nodes. Laboratory studies should include complete blood count, blood urea nitrogen (BUN), serum creatinine, liver panel, alkaline phosphatase, and serum lactate dehydrogenase. A chest x-ray or computed tomography (CT) scan of the chest is done to evaluate for pulmonary lesions. Elevation of liver function tests warrants CT scan of the liver. Elevation of alkaline phosphatase level or unexplainable bone pain suggests the need for bone scanning. Primary lesions equal to or thicker than 1.0 mm are at higher risk of regional lymph node involvement; therefore, the use of sentinel node surgery is recommended (see Section I.C).

C. Surgical treatment. The standard surgery for suspected melanoma lesions is excisional biopsy rather than incisional or "shave" biopsies. Importantly, a subsequent wide excision is required to provide adequate tumor-free margins as melanoma is notorious for local recurrences. Although there is some variation in recommendations, most would advocate a 1-cm

Table 15.1.   TNM classification for melanoma

T Status

Classification	Thickness (mm)	Ulceration
T1	≤1.0	a = No ulceration *and* Clark's level III or less
		b = With ulceration *or* Clark's level IV or V
T2	1.01–2.0	a = No ulceration
		b = With ulceration
T3	2.01–4.0	a = No ulceration
		b = With ulceration
T4	>4.0	a = No ulceration
		b = With ulceration

N status

Classification	Number of Lymph Nodes	Involvement
N1	1	a = Microscopic
		b = Macroscopic
N2	2–3	a = Microscopic
		b = Macroscopic
		c = "In-transit met" or "satellite" present but no lymph nodes involved
N3	≥4	Note: This classification also applies if "in-transit met" or "satellite" lesions present *with* metastatic nodes

M status

Classification	Metastatic Site	Serum LDH
M1a	Distant subcutaneous, skin, or node	Not elevated
M1b	Lung	Not elevated
M1c	All other visceral sites	Not elevated
M1c	Any	Elevated

LDH, lactate dehydrogenase.

tumor-free margin for melanomas less than 1 mm in thickness and 1- to 2-cm margins for deeper primary lesions if technically possible. Additionally, for primary lesions equal to or greater than 1 mm, sentinel node mapping is recommended. On the basis of work by Morton and others, lymph node "drainage areas" are assessed through a specific lymph node (sentinel node[s]—sometimes more than one) into which

Table 15.2. Clark's levels of invasion

Level	Description
I	Limited to the epidermis
II	Invades papillary dermis
III	Extends to papillary–reticular dermal junction
IV	Invades reticular dermis
V	Invades subcutaneous fat

lymph-borne metastases generally first occur. The absence of tumor involvement in this lymph node precludes the need for elective lymph node dissection. Although blue dye was originally used in this procedure, current refinements of this technique include the use of technetium-based radionuclides.

D. Adjuvant therapy. Eastern Cooperative Oncology Group (ECOG)1684 (protocol number) was a large randomized adjuvant trial of interferon α_{2b} (IFN-α_{2b}) in patients with deep primary lesions (>4 mm thick) or regional lymph node involvement that showed statistically significant improvement in overall survival in the treated group as compared to the observation group.

- **IFN** 20 MIU/m^2 IV 5 days/week for 4 weeks (as a "loading phase") followed by 10 MIU/m^2 SC 3 days/week for 48 weeks as a maintenance phase.

Table 15.3. Approximate survival in melanoma based on stage grouping

Stage	TNM (Pathologic)	5-year Survival (%)
IA	T1a	95
IB	T1b	90
	T2a	89
IIA	T2b	77
	T3a	
IIB	T3b	65
	T4a	
IIC	T4b	45
IIIA	N1a	53
	N2a	49
IIIB	N1b	51
	N2b	46
IIIC	N3	27
IV	M1a	19
All others	M	<10

From Balch CM, Buzaid AC, Soong SJ, et al. Final version of the American Joint Committee on Cancer staging system for cutaneous melanoma. *J Clin Oncol* 2001;19:3635–3648.

Toxicity (flu-like symptoms, hepatic dysfunction, and neurologic symptoms) was significant, but quality-of-life analysis demonstrated overall benefit. The follow-up study, ECOG 1690, also showed a significant disease-free survival advantage over the observation arm but not a benefit in overall survival. The difference between these two studies may be that patients on the observation arm in the subsequent trial (1,690) may have been treated with immunotherapy (including IFN or interleukin 2 [IL-2]) at the time of relapse. Given that it is clear that patients with deep cutaneous primaries and/or lymph node involvement are at high risk for metastatic recurrence and that most patients who suffer metastatic relapse will die of their disease, it is reasonable to treat such high-risk patients with either IFN or entrance into a clinical trial.

Chemotherapy as a single modality has not been shown to be more beneficial than observation alone, and high-dose IFN with chemotherapy confers no difference in relapse-free or overall survival between the single agent and combined therapy arms. An ongoing trial is examining the use of only the loading phase of IFN therapy in patients with lesions 1.5 to 4 mm Breslow depth or evidence of only microscopic lymph node involvement. A particularly fertile area of exploration is the administration of therapeutic vaccines. Granulocyte-macrophage colony-stimulating factor (GM-CSF) has been utilized by some investigators and warrants further examination. Regional perfusion chemotherapy in patients with high-risk extremity melanoma has been reported by the European Organisation for Research and Treatment of Cancer (EORTC)/World Health Organization (WHO), which found no substantial benefit.

E. Therapy of metastases
  1. **General considerations about systemic therapy**
     a. **Patient selection.** Although, in general, melanoma is considered relatively resistant to systemic therapy, certain favorable prognostic factors do lend themselves to a higher chance of response. These include ECOG performance status 0 or 1; subcutaneous, lymph node, or pulmonary metastasis; no prior chemotherapy; normal marrow, renal, and hepatic function; and absence of central nervous system (CNS) metastases. Some investigators have noted that women are more likely than men to respond to chemotherapy. The biologic basis for this finding has not been fully elucidated. Newer genomic and proteomic profiling may lead to a better understanding of prognostic factors. These response rates are highly dependent upon site of metastasis. When reviewing potential therapy for patients, patient characteristics as well as the natural history of the disease must be considered, including the median survival of patients in phase II studies that have 0% response rates can reach 7 months.
  2. **Biologic agents.** This class of agents, along with experimental therapy through clinical trials, represents the most significant hope for the future in the treatment of

this disease. Currently available agents in this class are as follows:

a. Interleukin 2 (IL-2; Proleukin, aldesleukin) appears to be the most active single agent for patients with visceral metastases. It is most commonly used in a "high-dose" regimen of **IL-2** at 600,000 IU/kg given in 15-minute IV infusions every 8 hours for a total of 14 doses.

This schedule produces responses in 15% to 20% of patients, many of long duration. A previous review of National Cancer Institute data showed a response rate of 50% in patients with disease limited to cutaneous/subcutaneous sites. Because this drug is associated with a capillary leak syndrome that can include hypotension, fluid retention, renal and hepatic hypoperfusion, and pulmonary edema, the dose and schedule mentioned in the preceding text require inpatient care. It should be used only by those experienced in its administration. Inpatient continuous-infusion schedules (18 MIU/m^2 given over 24 hour for up to 5 consecutive days) may also be administered. Patients receiving this dose must also be closely monitored. Moderate-dose IL-2 (22 MIU/m^2 given by 15-minute infusions for 5 consecutive days for 2 consecutive weeks) when given with low-dose cyclophosphamide (see Section I.E.6. and Table 15.4.) can be administered on an outpatient basis but requires significant premedication and daily physician examination. The role of low-dose SC administration of IL-2 is unclear; some investigators feel that such low-dose regimens are less likely to yield durable responses. It should be noted that the earlier literature may express IL-2 dosing in units other than International Units. Therefore, when comparing various studies, a "rule of thumb" for conversions is 1 mg = 3 $\times$ 10^6 Cetus Units = 6 $\times$ 10^6 Roche Units = 18 $\times$ 10^6 IU.

b. Interferon α_{2b} (Intron-A) and **interferon** α_{2a} (Roferon-A) have been examined with a wide range of doses, schedules, and routes from 3 to 50 $\times$ 10^6 IU/m^2 given SC, IM, or IV, administered three to five times per week. These agents have been found to have response rates of approximately 10% to 15% in a variety of studies. Additionally, some patients may have stable disease lasting many months or longer. In regards to dosing, some investigators believe that higher doses of IFN (20 MIU/m^2 IV, such as those given in adjuvant therapy) act more by inhibiting tumor cell proliferation, whereas lower doses of IFN ($\leq$5 MIU/m^2 SC) may be more immunostimulatory.

A recommended starting dose for subcutaneous IFN is **IFN** 3 MU SC three times per week.

c. Thalidomide, an inhibitor of angiogenesis, does not appear to be active as a single agent in melanoma but is being explored as an adjunct to temozolomide in brain metastases.

Table 15.4.   Multiagent systemic therapy for melanoma

Regimen	Drug Dosages
BCDT ("Dartmouth regimen")	BCNU (carmustine) 150 mg/m²/day on day 1 every 6 weeks
	Cisplatin 25 mg/m²/day on d 1–3 every 3 weeks
	DTIC (dacarbazine) 220 mg/m²/day on days 1–3 every 3 weeks
	Tamoxifen 20 mg PO daily
CVD	DDP (cisplatin) 20 mg/m²/day on days 1–4 every 3 weeks
	VLB (vinblastine) 2 mg/m²/day on days 1–4 every 3 weeks
	DTIC (dacarbazine) 800 mg/m² on day 1 only every 3 weeks
Biochemotherapy	Cisplatin 20 mg/m²/day on days 1–4
	Vinblastine 1.5 mg/m²/day on days 1–4
	Dacarbazine 800 mg/m² on day 1
	Interleukin-2 9 MIU/m² daily by continuous IV infusion on days 5–8 (96 hours) and 17–20 (96 hours)
	Interferon α-2b 5 MU/m² SC on days 5–9 and 17–21
	Cycles repeated every 3 weeks
	Maximum of 5 cycles for maximum of four cycles
Cyclophosphamide and moderate-dose interleukin-2	Cyclophosphamide 350 mg/m² IVPB on day 1
	Interleukin 2 22 MIU/m² IVPB on days 4–8, 11–15
	Repeat cycle every 21 days for three cycles. Thereafter give every 28–42 days

d. Tyrosine kinase inhibitors. These "small molecule" inhibitors, including sorafenib and sunitinib, of tumor angiogenesis are currently being investigated.

e. Combinations of biologic agents. The role of combinations of biologic agents remains an area of ongoing study. IL-2 and IFN-α have been utilized together, but most studies have found no advantage in response rates or response durations due to this combination as compared with IL-2 alone. The use of IFN following therapeutic vaccine therapy resulted in higher response rates than what is usually seen with IFN alone. Current studies are examining IFN and thalidomide in combination. A study utilizing histamine with low-dose subcutaneous IL-2 suggested improved survival in patients with liver metastases as compared to low-dose subcutaneous IL-2. A recent study combining the antihistamine famotidine and high-dose continuous infusion IL-2 also suggested activity in metastatic melanoma.

3. **Chemotherapy**

   a. **Single-agent chemotherapy.** Most cytotoxic agents commonly used in other tumor types are inactive in this disease. Several agents possess modest activity in melanoma with responses obtained primarily in lung and nonvisceral sites and typically in ambulatory patients with few or no symptoms of their disease.

      (1) **Dacarbazine (DTIC)** has historically been the most widely utilized single agent for the treatment of metastatic melanoma. The most commonly used doses are 200 mg/m^2 IV on days 1 to 5 every 3 weeks or 750 to 800 mg/m^2 IV on day 1 every 4 to 6 weeks. Most responses to this agent occur in subcutaneous or lymph node sites.

      (2) **Platinum-containing drugs.** Cisplatin 100 mg/m^2 IV every 3 weeks *or* carboplatin 400 mg/m^2 IV every 3 weeks appears to have similar efficacy.

      (3) **Taxanes.** Docetaxel 60 to 100 mg/m^2 is given in 1-hour IV infusions every 3 weeks, *or* paclitaxel 135 to 215 mg/m^2 is given in 3-hour IV infusions every 3 weeks.

      (4) **Temozolomide (an oral imidazole)** is an oral DTIC derivative with significant CNS penetrance and therefore the potential for clinical responses in the difficult subpopulation of patients with CNS metastases. Typical doses are 150 to 200 mg/m^2 PO daily for 5 days every 28 days.

      (5) **Vinca alkaloids** such as vinblastine and **nitrosoureas** such as carmustine have been used primarily in combinations.

   b. **Multiagent chemotherapy.** Despite decades of trials, no combination chemotherapy has emerged as a standard therapy. Whereas multiple regimens have shown high response rates in single-arm phase II or nonrandomized trials, there is no convincing randomized trial data to show statistically significant improvements in both response rate and median survival as compared with single-agent therapy (usually dacarbazine alone). In the 1990s, the "Dartmouth regimen" (dacarbazine, carmustine, cisplatin, and tamoxifen) was the most commonly employed chemotherapy regimen in stage IV melanoma. Whereas phase II studies suggested a higher response rate than dacarbazine alone, a phase III trial demonstrated no significant difference as compared to dacarbazine alone. Cisplatin, vinblastine, and dacarbazine currently comprise the most commonly used combination regimen (shown in Table 15.4).

4. **Hormones.** Although hormone receptors have been identified on some melanoma cell lines, these, unlike the ones seen in breast cancer, do not appear to be functional. Tamoxifen and megestrol acetate have no significant

antitumor activity when used alone in patients with metastatic disease. There has been some *in vitro* evidence and some indirect clinical evidence that these drugs may potentiate the activity of some cytotoxic agents.

5. Biochemotherapy. Three randomized studies have compared the combination of polychemotherapy (cisplatin, vinblastine, and dacarbazine) and the biologic agents IL-2 and IFN versus the chemotherapy regimen alone. The first published randomized comparison showed improved response rate and median time to progression (4.9 vs. 2.4 months) in favor of the combined chemotherapy with biotherapy. Unfortunately, confirmatory studies have shown no difference in median time to disease progression or median survival.

6. Other biochemotherapy regimens. An alternative approach involving biochemotherapy utilizes IL-2 with doses of chemotherapeutic agents that are chosen to theoretically augment an immune response. Cyclophosphamide, for instance, may increase lymphokine-activated killer (LAK) cell activity, decrease the dampening effect of regulatory T cells on the immune response, or allow for space in the bone marrow for repopulation by LAK cells. Mitchell et al. have shown activity of an outpatient combination of low-dose cyclophosphamide and IL-2 with an overall response rate (5% complete response [CR], 21% partial response [PR]) similar to those seen with high-dose inpatient IL-2 regimens. However, no randomized study data using this regimen has been published.

F. Regional therapy

1. Local perfusion. For patients with subcutaneous metastases limited to a single extremity, arteriovenous cannulation and perfusion of that limb with agents such as melphalan, cisplatin, or tumor necrosis factor α often with hyperthermia yield higher tissue concentrations of the drugs than what are achievable by IV administration. Phase II studies often show impressive response rates. Whether there is any survival advantage to this therapy as compared with systemic treatment remains controversial. Because of issues involving factors such as cost, the equipment required, and the physician training needed to implement this approach, its practicality is unclear. Hepatic arterial infusion therapy is theoretically appealing for ocular melanoma metastatic only to the liver. This therapy looks to be more active than systemic chemotherapy in ocular melanoma, although it is unclear that such an approach improves median survival.

2. Intralesional therapy with bacillus Calmette-Guérin (BCG), IFN-α, GM-CSF, and other agents has also been used with varying degrees of success.

3. Treatment of CNS metastases. Dexamethasone 10 mg IV followed by 6 mg every 6 hours IV or PO is given to reduce cerebral edema. As soon as possible, radiation should be started by either stereotactic, gamma knife, or three-dimensional conformal techniques. For solitary lesions, surgical resection followed by radiotherapy may yield a significant group of survivors over 1 year who experience good quality of life. The role of temozolomide needs to be further explored in this group of patients.

4. Radiotherapy is of variable efficacy in the treatment of the regional or bony metastases but sometimes may yield gratifying symptomatic benefit.

5. Surgery, when utilized judiciously, can result in long-term disease-free survivals of up to 20% in individuals with isolated metastatic sites. Special considerations for surgical resection of metastases include gastrointestinal metastases that threaten of significant morbidity such as impending bowel obstruction or even mortality due to perforation and single brain metastasis before the start of biologic therapy (as long-term steroid use, which is frequently needed in the setting of brain metastasis, is antagonistic with biologic agents). The role of adjuvant therapy in patients who have undergone metastatectomies needs to be elucidated. A reasonable approach is to treat such patients with IFN as described in the preceding text.

G. Experimental and future therapies are of great importance in this disease. Only a few salient approaches will be discussed here. A variety of references are available for further reading in the following text.

1. Therapeutic vaccines remain an area of intense interest, and much potential is expected in the coming years, although current clinical results have shown limited activity. In general, toxicity from vaccine therapy tends to be quite low, usually limited to local reactions to the vaccine or the immunologic adjuvant that may be combined with the antigenic stimulus. Most vaccine studies have dealt primarily with patients who have been rendered surgically free of all macroscopic disease. A purified ganglioside, GM-2KLH/QS-21, which demonstrated prolongation of survival of patients in whom the vaccine is optimally immunogenic, was tested in an adjuvant setting (ECOG E1694) but found to be inferior to IFN. Recently, an adjuvant phase III trial evaluating the Canvaxin polyvalent whole-cell vaccine in resected stage IV melanoma did not show significant benefit. Fewer studies have been done in patients with metastatic disease. A polyvalent melanoma cell vaccine and Melacine, a vaccine derived from allogeneic melanoma cell lines (approved for use in metastatic disease in Canada) are examples of vaccines that have achieved objective responses in patients with metastatic tumors. Vaccination with peptides derived from tumor-associated antigens specifically designed to associate with T cells in the context of major histocompatibility complex (MHC) class I or II molecules and vaccines based on vaccinia-infected melanoma cell lysates, are examples of other approaches of note. Potential advantages to vaccine-based therapy include relatively little toxicity, the possibility of long-term disease stabilization, and an immunologic effect that may continue long after dose administration.

2. Cellular therapy. The administration of *ex vivo* activated cells such as cytotoxic T cells theoretically specific for melanoma continues to be of interest. Currently, there is no evidence that the addition of bulk cultured T cells to

IL-2 therapy, for instance, is superior to IL-2 alone. The use of gene-modified T cells that might be more potent or cytotoxic T cells immunized to specific tumor epitopes offer theoretical potential. The addition of LAK cells to IL-2 has not been clearly shown to be better than IL-2 alone, although Rosenberg and colleagues identified a survival trend ($p = 0.064$) in favor of the LAK/IL-2 arm. Recent studies have examined the infusion of dendritic cells that have been pulsed with melanoma antigen.

II. Nonmelanoma skin cancer

A. Etiology and epidemiology. The American Cancer Society estimates that there were 1 million new cases of basal cell carcinoma (BCC) and squamous cell carcinoma (SCC) in the United States in 2006. These lesions occur twice as frequently in men as in women. BCC occurs four times more commonly than SCC (70%–80% vs. 10%–30%). Both are seen predominantly in the elderly. Risk factors for these two lesions include age more than 60, prior heavy sun exposure, fair complexion, and light-colored eyes or hair. Sun exposure, especially sunburns early in life, is the most important risk factor for development of these lesions. Other etiologic factors include prior irradiation to the skin for benign disorders, chronic inflammation, scarring or burns, and arsenic exposure. Patients who are chronically immunosuppressed such as in chronic lymphocytic leukemia and renal transplantation are also at increased risk, as are individuals with genetic disorders including xeroderma pigmentosum. There is evidence that human immunodeficiency virus infection may predispose to a clinically more aggressive SCC or BCC. Multiple BCCs or SCCs frequently occur in 30% to 50% of individuals.

B. Diagnosis and clinical features

1. Diagnosis of both SCC and BCC is made by biopsy, including incisional, excisional, or sometimes "shave," depending on the clinical situation. Staging systems are not typically utilized for these tumors as both have generally low potential for metastases. BCC originates in the basal layer of the epidermis and often presents as a nodular, ulcerative lesion ("rodent ulcer") with pearly or translucent edges and central ulceration. Approximately 30% of BCCs are found on the nose. Only approximately 0.1% of BCCs metastasize. Metastases typically occur when a long-standing lesion has been neglected. Lymph node metastases are the most common site (60%), with lung and bone metastases occurring less frequently. Despite being uncommon, once metastases occur survival is significantly decreased to 8 to 10 months.

SCCs often arise from crusty-appearing sun-damaged skin areas and demonstrate a higher rate of metastases (2%) than BCCs. Patients whose SCC arises from causes other than actinic damage (e.g., immunosuppression) may display a more rapid course with higher rates of metastases (20%–50%). Neglected lesions, large ulcerated lesions, and poorly differentiated histology are risk factors for metastases. Most metastases initially occur in lymph nodes (90%), with approximately 50% of patients developing metastases to other sites such as lung and bone.

SCCs may begin as premalignant lesions called *actinic keratoses* (AK) that are rough, pink or flesh-colored areas on sun-exposed skin. *In situ* SCC, known as *Bowen's disease*, exists before dermal invasion and appears as red-colored patches that are larger than AKs.

2. **Local treatment.** Surgical excision, electrodesiccation, curettage, Mohs micrographic surgery, radiation therapy, and cryotherapy all result in similar cure rates of approximately 95% when lesions are identified early. Treatment options are typically based on individual factors including the area involved, available treatment facilities, and physician skill. Surgical excision to attain margins of at least 3 to 10 millimeters is the preferred treatment in SCC because of the higher metastatic potential. BCC, which has a lower metastatic potential, can be treated with any of the techniques mentioned earlier as well as cryotherapy. Radiation therapy is the treatment of choice for areas where extensive surgical resection would result in poor cosmetic outcome, such as near eyelids, ear lobes, or tip of the nose.

Mohs micrographic surgery is an involved procedure in which thin layers are meticulously removed, chemically fixed, and immediately reviewed microscopically to be assured of clear margins. This allows for complete pathologic orientation of the tumor to ensure adequate local control. Mohs surgery is limited in its ability for local control if discontinuous areas of cancer involvement exist. Although this therapy is highly operator dependent, Mohs surgery currently has the highest 5-year cure rate and has become the standard of care for local primary or recurrent BCC and SCC lesions.

Topical treatment delivery of fluorouracil (5-FU) is used for AK and SCC *in situ* and is applied directly to the involved skin. It is not systemically absorbed, therefore no systemic toxicity is seen. Local side effects include red discoloration of the skin and photosensitivity. Imiquimod (Aldara) is U.S. Food and Drug Administration (FDA)-approved for local therapy of AKs and some small BCCs. It promotes immune system modulation by inducing IFN-α, IFN-γ, and interleukin-12 production. Both agents are used daily for several weeks.

Photodynamic therapy (PDT) has been used to treat AKs by topically applying a photosensitizing porphyrin or aminolevulinic acid (ALA) and then exposing the area to light. This process produces free radical oxygen species, which in turn cause tumor cell death. It has demonstrated effectiveness in less invasive BCCs and SCCs with a high cure rate in several studies. PDT is limited by the size of the lesion and significant photosensitivity after therapy. This therapy is still being evaluated for its future role in the treatment of skin cancers.

3. **Treatment of metastatic disease.** Metastases from either BCC or SCC may be treated with cisplatin-containing chemotherapy regimens. One of the more active regimens appears to be **cisplatin** 75 mg/m^2 IV and **doxorubicin** 50 mg/m^2 IV, both given on day 1 every 3 weeks.

Despite response rates as high as 70% with chemotherapy, once metastases have occurred cure is no longer possible and survival is typically less than 1 year.

C. Merkel cell carcinoma

1. **Etiology and epidemiology.** Merkel cell cancer is a rare cutaneous neuroendocrine tumor that arises in the basal layer of the epidermis. Approximately 500 cases are diagnosed yearly. Its microscopic appearance is that of small blue cells with scant cytoplasm and hyperchromatic nuclei ("small cell cancer of the skin"). Merkel cell cancer is 20 times more likely to occur in whites than nonwhites, occurs more frequently in men than in women, and affects persons at a median age of 65 to 70. Sun exposure is felt to be the major risk factor.

2. **Clinical features.** Initially, it may be seen as a blue or bluish red, nontender, firm skin lesion, starting as a nodule but increasing in size rapidly over weeks to months. The most commonly involved sites are the face and neck (50%) and the extremities (40%). There is no universally accepted staging system for this uncommon tumor; however, stage I is considered localized disease, stage II is involvement of regional lymph nodes, and stage III represents systemic metastases. In general, Merkel cell cancer has a tendency toward an aggressive, recurrent course similar in some ways to small cell lung cancer or melanoma. Most patients experience recurrence within 12 months of initial treatment. Fifty percent of patients experience local and regional nodal recurrences and one-third develop metastatic disease later. The most frequent distant metastatic sites are liver, lung, and bones. The overall 5-year survival rate for all stages is 50%.

3. **Treatment.** The rarity of this tumor precludes any prospective randomized treatment data. Standard therapy for this disease includes surgical resection with 2-cm margins when possible followed by lymph node dissection. Sentinel lymph node surgery has become the preferred technique since a negative lymph node precludes more extensive surgery.

Because of the risk of local recurrence, radiation therapy to the primary site and to the site of pathologically involved lymph nodes should be considered, especially in stage I disease. There has been no established role for adjuvant chemotherapy. High-risk patients may be offered chemotherapy; however, there is no data that it offers a survival advantage. For metastatic disease, the two most common regimens used have been cyclophosphamide, doxorubicin, and vincristine (CAV) or cisplatin and etoposide (EP) at doses utilized for small cell lung cancer. Response rates for these regimens are approximately 60%.

D. Mycosis fungoides (MF)

1. **Etiology and epidemiology.** MF is a cutaneous T cell–derived lymphoma with a CD4 T helper cell immunophenotype. It is an uncommon lymphoma, with just over 500 new cases diagnosed in the United States per year. It is seen predominantly in men with a median age of approximately 60 years. The lymphocytic infiltrate seen

in this disease is present in the upper aspect of the dermis, obscures the junction between the dermis and epidermis, and characteristically infiltrates the epidermis in clusters of cells that are called Pautrier's microabscesses. Involved lymph nodes have similar histologic findings. Biopsies early in the course of the disease (the "premycotic phase") may show nonspecific, nondiagnostic skin changes.

2. Clinical features. Patients with this disorder tend to display a skin rash that is erythematous, somewhat scaling, and pruritic. Over time, patches, plaques, and even ulcers can be seen. Patients may exhibit erythroderma and lymphadenopathy. Sézary's syndrome is a leukemic phase of MF with circulating lymphoma cells noted on peripheral smear. The course of MF can be variable, from a minority of patients having "skin-only" involvement to patients having extensive visceral metastases to the liver, lungs, spleen, and gastrointestinal tract. Staging is according to the TNM (B) system (Tables 15.5 and 15.6) and is based on the amount of skin involved and the presence of patches, plaques, or tumors. Patients with stage IA to IIA have an excellent prognosis with median survival greater than 11 years. Individuals with stage IIB to III disease have median survival of 3 to 4 years. Among patients with T4 lesions, a subgroup characterized by younger age (<65 years), less advanced stage (III), and no evidence of blood involvement has been shown to have a favorable prognosis with a median survival of approximately 10 years. Stage IVA/IVB has a poor prognosis with a median survival of less than 1.5 years. A subgroup of MF cases may undergo transformation to a large cell lymphoma characterized by CD30 positivity, which also heralds a poor prognosis.

3. Treatment. For individuals whose disease is confined only to the skin, electron beam radiation, PUVA (the combination of a photosensitizing substance such as psoralen and ultraviolet radiation), extracorporeal photopheresis, bexarotene gel, or topical application of nitrogen mustard or

Table 15.5. TNM (B) classes for Mycosis fungoides

T1	Limited patch/plaque lesions <10% of total skin surface
T2	Generalized patch/plaque lesion ≥10% of total skin surface
T3	Tumors
T4	Erythroderma, generalized skin involvement
N0	No clinically palpable lymph nodes
N1	Enlarged lymph nodes but microscopically negative
N2	Nonpalpable lymph nodes but microscopically involved
N3	Clinically palpable lymph nodes that are microscopically involved
M0	No visceral involvement
M1	Visceral involvement
B0	Absence of peripheral blood involvement
B1	Peripheral blood involvement

Table 15.6.   Clinical stages for mycosis fungoides

Stage	T	N	M
IA	T1	N0	M0
IB	T2	N0	M0
IIA	T1–2	N1	M0
IIB	T3	N0–1	M0
IIIA	T4	N0	M0
IIIB	T4	N1	M0
IVA	T1–4	N2–3	M0
IVB	Any	Any	M1

B symptoms have no specific bearing on this staging system.

carmustine can lead to CR of disease and potential for cure. Thick plaque disease may be better treated with electron beam therapy because PUVA and topical nitrogen mustard may be less able to penetrate the deep lesions. Imiquimod is being evaluated for this use as well. Patients who fail one of the local/topical therapies can be treated with a different type of local therapy and still have good control of the disease. For visceral disease or Sézary's syndrome, systemic therapy such as IFN-α 3 million units SC three times a week given continuously or gradually escalated to a cumulative weekly dose of 18 million units can yield response rates of over 60%. Combined regimens of IFN-α and retinoids such as bexarotene (150 mg/day) are being evaluated for enhanced immune modulation. "Traditional" antilymphoma chemotherapy agents such as cyclophosphamide, doxorubicin, vincristine, and prednisone (CHOP) appear less active in this type of lymphoma than in other non–Hodgkin's lymphomas and are typically reserved for those cases of MF that transform to large B-cell lymphomas or when disease becomes refractory to other systemic or local agents. Purine analogs such as fludarabine and pentostatin have some activity with response rates of 20% to 70%. Novel uses of gemcitabine (1,200 mg/m^2 weekly times 3 every 28 days) and liposomal doxorubicin (20 to 40 mg/m^2 every 2 to 4 weeks) used as single agents are being studied with reports of overall response rates of approximately 80% in refractory patients. Another agent, denileukin difitox (ONTAK, an IL-2–diphtheria toxin fusion protein) has been approved for refractory disease with response rates of 30% to 70%.

SUGGESTED READINGS

Melanoma

Agarwala SS, Glaspy J, O'Day SJ, et al. Results from a randomized phase III study comparing combined treatment with histamine dihydrochloride plus interleukin-2 versus interleukin-2 alone in patients with metastatic melanoma. *J Clin Oncol* 2002;20:125–133.

Atkins MB, Lee S, Flaherty LE, et al. A prospective randomized phase III trial of concurrent biochemotherapy with cisplatin, vinblastine, dacarbazine, IL-2 and interferon alpha-2b versus CVD alone in patients with metastatic melanoma (E3695): an ECOG-coordinated intergroup trial (abstr 2847). *Proc Am Soc Clin Oncol* 2003;22:708.

Bajetta E, Del Vecchio M, Nova P, et al. Multicenter phase III randomized trial of polychemotherapy (CVD regimen) versus the same chemotherapy (CT) plus subcutaneous interleukin-2 and interferon a-2b in metastatic melanoma. *Ann Oncol* 2006;17:571–577.

Balch CM, Buzaid AC, Soong SJ, et al. Final version of the American Joint Committee on Cancer staging system for cutaneous melanoma. *J Clin Oncol* 2001;19:3635–3648.

Brinkman JA, Fausch SC, Weber JS, et al. Peptide-based vaccines for cancer immunotherapy. *Expert Opin Biol Ther* 2004;4(2):181–198.

Chapman PB, Einhorn LH, Meyers ML, et al. Phase III multicenter randomized trial of the Dartmouth regimen versus dacarbazine in patients with metastatic melanoma. *J Clin Oncol* 1999;17(9):2745–2751.

Eton O, Legha SS, Bedikian AY, et al. Sequential biochemotherapy versus chemotherapy for metastatic melanoma: results from a phase III randomized trial. *J Clin Oncol* 2002;20:2045–2052.

Faries MB, Morton DL. Therapeutic vaccines for melanoma: current status. *BioDrugs* 2005;19(4):247–260.

Haluska FG, Hodi FS. Molecular genetics of familial melanoma. *J Clin Oncol* 1998;16:670.

Kim KS, Legha SS, Gonzalez R, et al. A phase III randomized trial of adjuvant biochemotherapy versus interferon alfa-2b in patients with high risk for melanoma recurrence. *J Clin Oncol* 2006;24(18s):453s.

Kirkwood JM, Ibrahim JG, Sosman JA, et al. High-dose interferon alfa-2b significantly prolongs relapse-free and overall survival compared with the GM2-KLH/QS-21 vaccine in patients with resected stage IIb–III melanoma: results of Intergroup Trial E1694/S9512/C509801. *J Clin Oncol* 2001;19:2370–2380.

Margolin K, Liu P-Y, Flaherty L, et al. Phase II study of BCNU, DTIC, cisplatin (DDP) and tamoxifen (Tam) in advanced melanoma: a Southwest Oncology Group study. *J Clin Oncol* 1998;16:664–669.

Meier F, Schittek B, Busch S, et al. The RAS/RAF/MEK/ERK and PI3K/AKT signaling pathways present molecular targets for the effective treatment of advanced melanoma. *Front Biosci* 2005;10:2986–3001.

Mitchell MS, Kempf RA, Harel W, et al. Low-dose cyclophosphamide and low-dose interleukin-2 for malignant melanoma. *Bull N Y Acad Med* 1989;65:128–144.

Morton DL, Foshag LJ, Hoon DSB, et al. Prolongation of survival in metastatic melanoma after active specific immunotherapy with a new polyvalent melanoma vaccine. *Ann Surg* 1992;216:463.

Morton DL, Wen DR, Wong JH, et al. Technical details of intraoperative lymphatic mapping for early stage melanoma. *Arch Surg* 1992;127:392.

Pollock PM, Trent JM. The genetics of cutaneous melanoma. *Clin Lab Med* 2000;20:667–690.

Quan W Jr, Ramirez M, Taylor WC, et al. Continuous infusion plus pulse interleukin-2 and famotidine in melanoma. *Cancer Biother Radiopharm* 2004;19(6):770–775.

Rosenberg SA, Lotze MT, Yang JC, et al. Prospective randomized trial of high-dose interleukin-2 alone or in conjunction with lymphokine-activated killer cells for the treatment of patients with advanced cancer. *J Natl Cancer Inst* 1993;85:622–632.

Nonmelanoma Skin Cancer

Aasi S, Leffell D. Chapter 27: cancer of the skin. In: DeVita VT, Hellman S, Rosenberg SA, eds. *Cancer: principles and practice of oncology*, 7th ed. Philadelphia: Lippincott Williams & Wilkins, 2005:1717–1744.

Fleming ID, Amonette R, Monaghan T, et al. Principles of management of basal and squamous carcinoma of the skin. *Cancer* 1995;75:699.

Foss F. Mycosis fungoides and the Sezary syndrome. *Curr Opin Oncol* 2004;16(5):421–428.

Goessling W, McKee PH, Mayer RJ. Merkel cell carcinoma. *J Clin Oncol* 2002;20:588–598.

Guthrie T Jr. Squamous cell and basal cell carcinoma of the skin. In: Foley JF, Vose JM, Armitage JO, eds. *Current therapy in cancer*, 2nd ed. Philadelphia: WB Saunders, 1999:255–257.

Guthrie TH Jr, Porubsky ES, Luxenberg MN, et al. Cisplatin-based chemotherapy in advanced basal and squamous cell carcinomas of the skin: results in 28 patients including 13 patients receiving multimodality therapy. *J Clin Oncol* 1990;8:342–346.

Marmur ES, Schmults CD, Goldberg DJ. A review of laser and photodynamic therapy for the treatment of nonmelanoma skin cancer. *Dermatol Surg* 2004;30(2):264–271.

Pectasides D, Pectasides M, Economopoulos T. Merkel cell cancer of the skin. *Ann Oncol* 2006;17:1489–1495.

Preston DS, Stern RS. Non-melanoma cancers of the skin. *N Engl J Med* 1992;327:1649.

Rupoli S, Barulli B, Guiducci B, et al. Low-dose interferon-alpha 2b combined with PUVA is an effective treatment of early stage mycosis fungoides: results of a multicenter study. Cutaneous-T Cell Lymphoma Multicenter Study Group. *Haematologica* 1999;84: 809–813.

Siegel RS, Pandolfino T, Guitart J, et al. Primary cutaneous T-cell lymphoma: review and current concepts. *J Clin Oncol* 2000;18: 2908–2925.

Szeimies RM, Calzavar-Pinton P, Karrer S, et al. Topical photodynamic therapy in dermatology. *J Photochem Photobiol* 1996;36: 213–219.

Vuyk HD, Lohuis PJFM. Mohs micrographic surgery for facial skin cancer. *Clin Otolaryngol* 2001;26:205–273.

CHAPTER 16

Primary and Metastatic Brain Tumors

April F. Eichler and Tracy T. Batchelor

I. Primary brain tumors (PBTs)

A. Incidence. There were 43,800 malignant and benign PBTs diagnosed in the United States in 2005. An estimated 18,500 new cases of malignant brain and central nervous system (CNS) tumors were diagnosed in 2005, representing 1.35% of all malignant cancers and accounting for 12,760 deaths in the same year. The age-adjusted 5-year relative survival for all malignant PBTs from 1995 to 2000 was 32%. The only established risk factor for PBT is ionizing radiation at high doses, which has been associated with an increased incidence of nerve sheath tumors, meningiomas, and gliomas. However, radiation-associated tumors account for only a small percentage of PBTs.

B. Gliomas. Gliomas account for 40% of all PBTs and include astrocytic, oligodendroglial, and ependymal tumors. Astrocytomas are the most frequent type, and these tumors manifest a wide spectrum of clinical behavior. The more malignant types—anaplastic astrocytoma and glioblastoma (GBM)—are not curable, although each may respond to radiation therapy (RT) and chemotherapy. Astrocytomas are graded based on the presence or absence of the following histologic features: nuclear atypia, mitoses, endothelial proliferation, and necrosis.

1. Grades I and II astrocytoma. Pilocytic astrocytomas are World Health Organization (WHO) grade I tumors that most commonly arise in the posterior fossa. These tumors are most common in the pediatric population and can be cured if a total resection is achieved. WHO grade II astrocytomas (low-grade astrocytomas) are most commonly observed in the third and fourth decades of life. This tumor typically appears as a nonenhancing, diffuse, hypointense mass on T1-weighted magnetic resonance imaging (MRI). Median survival is 7.5 years with a 5-year survival of 60%.

If feasible, a total resection should be performed and then the patient should be followed up regularly with serial MRI studies and clinical examinations. Randomized clinical trials have shown that there is no overall survival benefit when RT is given at the time of the original diagnosis, although progression-free survival may be improved with early RT. There is controversy regarding the management of WHO grade II astrocytoma in "high-risk" patients, for example, those of advanced age (>40 years) or with an elevated MIB-1 (a monoclonal antibody) labeling index (>3%–5%), as these tumors are more likely to progress rapidly. One option in this setting is to administer involved field radiation (IFR) up to 60 Gy.

In the event of tumor progression on computed tomography (CT) or MRI, further surgery, if possible, may be performed, and IFR is recommended. If, at the time of the recurrence, the histopathology demonstrates a higher-grade astrocytoma, chemotherapy can be initiated, which will be discussed in the next section on malignant astro-cytomas.

2. Grades III and IV Astrocytoma. Anaplastic astrocytoma (WHO grade III) occurs most commonly in the fourth and fifth decades, whereas GBM (WHO grade IV) occurs most commonly in the fifth and sixth decades. Median survival times are 24 to 36 and 9 to 12 months, respectively. These two types of tumors are indistinguishable by MRI, as both appear as diffuse hypointense lesions on T1-weighted images and both readily enhance after administration of intravenous contrast. These tumors are most commonly observed in the cerebral hemispheres and can have cystic or hemorrhagic components.

Histologic diagnosis is made by stereotactic biopsy or resection. Surgical debulking is the preferred initial treatment to minimize neurologic morbidity. Retrospective studies have suggested that gross total resection is associated with longer survival. Resection also relieves mass effect, which allows a patient to better tolerate subsequent IFR and often allows discontinuation of corticosteroids. Following surgery, IFR up to 60 Gy is given, usually in combination with chemotherapy. Positive prognostic factors include high Karnofsky performance score, gross total resection, and younger age.

a. Chemotherapy. Chemotherapy is now considered standard of care for glioblastoma since the publication of a European Organization for Research and Treatment of Cancer (EORTC) and National Cancer Institute of Canada (NCIC) randomized, multicenter trial of 573 patients comparing IFR (RT arm) with IFR plus concurrent temozolomide (TMZ) followed by 6 months of postradiation, monthly TMZ (chemoradiation arm). Patients treated with chemoradiation had a median survival of 14.6 months, as compared with 12.1 months in the RT arm. In addition, the 2-year survival rate was 26% in the chemoradiation group as compared with 10% in the RT group. On the basis of these results, concurrent TMZ/RT followed by monthly TMZ has become the standard of care for patients with newly diagnosed GBM. Patients with anaplastic astrocytoma could be treated similarly, although randomized data using TMZ/RT for newly diagnosed grade III tumors does not yet exist. One mechanism of resistance to alkylating agents is the deoxyribonucleic acid (DNA) repair enzyme O^6-methylguanine-DNA methyltransferase (MGMT). Multiple studies have shown that alkylating agents are more effective when MGMT is inactivated by promoter methylation. However, routine determination of MGMT methylation status has not yet achieved widespread acceptance.

b. Chemotherapy regimens. TMZ, an imidotetrazine analogue of dacarbazine (DTIC), acts by methylating DNA. It has excellent oral bioavailability and relatively good penetration of cerebrospinal fluid (CSF) (20%–30% of plasma levels). It is approved for the treatment of newly diagnosed GBM and recurrent anaplastic astrocytoma. The chloroethylnitrosoureas have been studied extensively for malignant glioma and include carmustine (BCNU) and lomustine (CCNU), typically given in combination with procarbazine and vincristine as PCV. BCNU and CCNU act by alkylating DNA and ribonucleic acid (RNA) and may also inhibit several key enzymatic processes by carbamoylation of amino acids in proteins. The following are regimens that have been used both in the adjuvant setting and for patients who have recurrence after surgery, IFR, or both.

(1) Temozolomide is administered differently depending upon whether it is being used in combination with IFR or not.

- **TMZ** is dosed at 75 mg/m^2 daily, 7 days/week, when given concurrently **with IFR,** for the entire duration of radiation.

  Trimethoprim–sulfamethoxazole should be administered thrice weekly with daily TMZ as prophylaxis against *pneumocystis jiroveci (formerly carinii)* pneumonia.

- **TMZ** is dosed at 150 to 200 mg/m^2 PO daily for 5 consecutive days in a 28-day treatment cycle when **given alone**.

  Administration of TMZ using a 21-day-on–7-day-off schedule, a strategy aimed at overcoming resistance by depleting MGMT, has not proved to be of benefit and might be more toxic.

(2) BCNU may be administered as adjuvant monotherapy and is given in either one dose or in 2 to 3 divided consecutive daily doses for a total of 150 to 200 mg/m^2 IV every 6 weeks.

(3) PCV is a combination of three antineoplastic agents given in a 6-week cycle:
Lomustine 110 mg/m^2 PO on day 1
Vincristine 1.4 mg/m^2 (maximum 2 mg) IV on days 8 and 29
Procarbazine 60 mg/m^2 PO days 8 through 21 of the 42-day cycle
    PCV is typically administered for 6 to 12 months or until tumor progression. PCV is associated with more myelotoxicity and neurotoxicity than other commonly prescribed chemotherapeutic drugs for malignant glioma.

(4) BCNU wafers are a depot source of BCNU that can be surgically implanted at the time of resection. The U.S. Food and Drug Administration (FDA) approved the 3.85% BCNU wafer for recurrent GBM after a phase III, double-blind, placebo-controlled clinical study involving 222 patients undergoing surgery for recurrent malignant glioma showed that BCNU wafers increased median survival from 20 to 28 weeks. A second randomized trial was conducted using BCNU wafers at the time of initial diagnosis of malignant glioma and led to FDA approval for newly diagnosed malignant glioma. This study showed a median survival of 13.9 months in the BCNU wafer group versus 11.6 months in the placebo arm. However, when anaplastic and nonglial histologies were excluded from the analysis, a survival advantage for patients with GBM was not observed.

Recurrent malignant astrocytoma may be treated by surgical debulking, radiosurgery, or chemotherapy. In general, recurrent malignant gliomas are resistant to most types of therapy, and consideration of treatment within the context of a clinical trial is appropriate.

3. **Oligodendroglioma (WHO grades II and III)**

a. **Characteristics.** Low-grade (WHO grade II) oligodendroglioma (LGO) and anaplastic (WHO grade III) oligodendrogliomas (AOs) are glial tumors that are found almost exclusively in the cerebral hemispheres and represent 4% to 15% of all gliomas. The peak incidence occurs in the fourth through sixth decades of life. Oligodendrogliomas have increased cellularity with homogeneous, hyperchromatic nuclei surrounded by clear cytoplasm: the classic "fried-egg" appearance. Allelic loss of the short arm of chromosome 1p and the long arm of chromosome 19q occurs in 50% to 70% of both AO and LGO and predicts better response to chemotherapy and longer survival. These tumors are hypointense on T1-weighted MRI scans and hyperintense on T2-weighted images and are located in the deep white matter. The median survival for WHO grade II oligodendrogliomas and WHO grade III oligodendrogliomas has been reported as 9.8 to 16.7 years and 3.5 years, respectively. However, these estimates do not stratify patients on the basis of the underlying status of chromosomes 1p and 19q.

b. **Treatment.** Although the optimal treatment for these tumors remains controversial, the general approach is similar to that for astrocytomas. In all cases, if a tumor is suspected, a stereotactic biopsy should be performed or confirmed tumors should be resected, if feasible. Residual or unresectable LGOs can be followed up with serial MRI studies and clinical examinations. As with low-grade astrocytomas, oligodendrogliomas with elevated MIB-1 labeling (>3%–5%) are considered higher risk and, therefore, are often treated like grade III tumors. Following the initial resection of an AO, RT has been a standard recommendation. However, since grade III tumors have shown 60% to 100% response rates to PCV, this form of chemotherapy or TMZ is administered either before IFR or in the postradiation period. PCV has been shown to prolong disease-free survival but not overall survival in two randomized phase III trials in patients with AO. TMZ has shown a 31% objective response rate as initial therapy for LGO in patients with clinical and/or radiographic progression and no prior therapy other than surgery.

C. Medulloblastoma (WHO grade IV)

1. **Characteristics.** Medulloblastomas are malignant embryonal tumors of the posterior fossa. Eighty percent are found in children younger than 15 years, and this neoplasm accounts for 20% of all pediatric brain tumors. Medulloblastomas represent 1% of tumors in patients older than 20 years. Histologically, the tumor is characterized by poorly differentiated, densely packed, hyperchromatic, nucleated, small, round, blue cells. Medulloblastomas are invasive and tend to metastasize through the CSF to the rest of the CNS. The staging evaluation for these patients should include contrast-enhanced MRI of the entire neuraxis (brain and spinal cord) and lumbar puncture for CSF cytopathology if the latter can be safely performed. If disseminated disease is found at the time of the diagnosis (poor-risk category), radical tumor resection confers little to no survival benefit.

2. **Treatment.** Treatment for local disease involves surgical resection, followed by craniospinal radiation (CSR) in adults to a dose of 36 Gy with a boost to the tumor bed to 54 Gy. In the average-risk patient, this treatment approach is associated with a 60% 5-year progression-free survival. In an attempt to minimize the long-term side effects of radiation in children, one study reported acceptable results with 23.4 Gy of CSR given, with a boost to the tumor bed to 55.8 Gy, followed by chemotherapy. This approach resulted in a 5-year progression-free survival of 79%.

There are multiple chemotherapy regimens for medulloblastomas, all of which were developed in the pediatric population. A common approach involves the use of the following drugs in combination: etoposide, cisplatin, cyclophosphamide, and vincristine. In patients with recurrent medulloblastoma, high-dose chemotherapy with autologous stem cell rescue may be beneficial.

D. Primary central nervous system lymphoma (PCNSL) in immunocompetent patients.

PCNSL is a diffuse large B-cell lymphoma arising within the CNS. This tumor accounts for 3.1% of all PBTs, and the median age at diagnosis is 60. Ocular involvement is seen in 5% to 20% of cases and leptomeningeal spread in 20% to 40% of cases. Sixty percent of tumors are supratentorial and commonly involve the periventricular regions and corpus callosum. Twenty-five percent to 50% of cases have multifocal disease at the time of diagnosis. The lesions are hypointense to isointense on T1-weighted MRI and enhance homogeneously on postgadolinium images. The tumors are responsive to corticosteroids, and as a result, these drugs should be avoided until a diagnosis has been established. The only role for surgery in PCNSL is to establish the diagnosis by biopsy. These tumors should not be resected except in the rare circumstance of brain herniation from mass effect.

Extent of disease evaluations for patients with PCNSL should include gadolinium-enhanced MRI of the brain and spine; CT scans of chest, abdomen and pelvis; ophthalmologic evaluation with slit lamp examination; lumbar puncture for CSF cytopathology, flow cytometry and IgH (immunoglobulin heavy) gene rearrangement testing; serum lactate dehydroge-nase level and a bone marrow biopsy. Patients should also be tested for the human immunodeficiency virus.

Whole-brain radiation therapy (WBRT) results in a 90% response rate, but the median survival with WBRT alone is less than 12 months. PCNSL is sensitive to many types of chemotherapy, with all successful regimens involving the use of high-dose methotrexate (3.5–8 g/m^2). Either alone or in com-bination with other chemotherapeutic drugs, methotrexate-based treatment is associated with radiographic response rates of 50% to 100% and survival durations of 40 to 90 months without the use of WBRT. Methotrexate is associated with potentially severe nephrotoxicity; so renal function must be closely monitored during methotrexate treatment.

II. **Brain metastases**

A. **Incidence.** Brain metastases are much more common than PBT in adults. The incidence is approximately 2.8 to 11.1/100,000 person-years in the United States. It is suspected that 20% to 25% of patients dying of cancer each year have brain metastases. Most commonly, cerebral metastases arise from cancer of the lung, breast, skin (melanoma), kidney, and colon.

B. **Treatment**

1. **Surgery.** Because metastatic cancers often do not ex-tensively infiltrate the surrounding normal brain paren-chyma, these tumors can usually be resected. However, this approach should be attempted only when the tumors are accessible and few in number, as revealed by CT or MRI, and when the patient's cancer is under good control systemically. In the 25% of brain metastases patients who have single or solitary lesions, surgery followed by WBRT results in longer survival than WBRT alone (40 vs. 15 weeks for cerebral metastases from lung cancer).

2. **Radiation therapy.** WBRT is recommended for pa-tients with brain metastases as micrometastatic disease is often present. Small brain metastases (generally less than 4 cm in diameter) that are solitary or persistent after WBRT may be treated with stereotactic radiosurgery (SRS) (linear accelerator, cobalt source/gamma knife, proton ra-diosurgery). This technique uses a stereotactic frame and specialized external-beam focusing. It permits a high dose of RT to be delivered to a small region in a single fraction. However, cerebral radiation necrosis is a potential com-plication and may necessitate either surgery or prolonged use of corticosteroids. The decision to proceed with either radiosurgery or resection should be individually tailored and based on status of the primary tumor, performance status, location of the tumor, and number of tumors. A ran-domized trial has shown that the addition of SRS to WBRT increases survival in patients with single brain metastasis and achieves effective palliation in patients with one to three brain metastases.

3. **Chemotherapy.** Chemotherapy has a limited role in the treatment of brain metastases. However, there are exceptions, as metastases from breast cancer occasionally respond well to the usual regimens for breast tumors.

Lymphomatous brain masses may also respond to methotrexate-based chemotherapy.

III. Leptomeningeal metastases. The treatment of leptomeningeal metastases includes RT to symptomatic areas of the CNS (e.g., to the base of the brain for cranial nerve dysfunction) and intrathecal (IT) chemotherapy with methotrexate, cytosine arabinoside (ara-C), or thiotepa.

   A. Chemotherapy regimens

   1. Methotrexate, 12 to 15 mg/dose, is the most commonly used IT chemotherapeutic agent. It is generally administered twice a week until the cytologic examination shows clearance of malignant cells from the CSF, and then once a month as maintenance.

   2. Cytarabine (ara-C) 50 mg is available in a sustained-delivery form (Depocyt, Depotec, depofoam) for IT administration that allows treatment every 2 weeks. This is an advantage over conventional IT drugs, which must be delivered two to three times each week. Concurrent administration of oral corticosteroids (dexamethasone 4 mg b.i.d. on days 1 to 5) is required with the sustained-release form of cytarabine as the main side effect from this medication is arachnoiditis. Nonliposomal ara-C can also be delivered intrathecally. The most common dose is 30 mg/m^2 given every 4 days until normalization of spinal fluid.

   3. Thiotepa 12 mg is a third IT chemotherapeutic agent that may be used if there is no response to methotrexate or cytarabine. However, the short CSF half-life of this agent may compromise its efficacy.

   B. Administration. All chemotherapeutic agents for IT administration should be freshly prepared in preservative-free diluent. Since drugs that are administered into the lumbar subarachnoid space result in lower concentrations of the drugs in the upper spine and brain, it is advisable to administer these drugs through an Ommaya reservoir, a device that is implanted under the scalp and connected by a catheter, through a burr hole, to the frontal horn of the lateral ventricle. This method allows more reliable delivery of drug to the CSF and better distribution of drug along CSF pathways and avoids the necessity of repeated lumbar punctures for the patient.

   C. Complications. Complications of IT chemotherapy include arachnoiditis and leukoencephalopathy. The latter is more likely to occur if the perforated tubing of the Ommaya catheter becomes lodged in brain tissue rather than in the lateral ventricle. Myelosuppression is not usually significant unless the patient undergoes spinal irradiation or systemic chemotherapy as well. Oral leucovorin is generally given after IT methotrexate (10 mg leucovorin PO every 6 hours for six to eight doses, starting 24 hours after the methotrexate) to prevent bone marrow toxicity.

IV. Treatment of cerebral edema

   A. Corticosteroids. These drugs are usually started soon after the diagnosis of a brain tumor is established. However, if PCNSL is suspected on the basis of CT or MRI, then corticosteroids should be withheld until after a biopsy has been done. In the rare patient with PCNSL who requires emergent antiedema measures, mannitol may be administered (see following text). **Dexamethasone 10 mg IV followed by 4 mg every 6 hours PO or IV** reduces or eliminates the lethargy, headaches, visual blurring, and nausea caused by cerebral edema and also often reduces some of the focal neurological signs and symptoms such as hemiparesis. The corticosteroid dose should be tapered and discontinued after a complete surgical resection has been performed or after radiation therapy has been completed and resumed if symptoms recur. The dose should be held at the lowest value that maximizes therapeutic benefit and minimizes side effects (e.g., gastric irritation, insomnia, mood swings, Cushingoid body features, increased appetite, and myopathy).

   B. **Treatment of refractory cerebral edema**
      1. **Increase dexamethasone.** When moderate doses of dexamethasone do not effectively control cerebral edema, the dose may be increased transiently up to 10 to 24 mg IV every 4 to 6 hours. This dose should usually not be maintained for longer than 48 to 72 hours.
      2. **An osmotic diuretic** in an urgent situation may act more rapidly than a corticosteroid. Mannitol 75 to 100 g IV (as a 15%–25% solution) is given by rapid infusion over 20 to 30 minutes and repeated at 6 to 8 hours intervals as needed. Careful monitoring of electrolytes, serum osmolarity, fluid intake and output, and body weight is essential to avoid dehydration. The osmotic diuresis may be discontinued when there is improvement in the signs and symptoms from cerebral edema and when the corticosteroids or other measures to reduce cerebral edema have taken effect.

V. **Treatment of seizures**
   A. **Seizures are a common presenting feature** in patients with brain tumors, with an incidence of approximately 20%. Prophylactic treatment for patients with brain tumors who have not had a seizure is not beneficial. However, it is common practice to administer a prophylactic anticonvulsant for a period of time after a biopsy or a craniotomy. If the patient has not had a seizure and has undergone only an uncomplicated biopsy or resection, the anticonvulsant may be discontinued after 4 to 8 weeks. If a patient does have a seizure and is to be placed on an anticonvulsant, phenytoin (Dilantin) at 300 mg/day is often recommended. Alternative monotherapies include carbamazepine, oxcarbamazepine, and valproic acid. Newer broad-spectrum anticonvulsants, such as levetiracetam (Keppra), are unproven for monotherapy but potentially of value in the future. If the patient has further seizures despite having sufficient serum levels of an anticonvulsant, then a second agent may be added. For those on long-term anticonvulsant therapy, it is important to check drug levels at intervals, especially after dosages of other medications have been changed or new medications have been added.
   B. **Common side effects** of anticonvulsant treatment include sedation, nausea, rash, diplopia, dysmetria, ataxia, and hepatic dysfunction. A rare but serious toxicity is Stevens-Johnson syndrome, which is an immune complex–mediated hypersensitivity disorder. There may be an increased risk of this complication in patients undergoing simultaneous cranial irradiation and corticosteroid taper. This may present as a

Table 16.1.   Antiepileptic drugs, enzyme-inducing versus nonenzyme-inducing

Enzyme-Inducing Antiepileptic Drugs (EIAED)	Non–Enzyme-Inducing Antiepileptic Drugs (NEIAED)
Phenytoin (Dilantin)	Valproic acid (Depakote)
Phenobarbital	Gabapentin (Neurontin)
Carbamazepine (Tegretol)	Lamotrigine (Lamictal)
Oxcarbazepine (Trileptal)	Levetiracetam (Keppra)
Primidone (Mysoline)	Topiramate (Topamax)
	Zonisamide (Zonegran)
	Tiagabine (Gabitril)
	Felbamate (Felbatol)

rash beginning as macules that may develop into papules, vesicles, bullae, urticarial plaques, or confluent erythema. A fever is present in 85% of cases.

C. Cytochrome P-450 induction. Several commonly used anticonvulsants (phenytoin, phenobarbital, carbamazepine) may induce the hepatic cytochrome P-450 enzyme system with potentially important clinical implications. This may result in increased metabolism and reduced plasma levels of chemotherapeutic drugs that undergo hepatic metabolism. This has been demonstrated in a trial of the topoisomerase I inhibitor irinotecan (CPT-11) in patients with recurrent malignant gliomas. It was found that the maximum tolerated dose of CPT-11 was approximately fourfold higher in patients taking cytochrome P-450–inducing anticonvulsants than in patients not on these drugs. This emphasizes the importance of using anticonvulsants only when clearly indicated. Non–enzyme-inducing antiepileptic drugs include valproic acid, gabapentin, lamotrigine, levetiracetam, topiramate, and zonisamide (Table 16.1).

SUGGESTED READINGS

Abrey LE, Batchelor TT, Ferreri AJ, et al. Report of an international workshop to standardize baseline evaluation and response criteria for primary CNS lymphoma. *J Clin Oncol* 2005;23:5034–5043.

Andrews D, Scott C, Sperduto P, et al. Whole brain radiation therapy with or without stereotactic radiosurgery boost for patients with one to three brain metastases: phase III results of the RTOG 9508 randomised trial. *Lancet* 2004;363:1665–1672.

van den Bent M, Chinot O, Boogerd W, et al. Second-line chemotherapy with temozolomide in recurrent oligodendroglioma after PCV (procarbazine, lomustine and vincristine) chemotherapy: EORTC Brain Tumor Group phase II study 26972. *Ann Oncol* 2003;14:599–602.

van den Bent M, Taphoorn M, Brandes A, et al. Phase II study of first-line chemotherapy with temozolomide in recurrent oligodendroglial tumors: the European Organization for Research and

Treatment of Cancer Brain Tumor Study Group 26971. *J Clin Oncol* 2003;21:2525–2528.

Brem H, Piantadosi S, Burger PC, et al. Placebo-controlled trial of safety and efficacy of intraoperative controlled delivery by biodegradable polymers of chemotherapy for recurrent gliomas. The Polymer–Brain Tumor Treatment Group. *Lancet* 1995;345: 1008–1012.

Cairncross J, Seiferheld W, Shaw E, et al. An intergroup randomized controlled clinical trial (RCT) of chemotherapy plus radiation (RT) versus RT alone for pure and mixed anaplastic oligodendrogliomas: initial report of RTOG 94–02. *J Clin Oncol* 2004;22:107s.

Glantz MJ, Cole BF, Forsyth PA, et al. Practice parameter: anticonvulsant prophylaxis in patients with newly diagnosed brain tumors—report of the Quality Standards Subcommittee of the American Academy of Neurology. *Neurology* 2000;54:1886–1893.

Hegi ME, Diserens AC, Gorlia T, et al. MGMT gene silencing and benefit from temozolomide in glioblastoma. *N Engl J Med* 2005;352:997–1003.

Hoang-Xuan K, Capelle L, Kujas S, et al. Temozolomide as initial treatment for adults with low-grade oligodendrogliomas or oligoastrocytomas and correlation with chromosome 1p deletions. *J Clin Oncol* 2004;22:3133–3138.

Hollerhage H, Zumkeller M, Becker M, et al. Influence of type and extent of surgery on early results and survival time in glioblastoma multiforme. *Acta Neurochir (Wein)* 1991;113:31–37.

Ino Y, Betensky R, Zlatescu M, et al. Molecular subtypes of anaplastic oligodendroglioma. *Clin Cancer Res* 2001;7:839–845.

Kleihues P, Cavenee WK. *WHO classification of tumors, pathology and genetics, tumours of the nervous system.* Lyon, France: IARC Press, 2000.

Langer C, Mehta M. Current management of brain metastases, with a focus on systemic options. *J Clin Oncol* 2005;23:6207–6219.

Medical Research Council Brain Tumor Working Party. Randomized trial of procarbazine, lomustine, and vincristine in the adjuvant treatment of high-grade astrocytoma: a medical research council trial. *J Clin Oncol* 2001;19:509–518.

Mrugala M, Kesari S, Ramakrishna N, et al.. Therapy for recurrent malignant glioma in adults. *Expert Rev Anticancer Ther* 2004; 4:759–782.

Packer RJ, Sutton LN, Elterman R, et al. Outcome for children with medulloblastoma treated with radiation and cisplatin, CCNU, and vincristine chemotherapy. *J Neurosurg* 1994;81:690–698.

Patchell RA, Tibbs PA, Walsh JW, et al. A randomized trial of surgery in the treatment of single metastases to the brain. *N Engl J Med* 1990;322:494–500.

Plotkin SR, Batchelor TT. Primary nervous-system lymphoma. *Lancet Oncol* 2001;2:354–365.

Stupp R, Mason WP, van den Bent MJ, et al. Radiotherapy plus concomitant and adjuvant temozolomide for glioblastoma. *N Engl J Med* 2005;352:987–996.

Wasserstrom WR, Glass JP, Posner JB. Diagnosis and treatment of leptomeningeal metastasis from solid tumors: experience with 90 patients. *Cancer* 1982;49:759.

Westphal M, Hilt D, Bortey E, et al. A phase 3 trial of local chemotherapy with biodegradable carmustine (BCNU) wafers (Gliadel wafers) in patients with primary malignant glioma. *Neuro-oncol* 2003;5: 79–88.

Yung WKA, Prados M, Yaya-Tur R, et al. Multicenter phase II trial of temozolomide in patients with anaplastic astrocytoma or anaplastic oligoastrocytoma at first relapse. *J Clin Oncol* 1999;17: 2762–2771.

CHAPTER 17

Soft Tissue Sarcomas

Robert S. Benjamin

I. **Classification and approach to treatment**
   A. **Types of soft tissue sarcomas.** The soft tissue sarcomas are a group of diseases characterized by neoplastic proliferation of tissue of mesenchymal origin. Thus, they differ from the more common carcinomas, which arise from epithelial tissue. Sarcomas can arise in any area of the body and from any origin; however, they most commonly arise in the soft tissue of the extremities, trunk, retroperitoneum, or head and neck area. There are more than 20 different types of sarcomas, classified according to lines of differentiation toward normal tissue. For example, rhabdomyosarcoma shows evidence of skeletal muscle fibers with cross-striations, liposarcoma shows fat production, and angiosarcoma shows vessel formation. Precise characterization of the types of sarcoma is often impossible, and these tumors are called *unclassified sarcomas*. All of the primary bone sarcomas may arise in soft tissue, leading to such diagnoses as extraskeletal osteosarcoma, extraskeletal Ewing's sarcoma, and extraskeletal chondrosarcoma. A common diagnosis in the recent past was malignant fibrous histiocytoma (MFH). This tumor is characterized by a mixture of spindle (or fibrous) cells and round (or histiocytic) cells arranged in a storiform pattern with frequent areas of pleomorphic appearance and frequent giant cells. There is no evidence of differentiation toward any particular tissue type. Many tumors previously called *pleomorphic fibrosarcoma, pleomorphic rhabdomyosarcoma*, and so forth were classified as MFH. As immunohistochemistry and molecular diagnostic techniques have improved, many of the tumors previously classified as MFH have been reclassified as pleomorphic something else. Furthermore, there are strong opponents of the term *MFH* since there is no evidence that the tumors have histiocytic origin, and pleomorphic tumors previously classified as MFH are now frequently referred to as *unclassified high grade pleomorphic sarcomas*.
   B. **Metastases.** Metastatic spread of all sarcomas tends to be through the blood rather than through the lymphatic system. The lungs are by far the most frequent site of metastatic disease. Local sites of metastasis by direct invasion are the second most common area of involvement, followed by bone and liver. (Liver metastases are common with intra-abdominal sarcomas, especially gastrointestinal stromal tumors [GISTs], however, and metastases to soft tissue are common with myxoid liposarcomas.) Central nervous system (CNS) metastases are extraordinarily rare except in alveolar soft-part sarcoma.
   C. **Staging.** Staging of sarcomas is complex and demands an expert sarcoma pathologist. Tumors have been staged

according to two systems: the American Joint Committee on Cancer (AJCC) staging system and the Musculoskeletal Tumor Society staging system. The new International Union Against Cancer (UICC)/AJCC staging system with international acceptance takes portions from each of the older systems and more appropriately identifies patients at increased risk of metastatic disease. Further revisions to this system are still under way, and a final, widely accepted system is still not in place. Since current and earlier publications still refer to the older systems, however, all will be included.

   1. **The old AJCC staging system**
      a. **Tumor grade.** The primary determinant of stage is tumor grade.

      Grade 1 tumors are stage I.
      Grade 2 tumors are stage II.
      Grade 3 tumors are stage III.
      Any tumor with lymph node metastases is automatically stage III.
      Any tumor with gross invasion of bone, major vessel, or major nerve is stage IV.

      b. **Stage.** Further divisions of stages I to III into A and B are based on tumor size.

      A = tumor smaller than 5 cm
      B = tumor size 5 cm or larger

      In stage III, lymph node metastases are classified as IIIC. In stage IV, local invasion is called IVA, and IVB represents distant metastases.
   2. **The Musculoskeletal Tumor Society staging system.** The Musculoskeletal Tumor Society stages sarcomas according to grade and compartmental localization. The Roman numeral reflects the tumor grade.

   Stage I: low grade
   Stage II: high grade
   Stage III: any-grade tumor with distant metastasis

      The letter reflects compartmental localization. Compartments are defined by fascial planes.

   Stage A: intracompartmental (i.e., confined to the same soft tissue compartment as the initial tumor)
   Stage B: extracompartmental (i.e., extending outside of the initial soft tissue compartment into the adjacent soft tissue compartment or bone)

      A stage IA tumor is a low-grade tumor confined to its initial compartment, a stage IB tumor is a low-grade tumor extending outside the initial compartment, and so forth.
   3. **The new AJCC staging system.** The stage is determined by tumor grade, tumor size, and tumor location relative to the muscular fascia. There are now four tumor grades.

   Grade 1: well differentiated
   Grade 2: moderately differentiated
   Grade 3: poorly differentiated
   Grade 4: undifferentiated

Tumor size is now divided as less than or equal to 5 cm or more than 5 cm (in the old AJCC system, it was less than 5 cm or more than or equal to 5 cm).

T1 = less than or equal to 5 cm
T2 = greater than 5 cm

Tumor status is subdivided by location relative to the muscular fascia.

Ta = superficial to the muscular fascia
Tb = deep to the muscular fascia

The AJCC stage grouping is as follows:

Stage I	T1a, 1b, 2a, 2b	N0	M0	G1–2
Stage II	T1a, 1b, 2a	N0	M0	G3–4
Stage III	T2b	N0	M0	G3–4
Stage IV	Any T	N1	M0	Any G
	Any T	N0	M1	Any G

The new staging system divides patients according to necessary therapy.

Stage I patients are adequately treated by surgery alone.
Stage II patients require adjuvant radiation therapy.
Stage III patients require adjuvant chemotherapy.
Stage IV patients are managed primarily with chemotherapy, with or without other modalities.

D. Evaluation. Patients are evaluated and followed up according to the plan in Table 17.1.
E. Primary treatment
  1. Surgery and radiotherapy. Treatment of the primary tumor involves surgery with or without radiation therapy. If radiation therapy is not used, surgery must be radical. Although this may often involve amputation or complete excision of the involved muscle group from origin to insertion, more and more frequently, wide local resection is performed, with or without adjuvant radiation, depending on stage and extent of negative margins.
  2. Adjuvant chemotherapy. The role of adjuvant chemotherapy remains controversial, with both positive and negative results reported. A meta-analysis of individual patient data indicated a highly significant decrease in the risk of disease recurrence (either local or distant) and death in patients treated with adjuvant chemotherapy; thus, *some investigators believe that adjuvant therapy is clearly indicated for patients whose histologic type, grade, or location is known to convey a poor prognosis.* The meta-analysis confirms a survival benefit for patients with primary sarcomas of the extremities as well as increased local or distant disease-free interval for all patients treated with doxorubicin (Adriamycin)-based adjuvant chemotherapy. A recent Italian cooperative group study using epirubicin and ifosfamide for patients with current stage III disease also demonstrated survival and disease-free survival advantage for patients treated with chemotherapy; however,

Table 17.1. Soft tissue sarcoma evaluation

Tests[a]	Initial	During Treatment	Follow-up (if no evidence of disease)
History and physical examination	X	Before each treatment	Year 1: q2 months; years 2, 3: q3 months; year 4: q4 months; year 5: q6 months; then yearly
CBC, differential, and platelet counts[b]	X	Twice weekly	Yearly
Electrolytes[b]	X	Before each treatment	—
Chemistry profile[b]	X	Before each treatment	q4 months
Urinalysis	If giving ifosfamide	As indicated by symptoms	—
PT, APTT, fibrinogen	X	—	—
Chest radiograph	X	Before each treatment	Same as for history and physical examination
CT scan chest	If chest radiograph appears normal	To confirm chest radiograph findings (if initially abnormal) or for surgical planning	If chest radiograph becomes equivocal
MRI primary (if not intra-abdominal), or	X	Preoperatively	—
Ultrasound primary	—	—	Year 1: q4 months; years 2, 3: q6 months

(continued)

Table 17.1.   *(Continued)*

Tests[a]	Initial	During Treatment	Follow-up (if no evidence of disease)
PET-CT	X	Every two to three cycles if preoperative therapy is given	—
CT of abdomen and pelvis	If myxoid liposarcoma or retroperitoneal or pelvic primary tumor	If baseline, every third cycle	If baseline, year 1: q4 months; years 2, 3: q6 months
ECG	If cardiac history	—	—
Cardiac nuclear scan (for ejection fraction)	If cardiac history	If doxorubicin dose is to exceed standard limits for schedule	Yearly for 2 years, then as clinically indicated
Central venous catheter	X	—	—
Bone marrow or screening MRI of spine and pelvis	If small cell tumor	—	—
Bone scan	If indicated by history	—	—
Plain film	If indicated by history	—	—

CBC, complete blood cell count; PT, prothrombin time; APTT, activated partial thromboplastin time; CT, computed tomography; MRI, magnetic resonance imaging; PET, positron emission tomography; ECG, electrocardiography; X, procedure to be done; —, procedure not needed.

[a]Tests may be ordered more frequently based on clinical indications.

[b]Required more frequently if patient is on a medical treatment program.

the statistical significance of the survival advantage was lost with further follow-up.

F. Prognosis. Prognosis is related to stage, with a 5-year survival rate of 99% for new AJCC/UICC stage I, 82% for stage II, and 52% for stage III. Corresponding rates of disease-free survival at 5 years are 78% for stage I, 64% for stage II, and 36% for stage III. Long-term results are still worse. The survival rate for stage IV disease is less than 10%; however, a definite fraction of patients in this category can be cured. Most patients with stage IV disease, if left untreated, die within 6 to 12 months; however, there is great variation in actual survival, and patients may go on with slowly progressive disease for many years.

G. Treatment response. Response to treatment is measured in the standard manner for solid tumors with the addition of tumor necrosis, both radiologically and pathologically, but there are increasing examples where good responses are missed by standard criteria, and newer approaches to computed tomography (CT) and magnetic resonance imaging (MRI) evaluation and the use of positron emission tomography (PET) are becoming more frequent.

1. Complete remission. This implies complete disappearance of all signs and symptoms of disease.

2. Partial remission. Standard response evaluation criteria in solid tumors (RECIST) criteria (Chapter 2, Section IV.B.1) are generally employed. This requires a 30% or greater decrease in measurable disease, calculated by comparing the sum of the longest diameters of all lesions before and after therapy. When disease can be followed objectively by MRI or CT, marked tumor necrosis attributable to chemotherapy demonstrated by imaging or pathology is considered at least the equivalent of a partial response by RECIST criteria.

3. Stable disease or improvement. Lesser degrees of tumor shrinkage are categorized by some physicians as stable disease and by others as improvement or minor response. Stable disease implies a less than 20% increase in disease for at least 8 weeks. There is increasing recognition that stable disease or improvement that persists for a minimum of 4 months is at least as meaningful for ultimate patient benefit as partial response. For all response categories, no new disease must appear during response.

4. Progression. New disease in any area or a 20% or more increase in measurable disease constitutes progressive disease.

5. Survival. All patients whose disease responds objectively to chemotherapy survive longer than patients with progressive disease, and the degree of prolongation of survival is directly proportional to the degree of antitumor response that can be measured.

II. Chemotherapy

A. General considerations and aims of therapy. Although there are numerous types of soft tissue sarcomas, there are few differences among them regarding responsiveness to a standard soft tissue sarcoma regimen. GISTs and alveolar soft-part sarcomas and, to a lesser extent, clear cell sarcomas and epithelioid sarcomas respond less frequently to standard regimens than do the other soft tissue sarcomas. GISTs, in particular, should not be treated with doxorubicin- and ifosfamide-based chemotherapy. GISTs are usually characterized by mutated *c-Kit* and have a high response rate with prolonged remissions after treatment with imatinib at 400 mg daily. Patients who do not respond or who have a relapse after initial therapy may respond to higher doses up to 800 mg in divided doses daily or to sunitinib. Angiosarcomas can respond to paclitaxel, while other sarcomas do not. Two tumors—Ewing's sarcoma and rhabdomyosarcoma—particularly in children, are responsive to dactinomycin, vincristine, or etoposide. The other tumors are not. The goal of therapy for patients with advanced disease is primarily palliative, although a small fraction (~20%) of patients who achieve complete remission are, in fact, cured. The first aim, therefore, is to achieve complete remission. Several investigators, including the author, have shown that the prognosis is the same whether complete remission is obtained by chemotherapy alone or by chemotherapy with adjuvant surgery, that is, surgical removal of all residual disease. Short of complete remission, partial remission causes some palliation, with relief of symptoms and prolongation of survival by approximately 1 year. Any degree of improvement or stabilization of previously advancing disease likewise increases survival.

B. Effective drugs. The most important chemotherapeutic agent is doxorubicin, which forms the backbone of all combination-chemotherapy regimens. Ifosfamide, an analog of cyclophosphamide that has documented activity even in patients who are refractory to combinations containing cyclophosphamide, is usually included in front-line chemotherapy combinations. It is always given together with the uroprotective agent mesna to prevent hemorrhagic cystitis. Dacarbazine (DTIC), a marginal agent by itself, adds significantly to doxorubicin in prolonging remission duration and survival as well as in increasing the response rate. Cyclophosphamide adds marginally, if at all, but is included in some effective regimens.

The key to effective sarcoma chemotherapy is the steep dose–response curve for doxorubicin. At a dose of 45 mg/m^2, the response rate is lower than 20% as compared with a 37% response rate at a dose of 75 mg/m^2. A similar dose–response relationship exists for ifosfamide and for combination chemotherapy, and the regimens with the best reported results are those using the highest doses.

C. Primary chemotherapy regimen (adjuvant or advanced). The most effective primary chemotherapy regimens include doxorubicin and ifosfamide (high-dose AI) or doxorubicin and dacarbazine (ADIC), with or without the addition of cyclophosphamide (CyADIC) or ifosfamide and mesna (MAID). The CyADIC regimen is a modification of the standard CyVADIC regimen, which includes vincristine. Because analysis has shown that vincristine makes no significant contribution and produces neurotoxicity, its addition at a dose of 2 mg maximum or 1.4 mg/m^2 weekly for 6 weeks and then once every 3 to 4 weeks is recommended only for treatment of rhabdomyosarcoma and Ewing's sarcoma.

By giving doxorubicin and dacarbazine by continuous 72- or 96-hour infusion, with the two drugs mixed in the same infusion pump, nausea and vomiting are markedly reduced, and the chemotherapy can be continued until a cumulative doxorubicin dose of 800 mg/m^2 is reached, with less cardiac toxicity than with standard doxorubicin administration and a cumulative dose of 450 mg/m^2.

 1. The high-dose AI regimen is as follows:

Doxorubicin by continuous 72-hour infusion at 75 mg/m^2 IV (25 mg/m^2/day for 3 days), *and*

Ifosfamide 2.5 g/m^2 IV over 2 to 3 hours daily for 4 days.

Vincristine 2 mg total dose is added on day 1 for small cell tumors such as rhadomyosarcoma, Ewing's sarcoma **(high-dose VAI)**.

Mesna 500 mg/m^2 is mixed with the first ifosfamide dose, and 1,500 mg/m^2 is given as a continuous infusion over 24 hours for 4 days in 2 L of alkaline fluid.

Filgrastim (granulocyte colony-stimulating factor) 5 µg/kg SC is given on days 5 to 15 or until granulocyte recovery to 1,500/µL. Alternatively, **Pegfilgrastim** at a dose of 6 mg is given on day 5.

Repeat cycle every 3 weeks.

 2. The continuous-infusion CyADIC regimen is as follows:

Cyclophosphamide 600 mg/m^2 IV on day 1, *and*

Doxorubicin, by continuous 96-hour infusion at 60 mg/m^2 IV (15 mg/m^2/day for 4 days), *and*

Dacarbazine by continuous 96-hour infusion at 1,000 mg/m^2 IV (250 mg/m^2/day for 4 days) mixed in the same bag or pump as the doxorubicin. Doses should be divided into four consecutive 24-hour infusions.

Repeat cycle every 3 to 4 weeks.

 3. The continuous-infusion ADIC regimen is as follows:

Doxorubicin by continuous 96-hour infusion at 90 mg/m^2 IV (22.5 mg/m^2/day for 4 days), *and*

Dacarbazine by continuous 96-hour infusion at 900 mg/m^2 IV (225 mg/m^2/day for 4 days) mixed in the same bag or pump as the doxorubicin. Doses should be divided into four consecutive 24-hour infusions.

Repeat cycle every 3 to 4 weeks.

 4. The MAID regimen is as follows:

Mesna by continuous 96-hour infusion at 8,000 mg/m^2 IV (2,000 mg/m^2/day for 4 days).

Doxorubicin by continuous 72-hour infusion at 60 mg/m^2 IV (20 mg/m^2/day for 3 days).

Ifosfamide by continuous 72-hour infusion at 6,000 mg/m^2 IV (2,000 mg/m^2/day for 3 days). Doses should be divided into three consecutive 24-hour infusions. (Some investigators prefer to infuse ifosfamide over 2 hours rather than over 24 hours because of higher single-agent activity with the shorter infusions.)

Dacarbazine by continuous 72-hour infusion at 900 mg/m^2 IV (300 mg/m^2/day for 3 days) mixed in the same bag or pump as the doxorubicin. Doses should be divided into three consecutive 24-hour infusions.

Repeat cycle every 3 to 4 weeks.

5. Dose modification. Doses of doxorubicin, cyclophosphamide, ifosfamide, and mesna should be increased by 25% and may be decreased by 20% for each course of therapy to achieve a lowest absolute granulocyte count of approximately 500/µL if growth factors are not used. *The maximum doxorubicin dose is limited to 600 to 800 mg/m^2*, depending on the duration (48–96 hours) of infusion, at which point, therapy should be discontinued unless cardiac biopsy specimens indicate that it is safe to continue. With Ewing's sarcoma and rhabdomyosarcoma, therapy may be continued, and dactinomycin 2 mg/m^2 in a single dose or 0.5 mg/m^2 daily for 5 days may be substituted for the doxorubicin, with continuation of the regimen for a total of 18 months.

6. An alternative regimen for children with rhabdomyosarcoma is an alternating regimen, using ifosfamide and etoposide alternating with the so-called VAdriaC regimen.

Vincristine 1.5 mg/m^2 is given weekly × 3 for the first two cycles of VAdriaC and then on day 1 only.

Doxorubicin is given at a dose of 60 to 75 mg/m^2 as a 48-hour continuous infusion, *and*

Cyclophosphamide 600 mg/m^2 is given daily for 2 days (with mesna).

After 3 weeks,

Ifosfamide is given at a dose of 1,800 mg/m^2 daily for 5 days (with mesna), *and*

Etoposide is given at a dose of 100 mg/m^2 daily for 5 days.

Chemotherapy cycles are alternated every 3 weeks for 39 weeks.

7. A less-intensive, older, but still effective regimen for children with good-prognosis rhabdomyosarcoma is the so-called pulse VAC regimen. Dactinomycin is given at a total dose of 2 to 2.5 mg/m^2 by divided daily injection over 5 to 7 days (e.g., 0.5 mg/m^2 daily for 5 days) repeated every 3 months for a total of five courses. Cyclophosphamide pulses of 275 to 330 mg/m^2 daily for 7 days are begun at the same time but are given every 6 weeks with vincristine 2 mg/m^2 on days 1 and 8 of each cyclophosphamide cycle. Cyclophosphamide cycles are terminated prematurely if the white blood cell counts fall below 1,500/µL. Chemotherapy continues for 2 years. (The necessity of the 2-year duration of the chemotherapy program is not certain.)

D. Secondary chemotherapy. Secondary chemotherapy for patients with sarcoma is relatively unrewarding, with response rates lower than 10% for almost all conventional drugs or regimens tested. The best commercially available drug is ifosfamide, which, if not used in primary treatment, produces a response in approximately 20% of patients. High-dose ifosfamide (12 g/m^2 or higher) may produce responses in patients resistant to lower doses in combination. Gemcitabine in our hands has a response rate of 18% and has become our standard drug for salvage therapy. Recent data indicate that the combination of gemcitabine and docetaxel (the **Gem-Tax regimen**) improves response rate, time to progression, and survival in a randomized comparison with gemcitabine alone.

The Gem-Tax regimen is as follows:

Gemcitabine 900 mg/m^2 over 90 minutes on days 1 and 8.

Docetaxel 100 mg/m^2 on day 8 only.

Filgrastim (granulocyte colony-stimulating factor) 5μg/kg SC is given on days 9 to 15 or until granulocyte recovery to 1,500/μL. Alternatively, **Pegfilgrastim** at a dose of 6 mg is given on day 9.

The duration of gemcitabine infusion is critical, since it can only be converted to its active metabolite, gemcitabine triphosphate, at a rate of 10 mg/m^2/minute. Doses are reduced by 25% to 675 mg/m^2 and 75 mg/m^2, respectively, for patients with extensive prior therapy or pelvic radiation. Dexamethasone 8 mg PO b.i.d. should be given for 3 days starting 1 day before docetaxel.

Methotrexate, with a response rate of approximately 15% regardless of schedule, is the only other active agent. Patients who do not respond to doxorubicin, ifosfamide, or gemcitabine-docetaxel should be entered in a phase II study of a new agent to see if some activity can be established because other reasonably good alternatives do not exist.

E. Complications of chemotherapy. Side effects of sarcoma chemotherapy can be classified into three categories: life threatening, potentially dangerous, and unpleasant.

    1. Life-threatening complications of chemotherapy are infection or bleeding. Thrombocytopenia lower than 20,000/μL occurs with this type of chemotherapy when growth factors are used to maintain dose intensity, but bleeding is rare and can be minimized by transfusing platelets at 10,000/μL. Approximately 20% to 40% of patients have documented or suspected infection related to drug-induced neutropenia at some time during their treatment course. These infections are rarely fatal if treated promptly with broad-spectrum, bactericidal antibiotics at the onset of the febrile neutropenia episode.

    2. Potentially dangerous side effects of chemotherapy include the following:

        a. Mucositis, which occurs in fewer than 25% of patients, may interfere with oral intake or may act as a source of infection.

        b. Granulocytopenia predisposes the patient to infection but, because of its brevity, rarely causes infection.

        c. Cardiac damage from doxorubicin rarely causes clinical problems at the doses recommended, with usually reversible congestive heart failure occurring in fewer than 5% of patients.

        d. Renal insufficiency is a rare complication of ifosfamide. Fanconi syndrome, particularly manifested by a significant loss of bicarbonate, is a dose-related complication of ifosfamide, occurring in 10% to 30% of patients at standard ifosfamide doses and in close to 100% of patients with high-dose regimens, the morbidity of which can be minimized by the routine use of alkaline infusions and correction of electrolyte levels with intravenous or oral replacement therapy. Only rarely does the nephrotoxicity progress to renal failure, often precipitated by dehydration or administration of minimally nephrotoxic drugs such as nonsteroidal anti-inflammatory drugs (NSAIDs). Patients treated with ifosfamide should be instructed to avoid NSAIDs, even years after chemotherapy!

e. CNS toxicity of ifosfamide is rarely a serious complication. Patients frequently demonstrate minor confusion, disorientation, or difficulty with fine movements. Somnolence and coma are rarely seen in patients without hypoalbuminemia and/or acidosis.

f. Hemorrhagic cystitis, a rare complication of cyclophosphamide therapy, used to be the dose-limiting toxicity of ifosfamide. It can be prevented in most cases by administration of another agent, mesna, before and after each ifosfamide dose, allowing higher doses of ifosfamide to be used.

g. Pulmonary toxicity, manifested by increasing dyspnea, is seen in less than 10% of patients treated with the gemcitabine–docetaxel combination, but occurs with about twice the frequency of that seen with gemcitabine alone. Careful attention to the possible occurrence of this problem and prompt treatment with high doses of corticosteroids can be life saving.

3. Unpleasant but rarely serious problems include nausea and vomiting (primarily from dacarbazine, ifosfamide, and docetaxel) and alopecia (from doxorubicin, cyclophosphamide, ifosfamide, and docetaxel). Gemcitabine, and to a greater extent, the gemcitabine–docetaxel combination, can cause profound fatigue. Gemcitabine can also cause drug fever and a rash (often confused for cellulitis) that can respond to corticosteroids.

F. Special precautions

1. Ifosfamide. Patients must be kept well hydrated with an alkaline pH to prevent CNS toxicity and minimize nephrotoxicity. Sodium bicarbonate or sodium acetate should be added to IV fluids at an initial concentration of 100 to 150 mEq/L, and fluid administration should be adjusted to produce a urine output of at least 2 L/day and to maintain the serum bicarbonate concentration at 25 mEq/L or higher. Other electrolytes should be adjusted as needed on a daily basis. Serum albumin should be kept within normal limits.

2. Doxorubicin. Avoid extravasation. Continuous infusions must (and short infusions should) be administered through a central venous catheter. Attention to cumulative dose administered (varying according to the schedule of administration) is critical to minimize the risk of cardiac toxicity.

SUGGESTED READINGS

Sarcoma meta-analysis collaboration. Adjuvant chemotherapy for localised resectable soft-tissue sarcoma of adults: meta-analysis of individual data. *Lancet* 1997;350:1647–1654.

Antman KH, Crowley J, Balcerzak SP, et al. An intergroup phase III randomized study of doxorubicin and dacarbazine with or without ifosfamide and mesna in advanced soft tissue and bone sarcomas. *J Clin Oncol* 1993;11:1276.

Antman KH, Montella D, Rosenbaum C, et al. Phase II trial of ifosfamide with mesna in previously treated metastatic sarcoma. *Cancer Treat Rep* 1985;69:499.

Benjamin RS, Legha SS, Patel RS, et al. Single agent ifosfamide studies in sarcomas of soft tissue and bone: the M.D. Anderson experience. *Cancer Chemother Pharmacol* 1993;31:S174–S179.

Demetri GD, von Mehren M, Blanke CD, et al. Efficacy and safety of imatinib mesylate in advanced gastrointestinal stromal tumors. *N Engl J Med* 2002;347:472–480.

Elias A, Ryan L, Sulkes A, et al. Response to mesna, doxorubicin, ifosfamide, and dacarbazine in 108 patients with metastatic or unresectable sarcoma and no prior chemotherapy. *J Clin Oncol* 1989;7:1208.

Fata F, O'Rielly E, Ilson D, et al. Paclitaxel in the treatment of patients with angiosarcoma of the scalp or face. *Cancer* 1999;86:2034–2037.

Frustaci S, Gherlinzoni F, De Paoli A, et al. Adjuvant chemotherapy for adult soft tissue sarcomas of the extremities and girdles: results of the Italian Randomized Cooperative Trial. *J Clin Oncol* 2001;19:1238–1247.

Greene FL, Page DL, Fleming ID, et al. for the American Joint Committee on Cancer. *AJCC cancer staging manual*, 6th ed. New York: Springer-Verlag, 2002.

Harrison L, Franzese F, Gaynor J, et al. Long-term results of a prospective randomized trial of adjuvant brachytherapy in the management of completely resected soft tissue sarcomas of the extremity and superficial trunk. *Int J Radiat Oncol Biol Phys* 1993;27:259–265.

Joensuu H, Roberts PJ, Sarlomo-Rikala M, et al. Effect of the tyrosine kinase inhibitor STI571 in a patient with a metastatic gastrointestinal stromal tumor. *N Engl J Med* 2001;344:1052–2056.

Lindberg RD, Martin RG, Romsdahl MM, et al. Conservative surgery and radiation therapy for soft tissue sarcomas. In: Martin RG, Ayala AG, eds. *Management of primary bone and soft tissue tumors*. Chicago: Year Book Publishing, 1977:289–298.

Maki RG, Hensley ML, Wathen JK, et al. A SARC multicenter phase III study of gemcitabine (G) vs. gemcitabine and docetaxel (G+D) in patients (pts) with metastatic soft tissue sarcomas (STS). (Abstract) *J Clin Oncol* 2006;24(18S):9514. ASCO Annual Meeting Proceedings Part I. (June 20 Supplement).

van Oosterom AT, Judson I, Verweij J, et al. Safety and efficacy of imatinib (STI571) in metastatic gastrointestinal stromal tumours: a phase I study. *Lancet* 2001;358:1421–1423.

Patel SR, Benjamin RS. Sarcomas: part I and II. *Hematol Oncol Clin North Am* 1995;9:513–942.

Patel SR, Gandhi V, Jenkins J, et al. Phase II clinical investigation of gemcitabine in advanced soft tissue sarcomas and window evaluation of dose-rate on gemcitabine triphosphate accumulation. *J Clin Oncol* 2001;19:3483–3489.

Patel SR, Vadhan-Raj S, Burgess MA, et al. Results of two consecutive trials of dose-intensive chemotherapy with doxorubicin and ifosfamide is highly active in patients with soft-tissue sarcomas. *Am J Clin Oncol* 1998;21:317–321.

Patel SR, Vadhan-Raj S, Papadopoulos N, et al. High-dose ifosfamide in bone and soft-tissue sarcomas: results of phase II and pilot studies. Dose response and schedule dependence. *J Clin Oncol* 1997;15:2378–2384.

Pisters P, Leung D, Woodruff J, et al. Analysis of prognostic factors in 1,041 patients with localized soft tissue sarcomas of the extremities. *J Clin Oncol* 1996;14:16799–11689.

Pollock RE. Soft tissue sarcoma. In: Greene FL, Page DL; Fleming ID, et al. eds. *AJCC cancer staging manual*, 6th ed. New York, NY: Springer-Verlag, 2002:193–197.

Therasse P, Arbuck SG, Eisenhauer EA, et al. New guidelines to evaluate the response to treatment in solid tumors. *J Natl Cancer Inst* 2000;92:205–216.

Verweij J, Casali PG, Zalcberg J, et al. Progression-free survival in gastrointestinal stromal tumours with high-dose imatinib: randomised trial. *Lancet* 2004;364:1127–1134.

Wunder J, Healey J, Davis A, et al. A comparison of staging systems for localized extremity soft tissue sarcoma. *Cancer* 2000;88:2721–2730.

Zalupski MM, Ryan J, Hussein M, et al. Defining the role of adjuvant chemotherapy for patients with soft tissue sarcoma of the extremities. In: Salmon SE, ed. *Adjuvant therapy of cancer VII*. Philadelphia: JB Lippincott Co, 1993:385–392.

CHAPTER 18

Bone Sarcomas

Robert S. Benjamin

There are four major sarcomas of bone, each differing somewhat in clinical behavior, chemotherapy responsiveness, and prognosis. All present as painful bony lesions, and all metastasize preferentially to lung and then to other bones. The prognosis of untreated sarcomas of the bone is inversely proportional to their chemotherapy responsiveness. The sarcomas are considered in order of greatest to least chemotherapeutic responsiveness: Ewing's sarcoma, osteosarcoma, malignant fibrous histiocytoma of bone, and chondrosarcoma.

Response to treatment is evaluated according to the usual criteria used for solid tumors and identical to that reported in Chapter 17. Angiography is particularly helpful in defining the response of primary bone tumors to chemotherapy, and the angiographic response correlates well with pathologic tumor destruction. Complete resection and examination of the total specimen are often required to determine response to therapy in a primary or even a metastatic lesion and to confirm complete remission.

I. **Staging.** Bone tumors are staged according to American Joint Committee on Cancer (AJCC) criteria as well as the criteria of the Musculoskeletal Tumor Society.

A. **The AJCC staging system.** The stage is determined by tumor grade, tumor size, and presence and sites of metastases. There are four tumor grades.

Grade 1: well differentiated—low grade
Grade 2: moderately differentiated—low grade
Grade 3: poorly differentiated—high grade
Grade 4: undifferentiated differentiated—high grade

Ewing's sarcoma is classified as G4

Tumor size is divided as less than or equal to 8 cm. Tumor size determines A and B substages of stages I and II, and stage III.

T1 = less than or equal to 8 cm
T2 = more than 8 cm
T3 = Discontinuous tumors in the primary bone site

Metastatic status is subdivided by presence and location of metastases.

M0 = No distant metastases
M1 = Distant metastases
    M1a = Lung
    M1b = Other distant sites, including lymph nodes

The AJCC stage grouping is as follows:

Stage IA	G1–2	T1	N0	M0
Stage IA	G1–2	T2	N0	M0
Stage IIA	G3–4	T1	N0	M0
Stage IIB	G3–4	T2	N0	M0
Stage III	Any G	T3	N0	M0
Stage IVA	Any G	Any T	N0	M1a
Stage IVB	Any G	Any T	Any N	M1b (includes N1)

B. The Musculoskeletal Tumor Society (MSTS) staging system. The Musculoskeletal Tumor Society stages sarcomas according to grade and compartmental localization.

The Roman numeral reflects the tumor grade.

Stage I: low grade
Stage II: high grade
Stage III: any-grade tumor with distant metastasis

The companion letter reflects **tumor compartmentalization.**

Stage A: confined to bone
Stage B: extending into adjacent soft tissue

C. Thus, a stage IA tumor is a low-grade tumor confined to bone, and a stage IB tumor is a low-grade tumor extending into soft tissue, and so forth. Patients are evaluated and followed up according to the plan in Table 18.1.

II. **Ewing's sarcoma**
  A. **General considerations and aims of therapy**
    1. **Tumor characteristics.** Ewing's sarcoma is a highly malignant, small, round-cell tumor of bone. It occurs most commonly in the second decade of life, and 90% of patients are younger than 30 years. There is a slight male predominance. The most common locations are the pelvis or the diaphysis of long tubular bones of the extremities. Often, systemic symptoms of fever and leukocytosis suggest infection. Radiographically, the predominant feature is osteolysis, although sclerosis does occur. Frequently, the periosteal reaction has the so-called onion skin pattern with layering of subperiosteal new bone, frequently with spicules radiating out from the cortex. Prognosis, until the era of modern chemotherapy, was extremely poor with a 5-year survival rate lower than 10% and almost half the number of patients dying within 1 year of diagnosis. Because Ewing's sarcoma is a high-grade tumor and, by definition, is almost always accompanied by a soft tissue mass, it is usually staged as AJCC stage IIB or IV depending on the demonstration of metastatic disease in lung (IVA), bone (IVB), or both. Bone metastases confer a markedly worse prognosis.
    2. **Primary treatment.** Because of the poor prognosis and because of the mutilative surgery involved in resection of the primary lesion, radiotherapy has been the primary modality for local tumor control. As techniques for limb salvage surgery have become more widely practiced, attempts

Table 18.1. Primary bone sarcoma evaluation

Tests[a]	Before Therapy	On Initial Treatment	Preoperative	On Subsequent Treatment	Follow-up
History and physical examination	X	Before each treatment	X	Before each treatment	Year 1: q2 months; years 2, 3: q3–4 months; year 4: q4 months; year 5: q6 months; then yearly
CBC, differential, and platelet counts[b]	X	Twice weekly	X	Twice weekly	Yearly
Chemistry profile[b]	X	Before each treatment	X	Before each treatment	Year 1: q4–6 months; then yearly
Calculated creatinine clearance	X	For methotrexate	—	For methotrexate	—
Electrolytes, Mg[b]	X	Before each treatment	X	Before each treatment	—
Urinalysis	If ifosfamide is given	As indicated by symptoms	X	Before each treatment	—
PT, APTT, fibrinogen	X	Before each IA treatment and daily while on IA treatment	X	—	—
Plain films of primary tumor	X	Every two cycles	X	q3 months	Year 1: q4–6 months; then yearly

(continued)

Table 18.1. *(Continued)*

Tests[a]	Before Therapy	On Initial Treatment	Preoperative	On Subsequent Treatment	Follow-up
CT of primary tumor	X	After two to four cycles	X	—	At end of treatment for head and neck or pelvic primaries
MRI of primary tumor	—	For surgical planning only	—	—	—
Bone scan	X				
PET-CT[c]	X	After two to four cycles	If needed to assess response	—	—
Chest radiograph	X	Before each treatment	X	Before each treatment	Year 1: q2 months; years 2, 3: q3–4 months; year 4: q4 months; year 5: q6 months; then yearly
Chest CT	X	If chest radiograph is equivocal, to assess response, or for surgical planning	—	If chest radiograph is equivocal, to assess response, or for surgical planning	If chest radiograph is equivocal or for surgical planning
Angiogram	—	Before each preoperative treatment	—	—	—

Bone marrow	Only for small cell ±tumors with metastases	—	—	—	—
ECG	If cardiac history is present	—	If cardiac history is present	—	—
Cardiac scan	If cardiac history is present	—	If doxorubicin dose exceeds standard limits for schedule	—	—
Central venous catheter	X	—	—	—	—
Bone tumor conference	X	—	—	—	If further multidisciplinary decisions are required

CBC, complete blood cell count; PT, prothrombin time; APTT, activated partial thromboplastin time; AI, intra-arterial; CT, computed tomography; MRI, magnetic resonance imaging; PET, positron emission tomography; ECG, electrocardiogram; X, procedure to be done; —, procedure not needed.

aTests may be ordered more frequently based on clinical indications.
bRequired more frequently if patient is on a medical treatment program.
cProcedure is suggested but optional.

to use surgery rather than radiation therapy are again increasing. There are indications that the use of surgery not only increases the rate of local control but may also improve overall prognosis. While this may, in fact, be the case, the conclusions need to be tempered by the fact that patients with the worst prognosis are not offered surgical resection.

B. Chemotherapy. The most effective primary chemotherapy regimens include vincristine, doxorubicin, and ifosfamide (high-dose VAI) or cyclophosphamide (VAdriaC), with or without the addition of dacarbazine (CyVADIC). In most cases where ifosfamide is not used in the primary treatment, ifosfamide and etoposide are added in an alternating fashion or after completion of the doxorubicin-based regimen.

　1. The high-dose VAI regimen is as follows:

Vincristine 2 mg total dose on day 1,

Doxorubicin (Adriamycin) by continuous 72-hour infusion at 75 mg/m^2 IV (25 mg/m^2/day for 3 days), *and*

Ifosfamide 2.5 g/m^2 IV over 2 to 3 hours daily for 4 days.

Mesna 500 mg/m^2 is mixed with the first ifosfamide dose, and 1,500 mg/m^2 is given as a continuous infusion over 24 hours for 4 days in 2 L of alkaline fluid.

Filgrastim (granulocyte colony-stimulating factor) 5 μg/kg SC is given on days 5 to 15 or until granulocyte recovery to 1,500/μL. Alternatively, **Pegfilgrastim** at a dose of 6 mg is given on day 5.

Repeat cycle every 3 weeks.

　2. CyVADIC regimen. Another good chemotherapeutic regimen for Ewing's sarcoma, particularly in adult patients, is the continuous-infusion CyVADIC regimen, which is mentioned in Chapter 17 (see Section II.C).

Cyclophosphamide 600 mg/m^2 IV on day 1.

Vincristine, 1.4 mg/m^2 (2 mg maximum) IV weekly for 6 weeks, then on day 1 of each cycle.

Doxorubicin (Adriamycin) 60 mg/m^2 IV by 96-hour continuous infusion through a central venous catheter (15 mg/m^2/day for 4 days).

Dacarbazine (DTIC) 1,000 mg/m^2 IV by 96-hour continuous infusion (250 mg/m^2/day for 4 days) mixed in the same bag or pump as the doxorubicin. Doses should be divided into four consecutive 24-hour infusions.

Repeat cycle every 3 to 4 weeks.

　Dose modifications. Courses are repeated with a 25% increase or decrease in the doses of cyclophosphamide and doxorubicin, depending on morbidity. Courses are repeated in 3 to 4 weeks as soon as recovery to 1,500 granulocytes/μL and 100,000 platelets/μL occurs. Complications are as described in Chapter 17 (see Section II.E), with the addition of peripheral neuropathy from vincristine. When the cumulative dose of doxorubicin has reached 800 mg/m^2, therapy is discontinued.

　3. Alternative regimens. Alternative regimens omit dacarbazine; vary doses of cyclophosphamide up to 4,200 mg/m^2; give dactinomycin with, or in place of, doxorubicin; and in some patients, add other drugs. The most common pediatric regimen at present alternates two regimens every 3 weeks: ifosfamide plus etoposide; and vincristine, doxorubicin plus cyclophosphamide, with dactinomycin substituted for doxorubicin after a cumulative (bolus) dose of 375 mg/m^2 (VAdCA). In a recent intergroup study, this regimen was superior to VAdCA alone. The schedule of drug administration is as follows:

a. Initial combination

Ifosfamide 1,800 mg/m^2 IV daily × 5 (with mesna), *and*
Etoposide 100 mg/m^2 IV daily × 5.

b. Three weeks later, start

Vincristine 1.5 mg/m^2 IV on day 1, *and*
Doxorubicin 75 mg/m^2 IV on day 1, *and*
Cyclophosphamide 1,200 mg/m^2 IV on day 1.

c. Three weeks later, return to the first regimen, and so forth. At a cumulative doxorubicin dose of 375 mg/m^2, substitute dactinomycin 1.25 mg/m^2. Chemotherapy continues for a total of 1 year.

d. Another version of the alternating regimen starts with an intensive VAdriaC regimen with the doxorubicin and vincristine given by 72-hour continuous infusion and the cyclophosphamide dose increased to 4,200 mg/m^2 divided into two equal doses on days 1 and 2.

4. Responses. Most patients with metastatic disease obtain complete remission; however, almost all patients, especially those with bone metastases, experience relapse and ultimately die of disease. When chemotherapy is used in the therapy of primary disease with surgery or radiation therapy, prognosis depends on the size and location of the primary tumor. Patients with large flat-bone lesions have a less than 30% cure rate as compared with a 60% to 70% cure rate for those patients with long-bone lesions, which are generally smaller. An alarming complication of the chemotherapy and radiation therapy combination is a high frequency of second malignancies in cured patients, with four of ten patients in one series developing secondary sarcomas within the irradiated fields. This complication is another reason for considering surgical intervention rather than radiation because chemotherapy is required for cure whether or not the primary lesion can be controlled with radiation.

5. Secondary chemotherapy. Occasional responses have been seen with etoposide (VP-16), topoisomerase I inhibitors, other alkylating agents (especially ifosfamide), the nitrosoureas, and cisplatin. A combination of etoposide and ifosfamide is now frequently used in patients for whom those drugs were not used in initial therapy. High-dose ifosfamide (14 g/m^2 divided over 3 to 7 days, either as a 2-hour infusion with each dose or as a continuous infusion) with mesna or high-dose doxorubicin (90 mg/m^2) plus dacarbazine (900 mg/m^2) as a 96-hour continuous infusion is occasionally effective in producing brief remissions in patients for whom these agents were not used or were used at substantially lower doses during initial therapy.

Nonetheless, secondary responses are extremely poor, and the survival of a relapsed patient with Ewing's sarcoma is measured in weeks.

6. High-dose chemotherapy. The standard chemotherapy used for Ewing's sarcoma is accompanied by severe but transient myelosuppression. The availability of hematopoietic growth factors to reduce infectious complications provides an added measure of safety but is not routinely required. Our policy has been to use growth factors for regimens known to cause febrile neutropenia in greater than or equal to 30% of patients or in patients who have had febrile–neutropenic episodes during a previous course of chemotherapy rather than to reduce the doses of the myelosuppressive drugs.

Bone marrow transplantation or peripheral stem cell rescue programs are still being investigated in patients presenting with poor prognostic features (large pelvic primary tumors, metastatic disease, poor response to induction chemotherapy) but have not yet been demonstrated to improve prognosis. Such regimens have been tried with negative results in patients relapsing after standard chemotherapy and have been demonstrated to have no significant benefit. Clearly, this approach should not be used in patients with relapse.

III. Osteosarcoma

A. General considerations. Osteosarcoma is a tumor with a poor prognosis in the absence of effective chemotherapy. It is the most common primary bone sarcoma. Frequently, it affects patients 10 to 25 years old and tends to be located around the knee in approximately two thirds of patients, with two thirds of those tumors involving the distal aspect of the femur. As with other sarcomas of bone, pulmonary metastases are most common, followed by bone metastases. Because conventional osteosarcoma is a high-grade tumor by definition and is accompanied by a soft tissue mass in 90% or more of patients, it is usually staged as IIB or IIIB, (MSTS), depending on the demonstration of metastatic disease in lung or bone.

B. Role of chemotherapy. Chemotherapy is usually employed in the neoadjuvant or adjuvant situation, and its value preoperatively has been conclusively demonstrated. Patients who show a complete response to preoperative chemotherapy with tumor destruction of at least 90% have significantly improved survival. Response rates in evaluable tumors range from 30% to 80%. Cure of primary disease with adjuvant chemotherapy is 50% to 80%.

C. Effective agents. The four major standard single agents in the treatment of osteosarcoma are cisplatin, doxorubicin, ifosfamide, and high-dose methotrexate. In addition, the combination of bleomycin, cyclophosphamide, and dactinomycin (BCD) has been effective.

D. Recommended regimen. A variety of regimens may be recommended based on preliminary or more extensive evaluation.

1. Doxorubicin and cisplatin

Doxorubicin 90 mg/m^2 IV by 96-hour continuous infusion through a central venous catheter, *and*

Cisplatin 120 mg/m^2 intra-arterially (for primary tumor) or IV on day 6.

Repeat every 4 weeks.

Three to four courses of therapy should be administered preoperatively. Postoperative therapy depends on the response of the primary tumor. Patients with tumor necrosis of 90% or more should continue on the same regimen for three to six postoperative courses or until a cumulative doxorubicin dose of 800 mg/m^2 is reached. If cisplatin must be discontinued earlier, decrease the doxorubicin dose to 75 mg/m^2 IV by 72-hour continuous infusion and substitute with ifosfamide 2,500 mg/m^2 IV over 3 hour daily for 4 days (the dose-intensive AI regimen for soft tissue sarcoma; see Chapter 17, Section II.C.1).

2. After primary chemotherapy, if there is less than 90% tumor necrosis at surgery, **switch to the alternative regimen** as follows:

a. High-dose methotrexate 12 g/m^2 IV every 2 weeks for 8 weeks with leucovorin rescue (see Section III.E.2).

b. Three weeks later, administer ifosfamide 2 g/m^2 IV over 2 hours for 5 consecutive days, with mesna 1,200 mg/m^2 IV in three divided doses each day (i.e., 400 mg/m^2 IV every 4 hours × 3) or by continuous infusion after a loading dose of 400 mg/m^2 mixed with the first ifosfamide dose plus doxorubicin 75 mg/m^2 IV by 72-hour continuous infusion. Three weeks later, repeat the course.

c. Three to 4 weeks later, repeat the entire cycle of four courses of methotrexate, and two courses of ifosfamide–doxorubicin. End with four more courses of high-dose methotrexate.

3. There are many alternative approaches to chemotherapy, adding high-dose methotrexate and/or ifosfamide to the induction regimen and continuing with the same three to four drugs postoperatively. The combination of bleomycin, cyclophosphamide, and dactinomycin (BCD) is rarely, if ever, used anymore.

E. Special precautions in administration

1. Cisplatin. Prehydration is necessary, with overnight infusion of IV fluids at 150 mL/hour or 1 L of fluid over 2 hours (for adults), followed by at least 6 L of fluid containing potassium chloride (KCl; at least 20 mEq/L) and magnesium sulfate (MgSO$_4$; at least 4 mEq/L) for the first 1 or 2 days or after cisplatin administration. The addition of mannitol (66 mL of a 15% solution) before cisplatin, followed by 266 mL of a 15% solution mixed with normal saline in a total volume of 1 L to run simultaneously with the cisplatin over 2 to 3 hours, is preferred by many investigators. Particular care in electrolyte balance, including frequent determinations of magnesium levels, is necessary. In the presence of severe hypomagnesemia, magnesium sulfate up to 1 to 2 mEq/kg may be infused over 4 hours.

2. High-dose methotrexate. The pretreatment-calculated creatinine clearance rate should be at least 70 mL/minute.

a. Methotrexate administration and alkalization of urine. Before administration of high-dose methotrexate, 0.5 mEq/kg of sodium bicarbonate is infused IV over 15 to 30 minutes in an attempt to create an alkaline urine. Allopurinol 300 mg/day for 3 days is given starting 1 day before the methotrexate infusion. Methotrexate is dissolved in no more than 1,000 mL of 5% dextrose in water, with a final concentration of approximately 2 g/100 mL. The total dose ranges from 8 g/m^2 for patients over 40 years to 12 g/m^2 for children and young adults. The dose should be increased on subsequent courses if an immediate postinfusion methotrexate level is less than 10^{-3} M. Sodium bicarbonate 50 mEq is added per liter of methotrexate solution, which is infused over 4 hours. After completion of the methotrexate infusion, 10 mL/kg of an IV infusion of 5% dextrose in water with 50 mEq/L of bicarbonate is given over 2 hours if the patient is unable to drink or if the 24-hour methotrexate levels of the previous high-dose methotrexate treatment have been higher than 1.5×10^{-5} M. The IV infusion is then discontinued, and the patient is encouraged to drink sufficient fluid to produce approximately 1,600 mL/m^2 of alkaline urine for the first 24 hours and 1,900 mL/m^2 daily for the next 3 days. Sodium bicarbonate 14 to 28 mEq PO every 6 hours is administered to ensure alkaline urine. The pH of the urine is measured, and if it is less than 7, an extra dose of bicarbonate is administered.

b. Leucovorin rescue. Twenty-four hours after the start of the methotrexate infusion, leucovorin 15 to 25 mg is administered PO every 6 hours for at least ten doses or IM if the oral medication is not tolerated.

c. Serum methotrexate levels. These levels should be followed up and should fall by approximately 1 log/day. When methotrexate concentration falls below 10^{-7} M, leucovorin may be safely discontinued. IV hydration is required whenever oral intake is inadequate to produce sufficient urine output as previously defined, for abnormal serum methotrexate concentration, for persistent vomiting, or for early toxicity.

3. Ifosfamide. Patients must be kept well hydrated with an alkaline pH to prevent central nervous system (CNS) toxicity and minimize nephrotoxicity. Sodium bicarbonate or sodium acetate should be added to IV fluids at an initial concentration of 100 to 150 mEq/L and fluid administration adjusted to produce a urine output of at least 2 L/day and to maintain the serum bicarbonate concentration at 25 mEq/L or higher. Other electrolytes should be adjusted as needed on a daily basis. Serum albumin should be kept within normal limits.

F. Complications. Complications of chemotherapy depend on the drugs. For doxorubicin, the major complication is infection owing to neutropenia. Other complications include stomatitis, nausea and vomiting, and delayed cardiac toxicity, as discussed in the management of soft tissue sarcomas (see Chapter 17, Section II.E). Ifosfamide produces myelosuppression, nausea and vomiting, and alopecia, similar to doxorubicin. Hemorrhagic cystitis, once the dose-limiting toxicity, is rarely seen because the use of mesna has become routine. The most serious toxicities of ifosfamide are nephrotoxicity and CNS toxicity. Nephrotoxicity in the form of Fanconi syndrome is a frequent problem, the morbidity of which can be minimized by the routine use of alkaline infusions and correction of electrolyte levels with intravenous or oral replacement therapy. Only rarely does the nephrotoxicity progress to renal failure, often precipitated by dehydration or administration of minimally nephrotoxic drugs such as nonsteroidal anti-inflammatory drugs (NSAIDs). Patients treated with ifosfamide should be instructed to avoid NSAIDs, even years after chemotherapy. Correction of acid–base balance and hypoalbuminemia can essentially prevent the CNS toxicity (see Chapter 17, Section II.E). Dactinomycin causes side effects similar to those of doxorubicin, but not cardiac toxicity. Methotrexate predominantly causes stomatitis, but it may cause myelosuppression and renal, hepatic, and CNS abnormalities. Cisplatin and dacarbazine cause severe nausea and vomiting. In addition, cisplatin nephrotoxicity is primarily a tubular defect, with hypomagnesemia as the most prominent manifestation, but hypocalcemia, hypokalemia, and hyponatremia also occur. Delayed cumulative nephrotoxicity can cause impaired glomerular function as well. Ototoxicity may occur but is less common. Delayed neurotoxicity also occurs. Both cisplatin and methotrexate can, by causing renal toxicity, exacerbate their other side effects.

G. Recurrence and treatment of refractory disease. Patients with osteosarcoma who are refractory to a combination of doxorubicin and cisplatin may respond to high-dose methotrexate; patients refractory to high-dose methotrexate may respond to doxorubicin plus cisplatin; and patients refractory to both may respond to ifosfamide or, rarely, to BCD. However, treatment of refractory disease is usually disappointing, and participation in studies of new agents is indicated for patients whose disease cannot be resected. Surgical resection of pulmonary metastases remains the only viable secondary therapy for most patients. For this reason, careful follow-up for detection of metastases while they are still at the stage of resectability is indicated.

H. High-dose chemotherapy. The standard chemotherapy used for osteosarcoma is accompanied by severe but transient myelosuppression. The availability of hematopoietic growth factors to reduce infectious complications provides an added measure of safety but is not routinely required. Our policy has been to use growth factors only for regimens known to cause febrile neutropenia in equal to or more than 30% of patients or in patients who have had febrile–neutropenic episodes during a previous course of chemotherapy rather than to reduce the doses of the myelosuppressive drugs.

Bone marrow transplantation or peripheral stem cell rescue programs have not been demonstrated to improve prognosis.

IV. Malignant fibrous histiocytoma of bone. This entity, characterized by a purely lytic lesion in bone, has an exceptionally poor prognosis when treated with surgery alone, although the number of reported patients is small. It may be extremely difficult to distinguish from fibroblastic osteosarcoma and may be best considered as a fibroblastic osteosarcoma with minimal (i.e., no detectable) osteoid production. The tumor responds well to the CyADIC regimen for soft tissue sarcomas, with more than half the number of patients obtaining at least partial remission. In addition, cisplatin at a dose of 120 mg/m^2 every 4 weeks has caused remissions, even in patients who did not respond to primary therapy. A particularly attractive approach for patients with large, unresectable primary tumors is the administration of cisplatin by the intra-arterial route. Complete tumor destruction in one patient and a good partial remission in a second patient are the reported results among three patients so treated. Systemic doxorubicin may be added, as for osteosarcomas (see Section III.D.1). Alternatively, responses have been seen after high-dose methotrexate-based regimens for osteosarcomas (see Section III.D.2). After local tumor destruction, surgery may be employed to remove residual disease. Because of the poor prognosis, adjuvant chemotherapy with the continuous-infusion CyADIC regimen is recommended until an 800-mg/m^2 cumulative doxorubicin dose has been reached.

V. Chondrosarcoma. The chemotherapy for chondrosarcoma is totally inadequate, and no regimen can be recommended except for the rare patients with mesenchymal chondrosarcoma, a subtype that may respond to CyADIC chemotherapy or cisplatin, or with dedifferentiated chondrosarcoma, which should be treated the same way as osteosarcoma. Most patients have conventional chondrosarcoma and are candidates only for surgical management. Metastatic disease should be treated with phase II protocols in an attempt to determine some effective type of chemotherapy that may be recommended in the future.

SUGGESTED READINGS

Bacci G, Briccoli A, Ferrari S, et al. Neoadjuvant chemotherapy for osteosarcoma of the extremity: long-term results of the Rizzoli's 4th protocol. *Eur J Cancer* 2001;37:2030–2039.

Bacci G, Ferrari S, Bertoni F, et al. Prognostic factors in nonmetastatic Ewing's sarcoma of bone treated with adjuvant chemotherapy: analysis of 359 patients at the Istituto Ortopedico Rizzoli. *J Clin Oncol* 2000;18:4–11.

Bacci G, Ferrari S, Bertoni F, et al. Neoadjuvant chemotherapy for peripheral malignant neuroectodermal tumor of bone: recent experience at the Istituto Rizzoli. *J Clin Oncol* 2000;18:885–892.

Bacci G, Ferrari S, Longhi A, et al. Neoadjuvant chemotherapy for high grade osteosarcoma of the extremities: long-term results for patients treated according to the Rizzoli IOR/OS-3b protocol. *J Chemother* 2001;13:93–99.

Benjamin RS, Murray JA, Carrasco CH, et al. Preoperative chemotherapy for osteosarcoma: a treatment approach facilitating limb salvage with major prognostic implications. In: Jones SE, Salmon SE, eds. *Adjuvant therapy of cancer*, Vol. IV. New York: Grune & Stratton, 1984:601–610.

Bone sarcoma. In: Greene FL, Page DL, Fleming ID, eds. *AJCC cancer staging manual*, 6th ed. New York, NY: Springer-Verlag, 2002:187–192.

Chawla SP, Benjamin RS, Abdul-Karim FW, et al. Adjuvant chemotherapy of primary malignant fibrous histiocytoma of bone: prolongation of disease free and overall survival. In: Jones SE, Salmon SE, eds. *Adjuvant therapy of cancer*, Vol. IV. New York: Grune & Stratton, 1984:621–629.

Gehan EA, Sutow WW, Uribe-Botero G, et al. Osteosarcoma: the M. D. Anderson experience, 1950–1974. In: Terry WD, Windhorst D, eds. *Immunotherapy of cancer: present status of trials in man*. New York: Raven Press, 1978.

Grier H, Krailo M, Link M, et al. Improved outcome in non-metastatic Ewing's sarcoma (EWS) and PNET of bone with the addition of ifosfamide (D) and etoposide (E) to vincristine (W), Adriamycin (Ad), cyclophosphamide (C), and actinomycin (A): a Children's Cancer Group (CCG) and Pediatric Oncology Group (POG) report. *Proc Am Soc Clin Oncol* 1994;13:A1443.

Kushner BH, Meyers PA, Gerald WL, et al. Very-high-dose short-term chemotherapy for poor-risk peripheral primitive neuroectodermal tumors, including Ewing's sarcoma in children and young adults. *J Clin Oncol* 1995;13:2796–2804.

Rosen G, et al. The successful management of metastatic osteogenic sarcoma: a model for the treatment of primary osteogenic sarcoma. In: van Oosterom AT, Muggia FM, Cleton FJ, eds. *Therapeutic progress in ovarian cancer, testicular cancer and the sarcomas*. Hingham: Leiden University Press, 1990:244–265.

CHAPTER 19

Acute Leukemias

Olga Frankfurt and Martin S. Tallman

I.   General features of acute leukemias. The acute leukemias are a heterogeneous group of disorders characterized by clonal proliferation and abnormal differentiation of neoplastic hematopoietic progenitor cells. Accumulation of immature hematopoietic cells, or blasts, in the bone marrow and peripheral blood, ultimately leads to inhibition of normal hematopoiesis. If left untreated, acute leukemias are rapidly fatal.

Over the last 40 years, significant therapeutic advances have been made, and many patients can now be cured of their disease. The general treatment approach for most patients with acute leukemia includes eradication of the leukemic clone with intensive systemic chemotherapy, followed by some form of consolidation and, in certain cases, maintenance therapy. Despite this strategy, many patients younger than 55 years and most of the older adults die from their disease.

Numerous questions regarding optimal therapeutic strategies for the patients with acute leukemia remain unanswered. Hence, all patients with acute leukemia ought to be considered candidates for clinical trials and should be treated in centers where appropriate intensive and comprehensive care can be provided.

    A. Epidemiology. The incidence of acute myeloid leukemia (AML) and acute lymphoblastic leukemia (ALL) is 2.7 and 1.5/100,000 population, respectively, and is slightly higher in men than in women. Sixty percent of ALL patients are children, with a peak incidence in the first 5 years of life. The second peak emerges after the age of 60 years. The incidence of AML rises exponentially after the age of 40 years, with the median age of disease presentation being 68 years. The median age of patients diagnosed with acute promyelocytic leukemia (APL), a distinct subtype of AML, is 40 years and the incidence of the disease does not increase with advanced age. While, in general, the incidence of acute leukemias is slightly higher in the populations of European descent, the incidence of APL is higher among patients of Spanish origin.

    B. Etiology and risk factors of acute leukemias. Although the association of the acute leukemias with various infectious, genetic, environmental, and socioeconomic factors has been evaluated extensively, the etiology remains obscure in most cases.

        1. Infection. There is a strong association between Epstein-Barr virus (EBV), a deoxyribonucleic acid (DNA) virus causing infectious mononucleosis, with Burkitt's lymphoma/leukemia.

        2. Genetic factors have been implicated in the pathogenesis of acute leukemia on the basis of epidemiologic studies showing the 25% increase risk of ALL within 1 year in a monozygotic twin of an affected infant. There is also a fourfold increase in the risk of developing leukemia in dizygotic siblings. The risk of developing acute leukemia is significantly higher in patients with Down and Klinefelter syndromes, and conditions with excessive chromosome fragility such as Fanconi's anemia, ataxia telangiectasia, and Bloom's syndrome.

3. Exposures to chemotherapy and radiation significantly increase the risk of developing acute leukemias. AML with chromosome 5 and/or 7 abnormality has been reported to occur 2 to 9 years after therapy with alkylating agents. Topoisomerase inhibitors have been linked to the development of AML and ALL with 11q23 aberration, characteristically 1 to 3 years after the exposure. An increased incidence of acute leukemias has been reported after the radiation exposure such as atomic bomb explosion, Chernobyl accident, and therapeutic radiation. Increased incidence of leukemia has been linked to the exposure to gasoline, benzene, tobacco, diesel, motor exhaust, and electromagnetic fields.

C. Clinical features of acute leukemias are shown in Table 19.1.

D. Diagnosis and classification. The acute leukemias are divided into AML and ALL, on the basis of the morphologic, immunohistochemical, and immunophenotypic characteristics of the stem cell of origin. Although the peripheral blood smear may be highly suggestive of the diagnosis, examination of the bone marrow aspirate and core biopsy is essential to confirm the diagnosis and to determine the extent of the disease. Cytogenetic analysis and molecular studies may aid in establishing an accurate diagnosis, estimate prognosis, and guide therapy.

    1. Acute myeloid leukemia (AML)

        a. Classification. Currently, two pathologic classifications are used to define AML. Morphology-based French–American–British (FAB) classification devised in 1976, utilizes cytochemical stains and, more recently, immunophenotyping by flow cytometry to differentiate myeloid from lymphoid blasts (Tables 19.2 and 19.3). According to FAB classification, eight subcategories of AML are established on the basis of the type of cell involved and the degree of differentiation (Table 19.4).

        A more recent World Health Organization (WHO) classification created in 1999 generated 17 subclassifications of AML, based on the presence of dysplasia, chromosomal translocations, and molecular markers (Table 19.4). Additional changes included decrease of the diagnostic threshold to 20% blasts (from the original FAB classification of 30%, hence eliminating RAEB-t category of myelodysplastic syndrome [MDS]) and the diagnosis of AML regardless of the percentage of marrow blasts in marrows with evidence of abnormal hematopoiesis and clonal cytogenetic abnormalities such as t(8;21), t(15;17), and t(16;16) or inv(16).

        b. Prognostic factors in AML. Cytogenetic information is the single most important prognostic factor for predicting the rate of remission, relapse, and overall survival (OS) (Table 19.5). On the basis of the recent

Table 19.1.   Clinical features of acute leukemias

Clinical and Laboratory Features	Signs and Symptoms
Anemia	Pallor, fatigue, exertional dyspnea, CHF
Neutropenia	Fever, infection
Thrombocytopenia	Petechiae, ecchymosis, retinal hemorrhages
Leukocytosis (10% of patients with WBC >100,000/μL)	Hepatomegaly, splenomegaly, lymphadenopathy (more common in ALL) Bone pain (40%–50% of children with ALL, 5%–10% of adults) Gingival hypertrophy (particularly M4, M5) Leukemia cutis Solitary mass or "granulocytic sarcoma" (<5% of AML at presentation), composed of leukemia myeloid cells in any organ, including bones, breast, skin, small bowel, and mesentery, and obstruction lesions of genitourinary and hepatobiliary tracts)
Leukostasis	Dyspnea, hypoxia, mental status changes
Mediastinal mass (80% of patients with T-cell ALL, rare in AML)	Cough, dyspnea, chest pain
CNS involvement (<1% in AML at presentation, 3%–5% of adult ALL)	Headache, diplopia, cranial neuropathies, particularly CN VI, VIII, papilledema, nausea, vomiting
Elevated PT, PTT, low fibrinogen	Intracranial bleeding, DIC (particularly in APL)
Acute renal failure (uncommon), acidosis, hyperkalemia, hyperphosphatemia, hypocalcemia, elevated LDH and uric acid levels	Tumor lysis syndrome

CHF, congestive heart failure; WBC, white blood cell; ALL, acute lymphoblastic leukemia; AML, acute myeloid leukemia; CN, cranial nerve; PT, prothrombin time; PTT, partial thromboplastin time; APL, acute promyelocytic leukemia; DIC, disseminated intravascular coagulation; LDH, lactate dehydrogenase.

Table 19.2. Antigens commonly demonstrated by flow cytometry techniques

Cell Lineage	Antigens
Lymphoid B	CD19, CD20, cytoplasmic CD22, CD23, CD79a
Lymphoid T	CD1, CD2, cytoplasmic CD3, CD4, CD5, CD7, CD8
Myelomonocytic	Myeloperoxidase, CD11c, CD13, CD14, CD33, CD117 (c-Kit)
Erythrocytic	Glycophorin A
Megakaryocytic	von Willebrand factor, GPIIb (CD41), GPIIIa (CD61)
NK cells	CD16, CD56
Nonlineage specific	TdT, HLD-DR

NK, natural killer; TdT, terminal deoxynucleotidyl transferase; HLD-DR, human leukocyte differentiation antigen-DR.

analysis of 1,213 patients with AML treated with Cancer and Leukemia Group B (CALGB) protocols, the 5-year survival for patients with favorable, intermediate, and poor risk cytogenetics was 55%, 24%, and 5%, respectively. *FLT3* gene aberrations, in the form of internal tandem duplication (ITD) or mutation at the activation loop position 835 (D835), are the most common genetic abnormality in AML, and has been reported to confer a poor prognosis. In the recent series, 5-year survival of patients with a normal karyotype *and* the presence of *FLT3* mutations was 20% as compared to that of 42% for patients with normal karyotype and absence of *FLT3* mutation. Although currently the information regarding *FLT3* status is unlikely to change the *initial* therapy, it may do so in the future, as FLT3 kinase inhibitors become part of the armamentarium of agents active against AML. ITD of the MLL (mixed lineage leukemia or myeloid–lymphoid leukemia) gene has also been associated with poor prognosis in patients with normal karyotype.

Additionally, advanced age, antecedent hematologic disorder, and prior exposure to chemotherapy/radiation are well-established factors associated with lower rates of

Table 19.3. Common histochemical stains that characterize the non–lymphoid cells

Sudan Black B (myeloblasts, promyelocytes)

Peroxidase (myeloblasts, promyelocytes)

Nonspecific esterases that are inhibited by sodium fluoride (monoblasts)

Periodic acid-Schiff (pronormoblasts in erythroleukemia)

Table 19.4. World Health Organisation classification of acute myeloid leukemia (AML) (simplified)

AML with recurrent cytogenetic translocations
- AML with t(8;21) (q22;22); AML1/ETO)
- Acute promyelocytic leukemia t(15;17)(q22;q12) (*PML / RAR*-α) and variants
- AML with abnormal bone marrow eosinophils inv(16)(p13q22) or t(16;16)(p13;q22); (CBFβ/MYH11)
- AML with 11q23 (MLL) abnormalities

AML with multilineage dysplasia
- With prior MDS
- Without prior MDS

AML and MDS, therapy related
- Alkylating agent related
- Epipodophyllotoxin related
- Other types

AML not otherwise categorized (correlated with FAB subtype)
- AML minimally differentiated (FAB M0)
- AML without maturation (FAB M1)
- AML with maturation (FAB M2)
- Acute myelomonocytic leukemia (FAB M4)
- Acute monocytic leukemia (FAB M5)
- Acute erythroid leukemia (FAB M6)
- Acute megakaryocytic leukemia (AmegL; FAB M7)
- Acute basophilic leukemia
- Acute panmyelosis with myelofibrosis

Acute biphenotypic leukemias

MDS, myelodysplastic syndrome; MLL, myeloid–lymphoid leukemia; FAB, French–American–British.

complete remission (CR) and long-term survival. Although 40% to 60% of older AML patients achieve a CR, only 5% to 16% are alive at 5 years.

2. **Adult ALL**

a. **The diagnosis and classification of ALL** are based on cell morphology, immunohistochemistry, as well as immunophenotypic and cytogenetic features. Marrow involvement with more than 25% lymphoblasts is used to differentiate ALL from lymphoblastic lymphoma, in which the preponderance of tumor bulk is in nodal structures. Approximately 70% to 75% of adult ALL cases are of precursor B-cell origin, 20% to 25% are of T-cell origin, and 5% are of mature B-cell origin (or Burkitt-type leukemia, FAB L3).

- **Precursor B-cell ALL** may be further subdivided into early precursors B-ALL, common ALL, and pre-B ALL. Precursor B-cell ALL cells are terminal deoxynucleotidyl transferase (TdT) positive and commonly express CD19, CD10 (the common ALL antigen or CALLA), and HLA-DR, but lack surface immunoglobulin.

Table 19.5. Acute myeloid leukemia prognostic groups based on cytogenetics at presentation[a]

Favorable
- t(15;17)—with any other abnormality
- inv(16) or t(16;16)[b] or del(16q)—with any other abnormality
- t(8;21)[b]—without del(9q) or complex karyotype

Intermediate
- +8[c], −Y, +6, del(12p) or normal karyotype

Unfavorable
- −5 or del(5q), −7 or del(7q), inv(3q), abnormalities of 11q23, 20q, 21q, del(9q), t(6;9), t(8;21) with del(9q) or with complex karyotype, t(9;22), abnormalities of 17p, complex karyotype (three or more abnormalities)

Unknown
- All other clonal chromosomal aberrations with less than three abnormalities

[a]Determined by conventional cytogenetic techniques, fluorescent *in situ* hybridization, or polymerase chain reaction.
[b]Karyotype in these two groups is part of "core-binding factor-type" acute leukemia.
[c]Some evidence suggests that trisomy 8 confers an unfavorable prognosis.

- **Mature B-cell ALL,** or Burkitt-cell leukemia, is associated with translocation of *c-myc* gene of chromosome 8 and the immunoglobulin heavy-chain gene on chromosome 14q32 in 80% of the cases or with the light-chain gene on the chromosome 2p11 or 22q11 in the other 20%. The recent increase in the incidence of Burkitt's leukemia/lymphoma is attributed to its association with human immunodeficiency virus (HIV) infection. Mature B-cell ALL cells are always positive for the membrane immunoglobulin with light chain restriction and commonly positive for CD10, CD19, CD20, CD22, and CD79b.
- **T-Cell ALL** arises from stage I (prothymocyte) and stage II thymocytes. Immunologic markers classically suggesting T-cell lineage are CD2 (sheep red blood cell receptor), CD3, CD7, CD38 (panthymocyte), and CD71 (transferrin receptor). The TdT can be demonstrated in T-cell (through thymocyte) lineage.

b. **Prognostic features in ALL**
   (1) **Clinical features.** Specific biologic and clinical features of ALL predict response to therapy, remission duration, and disease-free survival (DFS), and help determine the intensity of the induction and postremission therapy. In multivariate analysis, age older than 60 years is associated with a particularly poor prognosis, with shorter remission durations, and worse survival. Presenting white blood cell (WBC) counts of more than 30,000/μL is an adverse prognostic factor predicting shorter remission durations that

pertains more to precursor B-lineage ALL (threshold WBC count >50,000 to 100,000/μL may be important for T-cell ALL). Time required to achieve CR (>4 weeks) following induction chemotherapy has been demonstrated to be an adverse prognostic factor in some but not other clinical trials. A recent report from the GIMEMA (Gruppo Italiano per le Malattie Ematologiche dell'Adulto, [Italian Group for Adult Hematologic Diseases]) ALL group demonstrated that response (defined as peripheral blast count of > 1,000/μL on day 10) to 7 days of initial prednisone treatment before induction was prognostic in predicting disease favorable outcome in adult ALL patients.

The poor outcome associated with T-cell ALL and the expression of myeloid antigens on lymphoblasts, noted in 30% to 35% of adults with ALL, are overcome by the newer multiagent intensive induction regimens. In fact, the German Multicenter Studies for Adult ALL (GMALL) group has reported superior long-term event-free survival (EFS) of 50% to 60% for the group of T-ALL patients. **Favorable prognostic factors in T-lineage ALL** include mediastinal mass, younger age, and CD10 antigen expression. Earlier studies using immunophenotypic subclassification of leukemic cells had demonstrated mature B-cell ALL (FAB L3) to be associated with shorter remission rates and worse survival. Survival rates have improved significantly in adults with Burkitt's ALL through regimens adapted from childhood protocols using shorter, intensive, multiagent chemotherapy regimens, which have resulted in long-term survival rates of more than 50% in this group of patients.

(2) Cytogenetic abnormalities. Similar to AML, cytogenetic abnormalities are one of the most important factors predicting outcome in ALL. Approximately half the number of patients with ALL have cytogenetic abnormalities, which usually take the

Table 19.6. Adverse prognostic factors in B-lineage acute lymphoblastic leukemia (ALL)

Older age

High WBC

Cytogenetics: t(9;22), t(4;11), t(1:19), 9p21,11q23

Immunophenotype: mature B-ALL[a], null-cell ALL (non-T, non-CALLA)

Delayed time to CR (>4 weeks)[b]

WBC, white blood cell; CALLA, common ALL antigen; CR, complete remission.

[a] Has poor prognosis when treated with conventional ALL regimes. However, with modern regimens prognosis has improved.

[b] Was not shown to be a predictor of worse outcome in recent MRC UALL XII/ECOG E2993.

form of translocation rather than deletion as seen more commonly in AML (Table 19.6).

- **Philadelphia (Ph+) chromosome**. The t(9;22), one of the most ominous cytogenetic abnormalities in ALL, results in the formation of the *BCR / ABL* fusion gene with tyrosine kinase activity. This translocation, referred as *Philadelphia chromosome*, is the most common cytogenetic abnormality, found in up to 30% of adults with ALL, as compared with 5% of children. The BCR/ABL fusion protein in ALL is smaller with a molecular mass of 185 or 190 kDa as compared with the 210-kDa BCR/ABL protein seen in almost all chronic myelogenous leukemia (CML) patients (including blast crisis). The abnormal fusion protein upregulates tyrosine kinase activity and affects the downstream signaling pathways. In the recent update of the German ALL trials, 37% of patients were Ph+, with 77% showing the p190 and 23% showing p210 proteins. Although patients with Ph+ ALL may attain morphologic remission (82%) with conventional chemotherapy, most will have persistent molecular disease. The median survival of 6 to 14 months and long-term DFS of 0% to 10%, depend in part on intensity of induction and consolidation therapy. Patients who do achieve a molecular remission have longer remission duration (30 vs. 12 months).
- **Other translocations** associated with poor outcomes involve the mixed-lineage leukemia (*MLL*) gene on chromosome 11q23, partnered with several other chromosomes including 4q21, 9q22, and 19q13. Translocation t(4;11), the most common rearrangement of 11q23, occurs in approximately 10% of adult patients and is common among infants with ALL. Adults with this translocation tend to be older, have organomegaly, higher WBC count, and central nervous system (CNS) involvement.
- **Favorable cytogenetics.** ALL patients with t(10;14) karyotype (or other abnormality involving 14q (11–13)), Del (12p), or t(12p) (without associated Philadelphia chromosome) have a better prognosis, with long-term DFS rates exceeding 70% to 75%. Furthermore, rearrangement of the *TEL* gene (12q13) in children with precursor B-cell ALL was demonstrated to be a favorable genetic marker, with a 5-year DFS of 91% in one study.

3. Acute mixed-lineage and stem cell leukemias. With the expansion of immunophenotyping panels, use of electron microscopy and gene rearrangement studies for the characterization of acute leukemia, increasing degrees of infidelity of myeloid and lymphoid markers is demonstrated. Cases in which differentiation between AML and ALL is difficult are described by the WHO as "acute leukemia of ambiguous lineage" and are divided in three subgroups: *undifferentiated acute leukemia,* lacks all of the specific markers such as myeloperoxidase, CD3, cytoplasmic CD22, and cytoplasmic CD79a; *bilineal acute leukemia*, is characterized by dual blasts population, with each population expressing markers of a distinct lineage; and *biphenotypic acute leukemia*, characterized by blasts coexpressing lineage-*specific* antigens from two lineages. However, the coexpression of one or two lineage-*associated* antigens is not a sufficient criterion to diagnose biphenotypic leukemia and may produce well-defined syndromes that do not alter the basic cellular lineage (e.g., CD13/CD33 ALL, CD7 AML, TdT AML).

In stem cell leukemia, the cells express only rudimentary hematopoietic markers (e.g., Ia antigen, TdT, CD34). The identification of entities such as CD13/CD33 ALL and stem cell leukemia may be of prognostic importance and have therapeutic implications.

II.   Initial support. Once the diagnosis of acute leukemia has been established, the next 24 to 48 hours are spent preparing the patient for the initiation of cytotoxic chemotherapy. The following issues need to be addressed in almost all individuals facing induction chemotherapy.

A. Hyperleukocytosis, leukostasis, and leukapheresis. Hyperleukocytosis, defined as an absolute blast count of more than 100,000/μL, predisposes to rheologic complications. Leukostasis, manifesting as cerebral and cardiopulmonary dysfunction due to vascular obstruction and/or vessel wall necrosis with hemorrhage, occurs almost exclusively in AML and represents an oncologic emergency. Given the increased risk of early death with hyperleukocytosis, steps to rapidly reduce the blast counts should be undertaken as soon as the diagnosis is made. In the hemodynamically stable patient, leukapheresis is the most rapid way to lower the blast count. The goal of the leukapheresis session is to lower the blast count to less than 100,000/μL if possible. With very high blast counts (>200,000/μL), decreasing the blast count by 50% may have to be the initial goal because mathematic modeling suggests that prolonged leukapheresis after a "3-L exchange" does not significantly decrease the blast count further. Leukapheresis may be repeated daily. Systemic chemotherapy should be initiated immediately after emergent leukapheresis or if leukapheresis cannot be performed. Hydroxyurea 3 to 5 g/m^2/day split into three doses daily is most commonly used. Hydroxyurea is stopped at the time more specific induction chemotherapy is initiated. In patients presenting with hyperleukocytosis, an allopurinol dose of 600 mg b.i.d. is well tolerated for the first 2 days, followed by 300 mg b.i.d. for 2 to 3 days. Emergent cranial radiation for hyperleukocytosis and cranial nerve palsies is another treatment modality that may be used.

Blood transfusions in the anemic patient with hyperleukocytosis should be undertaken with great caution as aggressive packed RBC (PRBC) transfusion in such patients may precipitate symptoms of hyperviscosity. Unless the patient has symptoms due to anemia, a hematocrit of 20% to 25% is a reasonable goal.

B. Hydration and correction of electrolyte imbalance. Dehydration needs to be corrected and adequate urine output maintained to prevent renal failure due to the deposition of cellular breakdown products resulting from the tumor lysis syndrome (TLS). In the absence of cardiac disease, normal saline with or without 5% dextrose is infused to maintain the urine output at more than 100 mL/hour. The concomitant use of loop diuretics may be necessary in patients with congestive heart failure.

A variety of electrolyte abnormalities, such as hypocalcemia, hyperphosphatemia, and hyperkalemia may occur in patients with acute leukemia. Hypocalcemia may cause potentially lethal cardiac (ventricular arrhythmias, heart block) and neurological (hallucination, seizures, coma) complications. In an *asymptomatic* patient with laboratory evidence of hypocalcemia and hyperphosphatemia, calcium replacement is not recommended, because it may precipitate metastatic calcifications. However, in a patient with symptomatic hypocalcemia, calcium gluconate may be carefully administered to correct the clinical symptoms. Hyperkalemia, defined by a potassium level of greater than 6 mmoL/L, caused by massive cellular degradation, may precipitate significant neuromuscular (muscle weakness, cramps, paresthesias) and potentially life-threatening cardiac (asystole, ventricular tachycardia, and ventricular fibrillation) abnormalities. Patients should be treated with oral sodium–potassium exchange resin such as Kayexalate 15 to 30 g every 6 hours and combined glucose/insulin therapy.

Serum electrolytes, uric acid, phosphorus, calcium, and creatinine should be monitored several times a day, depending on the severity of the clinical condition and degree of metabolic abnormality. Early hemodialysis may be required in patients who develop oliguric renal failure or recalcitrant electrolyte disturbances. The electrocardiogram (ECG) should be obtained and cardiac rhythm monitored while these abnormalities are corrected.

C. Prevention of uric acid nephropathy. Hyperuricemia is common at presentation and may also occur with the tumor lysis caused by chemotherapy. Allopurinol is the mainstay of prevention of uric acid nephropathy. The usual initial adult dose is 300 mg (150 mg/m^2) twice a day for 2 to 3 days, which is then decreased to 300 mg once a day. Allopurinol should be stopped after 10 to 14 days to lessen the risk of rash and hepatic dysfunction. If chemotherapy needs to be initiated urgently, allopurinol at a dose of 600 mg twice a day is well tolerated for 1 to 2 days. With the advent of allopurinol, the role of urine alkalinization has become less clear. Although urine alkalinization increases uric acid solubility, it decreases the solubility of urinary phosphates and may promote phosphate deposition in patients susceptible to TLS (e.g., B-cell ALL and T-cell lymphoblastic leukemia). A commonly employed method of urine alkalinization is to hydrate the patient with D5W, to which two syringes of sodium bicarbonate (44 mEq of NaHCO$_3$ per syringe) have been added per liter.

Recombinant urate oxidase rasburicase, which recently became available in the United States, is a safe and effective alternative to allopurinol. Although the recommended dose of rasburicase is 0.15 to 0.2 mg/kg/day for 5 days, at our institution, an excellent control of hyperuricemia was achieved with a lower dose of 3 mg/day. Administration of 3 mg of rasburicase to 18 patients with hyperuricemia secondary to leukemia/lymphoma resulted in the normalization of the uric acid in 11 patients with just a single dose of rasburicase, in 6 patients with two doses and in 1 patient with three doses.

D. Correction of coagulopathy. Hemostatic defect secondary to thrombocytopenia may be potentiated by the presence of consumption coagulopathy, (disseminated intravascular coagulation [DIC]). Life-threatening bleeding complications are particularly common in patients with APL, due to the presence of DIC and primary fibrinolysis (see Section V.B.). Lysozyme released from monoblasts in M4 and M5 subtypes of AML may trigger a clotting cascade leading to consumption coagulopathy. In ALL, therapy with L-asparaginase may lead to DIC. Additionally, sepsis may contribute to coagulopathy in newly diagnosed patients with acute leukemias. Frequent monitoring of coagulation parameters and adequate replacement with cryoprecipitate or fresh frozen plasma products in appropriate patients is critical (see Chapter 29).

E. Blood product support. Most patients with acute leukemia present with evidence of bone marrow failure. Symptomatic anemia, hemoglobin less than 8 g/dL, thrombocytopenia less than $10,000/\mu L$, as well as signs of bleeding must be corrected. The threshold for platelet transfusion may be lower if conditions known to increase the risk of bleeding such as severe mucositis, fever, anemia, and coagulopathy are present. Blood products should be leucoreduced to decrease the risk of febrile nonhemolytic transfusion reaction, alloimmunization to human leucocyte antigens, which may lead to subsequent refractoriness to platelet transfusion, and transmission of cytomegalovirus (CMV). Additionally, blood products should be γ irradiated to reduce the risk of transfusion-related graft-versus-host disease (GVHD). Patients who are potential candidates for hematopoietic stem cell transplant (HSCT) should be screened for CMV and receive CMV-negative blood until CMV status is determined (see Chapter 29).

F. Human leukocyte antigen (HLA) typing. Patients who are candidates for HSCT should be HLA typed before the initiation of therapy, because chemotherapy-induced severe myelosuppression will not leave enough lymphocytes for HLA typing. However, occasionally an inadequate number of circulating lymphocytes and the presence of blast cells preclude the ability to carry out HLA typing before initial therapy. HLA-matched platelet transfusions may need to be administered to patients who develop alloimmunization and become refractory to pooled or single-donor platelets.

G. Fever or infection. Patients frequently have a fever or an infection at initial diagnosis. The approach to fever and infection is discussed in Chapter 28. The cardinal rule is that all patients with acute leukemia and fever are presumed to have an infection until proved otherwise. Given the additional myelosuppressive and immunosuppressive effects of chemotherapy, severe infections should be treated aggressively before initiating chemotherapy. However, the antibiotic treatment frequently needs to be administered concurrently with induction chemotherapy. Patients with acute leukemia need a careful physical examination daily. There should be close attention toward potential sites of infection, including the fundi, sinuses, oral cavity, intertriginous areas, perineum (attempts are made to avoid internal rectal examination during neutropenia), and catheter sites. A dental consultation at the time of diagnosis is often useful.

H. Vascular access. Because of the need for several sites of venous access for at least 1 month, a multiple-lumen implantable catheter (e.g., Hickman catheter or peripherally inserted central catheter [PICC] line) must be placed as soon as possible (except in patients suspected to have APL). An implantable port is not recommended for leukemic patients because there is higher risk of infection and hematoma at the access site. Because of the coagulopathy in patients with APL, the placement of a long indwelling catheter is avoided until the coagulopathy has been corrected. A risk of life-threatening bleeding in patients with APL is present even if most or all of the routine coagulation studies are normal.

I. Suppression of menses. A serum beta human chorionic gonadotropin (β-hCG) assay (pregnancy test) should be done in all premenopausal women before initiation of chemotherapy. It may be desirable to prevent menses during chemotherapy to avoid severe menorrhagia due to thrombocytopenia. Medroxyprogesterone (Provera) 10 mg twice a day may be started 5 to 7 days before the expected starting time of the next menstrual period. It may be increased to 10 mg three times a day or higher if breakthrough bleeding occurs. Depo-Provera is contraindicated in the thrombocytopenic and neutropenic patient.

J. Birth control and fertility. Given the potential teratogenic effects of cytotoxic chemotherapy, appropriate measures for preventing conception must be addressed with women of reproductive age undergoing chemotherapy. Although there are no clear data linking chemotherapy in the male partner to teratogenic effects in the fetus, it is prudent to suggest that appropriate birth control measures be undertaken in this situation as well. Late effects of chemotherapy, such as infertility, need to be considered in younger patients. Sperm cryopreservation should be offered to men of reproductive age before initiation of chemotherapy. Gonadal function in women seems to be less affected by cytotoxic chemotherapy. Cryopreservation of the *fertilized* eggs is currently available, whereas cryopreservation of *unfertilized* eggs may be conducted on an investigational basis. Treatment with a gonadotropin-releasing hormone (GnRH) agonist analog to induce a temporary prepubertal milieu is an additional option that may be considered in women of reproductive age.

K. Psychosocial support. Patients with acute leukemia are usually previously healthy individuals who have suddenly had to accept the possibility of their own imminent mortality. Intensive psychological and spiritual support by the health care team, family, and religious leaders is critical for maintaining the patient's sense of well-being (see Chapter 33).

III. Therapeutic principles and approach to therapy of acute leukemia

A. Therapeutic aim. The goals of chemotherapy are to eradicate the leukemic clone and to re-establish normal hematopoiesis in the bone marrow. Long-term survival is seen only in patients in whom a CR is attained. Although leukemia therapy is toxic and infection is the major cause of death during therapy, the median survival time of untreated (or unresponsive)

acute leukemia is 2 to 3 months, and most untreated patients
die of bone marrow failure and its complications. The doses
of chemotherapy are never reduced because of cytopenias, as
lowered doses still produce the unwanted side effects (further marrow suppression) without having as great a potential
for eradicating the leukemic clone and ultimately improving
marrow function.

B. Forms of chemotherapy

1. Induction chemotherapy is initial intensive chemotherapy given in an attempt to eradicate the leukemic clone
and to induce a complete remission (CR). The term *CR*
depicts patients who achieve recovery of normal peripheral
blood counts with recovery of bone marrow cellularity,
including the presence of less than 5% blast cells, in the
absence of extramedullary disease. The aim of induction
chemotherapy is to reduce the leukemia cell population by
several logs from the clinically detectable leukemia tumor
burden of 10^{11} to 10^{12} cells, commonly seen at diagnosis,
to *below* the morphologically detectable level of 10^9 cells.
It is important to note that because achievement of initial
CR represents only a 3- to 6-log leukemia cell reduction,
a substantial leukemia cell burden persists, and patients
usually relapse within months if further therapy is not
administered.

2. Postremission chemotherapy is administered subsequently to achieve a CR in a further attempt to eradicate
the residual, but often undetectable, leukemic clone. In a
younger patient population, considering the relatively high
rate of CR after the induction, future advances are likely to
be made through improved postremission therapy. Patients
older than 60 years, tend to achieve a suboptimal CR rate
of 40% to 60% and poor 5-year OS of approximately 10%,
and should be enrolled in investigational protocols aimed
at improving *induction and consolidation* therapy.

- **Consolidation** therapy involves repeated courses of the
  same drugs at similar or higher doses as those used
  to induce the remission, which are given soon after the
  remission has been achieved (2–3 weeks after the recovery of blood counts). Consolidation often requires further
  hospitalization.

- **Maintenance** therapy pertains primarily to ALL, and
  includes low doses of drugs designed to be administered
  on an outpatient basis for up to 2 years. In AML, this
  strategy applies only to APL.

3. Definition of response is based on the peripheral
blood counts and the status of the *recovered* bone marrow.
If the marrow is hypoplastic, it is imperative to repeat the
bone marrow biopsy to document remission upon recovery.

- **Complete response** (complete remission, CR) is the
  return of the complete blood count to a "normal" absolute neutrophil count (ANC) of more than $1,500/\mu L$
  and to a platelet count of more than $100,000/\mu L$ in conjunction with a normal bone marrow, that is, normal
  cellularity, less than 5% blasts or promyelocytes and
  promonocytes, an absence of obvious leukemic cells and

absence of extramedullary disease. Presence of minimal residual disease (MRD) as determined by flow cytometry or polymerase chain reaction (PCR) analysis is a predictor of the relapse. Relapse rates range from 0% in patients with less than 10^{-4} leukemic cells detected at the completion of the induction to 14% in those with 10^{-3} to 10^{-4} to 89% in patients with 1% residual disease.

- **Partial response (PR)** is the persistence of morphologically identifiable residual leukemia (5%–15% leukemic cells in the bone marrow).

IV. Therapy for adult AML (other than APL) (Table 19.7). The day that induction chemotherapy is started is arbitrarily called *day 1*. Bone marrow aspiration and biopsy are repeated on approximately days 10 to 14. If the bone marrow is severely hypoplastic with fewer than 5% residual blasts or if the bone marrow is aplastic, no further chemotherapy is given, and the patient is supported until bone marrow recovery occurs (usually 1–3 weeks). A bone marrow examination is repeated 2 weeks later (~days 26–28). Once a CR has been documented, the potential benefit of further consolidation therapy should be determined on an individual basis.

A. Induction therapy. Factors that influence the choice of the initial chemotherapeutic agents include the patient's age, cardiac function, and performance status. Age 60 has traditionally been considered a cut-off point for recommending the induction chemotherapy because of higher prevalence of unfavorable cytogenetics, antecedent myelodysplasia, expression of multidrug-resistant protein as well as frequency and severity of comorbid conditions affecting the ability to tolerate

Table 19.7. Therapeutic options for acute myeloid leukemia other than acute promyelocytic leukemia (outside of a clinical trial)[a]

Initial Cytogenetics	Induction Chemotherapy	Postremission therapy	
		HLA-Matched Donor	No Donor
Favorable	Standard 7 + 3[b]	HDAC × three to four cycles, *or* Two to three cycles followed by auto-HSCT	HDAC × three to four cycles, *or* two to three cycles followed by auto-HSCT
Intermediate	Standard 7 + 3	Allogeneic HSCT (Allo-HSCT) *or* HDAC × two to four cycles	HDAC × two to four cycles + auto-HSCT
Unfavorable	Standard 7 + 3	Allogeneic HSCT (Allo-HSCT)	HDAC × two to four cycles ± auto-HSCT

HLA, human leucocyte antigen; HDAC, high-dose cytarabine (ara-C); HSCT, hematopoietic stem cell transplantation;
[a] All individuals with acute leukemia should be treated in clinical trials.
[b] 7 + 3, cytarabine 100 mg/m^2 continuous infusion days 1–7 and anthracycline (e.g., daunorubicin 45–60 mg/m^2) by bolus infusion days 1–3.

intensive chemotherapy. The initial drug doses outlined in the following text are based on the presence of normal hepatic and renal functions and do not require modification for depressed (or elevated) peripheral blood counts.

1. "7 + 3"—Cytarabine and anthracycline induction. During the last 30 years, a series of clinical trials have identified an induction regimen of cytarabine (Ara-C) and anthracycline that is now considered standard **(Table 19.8)**. The most widely used combination includes cytarabine 100 mg/m^2 by continuous IV infusion for 7 days and daunorubicin (DNR) 45 to 60 mg/m^2/day IV for 3 days (known as 7 + 3). Although many investigators have strong personal biases regarding the choice of anthracycline or anthracenedione for induction therapy, we would consider daunorubicin, idarubicin, and mitoxantrone as essentially equivalent choices on the basis of current data. All three should be considered potentially cardiotoxic.

2. Dose intensification. The merit of cytarabine dose intensification has been explored in several clinical trials. On the whole, it appears that induction therapy with HDAC (high-dose Ara-C) plus DNR is associated with greater toxicity than SDAC (standard dose Ara-C) plus DNR, but *without* improvement in CR rate or survival. Hence, the addition of HDAC to induction regimens outside the clinical trial remains controversial.

3. Other regimens. Many permutations to the standard "7 + 3" regimen have been studied over the years in attempts to improve the CR rate of induction therapy and prolong survival. Except in the unfavorable subgroup of patients, defined by lactate dehydrogenase (LDH) values greater than 700 U/L, more than 40% blasts in the day-16 bone marrow, and unfavorable cytogenetics, in which TAD-HAM (thioguanine, cytarabine, and daunorubicin followed by HDAC and mitoxantrone) is associated with a

Table 19.8.   Commonly administered induction regimens in acute myeloid leukemia

"7 + 3" Cytarabine and anthracycline

> Cytarabine 100 mg/m^2/24 h continuous IV infusion on days 1–7 *and*
>
> Daunorubicin 45 to 60 mg/m^2 IV bolus on days 1–3 *or*
>
> Idarubicin 12 mg/m^2 IV bolus on days 1–3 *or*
>
> Mitoxantrone 12 mg/m^2 IV bolus on days 1–3

HDAC induction regimens for patients with cardiac disease

> Cytarabine 2–3 g/m^2 IV infusion over 1–2 h every 12 h for 12 doses, *or*
>
> Cytarabine 2–3 g/m^2 IV infusion over 2 h every 12 h on days 1, 3, 5

HDAC, high-dose cytarabine (ara-C).

higher CR rate (65% vs. 49%) and 5-year survival (25% vs. 18%), these permutations do not provide lasting benefit.

The use of an anthracycline or an anthracenedione is contraindicated **in patients with severe underlying cardiac disease**, particularly if the patient has had a recent myocardial infarction or has an ejection fraction of less than 50%. The choice of therapy in this situation is HDAC, although the optimum dose and schedule of HDAC therapy are not known (i.e., number of doses, dosage, and infusion rate) (see Table 19.8).

4. Residual disease. Patients who have residual disease at day 28 should be considered primary treatment failures and have alternative therapy initiated. If a significant response has been demonstrated at the day-10 to day-14 marrow (>50%−60% reduction in leukemic infiltration) but residual leukemia persists, a second course of similar chemotherapy (or an alternative regimen such as HDAC) is given. Patients with persistent significant involvement of leukemia on day 10 to 14 (<40%−50% leukemic reduction) should receive an alternative chemotherapy regimen. There is no dose modification for the second course based on blood cell counts. The doses of drugs may be decreased for the second cycle if the total dose of anthracycline would be cardiotoxic or hepatic dysfunction attributed to the chemotherapy develops.

5. Common HDAC toxicities. Neurotoxicity (cerebellar dysfunction, somnolence) occurs more frequently in older patients and as the number of doses of HDAC increases. Renal and hepatic dysfunction contributes to the development of neurotoxicity. One- to 2-hour infusions are generally recommended as opposed to the original infusion rate over 2 to 3 hours, as the neurotoxicity appears to be decreased with shorter infusion times.

Reducing the dose of cytarabine in the face of renal dysfunction may decrease the risk of neurotoxicity. The following schema has been suggested to decrease neurotoxicity in the face of renal dysfunction. For a baseline serum creatinine level of 1.5 to 1.9 mg/dL or an increase in serum creatinine of 0.5 to 1.2 mg/dL from baseline, reduce the cytarabine to 1 g/m^2/dose. For a baseline serum creatinine of more than 2 mg/dL or an increase of serum creatinine of greater than 1.2 mg/dL from baseline, reduce the cytarabine dose to 100 mg/m^2/day.

Because cytarabine is secreted in tears, ulcerative keratitis can be prevented by instilling eye drops (saline, methylcellulose, or steroid) every 4 hours while awake, and Lacri-Lube ophthalmic ointment (Allergan Pharmaceuticals) at bedtime, starting at the time HDAC is initiated and continuing for 2 to 3 days after the last dose of HDAC.

B. Postremission therapy. Despite attaining a CR, most patients with AML relapse, necessitating further therapy aimed at eradication of the residual yet undetected leukemic clone. There are three general treatment strategies for postremission therapy: consolidation chemotherapy, autologous hematopoietic stem cell transplantation (auto-HSCT), or allogeneic (allo) HSCT. Although the optimum postremission strategy remains

Table 19.9. High-dose cytarabine (ara-C) consolidation regimens

Cytarabine 3 g/m² IV infusion over 1–2 h every 12 h on days 1, 3, 5 (better tolerated) for 2- to 4-monthly courses, *or*

Cytarabine 3 g/m² IV infusion over 1–2 h every 12 h on days 1–6 for 1- to 3-monthly courses (most patients cannot tolerate more than one or two courses of standard HDAC), *or*

For patients older than age 60 and/or *patients with renal dysfunction (including creatinine <2.0 mg/dL)*, cytarabine 1.5 g/m² IV infusion over 1–2 h every 12 h on days 1, 3, 5 for 2- to 3-monthly courses

to be defined, almost all younger adults with AML benefit from further therapy. The type of postremission therapy should be determined on the basis of prognostic factors, particularly age and cytogenetics at diagnosis. Patients with AML in first CR should be considered candidates for experimental protocols examining postremission therapy options. For patients who cannot be enrolled in protocol studies, the approach to postinduction therapy used as a guide at Northwestern University is shown in Table 19.9. Consolidation should be initiated when the peripheral blood counts have returned to normal (ANC >1,500/μL and platelet count >100,000/μL), marrow cellularity is normal, infections have resolved, and mucositis has cleared.

1. AML with favorable cytogenetics, or so- called corebinding factor (CBF) leukemias, includes t(8;21), inv(16), and t(16;16) cytogenetics. There is increasing evidence that several courses of HDAC represent the best treatment option for this group of patients. The treatment-related mortality (TRM) of standard allo-HSCT makes this option currently prohibitive in this group of patients. Elevated WBC count (specifically, WBC index: WBC × [% of marrow blasts/100]) has been demonstrated to be an important prognostic factor in multivariate analysis for DFS and OS in t(8;21) AML. The French AML Intergroup reported the 3-year DFS and OS for t(8;21) patients with low WBC index (<2.5) to be 74% and 74%, respectively, as compared with the high WBC index (20 or above) group of 33% and 47%, respectively. Further clinical trials may identify a subset of AML patients with t(8;21), such as high WBC index, that may benefit from more intensive postremission therapy.

Current data suggest that HDAC offers a distinct advantage over standard-dose cytarabine consolidation in patients younger than 60 years. More than 40% to 50% of patients will be in a continuous CR 5 years after consolidation with HDAC.

2. AML with intermediate-risk cytogenetics. Long-term survival for patients presenting with intermediate cytogenetics is 40% to 45%. For patients younger than 60 years, data support the use of allo-HSCT as a postremission therapy. The largest collection of prospective cohort data in this subgroup by the Medical Research Council

(MRC) documented superior 3-year relapse rates of 18% for allo-HSCT, 35% for auto-SCT, and 55% for chemotherapy consolidation, and 3-year survival rates of 65%, 56%, and 48%, respectively. The U.S. Intergroup Study did not demonstrate advantage for allogeneic HSCT, although analysis was based on a much smaller cohort of patients. The optimal timing of allogeneic HSCT is yet to be established, although retrospective data collected from the International Bone Marrow Transplant Registry (IBMTR) demonstrated lack of additional benefit from receiving consolidation chemotherapy before matched sibling HSCT in first CR. In other words, patients in postinduction CR may proceed immediately to allogeneic HSCT.

Patients who do not have an HLA-identical sibling should receive consolidation chemotherapy incorporating HDAC or similar therapy. The optimal number and duration of HDAC has not been established, but 2 to 3 g/m^2 is recommended for two to four cycles in younger patients. In healthy patients, this may be followed by auto-HSCT. Autologous HSCT has been studied in this subgroup of patients but has not been shown to represent an advantage over consolidation chemotherapy alone in *randomized* studies conducted during the last decade.

3. AML with unfavorable cytogenetics. Despite the CR rates of up to 60%, this group of AML patients has the poorest long-term outcome, with reported 5-year OS of 11% (3%–20%) depending on the specific cytogenetic abnormality found at diagnosis (i.e., 3%–5% of patients with monosomy 5 and complex karyotype are alive at 3 years). The U.S. Intergroup Study demonstrated a significant long-term survival advantage for patients with unfavorable cytogenetics who received allo-HSCT for consolidation as compared with auto-HSCT or conventional chemotherapy. Although the total number of patients analyzed in this and similar trials has been small, matched-sibling allogeneic HSCT likely represents the therapy with the best current potential to prevent relapse. Moreover, select reports in younger patients have demonstrated long-term survival rates of 35% to 45% in patients undergoing mismatched-sibling allo-HSCT and matched unrelated donor (MUD) HSCT. Despite 100-day mortality rates of approximately 35% to 40%, these strategies may represent the best therapeutic choice for select patients because of the dismal long-term outcome with unfavorable cytogenetics. Low-intensity myeloablative or nonmyeloablative HSCT procedures have allowed less fit and older patients to proceed to allogeneic HSCT for consolidation, but these techniques should still be considered investigational. For less fit patients or patients without a suitable matched donor, enrollment in experimental clinical trials testing novel strategies should be aggressively pursued. Alternative-donor transplantation is an area of active investigation.

C. Acute megakaryocytic leukemia. AmegL (FAB M7) is a rare AML subtype (1%–2%) not encompassed in the "unfavorable" group that has very poor long-term outcome. The Eastern Cooperative Oncology Group (ECOG) described 20 AmegL cases out of 1,649 patients with newly diagnosed AML. The median age of patients described was 42 years, and 50% of patients entered CR with a median OS of 10.4 months (two patients remain alive). There have been only anecdotal reports of allo-HSCT for patients with AmegL. Novel therapeutic strategies are needed, including agents such as arsenic trioxide (As_2O_3), which has recently been demonstrated to inhibit growth and survival in megakaryocytic leukemia cell lines.

D. Relapsed AML. Significant number of patients with AML who achieve a remission will ultimately have a relapse. The goals of therapy for these patients vary from achievement of second CR with intensive chemotherapy and/or HSCT to best supportive care. The success of achieving a second CR varies greatly, depending less on cytogenetic characteristics but more on duration of first CR, age, and active comorbidities of the patient. The median duration of second CR is usually less than 6 months without HSCT, with long-term DFS rates of less than 10 months. Moreover, most standard salvage chemotherapy regimens induce significant toxicity. Survival is improved in patients who proceed to allo-HSCT with long-term OS rates that may approach 30% to 40%. Unfortunately, because of the lack of suitable availability of donors and patient morbidities, many patients are not eligible for allogeneic HSCT.

1. Options for the reinduction therapy include the immunoconjugate agent gemtuzumab ozogamicin (GO), intensive chemotherapy with conventional agents, investigational therapies on a clinical trial, immediate HSCT for the individual with a suitable allogeneic donor or cryopreserved autologous stem cells available, palliative-intent chemotherapy, or best supportive care. Individuals who relapsed after an allo-HSCT may be eligible for donor lymphocyte infusions as an immunologic maneuver to generate a graft-versus-leukemia (GVL) effect. The determination of the optimal therapy depends in part on the duration of the first remission, whether HSCT is planned, if a second CR is achieved, and the manner in which the relapse was detected. Individuals with remission less than 6 to 12 months in duration are best treated with investigational agents on clinical trials or, if feasible, immediate HSCT depending on the marrow blast percentage. Individuals with a remission greater than 18 to 24 months may be treated with more conventional salvage treatment that commonly includes a HDAC-containing regimen.

a. Gemtuzumab ozogamicin (GO), a recombinant humanized monoclonal anti-CD33 antibody conjugated to a highly potent antitumor antibiotic calicheamicin, is U.S. Food and Drug Administration (FDA) approved for the treatment of patients older than 60 years with $CD33^+$ AML in first relapse who are not candidates for cytotoxic therapy. Most AML blast cells (80%−90%) express the CD33 surface antigen, whereas pluripotent hematopoietic stem cells/tissues and nonhematopoietic cells do not. After administration, GO is believed to be internalized into lysosomes, where the calicheamicin dissociates from the antibody, migrates to the nucleus and causes double-stranded DNA breaks. Three multi-center trials demonstrated an overall response (OR) rate of 30% (16% CR with full platelet recovery) characterized by 5% or less blasts in the bone marrow, recovery of neutrophil count to $1,500/\mu L$, and RBC and platelet transfusion independence following two doses of GO. Median relapse-free survival (RFS) was 6.8 months, median survival was 5.9 months, 1-year OS was 31%, and no differences were noted in age or duration of first remission. (Of note, patients with myelodysplasia or first CR of less than 3 months were excluded from the study.) Additionally, there is data to suggest efficacy of GO in $CD33^-$ AML patients.

GO has been generally well tolerated with the most common side effect that patients experienced being a transient infusion-related syndrome (fevers, chills/rigors, nausea, pain, and hypotension). Notwithstanding, a significant minority of patients treated with GO have developed hepatic toxicity manifested as weight gain, ascites, jaundice, and abnormalities in the hepatic transaminases. A direct association of GO with liver injury may be confounded by prior and/or concomitant antileukemic cytotoxic therapies received by patients, but reports including patients who had received no prior antileukemic cytotoxic therapy (including patients who received single-agent GO) have infrequently documented significant liver injury. Results of liver histologic examination in five of seven patients who died with persistent liver dysfunction demonstrated sinusoidal injury with extensive sinusoidal fibrosis, centrilobular congestion, hepatocyte necrosis, and striking deposition of sinusoidal collagen, suggesting that GO targets $CD33^+$ cells residing in hepatic sinusoids.

The risk of veno-occlusive disease (VOD)–like syndrome appears to be higher in patients who proceed to allo-HSCT within 3 to 4 months of exposure to GO. Currently, the combination of GO with various chemotherapeutic and biologic agents as well as its role in eliminating MRD is being evaluated in clinical trials. Three recent studies, utilizing GO with intensive chemotherapy demonstrated a CR rate of approximately 85%.

b. Standard chemotherapy. The selection of conventional salvage therapy, the optimal dose of cytarabine, and the benefits of the addition of an anthracycline or other agents all remain important unanswered issues.

c. New agents and investigational strategies. Many new agents with diverse putative mechanisms of actions are currently evaluated in clinical trials.

- In phase I and II studies, a novel nucleoside analog *clofarabine*, induced a 16% CR rate in patents with relapsed AML. When clofarabine was combined with cytarabine, the OR rate was 32% with CR rate of 22%. When clofarabine was administered to previously untreated older patients with AML, the CR was 60%.

- *Farnesyl transferase inhibitors* (*FTI*), which interfere with retinoic acid syndrome (RAS) signaling pathway have activity in patients with newly diagnosed and refractory AML. In a recent study of older patients with newly diagnosed AML, orally administered FTI Zarnestra induced OR (CR + PR) of 39%, with CR 20% and median CR duration of 6.4 months.
- The protein kinase C active agent *bryostatin* is actively being evaluated before and after HDAC therapy.
- Internal tandem duplications (ITDs) of the receptor tyrosine kinase *FLT3* gene have been found in 20% to 30% of patients with AML and are believed to confer a poor prognosis. *Tyrosine kinase inhibitors that are active against FLT3* are being examined. So far, their success has been modest, with a 50% reduction in the peripheral blasts noted in 70% of patents and 50% bone marrow blast reduction in 10% of AML patients in one clinical trial. Some patients without ITD or activating loop mutation have responded to FLT3 inhibitors. Current clinical trials are evaluating FLT3 inhibitors in combination with chemotherapy.
- *Troxacitabine,* a novel dioxolane nucleoside analog was shown to induce 26% responses in patients with relapsed/refractory AML.
- Transcriptional therapy, histone deacetylase inhibitors (HDAC) and DNA hypomethylating agents are being studied in high-risk MDS and AML patients.
- The proteasome inhibitor *bortezomib* appears to have single agent activity in leukemia and has *in vitro* synergistic activity with HDAC inhibitors.
- Inhibition of P-glycoprotein (Pgp)-mediated cellular export of anthracyclines by *Zosuquidar* are being explored. The ECOG recently completed a prospective randomized trial of induction chemotherapy with and without Zosuquidar. Although addition of PSC-833, another multidrug resistance inhibitor, to anthracycline therapy provided no benefits over standard therapy, combination of Zosuquidar with GO in elderly patients who are not candidates for cytotoxic therapy is still being investigated.
- A high level of expression of antiapoptotic protein BCL-2, confers poor prognosis on AML patients. Addition of BCL-2 inhibitor Genasense to chemotherapy resulted in a 45% CR rate.

d. Options for reinduction therapy. Depending on prior therapy, age, and perceived ability to tolerate subsequent systemic treatment, chemotherapeutic options using *commercially available* drugs would include the following:

- **Gemtuzumab ozogamicin.** 9 mg/m^2 as a 2-hour IV infusion is used on days 1 and 15. No dose adjustments for anemia or thrombocytopenia should be made. Benadryl may be administered before infusion. Acetaminophen has the potential to contribute to hepatotoxicity (increased free radicals) and theoretically should be avoided.

- **"7 + 3."** Up to half of patients who undergo induction with the "7 + 3" regimen respond to a repeat course of "7 + 3." Patients who relapse within 6 to 12 months of the last chemotherapy are unlikely to respond to the same regimen again. Therefore, a different regimen should be considered.

- **HDAC.** Fifty percent to 70% of patients respond to HDAC. Although HDAC combination regimens may have a slightly higher response rate (RR), their increased toxicity may not make them significantly better than single-agent HDAC. Patients who relapse within 6 to 12 months of HDAC intensification are unlikely to have a significant response to further HDAC.
  1. **HDAC** (see Table 19.9)
  2. **HDAC plus anthracycline, for example, HDAC** 3 g/m^2 IV infusion over 2 hours every 12 hours on days 1 to 4, *plus* **mitoxantrone** 10 mg/m^2/day IV on days 2 to 5 or 2 to 6.

- **CAT**

  Cyclophosphamide 500 mg/m^2 IV every 12 hours on days 1 to 3,

  Topotecan 1.25 mg/m^2/day by continuous infusion on days 2 to 6, *and*

  Cytarabine 2 g/m^2 IV over 4 hours daily for 5 days on days 2 to 6.

- **MEC.** A variation of MEC currently used by the ECOG is as follows:

  Etoposide 40 mg/m^2/day IV infusion over 1 hour on days 1 to 5, *followed immediately by*

  Cytarabine 1 g/m^2/day IV infusion over 1 hour on days 1 to 5, *and*

  Mitoxantrone 4 mg/m^2/day IV sidearm push on days 1 to 5, given after completion of HDAC each day.

  MEC may produce significant gastrointestinal and cardiac toxicity. It is not recommended for patients older than 60 years or those with borderline cardiac function.

- **ME. Mitoxantrone** 10 mg/m^2/day IV on days 1 to 5 and **etoposide** 100 mg/m^2/day IV on days 1 to 5 represents an active and well-tolerated combination that is commonly used for relapsed or refractory leukemia.

- **High-dose etoposide** 70 mg/m^2/hour continuous IV infusion for 60 hours **and high-dose cyclophosphamide** 50 mg/kg (1,850 mg/m^2)/day IV infusion over 2 hours on days 1 to 4 is a highly toxic but active regimen that does not require bone marrow support. It is active against HDAC-resistant AML (30% CR). This regimen may be useful for young patients who are good candidates for allogeneic HSCT while waiting for an unrelated donor search to be completed.

E. CNS prophylaxis may be considered in patients at high risk of CNS recurrence such as patients with WBC more than 50,000/μL or those with myelomonocytic (FAB M4) or monocytic (FAB M5) differentiation. Patients treated with HDAC (>7.2 g/m^2) do not require intrathecal (IT) therapy as they achieve therapeutic drug level in the cerebrospinal fluid (CSF). If required, IT therapy with methotrexate (MTX) 12 mg or Ara-C 30 mg is used. For patients with CNS involvement (uncommon on presentation) chemotherapy should be administered through Ommaya catheter with 30 mg of hydrocortisone.

F. AML in older adults. AML is a disease of older adults as the median age of diagnosis is 68 years. Despite the refinements in supportive care and chemotherapy programs, the long-term survival rates have improved little over the last 30 years for patients older than 55 years. Standard remission-induction and postremission therapy result in median DFS of 10 months and rare long-term survival. Because of the effects of comorbid disease and age on normal physiology, older adults are less able to withstand the inherent toxicity of induction chemotherapy than young adults. There are also intrinsic differences in the biology of AML in older adults: a higher percentage of the leukemic cells express P-glycoprotein (Pgp) at diagnosis (71% vs. 35% in younger patients) and existence of an overt or covert antecedent hematologic disorder that predispose to drug resistance. Moreover, AML in older adults is associated with a greater number of high-risk cytogenetic abnormalities (i.e., abnormalities of chromosomes 5 and 7 and complex karyotypes). As reported by the MRC, the favorable cytogenetic risk group (see Table 19.5) was less common in patients older than 55 years (7% vs. 26% in patients younger than 55 years), whereas complex karyotypes were more common (13% vs. 6%). Furthermore, patients older than 55 years with complex karyotype predicted a poor outcome with OS of 2% at 5 years. The MRC recognized a predictive hierarchical cytogenetic classification for older adults similar to previous analysis for younger patients, although 5-year OS for favorable cytogenetic group patients older than 55 was 34% compared with 65% for younger patients (13% and 41%, respectively, for intermediate cytogenetic risk).

The decision to forgo therapy in an older patient with AML should not be made *a priori* based solely on age; rather, the decision to treat or not to treat should be based on more substantive factors such as the presence of comorbid disease, performance status before diagnosis, quality of life before diagnosis, and projected long-term survival.

1. Induction therapy. In older AML patients, only one randomized study has ever shown a survival advantage of remission-induction therapy as compared to low-dose therapy or supportive care. The survival advantage of 10 weeks was almost exactly the time of hospitalization required for the induction and one cycle of consolidation chemotherapy.

In general, 55% to 70% of elderly patients without complex karyotype cytogenetics can achieve a CR with induction chemotherapy (20%–30% for complex karyotypes). Although attenuated doses of "7 + 3" have been recommended in the past, full-dose therapy is now generally recommended in older adults without significant comorbidities, in part owing to improvements in supportive care. Continuous attempts have been made to improve the efficacy of this regimen by varying the doses of Ara-C and/or anthracycline; comparing one anthracycline or anthracenedione with another; combining with other chemotherapeutic agent; using growth factors as priming agents or as supportive care. Improved CR rates in many of the phase II studies were not confirmed in the randomized phase III trials.

- **Standard "7 + 3"**

  Cytarabine 100 mg/m²/day or 200 mg/m²/day IV continuous infusion on days 1 to 7, and
  Daunorubicin 45 to 60 mg/m²/day IV bolus for 3 days or
  Idarubicin 8 to 12 mg/m²/day IV bolus for 3 days.

- **Modified HDAC** decreases the cytarabine dose in an attempt to diminish the neurotoxicity that is dose-limiting in older adults. Modified HDAC is generally believed to be more toxic than the "7 + 3" regimen. We do not routinely recommend the use of HDAC for induction in older patients given the lack of data supporting improved remission rate and the significantly increased morbidity and mortality associated with HDAC during the induction period. In selected older patients with excellent performance status and a decreased ejection fraction, one can consider using modified HDAC. Although the optimum dose and schedule are not known, 1.5 to 2 g/m² IV over 2 hours every 12 hours for 8 to 12 doses may be used.

2. **Postremission therapy.** Older patients may tolerate one to two cycles of lower doses of HDAC (1.5 g/m² every 12 hours days 1, 3, and 5) than is usually given for younger adults, although a beneficial impact of HDAC consolidation chemotherapy on long-term outcome is not proved. The CALGB trial of varying doses of cytarabine (100 mg/m²/day, 400 mg/m²/day, and 3 g/m²) reported similar 5-year DFS and OS within each arm (each <15% and 8%, respectively). Other reports have demonstrated that prolonged consolidation courses (over four cycles) will likely not benefit long-term outcomes. Current experimental therapeutic strategies include incorporation of less intensive therapy, such as GO, FTIs, and *bcl-2* antisense oligonucleotides into consolidation (and induction) therapy. Autologous HSCT may be considered for fit patients, although, as in younger patients, the optimal timing of this therapy is not known. Low-intensity allogeneic HSCTs have been performed in older patients, but this modality should still be considered experimental in this setting. In a recent series of 122 patients with AML who underwent nonmyeloablative allogeneic HSCT, the 2-year DFS was 44% in related and 63% in unrelated donor transplant recipients. Outside of the clinical trial, treatment options include the following:

- **HDAC** 1.5 g/m² IV infusion over 1 to 2 hours every 12 hours on days 1, 3, and 5 (better tolerated) for one to two monthly courses (*with careful attention to cerebellar toxicity and to renal function; if either is noted to be apparent, HDAC should be immediately discontinued*).

- **Cytarabine** 100 mg/m^2/day for 5 days for two to three courses but there are no data to show that these strategies are effective.

Overall, there is no definitive data showing that postremission therapy benefits older adults.

3. **Newer therapeutic approaches** include GO, BCL-2 inhibitors, FLT3 inhibitors, and FTI inhibitors, hypomethylating agents, and histone deacetylase inhibitors. Older adults are increasingly offered an option of undergoing nonmyeloablative (mini)-HSCT as a postremission therapy. Although most of the studies evaluating mini-HSCT are limited to single-institution experience, they show feasibility of this potentially curative approach in the older patient population.

V.   Acute promyelocytic leukemia (APL). APL is a distinct subtype of AML, designated M3 by the FAB classification. It accounts for 10% to 15% of cases of adult AML in the general population and 20% to 25% of AML cases in Latin America. The median age at presentation (40 years) is significantly lower than that of patients diagnosed with other AML subtypes (68 years). Owing to the remarkable sensitivity of APL to anthracyclines, all-*trans* retinoic acid (ATRA), and arsenic trioxide (ATO), it has become the most curable acute leukemia in adults, with cure rates exceeding 80% with contemporary therapeutic strategies. Despite a good overall outlook in APL, several factors adversely affect the outcome in this disease:

- Age (>50–60)
- Male gender
- High WBC (>10,000/µL)
- CD56 expression (not in all the studies)

A. Cytogenetic abnormalities and prognostic factors. The characteristic molecular genetic abnormality in APL is the balanced reciprocal translocation between the gene for retinoic acid receptor α (RARα) located on chromosome 17 and the gene for the promyelocytic leukemia (PML) located on chromosome 15, resulting in 2 hybrid gene products PML-RARα and RARα-PML. PML-RARα fusion protein, detectable by PCR technique, is essential for the diagnosis and identification of MRD. Four alternative chromosomal translocations have been identified (PLZF-RARα, NPM-RARα, NuMA-RARα, STAT5b- RARα).

B. Management of coagulopathy in APL. Coagulopathy, a peculiar presenting feature of APL, must be managed aggressively at the *suspicion* of APL diagnosis, as it results in a high rate of spontaneous and potentially fatal hemorrhage. Pooled data through the late 1980s suggested that under the best of circumstances with cytotoxic induction chemotherapy, 5% of APL patients would die of CNS hemorrhage within the first 24 hours of hospitalization and another 20% to 25% would die of CNS hemorrhage during induction chemotherapy. With intensive supportive care and the introduction of all-*trans* retinoic acid (ATRA) therapy, the most recent studies suggest that less than 5% of patients will die of hemorrhage during induction chemotherapy, although overall induction mortality in APL remains approximately 10%. Regardless of clinical manifestations, essentially all patients with APL have laboratory features of DIC. **Management** guidelines for coagulopathy in APL:

- Initiate ATRA-based therapy at the *suspicion* of APL diagnosis.
- Monitor DIC panel at least daily.
- Maintain fibrinogen level at 100 to 150 mg/dL with cryoprecipitate transfusions.
- Maintain platelet count at 30 to 50,000/μL.
- Avoid central line placement.
- Avoid aminocaproic acid.

C. APL therapy. On the basis of cumulative experience of multiple cooperative groups, therapy for APL should **include simultaneous administration of ATRA and anthracycline-based chemotherapy for induction**, ATRA and chemotherapy for consolidation and a combination of ATRA and chemotherapy for maintenance (for high-risk subgroups of patients).

ATRA, a vitamin A derivative, is able to induce a high rate (85%) of short-lived clinical remissions by promoting cell maturation, differentiation, and apoptosis without producing marrow hypoplasia. Two large randomized clinical trials have demonstrated that the addition of ATRA to chemotherapy during induction results in improved EFS and OS, as compared with the use of chemotherapy alone. Additionally concomitant and extended administration of ATRA with chemotherapy resulted in superior CR rates (87% vs. 70%), reduced 4-year relapse rate (20% vs. 36%), and superior 4-year OS (71% vs. 52%) as compared to the sequential administration of ATRA and chemotherapy.

In patients with APL, anthracycline monotherapy can induce 50% to 99% CR with 50% to 60% relapse rate and 30% to 40% survival rate at 2 years. Although the choice of anthracycline is still debated, in the ATRA era, idarubicin is more frequently used as a monotherapy, whereas daunorubicin is mainly used in combination with other drugs (typically cytarabine). However, the *dose* of anthracycline appears to be important. A retrospective analysis by the Southwestern Oncology Group (SWOG) suggested that a higher dose of daunomycin (70 mg/m^2/day vs. 45 mg/m^2/day) resulted in improved CR rate, OS, and DFS.

The role of cytarabine in the induction and consolidation regimens for APL remains controversial, as several retrospective analyses failed to show the difference in the rate of CR with its addition. Long-term outcome data from the PETHEMA (Spanish Cooperative Group for the Study of Hematologic Malignancies) studies also suggested that cytarabine could be safely omitted during induction and consolidation with excellent CR, DFS, and OS rates. However, the recent trial conducted by the European APL Group aimed at comparing daunorubicin and ATRA with and without Ara-C was closed prematurely because of the increased rate of relapse in daunorubicin/ATRA arm. Hence, the role of Ara-C in induction and consolidation remains unclear, except for the patients with high-risk disease, where intermediate dose Ara-C appears important.

In the pre-ATRA era several studies showed a definitive benefit of maintenance chemotherapy. Since the ATRA became standard therapy, a combination of ATRA and low-dose chemotherapy was shown to be superior to ATRA alone, chemotherapy alone, and observation, in terms of relapse rate and DFS. However, two recent studies showed no advantage of maintenance therapy in patients who achieved a molecular remission after the 3-day cycle of consolidation. The optimal schedule, dose, and duration of maintenance therapy as well as a patient population most likely to benefit from maintenance are still under investigation.

1. **Induction**

- ATRA 45 mg/m²/day PO is divided into two doses with food given every day until CR (no longer than 90 days) plus an anthracycline, either daunorubicin 45 to 60 mg/m²/day for 3 days or idarubicin 12 mg/m² every other day for 4 days. In the modified regimen used by the PETHEMA group, the fourth dose of idarubicin was omitted in patients older than 70 years.

  It appears reasonable to initiate treatment with ATRA first for 2 to 3 days in patients with clinical evidence of bleeding to ameliorate the coagulopathy before initiating anthracycline-based therapy, provided the WBC count is not high (<10,000/μL). Otherwise, concurrent ATRA plus anthracycline-based therapy has been routine practice and may have the advantage of decreasing the incidence of *RAS* (see the following text). With ATRA and anthracycline, *hematologic* CR rate of greater than 90% are expected. Patients, who do not achieve a *hematologic* CR by 90 days, should be treated with alternative therapy. Presence of MRD (50% after induction) as determined by RT-PCR does not appear to have prognostic implications and does not warrant change in therapeutic approach. The role of cytarabine in induction remains unclear.

2. **Consolidation.** The goal of consolidation therapy is an achievement of molecular remission as determined by the RT-PCR, as it has been convincingly correlated with the improved outcome. Two to three cycles of anthracycline-based chemotherapy may be given, as in the North American Intergroup trial:

  a. **Daunorubicin** 50 to 60 mg/m²/day IV for 3 days, *or*

  b. **Idarubicin** 5 mg/m²/day on days 1 to 4 (consolidation no. 1), mitoxantrone 10 mg/m²/day on days 1 to 5 (consolidation no. 2), *and* idarubicin 12 mg/m² on day 1 only (consolidation no. 3), as in PETHEMA regimen *or*

  c. **Daunorubicin** 60 mg/m²/day IV for 3 days and Ara-C 200 mg/m²/day IV for 7 days, as in European APL 93 regimen

  The addition of ATRA may be considered, and if PCR-negative state is not achieved at the completion of consolidation, a salvage regimen should be initiated (HDAC or intermediate dose Ara-C, arsenic trioxide, GO or a clinical trial).

3. **Maintenance**

  a. ATRA 45 mg/m²/day PO, divided into two doses with food for 15 days every 3 months (or 7 days on/7 days off) *plus* 6-mercaptopurine 90 to 100 mg/m^2/day *plus* MTX 10 to 15 mg/m^2/week all for 2 years, *or*

b. ATRA 45 mg/m^2/day, PO, divided into two doses with food for 1 year, *or*

c. ATRA 45 mg/m^2/day, divided into two doses with food for 15 days every 3 months for 2 years.

Follow-up of PCR for *PML-RARα* every 3 to 6 months for 2 years and then every 6 months for 2 years has been considered in the past. However, because contemporary strategies now result in a relapse rate of only 5% to 20%, this schedule may not be necessary in all patients but can rather be carried out in high-risk patients.

4. Retinoic acid syndrome (RAS) is a complication of ATRA therapy, which manifests by unexplained fever, weight gain, respiratory distress, pericardial and pleural effusion, periodic hypotension, and acute renal failure. Typically, RAS occurs between the second day and the third week of ATRA therapy, with the incidence between 5% to 27% and a mortality (of those who develop RAS) between 5% and 29%. Although a rising WBC count may be a risk factor for RAS, it may occur with a WBC count below 5,000/μL. If the WBC count is more than 5,000 to 10,000/μL on presentation, ATRA and chemotherapy should be given concurrently. If the WBC count rises to more than 10,000/μL during ATRA monotherapy, induction chemotherapy should added. Regardless of the WBC count or the risk of neutropenic sepsis, at the first sign of RAS, dexamethasone (10 mg IV twice a day) should be initiated. If the symptoms are mild, ATRA may be continued concomitantly with steroids under careful observations. However, if the symptoms are severe or do not respond to steroid therapy, ATRA should be temporarily discontinued. Several uncontrolled trials reported a very low-mortality rate with the *prophylactic* corticosteroid therapy in patients with leukocytosis; however, no prospective randomized studies were conducted to address this issue.

5. Relapsed APL

a. Arsenic trioxide (ATO, As$_2$O$_3$). Approximately 10% to 30% of patients treated with a combination of ATRA and chemotherapy eventually relapse. Although second remissions with standard therapy are common, particularly if the last exposure to ATRA occurred more than 6 to 12 months before relapse, they are not durable. Several clinical trials show that ATO has remarkable activity in this patient population leading to its FDA approval in this setting. Preclinical mechanisms of action of ATO include apoptosis and APL cell differentiation. Chinese investigators demonstrated CR rates of at least 85% and 2-year DFS of 40% in patients with relapsed APL. A U.S. multicenter study of ATO for induction and consolidation therapy for relapsed APL confirmed the high CR rates and long-term survival, and most importantly, 85% rate of molecular remission after the completion of the consolidation therapy. Combination of arsenic trioxide with other active agents (ATRA, chemotherapy, GO) for the relapsed APL (induction and consolidation phases) are actively being studied.

ATO, either alone or in combination with ATRA, results in remission rates in excess of 90% in previously untreated patients. Incorporation of ATO into the consolidation regimen of first CR has been evaluated by the U.S. Intergroup APL trial (the results are pending). The most significant toxicities associated with ATO therapy include ventricular arrhythmia caused by the prolongation of QT interval, hyperleukocytosis, and APL differentiation syndrome.

b. Other therapies. Despite the high initial CR rates in relapsed disease, many patients relapse following arsenic-based treatment. Results of retrospective studies have demonstrated that HSCT may be an effective option at this point or upon achievement of second CR following ATO therapy, particularly autologous HSCT when molecular negative cells are harvested and reinfused.

A high rate of CD33 expression on the promyelocytes and *in vitro* activity of GO in ATRA and ATO-resistant leukemia cell lines provided a rationale for GO therapy in patients with APL. In patients with evidence of molecular relapse, single-agent GO reinstated the molecular remission in 14 out of 16 patients while 2 patients suffered from the disease progression. Combination of GO and ATRA in previously untreated patients resulted in 88% CR rate.

c. HSCT is routinely considered as a postconsolidation modality in second CR (CR2). However, most studies of HSCT in CR2 were conducted before introduction of ATO. Considering that most of the patients with relapsed and refractory disease can be successfully treated with ATO without introducing transplant-related toxicity, the optimal timing of the transplant is unclear.

d. Treatment regimens for relapsed APL

- **Arsenic trioxide**
  - **Induction**—0.15 mg/kg IV over 2 hours daily until bone marrow remission occurs, up to a cumulative maximum of 60 doses. Bone marrow biopsy should be obtained on or before day 28 of therapy, and subsequently weekly until CR.
  - **Consolidation**—start 3 to 4 weeks after completion of the induction therapy at 0.15 mg/kg IV over 2 hours daily for 5/7 days, for a cumulative total of 25 doses.

  Maintain potassium levels more than 4 mEq/L and magnesium levels more than 1.8 mg/dL. Monitor the heart frequently with an ECG. If QTc interval remains normal the ECG frequency may be reduced to once every 2 weeks. Monitor WBC count and for signs of APL syndrome. Institute steroids (dexamethasone 10 mg IV b.i.d.) at the earliest suggestion of the APL syndrome.

- **HSCT.** Patient should be referred for the evaluation for HSCT, with options being allo-HSCT if the patient fails to achieve a molecular remission and auto-HSCT if in a molecular remission.

VI.   Secondary AML. AML that develops after exposure to the alkylating agent is characterized by cytogenetic abnormalities involving chromosomes 5 and/or 7, a long latency (7–10 years), and, frequently, an antecedent MDS. Patients who develop AML following exposure to topoisomerase II inhibitors have a rearrangement of chromosome 11q23 (MLL), a relatively short latency period (2–3 years), and myelomonocytic or monocytic differentiation. High-dose chemotherapy with HSCT has been increasingly implicated in the pathogenesis of secondary leukemias. In one study, the estimated cumulative probability of developing therapy-related MDS or AML was approximately $8.6\% \pm 2.1\%$ at 6 years among 612 patients undergoing high-dose chemotherapy and HSCT for Hodgkin's disease and non–Hodgkin's lymphoma. The most important risk factor appears to be large cumulative doses of alkylating agents. However, patient age and previous radiotherapy, particularly total-body irradiation as part of the conditioning regimen, are additional risk factors.

Although up to 50% of patients with therapy-related AML may achieve a CR with chemotherapy, the median remission duration is approximately 5 months. Recent data suggest that secondary AML with favorable cytogenetics has an RR similar to that of *de novo* AML with the same cytogenetic features. Therapeutic options include supportive care, "7 + 3," HDAC, or other chemotherapy regimens. Younger patients with secondary AML should be considered for allo-HSCT in first remission. All patients should be treated on a clinical trial if at all possible. Amonafide, a topoisomerase II inhibitor that has shown promising activity in patients with AML, particularly AML arising on the background of MDS, is being evaluated in combination with ARA-C in clinical trials.

VII.   AML during pregnancy. The outcomes of both the mother and the fetus must be considered when discussing the therapeutic options for a pregnant woman who develops AML. Therapeutic abortion must be considered if AML develops during the first trimester. If therapeutic abortion is not an option or if AML develops during the second or third trimester, induction chemotherapy may be undertaken. Although there is a slightly increased risk of premature labor and fetal death, in most cases "7 + 3" appears to be well tolerated by both the patient and the fetus.

VIII.   Role of HSCT in AML (see also Chapter 5)

A.   Allogeneic. Matched-sibling allogeneic HSCT has emerged as an important and potentially curative postremission strategy for many AML patients. Initial studies in patients with relapsed and refractory disease have administered high-dose chemotherapy (cyclophosphamide and total-body irradiation) followed by the HLA-matched sibling bone marrow–derived stem cells, curing 10% to 15% of patients, who would otherwise have died of the disease. Similar studies conducted in patients in first CR increased cure rate to approximately 50% despite a treatment-related mortality (TRM) rate of approximately 20%. Multiple studies from single institutions and cooperative groups have confirmed these results. As discussed in Chapter 5, the important benefit attributable to the success of this strategy is the phenomenon of GVL effect whereby the donor cells recognize the recipient's cells, including leukemia cells, as foreign, with resulting cytotoxicity.

B. Autologous. The lack of a suitable HLA-matched donor and TRM limit the application of allogeneic transplantation. Alternatively, autologous HSCT is potentially available to all patients and has very low TRM rates (currently 3% or less in contemporary series and in a recent ECOG trial where there were no transplant-related deaths among 60 consecutive patients studied).

C. Matched unrelated donors (MUD). MUD transplant registries have grown, and this, coupled with more sensitive tissue-typing techniques, has become an effective approach for more patients. However, there are limitations to this strategy, including donor availability, length of time to identify the donor, and significant TRM (historically, approximately 30%–35%), and the exact role of MUD transplantation in patients with AML has not been established.

D. Haploidentical transplantation. Another alternative donor is a haploidentical family member. Almost every patient will have such a suitable donor available, and there is little reason for delay in proceeding to transplant beyond that present for an HLA-matched sibling donor transplant. This treatment is associated with delayed immune reconstitution and opportunistic infections, particularly CMV. Nevertheless, this approach is promising and warrants further research.

E. Umbilical cord transplants. Finally, hematopoietic stem cells procured from umbilical cords from related and unrelated donors can also restore hematopoiesis with acceptable risks of GVHD. This approach has been limited by the size of the recipient because it has often been difficult to collect enough stem cells. Simultaneous use of two umbilical cord transplants and *ex vivo* expansion of stem cells is an area of active research that may expand the application of umbilical cell transplantation.

F. Clinical trials of HSCT in AML. Several studies have compared prospectively the benefits of intensive consolidation with HDAC, autologous, and HLA-matched HSCT.

A recent European Organisation for Research and Treatment of Cancer (EORTC)/GIMEMA trial compared auto-HSCT with matched sibling HSCT for patients younger than 46 years, stratified by the cytogenetic risk. In the favorable risk group, the DFS for auto-HSCT and allo-HSCT were 66% and 62%, respectively, whereas treatment related mortality (TRM) was 6% and 17%, respectively. The outcome of patients treated with auto-HSCT was similar to the ones achieved with several cycles of HDAC. Hence, several cycles of consolidation HDAC chemotherapy is recommended for patients with favorable cytogenetics. Patients with intermediate cytogenetics achieved a 4-year DFS of 48.5% for allo-HSCT and 45% for auto-HSCT, similar to the 5-year DFS in patients treated with intermediate or high-dose cytarabine of 41%. For patients with high-risk cytogenetics or secondary AML, allo-HSCT produces DFS of 43%, similar to DFS for MUD HSCT reported by the IBMTR. In contrast the outcome of auto-HSCT was once again similar to the outcome of chemotherapy with poor DFS of 18%. Several clinical trials are exploring the utility of reduced intensity allogeneic HSCT as a consolidation strategy in patients older than 60 years.

IX.   Therapy for adult ALL (Tables 19.10 and 19.11). Over the last 30 years, significant advances have been made in the management of adult ALL. Current therapeutic strategies incorporate a more intensive induction and postremission regimens and take into account biologic and clinical features of the disease.

Table 19.10.   Initial therapeutic options for acute lymphoblastic leukemia outside a clinical trial[a]

Immunophenotype	Age (Years)	Therapy[b] (→ Postremission Therapy)
Precursor B-cell lineage Philadelphia+	<60	MRC/ECOG (Hoelzer/Linker)[c] → allo-HSCT (matched sibling *or* MUD if matched sibling is not available)
	>60	MRC/ECOG (Hoelzer/Linker) → intensification/consolidation/ maintenance
Philadelphia−	<60	MRC/ECOG (Hoelzer/Linker) → allo-HSCT[d] (matched sibling), *or* consolidation/ maintenance (if matched sibling not available)
	>60	MRC/ECOG (Hoelzer/Linker) → intensification/consolidation/ maintenance
T-cell lineage	<60	MRC/ECOG (Hoelzer/Linker) → allogeneic HSCT[d] (matched sibling), *or* consolidation/ maintenance (if matched sibling not available)
	>60	MRC/ECOG (Hoelzer/Linker) → intensification/consolidation/ maintenance
Mature B cell (Burkitt's, FAB L3)	<70	B-NHL 86, *or* hyper-CVAD (autologous or allogeneic HSCT in first CR should be considered experimental)
	>70	B-NHL 86, *or* R-hyper-CVAD

MRC, Medical Research Council; ECOG, Eastern Cooperative Oncology Group; HSCT, hematopoietic stem cell transplantation; MUD, matched unrelated donor; FAB, French–American–British.

[a] All individuals with acute leukemia should be treated in clinical trials.

[b] Intensive CNS treatment represents an integral component of all ALL protocols.

[c] CALGB 8811 represents an active regimen for precursor B-cell and T-cell ALL.

[d] Patients with very favorable cytogenetics (e.g., t[12p] without *BCR/ABL*) and patients with "thymic ALL" may be subgroups that do not benefit from allogeneic HSCT.

Table 19.11.   Examples of regimens frequently used for the management of acute lymphoblastic leukemia

Hoelzer/linker (MRC UKALLIIX/ECOG E2993)	CALGB 8811	Hyper-CVAD	MOAD ECOG
Induction (consists of two phases)	***Induction for patients <60 years***	***Odd cycles (1, 3, 5, 7)***	***Induction*** is given in sequential, 3–5, 10-day courses until CR is achieved, followed by two additional courses of MOAD
Phase I, weeks 1–4	Cyclophosphamide 1,200 mg/m² IV, day 1	Cyclophosphamide 300 mg/m² IV q12h, days 1–3	MTX 100 mg/m² IV, day 1 (increase by 50% courses 2 and 3 and by 25% each additional course until mild toxicity is achieved)
Vincristine[a] 1.4 mg/m² (maximum 2 mg) IV push, days 1, 8, 15, 22 Prednisone 60 mg/m² PO, days 1–28 (followed by 7 days' taper)	Daunorubicin 45 mg/m² IV, days 1–3	Mesna 600 mg/m²/day CI, days 1–3	
	Vincristine 2 mg IV, days 1, 8, 15, 22	Vincristine 2 mg IV, days 4 and 11	
	Prednisone 60 mg/m²/day PO, days 1–21	Doxorubicin 50 mg/m² IV, day 4	Vincristine 2 mg IV, day 2
Daunorubicin[b] 60 mg/m² IV push on days 1, 8, 15, 22	L-Asparaginase 6,000 IU/m² SC/IM, days 5, 8, 11, 15, 18, 22	Dexamethasone 40 mg/day, days 1–4; 11–14	L-Asparaginase 500 IU/kg (18,500 IU/m²), day 2
L-Asparaginase 10,000 U IV/IM, q.d., days 17–28.		***Even cycles (2, 4, 6, 8)***	Dexamethasone 6 mg/m²/day PO, day 1–10
Phase II, weeks 5–8 (postpone until the total WBC >3 × 10³ (μL)	***Induction for patients >60 years***	MTX 1 g/m² IV over 24 h, day 1 Leucovorin 50 mg IV to start 12 h after MTX, then 15 mg IV every 6 h until serum MTX less than 1 × 10⁻⁸ M, *and*	
Cyclophosphamide 650 mg/m² IV days 1, 15, 29,	Cyclophosphamide 800 mg/m², day 1 Daunorubicin 30 mg/m², days 1–3	Ara-C 3 g/m² IV infusion over 1 h q12h × four doses, days 2, 3 (reduce cytarabine dose to 1 g/m² for patients older than 60 years)	
Cytarabine 75 mg/m², 2 IV days 1–4, 8–11, 15–18, 22–25	Prednisone 60 mg/m²/day, days 1–7		
6-Mercaptopurine[c] 60 mg/m² PO once daily, days 1–28			

CNS treatment
MTX 12.5 mg, IT/IO, weekly until blasts are cleared form the CNS fluid
24-Gy cranial irradiation and 12 Gy to the spinal cord are administered concurrently with phase II induction
CNS prophylaxis
MTX 12.5 mg IT/IO[a] day 15 (phase I); days 1, 8, 15, 22 (phase II)

Intensification therapy
begins 4 weeks after the induction phase II and should be postponed until the WBC >3 × 10^3/μL

CNS prophylaxis and interim maintenance
Cranial irradiation 2,400 cGy, days 1–12
IT MTX 15 mg, days 1, 8, 15, 22, 29
6-Mercaptopurine 60 mg/m²/d PO, days 1–70
MTX 20 mg/m² PO, days 36, 43, 50, 57, 64

Early intensification (two cycles)
IT MTX 15 mg, day 1
Cyclophosphamide 1 g/m² IV, day 1

CNS prophylaxis and treatment
MTX 12 mg IT day 2 each course, *and*
Cytarabine 100 mg IT day 7 each course (if CNS leukemia is present, increase therapy to twice weekly until the CSF cell count normalizes).

(continued)

Table 19.11. *(Continued)*

Hoelzer/linker (MRC UKALLIIX/ ECOG E2993)	CALGB 8811	Hyper-CVAD	MOAD ECOG
MTX 3 g/m² IV, days 1, 8, 22 Leucovorin rescue starting at 24 h, 10 mg/m² PO/IV q6h × 12 or until the serum MTX concentration is <5 × 10⁻⁸M L-Asparaginase 10,000 U IV/IM, q.d., days 2, 9, 23 ***Consolidation therapy*** (for patients not proceeding to allogeneic HSCT). Given after intensification when the WBC is >3,000/µL and the platelet count is >100,000/µL ***Cycle I consolidation*** Cytarabine 75 mg/m² IV, days 1–5 Vincristine 2 mg IV, days 1, 8, 15, 22, Dexamethasone 10 mg/m² PO, days 1–28	6-MP 60 mg/m²/day PO, days 1–14 Ara-C 75 mg/m²/day SC, days 1–4, 8–11 Vincristine 2 mg IV, days 15, 22 L-Asparaginase 6,000 U/m² SC, days 15, 18, 22, 25 ***Late intensification*** Doxorubicin 30 mg/m² IV, days 1, 8, 15 Vincristine 2 mg IV, days 1, 8, 15 Dexamethasone 10 mg/m²/day PO, days 1–14 Cyclophosphamide 1 g/m² IV, day 29 6-Thioguanine 60 mg/m²/day PO, days 29–42 Ara-C 75 mg/m²/day SC, days 29–32; 36–39		***Consolidation therapy*** is repeated every 10 days for six courses. MTX (final dose from induction) IV, day 1 L-Asparaginase 500 IU/kg (18,500 IU/m²) IV infusion, day 2. ***Cytoreduction*** begins on day 30 of the last consolidation cycle; given monthly × 12 months. Vincristine 2 mg IV, day 1, 30 min before MTX

Etoposide 100 mg/m² IV, days
1–5

Cycle II consolidation (begins
4 weeks from day 1 of first
cycle or when WBC
>3,000/μL)

Cytarabine 75 mg/m² IV, days
1–5

Etoposide 100 mg/m² IV, days
1–5

Cycle III consolidation
(begins 4 weeks from day 1 of
second cycle or when WBC
>3,000/μL)

Daunorubicin 25 mg/m² IV on
days 1, 8, 15, 22

Cyclophosphamide 650 mg/m²
IV, day 29

Cytarabine 75 mg/m² IV, days
31–34, 38–41

6-Thioguanine 60 mg/m² PO,
days 29–42

MTX 100 mg/kg (3.7 g/m²) IV
infusion over 6 h, day 1, *and*

Leucovorin 5 mg/kg
(185 mg/m²) divided into 12
doses starting 2 h after the
MTX infusion, days 1–3

Dexamethasone 6 mg/m²/day
PO days 2–6

(continued)

Table 19.11. *(Continued)*

Hoelzer/linker (MRC UKALLIIX/ ECOG E2993)	CALGB 8811	Hyper-CVAD	MOAD ECOG
Cycle IV consolidation (begins 8 weeks from day 1 of 3-day cycle or when WBC >3,000/μL) Cytarabine 75 mg/m² IV, days 1–5 Etoposide 100 mg/m² IV, days 1–5			
Maintenance 6-Mercaptopurine 75 mg/m²/day PO Vincristine 2 mg IV every 3 months Prednisone 60 mg/m² PO for 5 days, q3 months with vincristine	***Prolonged maintenance*** (every month × 24 months from diagnosis) Vincristine 2 mg IV, day 1, Prednisone 60 mg/m²/day PO, days 1–5 MTX 20 mg/m² PO, days 1, 8, 15, 22	***Maintenance therapy*** *for 2 years.* 6-MP 50 mg PO t.i.d. MTX 20 mg/m²/week PO	***Maintenance*** begins on day 30 of the last course of cytoreduction. It is repeated monthly until relapse. Vincristine 2 mg IV, day 1 Dexamethasone 6 mg/m²/day PO, days 1–5

MTX 20 mg/m² PO or IV once/week (when the WBC >3,000/µL and the platelets >100,000/µL)

6-MP 60 mg/m²/day PO, days 1–28

6-Mercaptopurine 100 mg/m² PO daily, MTX 15 mg/m² PO weekly

MRC, Medical Research Council; ECOG, Eastern Cooperative Oncology Group; CI, continuous infusion; CR, complete remission; MTX, methotrexate; WBC, white blood cell; CNS, central nervous system; IO, intra-Ommaya reservoir; IT, intrathecal; HSCT, hematopoietic stem cell transplant.

[a] The vincristine dose should be modified to 50% for paresthesia proximal to the DIP (distal interphalyngeal) joints and stopped entirely for major muscle weakness, cranial nerve palsy, or severe ileus.

[b] Daunorubicin and vincristine doses should be modified on a weekly basis according to the serum bilirubin.

Direct bilirubin	Dose of vincristine to give	Dose of daunorubicin to give
2–3 mg/dL	100% calculated	50% calculated
>3 mg/dL	50% calculated	25% calculated

[c] Dose adjustments for hematologic toxicity from the MTX and 6-MP should be made on the basis of blood cell counts obtained before the start of each course

Dose	ANC (/µL)	Platelets (/µL)
100%	≥2,000	≥100,000
75%	1,500–1,999	75,000–99,999
50%	1,000–1,499	50,000–74,999
0%	<1,000	<50,000

Despite an excellent initial response to therapy (CR 80%–90%), the overall long-term DFS is 35% to 50% in adult patients with ALL. Most chemotherapeutic regimens for ALL have been developed as complete programs without testing the contributions of the individual components, and have not been compared with one another in a rigorous prospective randomized manner. All patients undergoing therapy for ALL should be enrolled in clinical trials.

The goals of intensified therapy are to eliminate leukemia cells, as determined by light microscopy and flow cytometry, before the emergence of drug-resistant clones, to restore normal hematopoiesis, and to provide adequate chemoprophylaxis for the sanctuary sites such as CNS. A typical ALL regimen consists of induction, consolidation/intensification, and maintenance; CNS prophylaxis is usually administered during induction and consolidation.

A. Induction. The addition of an anthracycline to the standard pediatric ALL induction regimen of vincristine, prednisone, and L-asparaginase increased CR rates in adults from 50–60% to 70–90% and median duration of the disease remission to approximately 18 months. In some studies dexamethasone has been substituted for prednisone because of its higher *in vitro* activity and better CNS penetration. Although L-asparaginase proved to be of value in the pre–anthracycline era, its role in anthracycline-based adult programs is unclear. Given the significant toxicity of L-asparaginase, many investigators no longer recommend its use, particularly in older patients.

Attempts to further improve the outcome of patients with ALL led to the incorporation of agents such as cytarabine, cyclophosphamide, etoposide, mitoxantrone, and MTX in the induction and postinduction therapy. It is unclear if intensification with additional agents or the use of multiple phases of induction therapy improved CR rates in the *unselected* patients; however, it may benefit certain subgroups.

The use of growth factors during induction may alleviate complications of prolonged bone marrow suppression and avoid delays in delivering dose-intensive chemotherapy. In a double-blind, randomized trial conducted by the CALGB, administration of granulocyte colony-stimulating factor (G-CSF) shortened the duration of neutropenia from 29 days in the placebo group to 16 days in the G-CSF group. The CR rates were higher with G-CSF (90% vs. 81%), whereas induction mortality was higher in the placebo group (11% vs. 4%).

B. Consolidation therapy typically includes three to eight cycles of non–cross-resistant drugs administered after remission induction. As mentioned in the preceding text, no randomized studies have compared the existing regimens.

C. Maintenance. The benefit of maintenance therapy in adult ALL patients is unclear. In patients with low-risk disease, who enjoy outcomes similar to pediatric patients, maintenance therapy appears to be justified. Considering that more than half the number of the high-risk patients have a relapse while undergoing maintenance therapy, alternative strategies of eradicating MRD are urgently needed. The utility of maintenance therapy has been questioned for T-cell ALL patients and it is not given for patients with mature B-cell ALL.

The traditional maintenance regimen is given for 2 to 3 years and includes daily doses of 6-mercaptopurine (6-MP), weekly doses of MTX, and monthly doses of vincristine and prednisone. Dose intensification or extension of maintenance beyond 3 years does not appear to be of benefit, whereas its omission has been associated with shorter DFS.

D. Minimal residual disease (MRD) in ALL. The aim of induction therapy in ALL is to reduce the leukemia cell population from 10^{11} to 10^{12} cells to below the cytologically detectable level of 10^9 cells. At this point, a substantial leukemia cell burden (i.e., MRD) persists and patients relapse within months without subsequent therapy. As described in the preceding text, standard ALL protocols require approximately 2 to 3 years of systemic therapy. Most ALL patients in continuous CR for 7 to 8 years are considered "cured," although late relapses have been reported. Various techniques such as flow cytometry and PCR, using either fusion transcript resulting from the chromosomal abnormalities or patient-specific junctional regions of rearranged Ig and TCR genes, can be used to detect approximately one to five blasts per 100,000 nucleated cells.

There is a significant correlation between the presence of MRD and early disease recurrence, particularly with greater than 10^{-2} residual blasts per 2×10^5 mononuclear bone marrow cells immediately after disease remission or greater than 10^{-3} at a later time. Although it is clear that MRD positivity is associated with increased rate of disease recurrence, large randomized studies are needed to incorporate MRD results into the treatment paradigm for adults with ALL.

E. CNS leukemia

1. CNS leukemia prophylaxis is an essential part of ALL therapy, as it has clearly been shown to reduce the incidence of CNS disease. Although uncommon at diagnosis (<10%), without CNS-directed therapy, 50% to 75% of patients will develop CNS disease. Depending on the protocol, CNS prophylaxis includes IT chemotherapy with MTX, Ara-C, and steroids, high-dose systemic chemotherapy with MTX, Ara-C, L-asparaginase, craniospinal irradiation (RT), or a combination of both. None of the combinations have been definitively proven to be superior to the others. The role of cranial RT has become controversial, because of the significant neurologic complications such as seizures, intellectual and cognitive impairment, dementia, and development of secondary CNS malignancy.

In adults, features that correlate with high-risk of development of CNS disease include mature B-cell ALL, serum LDH higher than 600 IU/L, and a proliferative index more than 14% (% S phase + G_2M phase).

2. The commonly used regimens for CNS prophylaxis include the following:

a. MTX, 12 mg/m^2 (maximum 15 mg), diluted in preservative-free saline, given IT once a week for 6 weeks. Some investigators also give 10 mg of hydrocortisone succinate IT to prevent lumbar arachnoiditis.

The IT MTX is given in an "in-and-out" manner. One to 2 mL of the MTX solution is injected into the spinal canal. Then, 0.5 to 1 mL of spinal fluid is withdrawn back into the syringe. This in-and-out process is repeated until all of the MTX has been given. This method is used to ensure that the MTX is actually given into the subarachnoid space. Leucovorin 5 to 10 mg may be given orally every 6 h for four to eight doses to ameliorate the mucositis, although this is usually not needed unless the patient is receiving concurrent systemic MTX. Complications of MTX include chemical arachnoiditis and leukoencephalopathy.

b. In the MD Anderson Hyper-CVAD regimen, IT **MTX** 12 mg on day 2 and **cytarabine** 100 mg on day 8 of each of eight cycles was administered to high-risk patients and on each of four cycles in low-risk patients.

c. Cranial irradiation with IT **MTX** has usually been initiated within 2 weeks of attaining a CR when classic maintenance is given. Cranial irradiation is usually given to the cranial vault (anteriorly to the posterior pole of the eye and posteriorly to C2) in 0.2 Gy fractions for a total of 18 to 24 Gy. The spine is not irradiated because marrow toxicity significantly limits the ability to give further chemotherapy. Common acute complications of radiation include stomatitis, parotitis, alopecia, marrow suppression, and headaches.

3. CNS leukemia therapy is similar to CNS prophylaxis.

a. Cranial irradiation is usually given to a total of 30 Gy in 1.5 to 2 Gy fractions.

b. IT chemotherapy is given in the manner described for CNS prophylaxis and is repeated every 3 to 4 days, with appropriate laboratory studies being done with each lumbar puncture (LP). When blast cells are no longer seen on the cytospin preparation, two more doses of IT drug are given, usually followed by a monthly "maintenance" IT injection.

Some investigators advocate either a simultaneous or alternating administration of IT Ara-C and MTX. The use of systemic therapy with high-dose cytarabine 1 to 3 g/m^2 IV infusion over 2 hours every 12 hours is also effective for the treatment of CNS leukemia. A practical approach is to initiate IT chemotherapy until the time that the HDAC is started. Further IT therapy can then be given on the basis of the results of subsequent CSF analysis after the HDAC is completed. A slow-release formulation of Ara-C (DepoCyt) that maintains cytotoxic concentrations for approximately 14 days has been demonstrated to be effective for the treatment of lymphomatous meningitis and solid tumors and is under evaluation in acute leukemia.

4. Guidelines for the management and prophylaxis of CNS disease. Obtain the diagnostic LP once the leukemic blasts are cleared from the peripheral blood (to preclude the CNS contamination in the event of traumatic LP). The first dose of IT chemotherapy could be given at the same time. Presence of lymphoblasts in the CSF

(>5 lymphocytes/μL and blasts on the differential or any lymphoblasts in the CSF) usually signifies CNS disease, although false-negative results are possible with predominantly cranial nerve involvement by leukemia. Patients presenting with clinical symptoms consistent with CNS involvement, such as headache, altered sensorium, and cranial nerve (particularly VI) palsy warrant an *immediate* CNS imaging and LP because neurologic dysfunction is most amenable to therapy within the first 24 hours. Infectious meningitis must also be excluded in the immunocompromised host. Consider Ommaya placement for patients with diagnosed CNS involvement or patients at high risk of developing CNS (as they will require longer CNS therapy). Isolated CNS relapse usually heralds bone marrow relapse if systemic therapy is not changed. Therefore, isolated CNS relapse is usually treated with systemic reinduction chemotherapy and IT chemotherapy, followed by cranial irradiation.

F. Precursor B-cell lineage and T-cell acute lymphoblastic leukemia (ALL). Although T-cell ALL previously had a poor prognosis with standard induction and maintenance chemotherapy, with the advent of more intensive chemotherapy regimens, RRs and long-term DFS are comparable with those for precursor B-cell ALL. RR of 100% and projected long-term DFS of 59% were demonstrated by the regimen devised by Linker et al. in 2002 for T-cell ALL. CALGB 8811 protocol produced a 100% CR rate with a 3-year RFS of 63% for a similar group of patients. Precursor B-cell and T-cell ALLs are treated with similar regimens in most contemporary protocols.

G. Mature (Burkitt) B-cell ALL is rare, constituting 2% to 4% of cases of adult ALL, and is associated with HIV syndrome. Characteristic clinical features include frequent CNS involvement, lymphadenopathy, splenomegaly, and high serum LDH levels. Current pediatric studies designed specifically for B-cell ALL, utilizing shorter duration, dose-intensive systemic chemotherapy and early CNS prophylaxis/treatment, have substantially improved the CR rate to approximately 90% and the DFS to 50% to 87%.

With the use of these therapeutic strategies in children as a template, clinical trials with young adults have demonstrated long-term survival rates of 70% to 80%. The German BFM group reported the improvement of CR rate from 44% to 74%, the probability of DFS from 0% to 71%, and the OS from 0% to 51% when the intensive treatment was compared with a standard ALL regimen. Hyper-CVAD regimen modeled by the MD Anderson Cancer Center after the total therapy B (see Hyper-CVAD, Table 19.11) induced a CR of 90% and cure rate of 70% in patients younger than 60, and a CR rate of 67% with cure rate of only 15% in older patients.

Addition of anti-CD20 antibody rituximab to the Hyper-CVAD regimen induced CR in 86% of patients, with 3-year OS, EFS, and DFS of 89%, 80%, and 88% respectively. Nine elderly patients achieved a CR with a 3-year OS rate of 89% (one patient died from infection in CR).

Hyper-CVAD therapy in combination with highly active antiretroviral therapy (HAART) regimen in HIV-positive patients resulted in a CR rate of 92%, with more than 50% of patients alive at 2 years after the diagnosis. The outcome appeared to be improved in patients taking HAART medications early in the course of the therapy.

Recommendations for management of mature B-cell ALL include

- R-Hyper-CVAD therapy *or*
- MRC/ECOG regimen, *or*
- CALGB regimen

One should also consider HIV testing and CNS prophylaxis.

H. Therapy for Ph+ ALL. Although the rates of CR in patients with Ph+ ALL are only slightly less than in those with Ph−disease (60%−80%), the long-term DFS is less than 10%. In the CALGB 8461 study, the CR rate in Ph+ ALL was 79% and 5-year remission duration was 8% (vs. 38% in diploid ALL). Currently, allo-HSCT is recommended for Ph+ ALL patients in first remission as the only modality shown to provide long-term DFS. The MRC/ECOG international prospective ALL group compared the outcomes of Ph+ ALL patients treated with matched sibling allo-HSCT, matched unrelated allo-HSCT, auto-HSCT, and consolidation/maintenance chemotherapy. The 5-year RR was lower in allo-HSCT group (29%) than with auto-HSCT/chemotherapy group (81%), whereas the 5-year survival rates were 43% and 19%, respectively. The treatment-related mortality (TRM), not surprisingly, was higher in the patients undergoing allo-HSCT; 43% for matched unrelated allo-HSCT; 37% for matched sibling HSCT; 14% for auto-HSCT; and 8% for chemotherapy.

Imatinib mesylate (Gleevec), a potent selective inhibitor of the *bcr-abl* tyrosine kinase, has been shown in phase I and II clinical trials to have substantial (CR 20%−58%), albeit non-sustained (42−123 days) activity in patients with relapsed and refractory Ph+ ALL. Administration of imatinib to 20 patients with Ph+ ALL relapsed after the allo-HSCT induced a CR in 55%. Incorporation of imatinib in the first-line chemotherapy regimen, such as Hyper-CVAD, is associated with the hematologic CR rates consistently higher than 90%, with concurrent administration resulting in greater antileukemic efficacy. Of interest, imatinib *monotherapy* in previously untreated patients results in the CR rate of approximately 95%, without the associated toxicity of chemotherapy.

Dasatinib (BMS-354825, Bristol-Myers Squibb) is a novel, oral kinase inhibitor that targets bcr-abl and SRC kinases, shows activity in Gleevec resistant Ph+ ALL, and had recently been FDA approved for CML. In a resent study 70% (seven out of ten) of patients with Ph+ ALL and CML with lymphoid blast crisis achieved a major hematologic response with dasatinib. Dasatinib is currently being evaluated in combination with chemotherapy for patients with Ph+ ALL.

I. ALL in older adults. The therapeutic advances and improved outcomes in children and young adults with ALL did not occur in older ALL patients. Likely reasons include fundamental biologic differences in the spectrum of ALL in this patient population, presence of coexisting medical conditions and decreased ability to tolerate intensive chemotherapy.

Additionally, older patients have been frequently excluded from the clinical trials. The outcomes of older ALL patients treated on the five sequential CALGB studies as compared to their younger counterparts have been demonstrated. The CR rate decreases from 90% in patients younger than 30 years to 81% in patients between 30 and 59 years, and to 57% in those older than 60 years; the 3-year OS is estimated to be 58%, 38%, and 12%, respectively. On the basis of the data provided by the Hoelzer and Pagano et al., from 1990 to 2004, for patients older than 60 years treated with intensive chemotherapy, the weighted mean CR rate was 56%; 23% suffered from early mortality and 30% had primary refractory disease.

In a randomized clinical trial evaluating the use of growth factors during chemotherapy for ALL, older patients enjoyed the greatest benefit. Therefore, it is recommended to administer growth factors during ALL treatment in older adults.

Full doses of VPD-based induction protocols are used in elderly patients with ALL. Some investigators decrease the dose of vincristine by 50%. The MRC UKALLIIX/ECOG E2993 and CALGB 8811 regimens should be considered for patients who are thought to be able to tolerate more intensive therapy.

Underlying cardiac disease may preclude the use of an anthracycline for induction therapy. An active program is **MOAD**, which is given in sequential 10-day courses (minimum three, maximum five) until remission is achieved (see Table 19.11) Once a CR has been attained, two additional courses of MOAD are given.

J. Salvage therapy for ALL. Although a second remission can usually be achieved in 10% to 50% of adults with ALL, it tends to be short lived (6–7 months). If a second remission can be attained, suitable patients with relapsed ALL should be evaluated for the HSCT. Salvage therapies typically include combinations of vincristine, steroids, and anthracyclines; combinations of MTX and L-asparaginase; and HDAC-containing regimens. Novel agents are incorporated into the salvage regimens continuously. None of the programs used for relapse is distinctly superior to the others, and any perceived differences are likely attributable to the usual biases of study selection.

1. "7 + 3" (cytarabine and daunorubicin) as used for the induction of AML is active in ALL. Vincristine and prednisone may be added.

2. Etoposide and cytarabine are given every 3 weeks for up to three courses until marrow hypoplasia and remission are achieved. They are then repeated monthly until relapse.

Etoposide 60 mg/m^2 IV every 12 hours on days 1 to 5, *and* Cytarabine 100 mg/m^2 IV bolus every 12 hours on days 1 to 5.

HDAC-based regimens have been reported to induce CR rates in 17% to 70% of patients.

3. HDAC as a single agent has modest activity in ALL, with a CR rate of approximately 34% and a median remission duration of 3.6 months. The addition of idarubicin or mitoxantrone increases the RR to 60%, but the median response time remains 3.4 months.

4. Cytarabine and fludarabine comprise an active *non-cardiotoxic* combination. The median response duration is 5.5 months. Neurotoxicity is low. A second course can be given in 3 weeks if needed.

a. Induction

Cytarabine 1 g/m^2/day IV over 2 hours on days 1 to 6, *and*

Fludarabine 30 mg/m^2/day IV over 30 minutes, 4 hours before cytarabine on days 2 to 6.

b. Consolidation is given monthly for two to three courses.

Cytarabine 1 g/m^2/day IV over 2 hours on days 1 to 4, *and*

Fludarabine 30 mg/m^2/day IV over 30 minutes, 4 hours before cytarabine on days 1 to 4.

c. Maintenance

6-Mercaptopurine 50 mg PO t.i.d., *and*
MTX 20 mg/m^2/week PO.

5. FLAG-IDA (fludarabine, cytarabine, G-CSF, and idarubicin) induced a 39% CR rate in patients with relapsed/refractory ALL. The responders have received the second cycle followed by allo-HSCT and achieved a DFS of 6 months (7–38 months) and OS of 9 months (7–38 months).

- Fludarabine 30 mg/m^2/day IV over 30 minutes on days 1 to 5, *and*
- Cytarabine 2 g/m^2/day IV over 4 hours on days 1 to 5, *and*
- Idarubicin 10 mg/m^2/day days 1 to 3, *and*

G-CSF 5 µg/kg SC 24 hours after the completion of chemotherapy and until neutrophil regeneration.

6. Hyper-CVAD (**see Table** 19.11) therapy achieves CR rates similar to a combination of HDAC, mitoxantrone, and granulocyte-macrophage colony-stimulating factor (GM-CSF) (44% vs. 30%); however the survival is improved.

L-asparaginase was administered in combination with MTX, anthracyclines, vinca alkaloids, and prednisone with RR ranging from 33% to 79% and median DFS from 3 to 6 months.

7. Sequential MTX and L-asparaginase resulted in significant stomatitis (dose-limiting toxicity); 23% of treated patients had allergic reactions to L-asparaginase.

a. Induction

MTX 50 to 80 mg/m^2 IV on day 1, *and*
L-Asparaginase 20,000 IU/m^2 IV 3 hours after MTX on day 1, *followed by*
MTX 120 mg/m^2 IV on day 8, *and*
L-Asparaginase 20,000 IU/m^2 IV on day 9.

Repeat day 8 and 9 doses for MTX and L-asparaginase every 7 to 14 days until remission is attained.

b. Maintenance is repeated every 2 weeks.

MTX 10 to 40 mg/m^2 IV on day 1, *and*
L-Asparaginase 10,000 IU/m^2 IV on day 1.

K. Hematopoietic stem cell transplantation in acute lymphoblastic leukemia (ALL)

1. **Autologous hematopoietic stem cell transplantation** for patients in first remission appears to offer no advantage over chemotherapy, on the basis of the data from the small prospective trials reported to date and preliminary prospective randomized MRC/ECOG ALL data, because of high rates of relapse.

2. **Allogeneic matched-sibling hematopoietic stem cell transplantation.** Patients receiving matched sibling HSCT in first CR reach a survival rate of 50% (20%–81%). Prior studies have not demonstrated an advantage with allogeneic HSCT as compared to standard chemotherapy for ALL patients *without* high-risk features in first CR. However, many of these trials have lacked sufficient numbers of patients, have used varied patient selection criteria, or did not allow for direct, prospective comparisons.

According to the data collected by the IBMTR 9-year DFS was not different for patients treated with chemotherapy and allo-HSCT (32% vs. 34%). High treatment-related mortality (TRM) in HSCT group was the main reason for poor outcome, whereas recurrence rate was twice as high in the chemotherapy group (66% vs. 30%).

The benefit of allo-HSCT in *high-risk* ALL patients was shown by a large French multicenter trial (LALA87) that compared the allo-HSCT with chemotherapy or auto-HSCT in first CR. Although 5-year OS was not significantly different (48% vs. 35%, $p = 0.08$) for patients with high-risk disease, both 5-year OS (44% vs. 22%) and DFS (39% vs. 14%) were significantly better with allo-HSCT. Similarly, the 10- year OS for high-risk group was 44% with allo-HSCT and only 11% in the chemo/auto-HSCT arm, whereas in the standard-risk population the corresponding numbers were 49% and 39% ($p = 0.6$), respectively.

Results from the prospective International MRC/ECOG ALL Trial have demonstrated favorable results for Ph-negative patients treated with matched-sibling allo-HSCT as compared with a combined cohort of auto-HSCT and consolidation chemotherapy. The actuarial 5-year EFS for the allo-HSCT is 54% as compared with 34% for the chemotherapy/auto-HSCT group (100-day mortality for Ph-negative patients in allo-HSCT arm was 21%). This survival advantage for allo-HSCT included patients with *standard-risk* ALL disease (defined as Ph negative, younger than 36 years, time to CR <4 weeks, and WBC count <30,000/µL for B-cell lineage and <100,000/µL for T-cell lineage) with 5-year EFS rates and 5-year relapse rates of 66% and 17%, respectively, versus 45% and 50%, respectively, for the chemotherapy/auto-HSCT group. Particular subgroups of patients with good long-term EFS such as chromosome 12 and 14 abnormalities (and possibly thymic ALL patients) may not benefit from allo-HSCT in first CR. Further evaluation is warranted to determine the optimal intensity of postremission therapy for this patient population. Despite the high risk of early toxicity, matched-sibling allo-HSCT should be considered for most ALL patients in first CR, including standard-risk patients.

3. Matched unrelated donor (MUD) hematopoietic stem cell transplantation. As less than 30% of suitable ALL patients have an HLA-matched sibling donor, MUD HSCT is a viable option available to younger (40–50 years old) patients. Although treatment-related mortality (TRM) remains unacceptably high (40%–50% at 100 days), the outcomes have been improving, in part through the use of better matching at the HLA loci with molecular rather than serologic methods. The National Marrow Donor Program reported on 127 high-risk, defined as presence of t(9;22), t(4;11), or t(1;19), ALL patients, who received a MUD HSCT between 1988 and 1999. The cumulative TRM incidence at 2 years was 61% (54% in first CR, 75% in second CR, and 64% in primary induction failure), whereas the OS at 2 years from transplant was 40%, 17%, and 5%, respectively. The DFS for patients transplanted in CR1 is 32% at 4 years with a 13% cumulative incidence of relapse.

On the basis of the available data, we advocate the use of MUD HSCT for physically fit Ph-positive patients in first CR, if a matched-sibling donor is not available.

4. Alternative-donor hematopoietic stem cell transplantation. Mismatched family member and haploidentical HSCTs have been evaluated and are options, but these procedures should still be considered experimental in ALL.

L. Novel and experimental strategies for the therapy of ALL. It is unlikely that altering the sequence of currently available chemotherapeutic agents or increasing their intensity will produce a qualitative improvement in the outcome of adult patients with ALL. A number of experimental approaches that are currently being evaluated in clinical trials include monoclonal antibodies, farnesyl transferase inhibitors, tyrosine kinase inhibitors, antimetabolites, and other agents.

SUGGESTED READINGS

Amadori S, Suciu S, Stasi R, et al. Gemtuzumab ozogamicin (Mylotarg) as single-agent treatment for frail patients 61 years of age and older with acute myeloid leukemia: final results of AML-15B, a phase 2 study of the European Organisation for Research and Treatment of Cancer and Gruppo Italiano Malattie Ematologiche dell'Adulto Leukemia Groups. *Leukemia* 2005;19:1768–1773.

Andersen MK, Larson RA, Mauritzson N, et al. Balanced chromosome abnormalities inv(16) and t(15;17) in therapy-related myelodysplastic syndromes and acute leukemia: report from an international workshop. *Genes Chromosomes Cancer* 2002;33:395–400.

Annino L, Vegna ML, Camera A, et al. Treatment of adult acute lymphoblastic leukemia (ALL): long-term follow-up of the GIMEMA ALL 0288 randomized study. *Blood* 2002;99:863–871.

Bishop JF, Matthews JP, Young GA, et al. Intensified induction chemotherapy with high dose cytarabine and etoposide for acute myeloid leukemia: a review and updated results of the Australian Leukemia Study Group. *Leuk Lymphoma* 1998;28:315–327.

Blume KG, Forman SJ, Snyder DS, et al. Allogeneic bone marrow transplantation for acute lymphoblastic leukemia during first complete remission. *Transplantation* 1987;43:389–392.

Byrd JC, Mrozek K, Dodge RK, et al. Pretreatment cytogenetic abnormalities are predictive of induction success, cumulative incidence of relapse, and overall survival in adult patients with de novo acute myeloid leukemia: results from Cancer and Leukemia Group B (CALGB 8461). *Blood* 2002;100(13):4325–4336.

Cave H, van der Werff ten Bosch J, Suciu S, et al. Clinical significance of minimal residual disease in childhood acute lymphoblastic leukemia. European Organization for Research and Treatment of Cancer–Childhood Leukemia Cooperative Group. *N Engl J Med* 1998;339:591–598.

Chessells JM, Hall E, Prentice HG, et al. The impact of age on outcome in lymphoblastic leukaemia; MRC UKALL X and XA compared: a report from the MRC Paediatric and Adult Working Parties. *Leukemia* 1998;12:463–473.

Cortes J, Thomas D, Rios A, et al. Hyperfractionated cyclophosphamide, vincristine, doxorubicin, and dexamethasone and highly active antiretroviral therapy for patients with acquired immunodeficiency syndrome-related Burkitt lymphoma/leukemia. *Cancer* 2002;94:1492–1499.

Dombret H, Gabert J, Boiron JM, et al. Outcome of treatment in adults with Philadelphia chromosome-positive acute lymphoblastic leukemia–results of the prospective multicenter LALA-94 trial. *Blood* 2002;100:2357–2366.

Durrant IJ, Prentice HG, Richards SM. Intensification of treatment for adults with acute lymphoblastic leukaemia: results of U.K. Medical Research Council randomized trial UKALL XA. Medical Research Council Working Party on Leukaemia in Adults. *Br J Haematol* 1997;99:84–92.

Faderl S, Gandhi V, O'Brien S, et al. Results of a phase 1–2 study of clofarabine in combination with cytarabine (ara-C) in relapsed and refractory acute leukemias. *Blood* 2005;105:940–947.

Faderl S, Jeha S, Kantarjian HM. The biology and therapy of adult acute lymphoblastic leukemia. *Cancer* 2003;98:1337–1354.

Faderl S, Kantarjian HM, Talpaz M, et al. Clinical significance of cytogenetic abnormalities in adult acute lymphoblastic leukemia. *Blood* 1998;91:3995–4019.

Foroni L, Coyle LA, Papaioannou M, et al. Molecular detection of minimal residual disease in adult and childhood acute lymphoblastic leukaemia reveals differences in treatment response. *Leukemia* 1997;11:1732–1741.

Goldman SC, Holcenberg JS, Finklestein JZ, et al. A randomized comparison between rasburicase and allopurinol in children with lymphoma or leukemia at high risk for tumor lysis. *Blood* 2001;97(10):2998–3003.

Goldstone A, Prentice HG, Durant J. Allogeneic transplant (related or unrelated donor) is the preferred treatment for the adult Philadelphia chromosome positive (Ph+) acute lymphoblastic leukemia (ALL). Results from the International ALL trial (MRC UKALLXII/ECOG E2993). *Blood* 2001;98:856a.

Harris NL, Jaffe ES, Diebold J, et al. World Health Organization classification of neoplastic diseases of the hematopoietic and lymphoid tissues: report of the Clinical Advisory Committee meeting-Airlie House, Virginia, November 1997. *J Clin Oncol* 1999;17:3835–3849.

van der Holt B, Lowenberg B, Burnett AK, et al. The value of the MDR1 reversal agent PSC-833 in addition to daunorubicin and cytarabine in the treatment of elderly patients with previously untreated acute myeloid leukemia (AML), in relation to MDR1 status at diagnosis. *Blood* 2005;106(8):2646–2654.

Ichimura M, Ishimura T, Belsky JL. Incidence of leukemia on atomic bomb survivors belonging to fixed cohort in Hiroshima and Nagasaki,1950–1971: radiation dose, years after exposure, age at exposure, and type of leukemia. *J Radiat Res* 1987;19:262–282.

Kantarjian H, Giles F, Wunderle L, et al. Nilotinib in imatinib-resistant CML and Philadelphia chromosome-positive ALL. *N Engl J Med* 2006;354:2542–2551.

Kantarjian HM, O'Brien S, Smith TL, et al. Results of treatment with hyper-CVAD, a dose-intensive regimen, in adult acute lymphocytic leukemia. *J Clin Oncol* 2000;18:547–561.

Kell WJ, Burnett AK, Chopra R, et al. A feasibility study of simultaneous administration of gemtuzumab ozogamicin with intensive chemotherapy in induction and consolidation in younger patients with acute myeloid leukemia. *Blood* 2003;102:4277–4283.

Koller CA, Kantarjian HM, Thomas D, et al. The hyper-CVAD regimen improves outcome in relapsed acute lymphoblastic leukemia. *Leukemia* 1997;11:2039–2044.

Larson RA, Dodge RK, Burns CP, et al. A five-drug remission induction regimen with intensive consolidation for adults with acute lymphoblastic leukemia: cancer and leukemia group B study 8811. *Blood* 1995;85:2025–2037.

Mortuza FY, Papaioannou M, Moreira IM, et al. Minimal residual disease tests provide an independent predictor of clinical outcome in adult acute lymphoblastic leukemia. *J Clin Oncol* 2002;20:1094–1104.

Ottmann OG, Druker BJ, Sawyers CL, et al. A phase 2 study of imatinib in patients with relapsed or refractory Philadelphia chromosome-positive acute lymphoid leukemias. *Blood* 2002;100: 1965–1971.

Ottmann O, Wassmann B, Gokbuget N, et al. A randomized phase II study comparing Imatinib with chemotherapy as induction therapy in elderly patients with newly diagnosed Philadelphia-positive acute lymphoid leukemia(Ph+ ALL). *Hematol J* 2004;5:S112.

Ottmann O, Wassmann B, Pfeifer H. Activity of the ABL-tyrosine kinase inhibitor Gleevec (STI571) in Philadelphia chromosome positive acute lymphoblastic leukemia (Ph+ ALL) relapsing after allogeneic stem cell transplantation (allo-SCT). *Blood* 2001;98:589.

Robison LL, Neglia JP. Epidemiology of Down Syndrome and childhood acute leukemia. *Prog Clin Biol Res* 1987;246:19–32.

Rowe JM, Buck G, Burnett AK, et al. Induction therapy for adults with acute lymphoblastic leukemia: results of more than 1500 patients from the international ALL trial: MRC UKALL XII/ECOG E2993. *Blood* 2005;106:3760–3767.

Rowe JM, Neuberg D, Friedenberg W. A phase 3 study of three induction regimens and of priming with GM-CSF in older adults with acute myeloid leukemia: a trial by the Eastern Cooperative Oncology Group. *Blood* 2004;103:479–485.

Rowe JM, Tallman MS. Intensifying induction therapy in acute myeloid leukemia: has a new standard of care emerged? *Blood* 1997;90:2121–2126.

Sebban C, Lepage E, Vernant JP, et al. Allogeneic bone marrow transplantation in adult acute lymphoblastic leukemia in first complete remission: a comparative study. French Group of Therapy of Adult Acute Lymphoblastic Leukemia. *J Clin Oncol* 1994;12:2580–2587.

Sievers EL. Efficacy and safety of gemtuzumab ozogamicin in patients with CD33-positive acute myeloid leukaemia in first relapse. *Expert Opin Biol Ther* 2001;1:893–901.

Slovak ML, Kopecky KJ, Cassileth PA, et al. Karyotypic analysis predicts outcome of pre-remission and post-remission therapy in adult acute myeloid leukemia: a Southwest Oncology Group/Eastern Cooperative Oncology Group Study. *Blood* 2000;96:4075–4083.

Specchia G, Pastore D, Carluccio P, et al. FLAG-IDA in the treatment of refractory/relapsed adult acute lymphoblastic leukemia. *Ann Hematol* 2005;84(12):792–795.

Suki S, Kantarjian H, Gandhi V, et al. Fludarabine and cytosine arabinoside in the treatment of refractory or relapsed acute lymphocytic leukemia. *Cancer* 1993;72(7):2155–2160.

Tallman MS, Neuberg D, Bennett JM, et al. Acute megakaryocytic leukemia: the Eastern Cooperative Oncology Group experience. *Blood* 2000;96(7):2405–2411.

Tallman MS, Rowlings PA, Milone G, et al. Effect of postremission chemotherapy before human leukocyte antigen-identical sibling transplantation for acute myelogenous leukemia in first complete remission. *Blood* 2000;96(4):1254–1258.

Talpaz M, Shah NP, Kantarjian H, et al. Dasatinib in imatinib-resistant Philadelphia chromosome-positive leukemias. *N Engl J Med* 2006;354(24):2531–2541.

Thiebault A, Vernant JP, Degos L, et al. Adult acute lymphocytic leukemia study testing chemotherapy and autologous and allogeneic transplantation. A follow-up report of the French protocol LALA 87. *Hematol Oncol Clin North Am* 2000;14:1353–1366.

Thiede C, Steudel C, Mohr B, et al. Analysis of FLT3-activating mutations in 979 patients with acute myelogenous leukemia: association with FAB subtypes and identification of subgroups with poor prognosis. *Blood* 2002;99:4326–4335.

Thomas X, Boiron JM, Huguet F, et al. Outcome of treatment in adults with acute lymphoblastic leukemia: analysis of the LALA-94 trial. *J Clin Oncol* 2004;22(20):4075–4086.

Thomas D, Cortes J, Giles FJ. Combination of Hyper-CVAD with imatinib mesylate (STI571) for Philadelphia (Ph-) positive adult lymphoblastic leukemia (ALL) or chronic myelogenous leukemia in lymphoid blasts phase (CML-LBP). *Blood* 2001;98:803a.

Tilly H, Castaigne S, Bordessoule D, et al. Low-dose cytarabine versus intensive chemotherapy in the treatment of acute nonlymphocytic leukemia in the elderly. *J Clin Oncol* 1990;8(2):272–279.

Trifilio S, Tallman M, Singhal S, et al. Low-dose recombinant urate oxidase (Rasburicase) is effective in hyperuricemia. *Blood* 2004;104:3312 (American Society of Hematology Annual Meeting abstracts.) San Diego.

Vignetti M, Fazi P, Meloni G, et al. Dramatic improvement in CR rate and CR duration with Imatinib in adult and elderly Ph+ ALL patients: results of the GIMEMA Prospective Study LAL0201. *Blood* 2004;104:2739 (American Society of Hematology Annual Meeting abstracts) San Diego.

Wadleigh M, Richardson PG, Zahrieh D, et al. Prior gemtuzumab ozogamicin exposure significantly increases the risk of veno-occlusive disease in patients who undergo myeloablative allogeneic stem cell transplantation. *Blood* 2003;102(5):1578–1582.

Wassmann B, Pfeifer H, Goekbuget N, et al. Alternating versus concurrent schedules of imatinib and chemotherapy as front-line therapy for Philadelphia-positive acute lymphoblastic leukemia (Ph+ALL). *Blood* 2006;108:1469–1477.

Weick JK, Kopecky KJ, Appelbaum FR, et al. A randomized investigation of high-dose versus standard-dose cytosine arabinoside with daunorubicin in patients with previously untreated acute myeloid leukemia: a Southwest Oncology Group Study. *Blood* 1996;88(8):2841–2851.

Wetzler M, Dodge RK, Mrozek K, et al. Prospective karyotype analysis in adult acute lymphoblastic leukemia: the cancer and leukemia Group B experience. *Blood* 1999;93(11):3983–3993.

CHAPTER 20

Chronic Leukemias

Peter White and Paul R. Walker

The chronic leukemias have traditionally been grouped together to underscore their differences from the more aggressive acute leukemias, but their course is not necessarily indolent; paradoxically, the possibility for achieving cure of these disorders has been more limited than with some acute leukemias. There have been two recent advances that have greatly impacted the understanding and treatment of the chronic leukemias. First is the recognition that treating to an absent (negative) minimal residual disease (MRD) state, as assessed by either polymerase chain reaction (PCR) in chronic myelogenous leukemia (CML) or flow cytometry in chronic lymphocytic leukemia (CLL), has improved durability of response as compared to just traditional morphologic responses and remissions. CML patients are best served when treated to and monitored for negative MRD, and the same may prove true for CLL as well. Second is the sobering understanding that the stem cell population of the chronic leukemias appear to be differentially resistant to treatment that is very effective in the progeny population. This resistance of the often dormant stem cell population limits treatment effectiveness of control, and is a barrier to cure.

I. **Chronic myelogenous leukemia.** CML is a relatively uncommon disorder, accounting for 15% of adult leukemias in the United States. The median age at diagnosis is 53 years. Less than 10% of cases are under 20 years of age. There is a slight male predominance. Ionizing radiation is the only known causative factor. There are no known genetic susceptibility factors.

The pathognomonic finding is the Philadelphia (Ph) chromosome, involving a reciprocal translocation between chromosomes 9 and 22, t(9;22) (q34;q11), resulting in a hybrid *BCR-ABL* gene. The BCL-ABL fusion protein encoded by this gene results in permanently switched-on tyrosine kinase signaling activity and in leukemogenesis. The activated BCR-ABL tyrosine kinase becomes both the cause and perpetuator, allowing unregulated proliferation of the CML clone. It is not the sole factor, however. A multitude of other secondary and associated BCR-ABL-induced abnormalities in CML cells affect proliferation and differentiation; activation of mitogenic signaling pathways; altered cellular adhesion; inhibition of apoptosis; and downstream Ras, mitogen-activated protein kinase (MAPK), Myc, Phosphatidylinositol 3 (PI-3) kinase, and Janus kinase signal transducer and activator of transcription (STAT) pathways. It is now recognized that there are two distinct compartments of CML cells. Myeloid progeny, including erythroid-megakaryocyte-granulocyte lineages, carry the Ph chromosome (Ph+) and actively proliferate. There is also a Ph+ stem cell population of pluripotential myeloid progenitor cells. This stem cell population is often dormant and resistant to treatment, but must be eradicated, or at least kept dormant, to cure CML.

A. Diagnosis. The typical clinical picture is of a middle-aged patient with a total white blood cell (WBC) count more than 25,000 and peripheral smear differential spectrum of circulating immature and mature granulocytic progeny (the peripheral blood will look like bone marrow) with basophilia and palpable splenomegaly. Splenic and/or constitutional symptoms may be present. Palpable lymphadenopathy is absent. The bone marrow is hypercellular with myeloid hyperplasia. Dysplastic changes are minimal. Mild increased reticulum can be seen.

Diagnosis requires identification of either the Ph chromosome or the BCR-ABL fusion product. The neutrophil leukocyte alkaline phosphatase (LAP) score is low in CML; in contrast, it is elevated in leukemoid reactions and other reactive leukocytosis states. If there are no other clinical or hematologic findings to suggest CML, LAP can be helpful as a negative discriminator. However, it is never absolute or diagnostic.

The Ph chromosome can be identified in 95% of CML patients by standard bone marrow cytogenetic techniques or by fluorescence *in situ* hybridization (FISH) (which does not require dividing cells) of bone marrow or peripheral blood. An initial bone marrow is recommended for diagnostic confirmation and assessment of additional cytogenetic abnormalities. Assessing the BCR-ABL transcript in peripheral blood by PCR techniques can identify the small fraction of patients who are Ph-negative by routine cytogenetics. PCR has evolved into a very important way to assess and monitor response to treatment.

The differential diagnosis does include a heterogeneous group of typical clinical picture but Ph chromosome−/BCR-ABL−negative patients including some with chronic myelomonocytic leukemia and chronic neutrophilic leukemia. The latter is a rare clonal myeloproliferative disorder of the elderly. In contrast to CML, these Ph⁻ patients lack basophilia and also have elevated LAP scores.

B. Classification. CML is characterized by three evolutionary phases, each carrying a different clinical and hematologic picture, natural history, and treatment outcome.

    1. Chronic phase is the usual initial presentation of CML. 85% of patients present at diagnosis in the chronic phase. This is marked by immature myeloid cells in the peripheral blood and marked granulocytic hyperplasia in the marrow, but myeloblasts are less than 10% in both peripheral blood and bone marrow. Absolute eosinophilia and basophilia are typically present (in contrast to reactive leukocytosis). The chronic phase will typically run an indolent course of 3 to 5 years before progressing to the accelerated phase, even without treatment.

    2. Accelerated phase is a transition process to the blast phase. It is poorly defined but is usually marked by loss of previously controlled WBC counts and clonal evolution with the development of new chromosomal abnormalities in addition to the persisting or reemerged Ph chromosome. Peripheral blood counts show one or more of the following: blasts equal to or more than 15%, blasts plus promyelocytes equal to or more than 30%, basophils more than 20%, or fall in platelet count to less than or equal to 100,000/μL, unrelated to ongoing treatment. These laboratory findings are often accompanied by the reemergence or progression of symptoms such as fever, bone pain, and fatigue, or worsening splenomegaly. Median survival before imatinib was just 18 months, but now with imatinib it can exceed 4 years.

3. Blastic phase, also called "blast crisis," is the progressed transformation of CML to acute leukemia. It is defined by the acute leukemia criteria of more than 20% marrow blasts. However, patients with 20% to 29% blasts seem to carry a better prognosis than those meeting the older criteria of more than 30% blasts. The majority, 50% to 70% of cases, will show a myeloid phenotype (acute myelogenous leukemia [AML]), but 25% lymphoid (acute lymphocytic leukemia [ALL]), and 5% an undifferentiated phenotype. Recent studies have identified BCR-ABL kinase domain mutations in 30% to 40% of these patients. Persistence of the Ph chromosome including additional Ph chromosomes and other cytogenetic abnormalities will be present. Extramedullary tumor masses (chloromas) can occur in both the accelerated and blastic phases. Durable response to chemotherapy, using various acute leukemia regimens, is typically poor, and median survival in blast phase is 3 to 6 months. ALL will respond better and has a better prognosis than AML evolutions. A chronic phase remission can occur with treatment as the blastic progeny clone is eradicated but the chronic phase Ph + stem cell persists.

C. Prognosis. Separation of these three stages is imprecise, and approximately 25% of patients progress directly from chronic phase to blast phase. Moreover, the duration of the chronic phase is difficult to predict, although a number of factors indicate an increased risk for progression, including greater age, splenomegaly, elevated platelet counts, and higher numbers of peripheral blood myeloblasts, eosinophils, or basophils. The Sokal prognostic system and the Hasford classification utilize a formula factoring in age, spleen size, and the hematologic picture to assign three risk (low-intermediate-high) groups of differing prognosis with 5-year survivals of 76%, 55%, and 25%. Both were developed in patient cohorts treated with interferon, however. No prognostic system has been validated in the imatinib era, limiting their usefulness. Regardless of pretreatment characteristics, the most important and best prognostic predictor is the quality of the MRD response to treatment, as measured by the degree of cytogenetic and molecular response.

D. Therapy. The "imatinib/gleevec era" has revolutionized the treatment of CML but also ushered in some questions of treatment uncertainty. Targeting and inhibiting the BCR-ABL mitogenic pathway with imatinib has achieved dramatic cytogenetic and molecular levels of responses with prolonged disease control never before seen in CML. However, it still appears that imatinib can just control, but not completely eradicate and cure, the stem cell clone. This leaves open the question of on whom and when the transplant should be done. It is clear that imatinib is the starting point in treating chronic phase CML and that close molecular monitoring of the

BCR-ABL transcript is important to best manage an individual with CML.

1. Imatinib (Gleevec) is a small molecule inhibitor of the BCR-ABL tyrosine kinase. In interferon-refractory patients, the rate of complete cytogenetic responses at 40 months was 52%. In the landmark phase III IRIS study in newly diagnosed patients comparing 400 mg imatinib to the then standard interferon/cytarabine, 96% of the imatinib-treated patients had complete hematologic response, 76% a complete cytogenetic response, and 43% major molecular responses with a 3-log decrease in BCR-ABL messenger ribonucleic acid (mRNA) transcripts; all of these are far better than the interferon combination, demonstrating convincing superiority of imatinib. As the imatinib experience grows, several initial unknowns are becoming clear. Dose can be an issue. 800 mg does seem to achieve a more rapid BCR-ABL molecular response; 60% versus 39% 3-log reduction, and 26% as compared to 4% complete molecular response with the 800 mg as compared to 400 mg dosing in early follow-up. However, a recent update from the IRIS trial indicates that with ongoing time and treatment the major molecular response rate increased to 75% at 49 months median follow-up in those patients achieving a complete cytogenetic response at 12 months. It is not clear if the 800-mg dose is ultimately superior to 400 mg. A phase III trial of this dosing comparison is ongoing. A 3-log BCR-ABL mRNA response by quantitative PCR does translate into more durable disease control as compared to less than a 3-log decrease. The deeper the molecular response, the longer the clinical response. Additional kinase mutations or other constitutive pathway stimulation can cause imatinib resistance. It is now known that imatinib has limited effectiveness on the dormant stem cell. Durable control but not cure is the treatment goal with imatinib. The exact median time frames of disease control and overall survival (OS) with imatinib are unknown. It remains hopeful that survival will exceed 15 years in responding patients, and ongoing advances in therapy may push that even longer.

a. The initial management of early phase CML:

- **Imatinib** 400 mg oral daily is the standard initial dosing in chronic phase disease; 800 mg is the standard dose in accelerated phase.

  Treatment is best given continuously, and dosing lower than 300 mg daily is ineffective.

- **Hydroxyurea** 1 to 2 g daily is given as well if the WBC count is more than $100,000/\mu L$ or massive splenomegaly is present.

- **Allopurinol** 300 mg daily is often used until counts normalize.

  Imatinib is overall well tolerated. Nausea, peripheral and periorbital edema, muscle cramps, diarrhea, weight gain, and fatigue can occur, but all usually grade 1 to 2. Nausea can be lessened by taking the drug with a large glass of water and a full meal. Muscle cramps can be lessened by tonic water and calcium. Imatinib inhibits and is metabolized through the CYP450 pathway causing potential drug interactions. Liver toxicity can also occur. Myelosuppression is the most common grade 3 to 4 toxicity with neutropenia and thrombocytopenia forcing treatment interruption or dose reduction at times, in particular during the first few months of treatment. Granulocyte colony-stimulating factor (G-CSF) can be used to maintain adequate dose intensity in the face of grade 3 or 4 neutropenia. Congestive heart failure is rare. It may be related to imatinib inhibition of Abl, which may be related to mitochondrial function in the heart.

Maintaining imatinib dosing at higher than 300 mg daily is pharmacologically important to achieve effective inhibitory plasma concentrations.

b. Treatment and disease monitoring is used to assess for early hematologic treatment toxicity and to evaluate the ongoing and ultimate disease response, with the treatment goal of MRD measured by a complete cytogenetic response and a 3-log reduction molecular response. A reasonable approach, modifiable to an individual patient and case, is:

(1) Complete blood cell count (CBC) weekly until stable, then every 4 to 6 weeks.

(2) Marrow cytogenetics at diagnosis, at 6 and 12 months of initial treatment, and yearly with ongoing treatment.

(3) Peripheral blood quantitative reverse transcriptase PCR(RT-PCR) for BCR-ABL mRNA at diagnosis and every 3 months with ongoing treatment.

The timing and level of response are important management milestones. The earlier a cytogenetic and molecular response, the better and longer the ultimate response will be. A partial cytogenetic response (1%–35% Ph positive metaphases) by 3 to 6 months predicts an 80% to 95% likelihood of achieving an eventual complete cytogenetic response. Quantitative PCR on peripheral blood is the monitoring method of choice. There is a significant correlation between the molecular response at 3 months and cytogenetic response at 12 months. At 42 months of follow-up, those patients with a complete cytogenetic response by 12 months and a major molecular response (>3-log reduction in BCR-ABL mRNA) had a progression-free survival of 98% as compared to 90% if less than 3-log reduction and 75% for patients without a complete cytogenetic response. There is no absolute latest point in time at which a patient should have a complete cytogenetic response before considering an altered treatment approach. That must be individualized based up age and other viable treatment options available. In a young patient who is a transplant candidate, if there is not an early optimal response within 6 to 12 months, consideration of this alternative therapy is appropriate.

c. Imatinib resistance can either be primary or secondary. Primary hematologic resistance without a complete hematologic response occurs in approximately 5% of patients. Primary cytogenetic resistance, failing to achieve a partial cytogenetic response at 6 months or complete cytogenetic response at 12 months, will occur in 15% of patients. After 42 months of follow-up, 16% of patients treated on the IRIS study developed secondary resistance or progressed overtly. In patients previously treated with interferon, 26% in chronic phase developed resistance or progression. Imatinib resistance is much higher in accelerated (73%) and blast phases (95%). Causes of resistance can either be BCR-ABL dependent or independent. Acquired kinase domain mutation in BCR-ABL is the most frequent mechanism, preventing the conformal binding of imatinib to the ABL kinase domain, and causing BCR-ABL reactivation. A small number of cases can be due to BCR-ABL overproduction, overcoming the imatinib inhibition effect. The BCR-ABL–independent resistance develops through alternate pathways with SRC activation implicated in some cases. Imatinib resistance will be identified by either overt hematologic progression or now more frequently by a 1-log increase in the BCR-ABL q-PCR result of the peripheral blood. At that time, a repeat bone marrow with cytogenetics and screening for the new kinase mutations, if that technology is available, should be performed. At this time, the main purpose outside of a clinical trial would be to identify the T315I mutation that does not respond to alternative kinase inhibitors.

The management of imatinib resistance has no single strategy. Just changes in mutation alone may not absolutely warrant a change in therapy in circumstances when a different therapy may be more toxic or not accessible. Overt phase progression forces a treatment change, as the current therapy is ineffective. Mutation changes are clearly a harbinger of phase progression but in a variable time frame. Optimal control has been lost but just at a biologic and not yet clinical level. Imatinib dose escalation up to 800 mg can be undertaken; however, tolerance and durability are limiting factors. The addition of a conventional agent, either interferon or cytarabine, could also be undertaken but this is best utilized if just a suboptimal initial response has occurred. An allogeneic stem cell transplant in a transplant candidate would remain an option.

d. Imatinib alternatives. The best approach for patients resistant to imatinib seems to be the new small molecule ABL kinase inhibitors, dasatinib (BMS-354825) and AMN107. Both are being actively investigated with exciting preliminary results. AMN107 is a derivative of imatinib and has shown 40% overall and 13% cytogenetic responses in resistant chronic phase and accelerated phase disease but is less effective in blastic phase. Dasatinib, structurally unrelated to imatinib, binds both the

ABL kinase domain and also inhibits SRC family kinases. Dasatinib has been granted U.S. Food and Drug Administration (FDA) approval for second-line use in CML. Single-arm studies of extensively pre-treated patients have shown major cytogenetic responses in 45% of chronic phase disease and major hematologic responses in 59% accelerated phase and 31% blast phase CML. It is premature to know response durability.

- **Dasatinib (Sprycel)** is given as 70 mg PO twice daily for initial dosing. Doses are adjusted up or down in 20-mg increments as needed; doses above 90 to 100 mg b.i.d. have not been investigated in clinical trials. Fluid retention including pleural and pericardial effusions, bleeding, febrile neutropenia, and diarrhea are the most frequent grade 3/4 adverse events.

2. Allogeneic stem cell transplant. This remains the only known curative treatment for CML. A current debate and dilemma is on whom and when the transplant should be done. The earlier the disease at the time of transplant, the better the outcome: 5-year survival rates will range from 60% to 80% in chronic phase disease to 25% to 40% in accelerated phase, and 10% in blastic phase. "Early" chronic phase is better than the "late" phase In the interferon era, transplanting within 12 months of diagnosis was the aim. Now with the better responses and tolerance of imatinib, that is not as clear. Recent data from the Fred Hutchinson transplant experience indicates that transplanting within 24 months of diagnosis maintains a maximal outcome. A younger age is also better but even this is in flux with reduced-intensity conditioning transplant regimens increasing the age of potential transplant recipients. Treatment-related mortality, let alone the tremendous morbidities, does increase with age. Graft-versus-leukemia effect appears crucial to achieve a cure, indicating the need for immune effects to eradicate the CML stem cell. For those transplant candidate patients not achieving an optimal cytogenetic and molecular response, the decision to transplant is easy, with no other hope of durability, let alone curability. Likewise in potential transplant candidates who relapse on imatinib, stepping to transplant is an easy decision. However, there is still significant mortality and morbidity even in young patients and the disease is less curable as time goes on. There are no absolute guidelines at this point in time. As the imatinib experience extends, clearer guidelines and direction may identify those who should be transplanted at initial diagnosis. In patients younger than 30 years, this should still be a prime consideration even in the imatinib era. The Gratwohl score (Table 20.1) can give a sense of the outcome and mortality of a transplant in groups by factoring in disease stage, age, donor type and gender, and timing with transplant-related mortality ranging from 20% in favorable groups but more than 50% in unfavorable settings. However, as with all of the prognostic models, these were developed in the pre-imatinib era, limiting applicability, particularly in

Table 20.1. Gratwohl score for predicting transplant outcome

Score	0		1		2	
Donor type	Related		Matched, unrelated		—	
Disease state	Chronic		Accelerated		Blastic; second chronic	
Age	<20 year		20–40 year		>40 year	
Donor/recipient gender	M/M; F/F; M/F		F/M		—	
Time from diagnosis	<12 months		>12 months		—	
Score	0	1	2	3	4	5	6
Survival at 5 years (%)	72	70	62	48	40	18	22
Transplant mortality (%)	20	23	31	46	51	71	73

patients achieving a major or complete molecular response with imatinib. Only with a full and candid discussion with the patient regarding currently available data—imatinib does not appear to eradicate the CML stem cell; it can only be viewed as control, although durable, and not curative therapy; and upon disease progression the cure rate of transplant does decrease—can the best decision for an individual be made. Early referral to a transplant center of all potential transplant candidates can help the initial understanding of the rigors of a transplant and also best facilitate the timeliness of implementation.

Treatment of relapse after a transplant can still be successful with augmentation of the graft-versus-leukemia effects with donor lymphocyte infusions. Recent use of imatinib in this setting has also been effective, suggesting a certain degree of potential synergism between imatinib and the graft-versus-leukemia effect.

Autologous stem cell transplants, just utilizing high-dose cytotoxic chemotherapy and a marrow rescue without any graft-versus-leukemia effects, have not shown any durable benefit. Nonmyeloablative stem cell transplants with reduced-intensity conditioning are an expanding option for the older population but are still fraught with significant mortality and graft-versus-host disease.

3. Interferon and cytarabine no longer have a role as primary therapy in CML given the results of the IRIS trial and availability of imatinib. However, studies of combination regimens of imatinib and either interferon and/or cytarabine are ongoing with early phase II studies showing significant molecular responses. A differential mechanism of effect of interferon as compared to imatinib may be on the stem cell.

4. Accelerated phase CML may still respond to higher (800 mg) dosing of imatinib; however, it is usually much less responsive, and with higher resistance and progression than chronic phase disease. An allogeneic stem cell transplant is arguably the only chance of prolonged survival. Clinical trials should be utilized if accessible.

5. **Blastic phase CML** is notoriously resistant to any treatment including allogeneic stem cell transplants. Determining whether the blastic phase conversion is to AML or ALL will direct the induction chemotherapy approach. Continuing imatinib with either the ALL or AML induction regimen is safe and well tolerated and appears to improve durability. Clinical trials, if available, should be offered to the patient.

II. **Chronic lymphocytic leukemia (CLL).** CLL is marked by the accumulation of a clone of morphologically mature but immunologically nonfunctional or aberrant B lymphocytes in the peripheral blood, bone marrow, spleen, and lymph nodes. Unlike CML, failure of apoptosis rather than cell proliferation accounts for most of this excess accumulation. Over 90% of CLL lymphocytes are in a quiescent G_0 phase of the cell cycle, and the doubling time for circulating lymphocytes is prolonged. The clinical course is typically indolent, and median survival time is in excess of 10 years for patients presenting with early-stage disease. Stage alone does not reliably predict survival for individual patients, however, and characteristics such as abnormal karyotype and unmutated state of immunoglobulin heavy chain genes may foretell more rapid progression.

CLL is the most common form of leukemia in Western societies (though not in Asia), with an annual incidence in the United States of 2.7 cases/100,000 individuals. Incidence in males is twice that in females. Owing to unidentified hereditary factors, relatives of CLL patients have a threefold increased risk of developing CLL or similar lymphoid neoplasms. Median age at diagnosis in the United States is over 70 years; approximately 10% of patients are younger than 50 years.

A. **Diagnosis.** Accepted diagnostic criteria require (1) sustained lymphocytosis—equal to or more than 5,000/μL; (2) marrow lymphocytosis—equal to or more than 30% of nucleated cells; and (3) phenotypic demonstration of monoclonality, with lymphocytes typically positive for CD5, CD19, CD20 (weak), and CD23, but negative for CD10. Surface Ig is demonstrable but dim on flow cytometry, with monoclonality for either κ or λ light chains. Marrow evaluation is not required if (1) and (3) are fulfilled, but it provides a baseline for evaluation of treatment, and the pattern of infiltration has prognostic import (nodular or interstitial good, diffuse bad). The lymphocytes in CLL are morphologically mature and virtually indistinguishable from normal lymphocytes, although a few prolymphocytes with a prominent nucleolus may be found. Numerous prolymphocytes suggest transformation to prolymphocytic leukemia (seen in ~10% of advanced-stage CLL cases) or de novo prolymphocytic leukemia, a separate group of B-cell and T-cell neoplasms. Differential diagnosis of CLL also includes other lymphoid neoplasms such as hairy cell leukemia (HCL), mantle cell lymphoma, large granular lymphocytic leukemia, adult T-cell leukemia/lymphoma, follicle center cell lymphoma, and Sézary syndrome. Morphologic

Table 20.2.   Modified Rai Staging System for chronic lymphocytic leukemia

Stage (risk)	Criteria	Median Survival Time (years)
0 (low risk)	Lymphocytosis only (in blood and bone marrow)	>10
I, II (intermediate risk)	Lymphocytosis plus adenopathy or lymphocytosis plus splenomegaly or hepatomegaly	6
III, IV (high risk)	Lymphocytosis plus anemia (hemoglobin <11 g/dL) or thrombocytopenia (platelets <100 × 10^3/μL)	<2

features and phenotypic patterns on flow cytometry are the key to separating these entities.

B. Staging and prognosis. Clinical stage is prognostically important, and should be assessed in all patients at diagnosis, utilizing either the five-tier Rai system or the three-tier Binet system (see Tables 20.2 and 20.3). Initial evaluation should also include serum lactate dehydrogenase (LDH) and β_2-microglobulin (elevations unfavorable) and quantitation of serum Ig levels (hypogammaglobulinemia develops in 70% of patients as CLL evolves).

Independent of stage, the following features also carry unfavorable prognostic import: diffuse pattern of marrow infiltrate; doubling time of peripheral blood lymphocytes less than 1 year; expression of CD38 and/or zeta-associated protein 70 (ZAP-70) by lymphocytes; and unmutated state of Ig variable-region genes. Abnormal karyotype is frequently demonstrable by cytogenetics or FISH (conveniently performed on peripheral blood); trisomy 12, 17p⁻, and 11q⁻ are unfavorable; normal

Table 20.3.   Binet Staging System for chronic lymphocytic leukemia

Stage	No. of Lymphoid Areas Involved[a]	Anemia or Thrombocytopenia[b]	Median Survival (years)
A	0–2	No	>7
B	3–5	No	<5
C	0–5	Yes	<3

[a] Five areas are designated: cervical, axillary, inguinal, spleen, and liver. Bilateral involvement of regional nodes does not increase the number of areas designated.
[b] Anemia is defined as hemoglobin <10 g/dL, platelets <100 × 10^3/μL.

karyotype is neutral; and 13q⁻ is favorable. Testing for these risk factors is not considered essential, and their role as guides to management decisions is not yet clear.

C. Approach to therapy. The standard approach is to withhold treatment in asymptomatic early-stage patients. Conventional chemotherapy in this setting confers no survival advantage over a watch-and-wait strategy. Indications to initiate treatment include systemic symptoms (fatigue, weight loss, night sweats, recurrent infections), significant cytopenias due to marrow suppression or autoimmune processes, symptomatic or progressive lymphadenopathy, marked splenomegaly, rapid lymphocyte-doubling time (<6 months), and extreme lymphocytosis. There is no firm consensus, but a lymphocyte count of equal to or greater than 150,000/μL is frequently used as a treatment threshold. Hyperviscosity or leukostasis syndromes are rare under 800,000/μL, however. Duration of treatment depends on response, but in most cases treatment is discontinued after clinical control of the disease is achieved. There is no evidence that prolonged maintenance therapy improves OS.

Standardized criteria, developed by a National Cancer Institute (NCI) Working Group, to classify response are as follows:

   1. Complete remission (CR). No evidence of clinical disease for more than 2 months. Requires CBC with lymphocytes less than 4,000/μL, neutrophils equal to or more than 1,500/μL, platelets equal to or more than 100,000/μL, hemoglobin equal to or more than 11 g/dL; marrow lymphocytes less than or equal to 30% with no lymphoid nodules; and no constitutional symptoms, hepatosplenomegaly, or palpable lymphadenopathy.

   2. Partial remission (PR). 50% or greater reduction in peripheral blood lymphocytes, 50% or greater reduction in adenopathy and/or hepatosplenomegaly plus at least one of the following: (a) 50% or greater improvement in platelet and hemoglobin levels, (b) platelets 1,000/microliter or higher, or (c) hemoglobin 11 g/dL or higher. Improvement in clinical stage (e.g., from Binet C to B) may also be considered a PR. Patients who achieve CR except for persistence of lymphoid nodules in marrow are classified as "nodular PR."

   3. Stable disease. Patients who fail to meet the criteria for PR but do not show evidence of progression (e.g., no increasing lymphadenopathy) are considered to have stable disease.

D. Specific regimens
   1. Nucleosides
      a. Fludarabine. This nucleoside analog is now commonly used as first-line therapy. In a large trial of intermediate- and high-risk (Rai stage I to IV) CLL patients, fludarabine gave 20% CR and 43% PR versus 4% CR and 33% PR for chlorambucil, formerly regarded as the standard agent. Time to progression was also longer following fludarabine: 25 versus 14 months. Importantly, however, there was no OS advantage for fludarabine, which also causes greater myelotoxicity and immunosuppression (with prolonged decreases in

CD4 lymphocytes). Chlorambucil thus continues to be considered appropriate for first-line treatment. For chlorambucil failures, fludarabine provides effective salvage, with 46% response rate, in contrast to 7% response to chlorambucil given after fludarabine failure. Patients with fludarabine-induced remissions lasting for equal to or greater than 12 months show reasonable response rates if retreated with fludarabine upon relapse, but combination therapy (see following text) is generally more effective. The recommended regimen for monotherapy is as follows:

- **Fludarabine** 25 mg/m^2/day IV (10- to 30-minute infusion) on days 1 to 5, every 28 days, repeated for six to ten cycles. Dose reductions for renal impairment are required (see Chapter 4). Patients with no response after two cycles should be considered for alternative therapies. Allopurinol is given for 10 to 14 days in advanced-stage patients; patients with very high tumor mass are monitored for tumor lysis syndrome. Cytopenias and immunosuppression are major side effects. Reversible neurologic toxicity is occasionally seen. To avoid transfusion-related graft-versus-host disease, blood products should be irradiated. Prophylaxis against Pneumocystis and *Mycobacterium tuberculosis* should be considered in selected patients.

b. Cladribine. This nucleoside is approved for use in HCL (see following text). Its efficacy in CLL seems comparable to that of fludarabine, with 40% to 60% response rates in previously untreated patients. It is of little benefit in fludarabine-refractory patients. Recommended dose is

- **Cladribine** 0.12 to 0.14 mg/kg ($\sim$5 mg/m^2) IV as a 2-hour infusion on days 1 to 5; repeat every 4 weeks. As with fludarabine, discontinue if no response is seen after two cycles. Toxicity is similar to that of fludarabine, including prolonged immunosuppression.

c. Pentostatin. Approved for hairy cell leukemia, this nucleoside appears to have efficacy similar to the other nucleosides in CLL, and may be less myelotoxic. Recommended dose is

- Pentostatin 4 mg/m^2 by IV bolus or by 20- to 30-minute infusion, given weekly × 3, then every 2 weeks × 3, then once a month. Precautions regarding immunosuppression apply as with fludarabine and cladribine. Do not use with fludarabine.

2. **Alkylating agents**
   a. Chlorambucil is still considered an appropriate first-line treatment, especially in the frail elderly. It is well tolerated, with minimal nausea and no alopecia; reversible myelotoxicity is the major side effect. Prolonged use may lead to myelodysplastic syndromes. Palliative responses will be seen in most CLL patients, though not necessarily meeting the criteria for PR as detailed in the

preceding text; CR occurs in a modest percentage. It is not effective for salvage after fludarabine or cladribine failure. Dosing schedule may be either continuous or intermittent:

- **Chlorambucil** 2 to 6 mg PO daily, with adjustments according to biweekly CBC, *or*
- **Chlorambucil** 0.4 to 0.7 mg/kg (15–26 mg/m^2) PO given as single dose on day 1, or divided over days 1 to 4. Repeat treatment every 2 to 4 weeks depending on myelotoxicity. The intermittent schedule may be less myelotoxic and have better patient compliance. Combination of chlorambucil with prednisone, once popular, is of questionable benefit.

b. Cyclophosphamide is equally effective as chlorambucil but carries risks of cytopenias, nausea, alopecia, and hemorrhagic cystitis.

- Continuous dose is 50 to 100 mg PO daily;
- Intermittent dose is 500 to 750 mg/m^2 PO or IV every 3 to 4 weeks.

To avoid cystitis, morning dosing and 2 to 3 L of daily PO fluid intake are indicated.

3. Steroids

- **Prednisone 40 to 80 mg daily for 5 to 7 days, repeated every 4 weeks** may be useful in patients who cannot tolerate myelotoxic agents, and is also used routinely for autoimmune complications. The preferred schedule is intermittent dosing, but continuous maintenance dosing is often needed for control of autoimmune hemolysis or thrombopenia. Hyperglycemia, psychiatric reactions, osteoporosis, and immunosuppression are hazards. A transient initial rise in lymphocyte count is not unusual, followed by a fall, with subsequent improvement in lymphadenopathy and splenomegaly.

4. Monoclonal antibodies

    a. Rituximab is a chimeric (mouse–human) monoclonal antibody specific against CD20, a surface glycoprotein present on neoplastic and on mature normal B lymphocytes. It is thought to cause cell lysis through complement and antibody-dependent cellular cytotoxicity. CD20 expression on CLL lymphocytes is typically weak, but responses (usually PR) have been reported in 25% of patients previously treated with fludarabine or chlorambucil, utilizing standard rituximab doses. Escalated dosing may produce higher responses, but expense is significant. Rituximab is also utilized in combination with fludarabine, cyclophosphamide, and other agents for salvage therapy. The standard dosage is as follows:

- **Rituximab** 375 mg/m^2 IV weekly × 4 (or 4 to 8). Infusions are started at 50 mg/hour for the first hour and then escalated at 50 mg/hour increments every 30 minutes as tolerated up to 400 mg/hour.

Infusion reactions are routinely seen, consisting of transient chills and fever, often accompanied by nausea, dyspnea, or flushing; hypotension occurs in approximately 10% of patients. Interrupting the infusion, until symptoms subside, will usually allow infusion to be resumed at half the previous rate, and then slowly escalated to complete the scheduled dose. Subsequent infusions can usually be given at an initial rate of 100 mg/hour, with 100-mg/hour increments at 30-minute intervals, up to 400 mg/hour. Pretreatment with acetaminophen and diphenhydramine is recommended, and epinephrine should also be on hand to treat rare anaphylactic reactions. With high tumor burden, a more ominous syndrome with vomiting, hypotension, and dyspnea may be seen, because of massive release of cytokines from damaged lymphocytes. Rarely, tumor lysis syndrome has also occurred. To minimize these problems, patients with lymphocyte counts more than $50,000/\mu L$ may be given 50 mg rituximab on day 1, a dose of 150 mg on day 2, and the remaining on day 3, to total 375 mg/m^2. When feasible, lymphocyte count should be reduced by other agents before rituximab. Myelotoxicity with rituximab is minimal, and severe cytopenias are rare. Circulating normal B lymphocytes are depleted, but not T lymphocytes; immunosuppression has not been a major problem.

b. Alemtuzumab (Campath-1H). This is a humanized chimeric monoclonal antibody targeted against CD52, a surface glycoprotein expressed on normal and neoplastic B and T lymphocytes. Cell death results from apoptosis, complement activation, and antibody-dependent cell-mediated cytotoxicity. Alemtuzumab induces profound immunosuppression, with gradual return of CD4 lymphocytes over many months; opportunistic infections are common, including cytomegalovirus (CMV) and fungi. Severe anemia, neutropenia, and/or thrombocytopenia are seen in 50% to 70% of cases, with recovery typically in 3 to 4 weeks; rare cases of fatal pancytopenia are reported. As with rituximab, infusion-related chills, fever, and nausea are common; pretreatment with acetaminophen/diphenhydramine is recommended. Anti-infection prophylaxis with trimethoprim–sulfa DS b.i.d. 3 days/week and famciclovir 250 mg b.i.d. or valacyclovir 500 mg b.i.d. daily should accompany alemtuzumab treatment and be continued until CD4 T-cell count is equal to or more than $200/\mu L$, or for a minimum of 2 months after therapy. All blood products for transfusion should be irradiated. Monitoring CMV antigen blood levels may be advisable. Alemtuzumab is indicated for use in patients with fludarabine-refractory CLL. In a pivotal trial, response rate was 33% (2% CR, 31% PR); median time to progression was 9.5 months for responders. Recommended schedule is

- **Alemtuzumab** 3 mg as a 2-hour IV infusion is given on day 1 with close monitoring of vital signs. Repeat 3 mg daily until infusion reaction is minimal, then escalate to 10 mg; repeat 10 mg daily until tolerated, then escalate to 30 mg (30 mg level usually reached within 7 days); continue 30 mg three times weekly (Monday, Wednesday, Friday). Total weekly dose should not exceed 90 mg. Continue up to 12 weeks depending on clinical response; discontinue after achieving CR (marrow reassessment needed), or for serious toxicity, for progressive disease, or if disease is stable for more than 4 to 6 weeks. Off-label use of subcutaneous alemtuzumab (dose: 30 mg SC, 3 × weekly) may be useful in patients intolerant of infusions; minor injection-site reactions are common. Alemtuzumab may also be appropriate as first-line therapy for selected patients with 17p⁻ or p53 mutations, who respond poorly to fludarabine and alkylators. Its use in CR patients to clear the marrow of MRD is under study, and may improve OS.

5. Combination chemotherapy. Enthusiasm has waned for the use of steroids combined with chlorambucil or fludarabine, and little advantage has been found in utilizing lymphoma regimens such as COP or CHOP. There is currently great interest, however, in various combinations involving rituximab, alemtuzumab, fludarabine, pentostatin, and cyclophosphamide. These combinations have resulted in significantly higher percentages of CR, when used either as first-line therapy or as salvage for relapsing or refractory CLL. Progression-free survival is lengthened, and evidence suggests that OS is improved in patients achieving CR, when marrow is negative for MRD by molecular or cytofluorometric techniques. Options include the following:

a. Fludarabine 30 mg/m^2 IV on days 1 to 3 and **cyclophosphamide** 250 mg/m^2 IV on days 1 to 3 (both given as separate 30-minute infusions); cycle repeated every 28 days, up to six cycles, depending on response. As first-line treatment in a phase III trial of younger (<66 years) CLL patients, this combination gave 24% CR versus 7% CR for fludarabine alone.

b. Fludarabine 25 mg/m^2 IV on days 1 to 3; **cyclophosphamide** 200 mg/m^2 IV on days 1 to 3; and **mitoxantrone** 6 mg/m^2 IV on day 1; given every 4 weeks for up to six cycles. In a small phase 2 study of relapsed and refractory CLL, CR was 50% (including 17% MRD-negative) and PR 28%.

c. Fludarabine 25 mg/m^2 IV on days 1 to 5 of each cycle plus **rituximab** 375 mg/m^2 IV on days 1 and 4 of cycle one, and on day 1 only of cycles two to six; repeat every 28 days for six cycles, followed by consolidation (after 2-month observation interval) with rituximab 375 mg/m^2 IV once weekly × 4. In a recent phase 2 study of treatment-naive patients, this concurrent schedule gave 47% CR versus 28% CR in patients treated sequentially (rituximab given only after completion of the fludarabine).

d. Fludarabine 25 mg/m^2 IV on days 2 to 4 and **cyclophosphamide** 250 mg/m^2 IV on days 2 to 4, plus **Rituximab** 375 mg/m^2 IV on day 1, in cycle one. In subsequent cycles (every 28 days), rituximab dose is

500 mg/m^2 on day 1, with fludarabine 25 mg/m^2 on days 1 to 3 and cyclophosphamide 250 mg/m^2 on days 1 to 3. In previously untreated CLL, this combination has been reported to produce CR in 70%, nodular PR in 10%, and PR in 15% of patients. In previously treated patients, CR was 25%, nodular PR was 16%, and PR was 32%. A significant percentage of patients in CR have no MRD detectable by molecular techniques. The impact of these responses on OS is unknown as yet.

e. **Fludarabine** plus **alemtuzumab.** Cycle 1: after dose escalation of alemtuzumab to 30 mg (see Section II.D.4.b), fludarabine 30 mg/m^2 IV over 15 to 30 minutes on days 1 to 3, plus alemtuzumab 30 mg IV over 2 hours on days 1 to 3. Subsequent cycles (every 28 days, up to a total of 6, as tolerated): fludarabine 30 mg/m^2 on days 1 to 3, plus alemtuzumab 30 mg over 4 hours on day 1 (no preceding lead-in escalation), then 30 mg over 2 hours on days 2 and 3. In a phase 2 study of 36 relapsed or refractory subjects, CR rate was 30% and PR was 53%, with acceptable toxicity.

f. Pentostatin 2 mg/m^2, cyclophosphamide 600 mg/m^2 and rituximab 375 mg/m^2 each given once every 21 days for 6 cycles (except cycle 1 when rituximab is given at 100 mg/m^2 day 1 and 375 mg/m^2 on days 3 and 5 of the first week of therapy) has yielded 91% response rate with 41% complete responses.

6. **Transplantation.** The role of SCT for CLL is in a state of flux. There is suggestive evidence that a significant fraction of patients may be cured following allo-SCT, since survival plateaus can be seen in various series, but transplant-related mortality, mostly due to graft-versus-host disease, has been in the 25% to 50% range. Graft-versus-leukemia effect is important in achieving CR, and detection of MRD after transplant does not necessarily predict for clinical relapse. Nonmyeloablative SCT allows for allografting at more advanced age and with low transplant-related mortality, and currently seems preferable to myeloablative regimens, especially if there are multiple comorbidities. Autologous SCT appears feasible even in patients older than 70 years and achieves approximately 80% CR, with 40% to 70% OS at 4 years, but relapse rate is high and there is no plateau in the survival curve, suggesting that cure is not achievable with current techniques. Improved purging methods to remove CLL cells contaminating the harvested stem cells may be helpful, but the absence of graft-versus-leukemia effect will likely remain an obstacle to long-term success for autografting.

7. **Radiation therapy.** For patients with refractory cytopenias or abdominal symptoms attributable to massive splenomegaly, low-dose radiation (e.g., 10 Gy delivered in multiple fractions) provides improvement in most patients, though sometimes with significant worsening of cytopenias because of poorly understood remote suppression of bone marrow. Median duration of responses has been reported as 12 months. Radiation is also occasionally indicated for

bulky lymphadenopathy with compression of veins, nerve roots, ureters, and so on.

8. Splenectomy. On rare occasions, splenectomy is indicated for relief of cytopenias or abdominal symptoms. Operative mortality historically has been approximately 10%, but may be lower with laparoscopic techniques. Response is unpredictable, but significant improvement in platelet count is seen in most patients.

9. New therapies. Lenolidomide 25 mg daily has been reported to result in clinical response in over half of treated patients with relapsed or refractory CLL.

E. Complications

1. Autoimmune syndromes. Despite hypogammaglobulinemia and a poor antibody response to vaccines, approximately 15% of CLL patients develop autoimmune hemolytic anemia, and an equal number have a positive Coombs test without overt hemolysis. The antibodies are typically polyclonal immunoglobulin G (IgG), of indeterminate specificity. Hemolytic anemia is an indication for chemotherapy of the CLL, regardless of stage. Alkylating agents are considered preferable to fludarabine, and steroids are routinely given (e.g., prednisone 1 mg/kg PO daily initially). Recent reports indicate a role for rituximab as well. The following combination seems reasonable:

- **Rituximab** 375 mg/m^2 on day 1, *and* **Cyclophosphamide** 750 to 1,000 mg/m^2 IV on day 2, *and* **Dexamethasone** 12 mg IV on days 1 and 2, and then 12 mg PO on days 3 to 7; repeat monthly.

Antibody-mediated thrombopenia occurs in approximately 2% of CLL patients. Steroids and alkylating agent are recommended, with or without rituximab. Pure red cell aplasia is another autoimmune entity occasionally seen in CLL. Steroids and cyclosporine are recommended.

2. Infections. Hypogammaglobulinemia contributes to recurrent infections in CLL, typically with streptococci, staphylococci, and other pyogenic organisms. In patients further immunosuppressed by chemotherapy, organisms such as fungi, Pneumocystis, Listeria, Mycobacteria, and CMV can pose formidable problems. Replacement therapy with pooled γ globulin has been controversial, in part due to expense, but its use seems justifiable in patients who have had recurrent and/or life-threatening infections. The dose is as follows:

- γ **Globulin** 400 mg/kg IV every 3 to 4 weeks; lower doses of 200 to 250 mg/kg every 4 weeks may also provide protection at more acceptable costs.

Immunizations utilizing dead vaccines (e.g., antipneumococcal vaccine) are appropriate but usually elicit poor antibody responses.

3. Transformations. Unlike CML, CLL only rarely evolves to acute leukemia. Instead, up to 10% of CLL patients develop an aggressive large cell lymphoma or immunoblastic lymphoma, arising either *de novo* or from the original CLL clone. This is referred to as *Richter's syndrome*. Onset of fever and other systemic symptoms, rising LDH, and localized enlargement of lymph nodes often herald this ominous situation. Node biopsy is usually required to confirm the diagnosis. Chemotherapy utilizing regimens for intermediate- or high-grade lymphoma is appropriate but usually of marginal benefit. Median survival is approximately 5 months following recognition of Richter's syndrome.

Another 10% of CLL cases evolve into the picture of prolymphocytic leukemia, showing larger, less mature lymphocytes with a prominent nucleolus. Chemotherapy is generally unsatisfactory, with reported median survival of 9 months. Distinction must be made between (a) CLL undergoing prolymphocytic transformation and (b) de novo prolymphocytic leukemia, a heterogeneous group of B-cell and T-cell neoplasms showing characteristic immunophenotypes on flow cytometry. By convention, diagnosis of de novo prolymphocytic leukemia requires more than 55% prolymphocytes. These patients respond poorly to chemotherapy, although some success is seen with nucleosides or with CHOP as used in non–Hodgkin's lymphoma. Alemtuzumab shows promising response rates in T-cell prolymphocytic leukemia.

III. Hairy cell leukemia (HCL). HCL is an uncommon B-cell neoplasm characterized by mononuclear cells with villiform cytoplasmic projections, usually visible in peripheral blood smears and in marrow aspirates, though increased marrow reticulin often results in a "dry tap." There is a strong male predominance; median age at presentation is in the sixth decade.

A. Diagnosis. Pancytopenia is present in approximately 50% of patients and cytopenia of at least one element in virtually all. Neutropenia and monocytopenia can be profound, leading to recurrent infections by a wide variety of organisms including Mycobacteria and fungi. Splenomegaly is present in 90% of patients and may be massive; palpable lymphadenopathy is uncommon.

Characteristic morphology and flow cytometry pattern (monoclonality for κ/λ light chains; positivity for CD11c, CD20, CD22, CD25, and CD103), plus strong positivity for tartrate-resistant acid phosphatase (TRAP), establish the diagnosis and distinguish HCL from the similar entity of splenic lymphoma with villous lymphocytes, and from B-cell prolymphocytic leukemia. A "variant" form of HCL may also cause confusion. This presents with cells that are negative for CD25 and CD103, negative or weakly positive for TRAP, and have prominent nucleoli; this variant group responds less well to treatment.

B. Therapy. Some patients remain asymptomatic and do not initially require treatment. Indications for initiating chemotherapy include marked cytopenias, recurrent infections, symptomatic splenomegaly, or other systemic complications.

1. Splenectomy will reverse cytopenias but is reserved for urgent situations such as uncontrolled infection, severe refractory cytopenias, and unresponsive splenic pain.

2. Interferon α (IFN-α) produces a response in the majority of patients, but CRs are uncommon, response is slow, and relapse is frequent. IFN-α is largely superseded by purine analogs.

3. Cladribine is a nucleoside or purine analog, currently considered the treatment of choice, with 75% to 90% CR following one cycle of treatment. However, MRD can be detected in 25% to 50% of patients in CR, and relapse rate is approximately 35%. Median time to relapse for all responders (PRs and CRs) was 42 months in a recent Scripps Clinic follow-up. Retreatment with cladribine gives approximately 60% second CR. OS at 10 years is approximately 90%. It is not yet clear if permanent cure is achieved. Standard dosage is as follows:

- **A single cycle of cladribine** 0.1 mg/kg/day as continuous IV infusion over 7 days. Alternatively, a 5-day regimen may be used:
- **Cladribine** 0.12 to 0.14 mg/kg (~5 mg/m^2) IV as a 2-hour IV infusion days 1 to 5.

Cytokine fever and worsening of cytopenias may accompany treatment. Prolonged immunosuppression is to be expected, and CD4 T-cells remain low over many months.

4. Pentostatin is also a nucleoside analog with response rates comparable to cladribine, but multiple cycles are required to reach CR. Cytopenias, fever, and immunosuppression are major side effects. Recommended dose is as follows:

- **Pentostatin** 4 mg/m^2 by IV bolus every 2 weeks until CR (median eight courses required).

5. Rituximab. Hairy cells strongly express CD20, and respectable response rates are reported in both relapsing and previously untreated HCL. Four to eight infusions of rituximab 375 mg/m^2 weekly have been utilized. CRs with a strikingly high percentage of negative MRD have recently been reported in a small series of HCL patients (most previously untreated) who received cladribine followed by rituximab. It is not yet clear how this impacts survival.

6. BL-22 is a recombinant immunotoxin containing an anti-CD22 immunoglobulin variable domain fused to truncated pseudomonas exotoxin. Both classic and variant HCL cells are CD22$^+$. An NCI study of cladribine-resistant patients had a 69% CR. This is available through the NCI for compassionate use.

7. Relapsed disease. There is no absolute paradigm, and second-line treatment must be individualized. In purine analog-sensitive disease, retreatment with cladribine or pentostatin can still be very effective. Primary or consolidation use of rituximab would be a strong consideration. In cladribine-resistant disease, the BL-22 immunotoxin would be the best option.

SUGGESTED READINGS

Chronic Myelogenous Leukemia

Deininger MW. Chronic myeloid leukemia—management of early stage disease. *Hematology (American Society of Hematology Education Program)* 2005:174–182.

Goldman JM, Hughes T, Radich J, et al. Continuing reduction in level of residual disease after 4 years in patients with CML in chronic phase responding to first-line imatinib in the IRIS study. *Blood* 2005;106:163a.

Goldman JM, Melo JV. Chronic myeloid leukemia—advances in biology and new approaches to treatment. *N Engl J Med* 2003;349: 1451–1464.

Gratwohl A, Hermans J, Goldman JM, et al. Risk assessment for patients with chronic myeloid leukaemia before allogeneic blood or marrow transplantation. Chronic leukemia working party of the European group for blood and marrow transplantation. *Lancet* 1998;352:1087–1092.

Hughes TP, Kaeda J, Branford S, et al. Frequency of major molecular responses to imatinib or interferon alfa plus cytarabine in newly diagnosed chronic myeloid leukemia. *N Engl J Med* 2003;349: 1423–1432.

Shah NP. Chronic myeloid leukemia—loss of response to imatinib: mechanisms and management. *Hematology (American Society of Hematology Education Program)* 2005:183–187.

Talpaz M, Silver RT, Druker BJ, et al. Imatinib induces durable hematologic and cytogenetic responses in patients with accelerated phase chronic myeloid leukemia: results of a phase II study. *Blood* 2002;99:1928–1937.

Chronic Lymphocytic Leukemia and Hairy Cell Leukemia

Byrd JC, Rai K, Peterson BL, et al. Addition of rituximab to fludarabine may prolong progression-free survival and overall survival in patients with previously untreated chronic lymphocytic leukemia. *Blood* 2005;105:49–53.

Chadha P, Rademaker AW, Mediratta P, et al. Treatment of hairy cell leukemia with 2-chlorodeoxyadenosine (2-CdA): long-term follow-up of the Northwestern University experience. *Blood* 2005;106: 241–246.

Cheson BD, Bennett J, Grever M, et al. National Cancer Institute Sponsored Working Group guidelines for chronic lymphocytic leukemia: revised guidelines for diagnosis and treatment. *Blood* 1996;87:4990–4997.

Eichhorst BF, Busch R, Hopfinger G, et al. Fludarabine plus cyclophosphamide versus fludarabine alone in first-line therapy of younger patients with chronic lymphocytic leukemia. *Blood* 2006; 107:885–891.

Keating MJ, Flinn I, Jain V, et al. Therapeutic role of alemtuzumab (Campath-1H) in patients who have failed fludarabine: results of a large international study. *Blood* 2002;99:3554–3561.

Keating MJ, O'Brien S, Albitar M, et al. Early results of a chemoimmunotherapy regimen of fludarabine, cyclophosphamide, and rituximab as initial therapy for chronic lymphocytic leukemia. *J Clin Oncol* 2005;23:4079–4088.

Rai KR, Peterson BL, Appelbaum FR, et al. Fludarabine compared with chlorambucil as primary therapy for chronic lymphocytic leukemia. *N Engl J Med* 2000;343:1750–1757.

CHAPTER 21

Myeloproliferative Diseases and Myelodysplastic Syndromes

Peter White and Paul R. Walker

I. Myeloproliferative diseases. The myeloproliferative diseases (MPDs) are clonal disorders of pluripotent hematopoietic stem cells or of lineage-committed progenitor cells. MPDs are characterized by autonomous and sustained overproduction of morphologically and functionally mature granulocytes, erythrocytes, or platelets. Although one cellular element is most strikingly increased, it is not uncommon to have modest or even major elevations in other myeloid elements (e.g., thrombocytosis and leukocytosis in polycythemia vera [P. vera]). Bone marrow aspirates and biopsy specimens typically show hyperplasia of all myeloid lineages (panmyelosis). Morphologic maturation and cellular function are essentially normal, although platelet dysfunction occasionally contributes to bleeding. The overproduction of blood elements in the MPDs now appears related to "switched-on" tyrosine kinase signaling pathways. For chronic myelogenous leukemia (discussed in Chapter 20), this arises from the t(9;22) translocation and the BCR-ABL gene product. For the MPDs discussed in this chapter, a single nucleotide mutation in the gene for JAK2, a tyrosine kinase normally activated by erythropoietin and other cytokines, plays an analogous role. JAK2 V617F is present in 74% to 97% of P. vera patients, and in 30% to 50% of patients with essential thrombocythemia (ET) and idiopathic myelofibrosis (IMF). Positivity for JAK2 V617F gives important diagnostic confirmation for MPD, though negative results do not exclude MPD.

    A. Polycythemia vera (P. vera)

        1. Diagnosis. P. vera must be distinguished from relative or spurious polycythemia (normal red blood cell [RBC] mass, decreased plasma volume) and from secondary erythrocytosis (increased RBC mass due to hypoxia, carboxyhemoglobinemia, inappropriate erythropoietin syndromes with tumors or renal disease, etc.).

        Proper formulation of major and minor criteria to establish the diagnosis of P. vera is a topic of some discussion at present. Proposed modifications of the original criteria of the Polycythemia Vera Study Group incorporate the following elements:

        A1. Increased RBC mass: more than 125% of predicted normal by direct measurement of blood volume; or by inference if hematocrit is more than 60% for men or more than 56% for women, or if multiple phlebotomies are required to lower hematocrit to normal range

        A2. Normal arterial O_2 saturation ($\geq$92%)

        A3. Splenomegaly

A4. Abnormal karyotype (other than t9;22), JAK2 V617F, or other clonality marker

B1. Thrombocytosis more than 400,000/µL

B2. Neutrophilic leukocytosis more than 10,000/µL

B3. Hypercellular bone marrow with panmyelosis

B4. Subnormal serum erythropoietin level and/or no rise following phlebotomy

B5. Spontaneous growth of erythroid colonies *in vitro* in the absence of erythropoietin (test is expensive and not widely available)

A1 + A2 + either A3 or A4 establishes diagnosis of P. vera

A1 + A2 + two or more B criteria establishes diagnosis of P. vera

An erythropoietin level in the low normal range showing no rise after phlebotomy is consistent with P. vera. An elevated erythropoietin level at presentation is strong evidence against P. vera. Splenomegaly is present in 70% of P. vera cases, but borderline enlargement on ultrasound is of questionable significance. Panmyelosis (hyperplasia of all nonlymphoid marrow elements) is present in 80% of cases but may be difficult to quantify; clusters of megakaryocytes strengthen the case for P. vera (or other MPD). Marrow karyotype is abnormal in 10% to 20% of patients at diagnosis; iron stores are typically absent.

2. Aims of therapy. Thrombosis (stroke, myocardial infarct, and deep venous thrombosis [DVT]) is a major cause of morbidity in P. vera, due to increased blood viscosity and other factors. Lowering the hematocrit to 40% to 45% by phlebotomy reduces the risk of thrombosis; concomitant use of phlebotomy and hydroxyurea or other myelosuppressive agents may be advisable, particularly if platelet counts are markedly elevated. It is especially important to maintain good long-term control of hematocrit and platelets in the elderly and in those with a history of thrombosis. Control of hypertension and diabetes, and avoidance of smoking are also important.

3. Treatment regimens

a. Phlebotomy. Removal of 350 to 500 mL of blood every 2 to 4 days (less often in the elderly or in patients with cardiac disease) is the standard initial approach; goal is to lower hematocrit to 40% to 45%. The blood count is then checked monthly, and phlebotomy is repeated as needed to maintain the hematocrit at less than or equal to 45%. Rapid lowering of the hematocrit may also be achieved in emergency situations by erythroapheresis. Elective surgery should be deferred until the hematocrit has been stable at less than or equal to 45% for 2 to 4 months. Platelet function should be evaluated before surgery or invasive procedures.

b. Antithrombotic therapy. Concomitantly with phlebotomy, use of low-dose aspirin is now widely regarded as standard therapy, following a large European study, the ECLAP (European collaboration on low-dose aspirin in polycythemia) trial that showed approximately 60% reduction in thrombotic events utilizing 100 mg ASA daily. Higher doses of aspirin (325 mg daily) carry risk of bleeding, especially in patients with platelet counts more than $1.5 \times 10^6/\mu$L, in whom acquired von Wille-brand's disease may be seen. The exact thrombogenic role of platelets in MPDs is not clear, but hydroxyurea and anagrelide have been shown to lower platelet counts and reduce the risk of thrombosis.

c. Myelosuppressive agents. Myelosuppressive agents are indicated in conjunction with phlebotomy for persistent thrombocytosis, recurrent thrombosis, enlarging spleen, or similar problems. They may also reduce the risk of progression to myelofibrosis as compared with phlebotomy alone. Most alkylating agents carry a high risk of producing myelodysplastic syndrome (MDS) or leukemia and should no longer be used. Currently recommended choices are as follows:

(1) Hydroxyurea 10 to 30 mg/kg PO daily. Weekly blood cell counts are required initially, with dose adjustments to maintain the hematocrit at less than or equal to 45%, the platelet count at 100,000 to $500,000/\mu$L, and the white blood cell (WBC) count at more than $3,000/\mu$L. Side effects are usually minimal, but long-term use may cause painful leg ulcers and aphthous stomatitis. The risk of leukemia may be slightly increased as well. For younger patients and cases difficult to control with hydroxyurea, acceptable alternatives include the following:

(2) Interferon α is usually effective in controlling hematocrit, platelet count, and splenomegaly and in relieving pruritus. The starting dose is 1 to 3×10^6 U/m^2 three times weekly (pegylated interferon once weekly may also be an option – see Section I.B.2.c.). Common side effects include myalgia, fever, and asthenia, usually controlled with acetaminophen. Leukemogenic effects are presumably absent, but high cost is a deterrent to long-term use.

(3) Radioactive phosphorus (^{32}P) 2.3 mCi/m^2 IV (5 mCi maximum single dose). Repeat in 12 weeks if the response is inadequate (25% dose escalation optional). Lack of response after three doses mandates a switch to other forms of therapy. Use of ^{32}P entails approximately 10% risk of leukemia by 10 years, and it is best reserved for the elderly and patients refractory to other modalities. Supplemental phlebotomies may be required for patients with satisfactory platelet and WBC counts but with rising hematocrit levels.

(4) Busulfan appears to have less leukemogenic potential than other alkylating agents and is appropriate in patients whose disease is not controlled by other treatments or in the elderly. It is best given in short courses over several weeks (to avoid prolonged marrow suppression) at 2 to 4 mg/day.

(5) Anagrelide selectively inhibits platelet production, and platelets start to fall in 7 to 14 days. The WBC count is unaffected; hemoglobin may fall slightly. Responses to anagrelide have been reported in more than 80% of patients with all MPDs, and thrombotic risk is reduced. Recommended starting dose is 0.5 mg PO q.i.d. Average dose for control is 2.4 mg daily. Side effects include headache (44%), palpitations, diarrhea, asthenia, and fluid retention. It should be used with caution in cardiac patients and is contraindicated in pregnancy.

d. Ancillary treatments. To control **hyperuricemia**, allopurinol 300 mg/day is usually effective. **Pruritus** is a frequent problem, but usually abates with myelo-suppressive therapy. Cyproheptadine 5 to 20 mg/day or paroxetine 20 mg/day may be helpful; interferon α is also frequently effective. Aspirin is often helpful for **erythromelalgia** (hot, red, painful digits) and is commonly used to prevent thrombosis.

4. Evolution and outcome. The median survival time for patients with P. vera is approximately 10 years. One third of deaths is caused by thrombosis. The risk of leukemia is low (~1.5%) in patients treated by phlebotomy alone. Many patients progress to a "spent phase," with increasing splenomegaly and stable or falling hematocrit, or develop postpolycythemic myelofibrosis. The risk of leukemia is markedly elevated in such patients.

B. Essential thrombocythemia (ET)

1. Diagnosis. Diagnosis of ET requires a persistent elevation of the platelet count above 600,000/μL plus the absence of known causes of reactive or secondary thrombocytosis (e.g., iron deficiency, malignancy, chronic inflammatory disease). To exclude other MPDs, hematocrit and RBC mass should be normal, myelofibrosis absent and t(9;22) absent. Marrow aspiration and biopsy should be performed to assess hyperplasia of megakaryocytes, evaluate iron stores and fibrosis, and exclude MDS, in particular 5q- syndrome. Overall cellularity is clearly increased in approximately 70% of patients, and marked megakaryocytic hyperplasia is seen in 65%. Abnormal karyotype is found in less than 10% of patients. Approximately 50% have the JAK2 V617F mutation, and these patients may closely resemble P. vera clinically. Moderate leukocytosis is common. Palpable splenomegaly is present in less than 50% of patients. Platelet function studies may show either spontaneous aggregation or impaired response to agonists. Microvascular occlusion may cause digital gangrene, transient ischemic attacks, visual complaints, and paresthesias. Large-artery thrombotic episodes are also common. DVT is uncommon. The risk of hemorrhagic problems is significant, particularly with platelet count more than $1.5 \times 10^6/\mu L$.

2. Treatment regimens. Observation alone or low-dose ASA is considered a reasonable course in younger, symptom-free patients with less than 1×10^6 platelets/μL. Therapy to lower platelet count to less than $400 \times 10^3/\mu L$ should be undertaken in the elderly and in patients otherwise at increased risk for hemorrhagic or thrombotic complications. Options include the following:

a. Hydroxyurea 10 to 30 mg/kg PO daily, with dosage adjustments on the basis of weekly blood counts, should give satisfactory response in 2 to 6 weeks. Its use in combination with low-dose ASA may give optimal protection against arterial thrombosis and evolution to myelofibrosis. Possible teratogenic and leukemogenic effects should be kept in mind.

b. Anagrelide (see Section I.A.3.c.5) can be a reasonable alternative to hydroxyurea, and is perhaps preferable in younger patients. Anagrelide plus ASA was inferior to hydroxyurea plus ASA in a large recent trial, however. This agent should not be used in pregnancy.

c. Interferon α. Most ET patients respond to this agent, at an initial dose of 3×10^6 U/day SC. Maintenance doses of 3×10^6 U three times weekly usually suffice. Pegylated interferon at an initial dose of 1.5 to 4.5 μg/kg/week SC seems comparable in efficacy and side effects. Use of interferon in pregnancy is considered safe. As noted in Section I.A.3.c.2, side effects and expense are potential problems. Effectiveness in reducing thrombosis is uncertain.

d. Platelet apheresis. Platelet apheresis may be indicated in emergent situations (e.g., cerebral ischemia), but the effect is usually short-lived.

e. ^{32}P and alkylating agents. These agents are effective but carry increased risk of secondary leukemia. Nitrogen mustard (mechlorethamine 0.15 to 0.3 mg/kg [6 to 12 mg/m^2] IV) can be helpful when rapid reduction in platelet count is needed. Busulfan 2 to 4 mg/day initial dose is appropriate in selected elderly patients resistant to other agents.

f. Aspirin (ASA) 81 to 325 mg/day may control erythromelalgia and similar vaso-occlusive problems but is contraindicated in patients with a history of hemorrhagic symptoms, and with platelet counts more than $1 \times 10^6/\mu L$. ASA may be useful in pregnant patients in whom the preceding agents are contraindicated. Its routine use in ET is a matter of debate.

g. Stem cell transplantation (SCT). Experience with this modality is quite limited, but transplant may be a consideration in a young patient with poor control and major complications.

3. Evolution and outcome. The course of essential thrombocythemia is often indolent, particularly in young patients. The median survival exceeds 10 years, and some patients appear to have normal life expectancy. Transformation to myelofibrosis, MDS, or acute leukemia occurs in 5 to 10%. Thrombosis is the major cause of ET-related death.

C. Idiopathic myelofibrosis (IMF) also called *agnogenic myeloid metaplasia*

1. Diagnosis. This is a clonal disorder of the hematopoietic stem cell, marked by an intense reactive (nonclonal) fibrosis of the marrow; splenomegaly (frequently massive), reflecting ectopic hematopoiesis in the spleen and portal hypertension; and the presence of immature granulocytes and nucleated RBCs in the peripheral blood (leukoerythroblastic blood picture) plus teardrop RBCs and giant platelets. Mild to moderate elevations of WBC and platelet counts are common initially; cytopenias dominate later on. JAK2 V617F mutation is present in approximately 50% of IMF patients. An abnormal karyotype is also demonstrable in approximately 50%, and connotes shortened survival time. Other adverse prognostic factors include advanced age, anemia, WBC less than 4,000/µL or more than 30,000/µL, thrombocytopenia, blasts in peripheral blood, and hypercatabolic symptoms (weight loss, night sweats, fever). Major causes of death in IMF include marrow failure, infection, portal hypertension, and leukemic transformation. Diseases causing secondary marrow fibrosis, such as metastatic carcinoma, hairy cell leukemia, and granulomatous infections, must be excluded. Cases of MDS with marrow fibrosis are easily confused with IMF. Post-polycythemic myelofibrosis is clinically indistinguishable but carries a poor prognosis, evolving into acute leukemia in 25 to 50% of patients (as compared to 5%–20% for *de novo* IMF). Acute megakaryoblastic leukemia (M7) may also present with a myelofibrotic picture and be confused with IMF.

2. Treatment regimens. The median survival time is 5 years, but symptom-free patients may do well without treatment for a number of years. Intervention is indicated in the following situations:

    a. Anemia. Androgens (e.g., testosterone enanthate 600 mg IM weekly or fluoxymesterone 10 mg PO b.i.d. or t.i.d. for men; danazol 400 to 600 mg PO daily for women) are recommended and they reduce transfusion requirements in 30 to 50% of patients. Corticosteroids (e.g., prednisone 40 mg/m² PO daily) should be tried if overt hemolysis is present. Erythropoietin is helpful in a small percentage of patients but requires large doses; response is unlikely if serum erythropoietin level is more than 200 mU/mL. In limited studies, improvement in cytopenias or transfusion requirements has been reported in 20 to 50% of IMF patients receiving low-dose thalidomide (50 mg/day) or lenalidomide (5–10 mg/day).

    IMF patients routinely become transfusion-dependent; early institution of iron-chelating agents is advisable (see discussion under Section II.D.8.).

    b. Splenomegaly. Massive splenomegaly may lead to cytopenias, portal hypertension, variceal bleeding, abdominal pain, or compression of adjacent organs. Anorexia, fatigue, and hypercatabolic complaints may be prominent. First option for control by myelosuppressive therapy is hydroxyurea, given as for P. vera (see Section I.A.3.c). Melphalan (2.5 mg PO three times weekly, with escalations up to 2.5 mg daily as tolerated), and busulfan (2 mg/day in older patients) can also be considered. Interferon α produces responses in some cases, but its role is not clearly established in IMF.

    Radiation, 50 to 200 cGy, is effective in improving splenomegaly but causes cytopenias in 40% of patients. Radiation is occasionally indicated for extramedullary hematopoietic tumors causing compression syndromes or for bone pain. Splenectomy is indicated in carefully selected cases but carries significant perioperative mortality and morbidity from bleeding, sepsis, and postoperative thrombocytosis. Splenectomy may also increase the risk of blast transformation.

c. Curative intent. Myeloablative allogeneic marrow or stem cell transplantation (SCT) from appropriately matched donors appears to be potentially curative, but transplant-related mortality is high in IMF patients older than 45 years. Younger patients with an expected survival of less than or equal to 5 years may be reasonable candidates. Engraftment rates are equal to those in other hematologic disorders, and "graft vs myelofibrosis" effect has been demonstrated. Encouraging early results with nonmyeloablative SCT suggest that this modality may be the most appropriate option, and that it is feasible in older IMF patients.

II. Myelodysplastic syndromes (MDS). This is a diverse group of hematopoietic stem cell clonal neoplasms that is characterized by ineffective hematopoiesis and dysplastic morphologic changes in one or more lineages. The disease has a median age of 65 to 70 years, is the most frequent hematologic malignancy in the over-65 age-group, and affects 20,000 to 30,000 cases annually in the United States. For the population over 60 years of age, the incidence is 1 in 500. Eighty percent of cases occur *de novo* and have no specific etiology or known cause. In the remaining 20% of cases, an association with prior chemotherapy use can be identified, most frequently high-dose alkylator or topoisomerase-II inhibitor-based regimens, or exposure to radiation. Whether a specific inciting cause can be identified or not, the pathophysiologic process of MDS is deoxyribonucleic acid (DNA) damage in a pluripotential bone marrow stem cell with a dynamic balance of secondary and associated changes in proliferation, differentiation, and apoptosis intrinsic cellular pathways along with extrinsic marrow microenvironment, angiogenic, cytokine, and immune effects. Clonal cytogenetic abnormalities can be identified in 40% to 50% of de novo cases, most typically a loss of chromosome material involving chromosomes 5, 7, 11, 20, or Y; or trisomy of chromosome 8. Cytogenetic abnormalities in chromosomes 5 or 7 will be identifiable in 95% of therapy-related cases, with one half also having complex cytogenetic changes involving three or more chromosomes.

A. Diagnosis. The typical clinical picture is of an elderly patient with macrocytic anemia, with or without thrombopenia and neutropenia. Initial diagnostic studies needed are complete blood count (CBC) with differential and peripheral smear review, bone marrow aspirate and biopsy with cytogenetics, reticulocyte count, serum erythropoietin level before transfusion, serum iron-TIBC-ferritin, B12 and folate levels, along with human immunodeficiency virus (HIV) status if there is clinical concern, and human leukocyte antigen (HLA) typing in young patients if the patient is a candidate for transplant or aggressive immunosuppressive therapy. There is no single diagnostic test, however. A confirmed diagnosis is made from the hematologic picture of cytopenias and dysplastic lineage morphology supported by associated marrow cytogenetic findings, if abnormal. The typical dysplastic features seen in the marrow and peripheral blood include megaloblastoid precursors, budding and irregular nuclear outline of normoblasts, hypochromia and basophilic stippling of RBCs, iron-laden sideroblasts, hyposegmentation (bilobed Pelger-Huet–like forms are characteristic) and hypogranularity of neutrophils, hypolobar and/or micromegakaryocytes, and hypogranular platelets. Platelet and neutrophil functional abnormalities exist, further contributing to the symptomatic cytopenias. The bone marrow is most often hypercellular (but 10%–20% will be hypocellular) with a low reticulocyte count. Abnormal localization of immature precursors (ALIP) is often seen on the marrow core biopsy. A variable number of myeloblasts will be seen from less than 5% up to 20%. Differential diagnosis includes B_{12} and folate deficiency, lead poisoning, and alcohol abuse in patients with sideroblastic anemia, aplastic anemia in patients with hypoplastic marrows, IMF (ideopathic myelofibrosis or agnogenic myeloid metaplasia) if marrow fibrosis is present, and paroxysmal nocturnal hemoglobinuria (PNH).

B. Classification. The French-American-British (FAB) classification for MDS put forth in 1982 continues to be useful (Table 21.1). More recently the World Health Organization (WHO) modified this classification to better correlate with more homogeneous subsets and natural histories (Table 21.2). The major changes (1) lowered the percentage of marrow blasts to

Table 21.1. Myelodysplastic Syndrome subtypes: French-American-British classification

FAB Subtype	% Marrow Blasts	% Peripheral Blood Blasts	Other Findings	Median Survival (months)
Refractory anemia (RA)	<5	≤1	—	43
Refractory anemia with ring sideroblasts (RARS)	<5	≤1	≥15% ring sideroblasts	73
Refractory anemia with excess blasts (RAEB)	5–20	<5	—	12
Refractory anemia with excess blasts in transformation (RAEB-t)[a]	20–30 *or*	≥5 *or*	Presence of Auer rods	5
Chronic myelomonocytic leukemia (CMML)	≤20	<5	Monocytes >1,000/μL	20

[a] In a subsequent revised scheme, RAEB-t cases are reclassified as acute leukemia.

**Table 21.2. World Health Organization classification
of myelodysplastic syndrome and pertinent features**

Subtype	Blood Findings	Bone Marrow Findings
RA	Anemia; no blasts	Erythroid dysplasia only; <5% blasts
RARS	Anemia; no blasts	RA + 15% or greater ringed sideroblasts
RCMD	Bi- or pancytopenia; no blasts	Dysplasia in >10% cells in two or more lineages
RCMD-RS	RCMD	RCMD + 15% or greater ringed sideroblasts
RAEB		Uni- or multilineage dysplasia plus
RAEB-1	No Auer rods and <5% blasts;	No Auer rods and 5–9% blasts
RAEB-2	Auer rods or 5–19% blasts	Auer rods or 10–19% blasts
MDS-U	Cytopenias; no blasts	Unilineage dysplasia in granulocytes or megakaryocytes; <5% blasts
MDS with isolated del(5q-)	Anemia; <5% blasts	Normal to increased megakaryocytes

RA, refractory anemia; RARS, refractory anemia with ringed sideroblasts; RCMD, refractory cytopenia with multilineage dysplasia; RCMD-RS, refractory cytopenia with multilineage dysplasia and increased ringed sideroblasts; RAEB, refractory anemia with excess blasts; MDS-U, myelodysplastic syndrome, unclassified.

define full blown acute myelogenous leukemia at less than or equal to 20%, removing refractory anemia with excess blasts in transformation (RAEB-t) as a category; (2) separated out the 5q- syndrome, given its different clinical picture and treatment; and (3) moved chronic myelomonocytic leukemia to a separate category of myelodysplastic/myeloproliferative disease.

C. Prognosis. Acute leukemia transformation potential and survival correlate to some degree with both the FAB and WHO classifications, but even more so with the International Prognostic Scoring System (IPSS). The IPSS (Table 21.3) assigns a score based on the percentage of marrow blasts, initial marrow cytogenetics, and the number of peripheral cytopenias to provide a better prognostic risk stratification for an individual; the IPSS can be very helpful in guiding management decisions. Although not included in the IPSS, age of the patient is also of major prognostic impact (e.g., median survival for low-risk patients is 11.8 years for age less than 60 years vs. 3.9 years for age more than 70 years). The natural history is one of ultimate transformation to acute myeloblastic leukemia (AML) or progressive bone marrow failure fraught with refractory symptomatic cytopenia-related complications.

Table 21.3.   International Prognostic Scoring System (IPSS) for myelodysplastic syndrome

Prognostic Factor	Score Value				
	0	0.5	1.0	1.5	2.0
% Marrow blasts	<5	5–10	—	11–20	21–30
Karyotype[a]	Good	Intermediate	Poor	—	—
Cytopenias[b]	0–1	2–3	—	—	—

Risk category	Total score	Median survival (years)
Low	0	5.7
Intermediate-1	0.5–1.0	3.5
Intermediate-2	1.5–2.0	1.2
High	2.5	0.4

Note that the IPSS conforms to the French-American-British classification and includes refractory anemia with excess blasts in transformation patients who would be classified as acute myeloblastic leukemia under the WHO system.

[a] Good, normal karyotype, −Y, 5q−, or 20q−. Poor, chromosome 7 abnormal (monosomy, 7q−, etc.); or complex (three separate abnormalities). Intermediate, all other abnormal karyotypes.

[b] Cytopenias defined by hemoglobin <10 g/dL, neutrophils <1,500/μL, and platelets <100,000/μL.

D. Therapy. The management of MDS is guided by the patient's age, IPSS category, serum erythropoietin level, cytogenetics if 5q- is present, and by assessing HLA status in a candidate for stem cell transplant or immunosuppressive therapy. All patients should receive appropriate blood product transfusion support.

   1. **General approach**
      a. **Low-risk patients** (IPSS low and intermediate-1):
      - If serum erythropoietin level is less than 500 mU/ml, treat with growth factors (erythropoietin analog, adding granulocyte colony-stimulating factor (G-CSF) if no hematocrit response)
      - Azacytidine, decitabine, or lenalidomide if no clinical response to growth factors

      b. **High-risk patients** (IPSS Intermediate-2 and higher):
      - If young and a donor available, allogeneic stem cell transplant
      - If not a transplant candidate, azacytidine, decitabine, or lenalidomide

      c. **5q- cytogenetics** Lenalidomide

      d. **HLA-DR 15 positive** (younger patients with a hypoplastic marrow):
      - ATG (antithymocyte globulin) or
      - Cyclosporine A

2. Growth factors. Erythropoietin analogs, either epoetin or darbepoetin, can effectively achieve a meaningful hemoglobin improvement in 15% to 25% of patients. In patients with a serum erythropoietin level less than 500 mU/mL, a trial of an erythropoietin analog is indicated. Low-risk patients do respond better than high-risk patients. Usually higher dosing than used in chemotherapy-associated anemias is needed. An adequate therapeutic trial of 8 to 12 weeks is appropriate. G-CSF can be synergistic with erythropoietin therapy, enhancing the erythroid response rate potential up to 40%. This synergism is particularly effective in patients with more than 15% ringed sideroblasts. These growth factors need to be continued to maintain the achieved benefit.

    a. Recombinant human erythropoietin 40,000 to 60,000 units SC 2 to 3 times weekly; taper to least effective dosing schedule if response, and continue, or darbepoetin 150 to 300 μg/kg SC weekly. If there is an inadequate or no response to the erythropoietin analog alone and if still indicated clinically, add G-CSF (granulocyte colony-stimulating factor)

    b. G-CSF (filgrastim) 1 to 2 μg/kg subcutaneously 2 to 3 times weekly, with the erythropoietin analog

3. Specific Agents

    a. Azacytidine is a hypomethylating agent inhibiting DNA methyltransferase reversing the epigenetic silencing of gene transcription. The exact mechanism of action in MDS is most likely multifactorial. In a landmark phase III trial compared azacytidine to supportive care only, azacytidine showed a 60% hematologic response rate, prolonged the time to leukemic transformation or death (21 vs. 13 months), and improved quality-of-life parameters. It is now approved by the U.S. Food and Drug Administration (FDA) for use in all types of MDS.

    • **Azacitidine 75 mg/m^2 SC daily for 7 days every 28 days** continuing treatment as long as a favorable benefit/tolerance balance. Increase to 100 mg/m^2/day can be considered if there is no response. The most common toxicity is myelosuppression with a 20% treatment-related infection rate. It is generally very well tolerated and can be administered as an outpatient.

    b. Decitabine (Dacogen) is another hypomethylating agent DNA methyltransferase inhibitor that has shown significant activity in MDS. Initial European phase II studies showed 50% hematologic response rates, notably even higher in IPSS high-risk patients. A landmark phase III trial that compared decitabine to supportive care confirmed significant response rates (17% complete response (CR) or partial response (PR) by International Working Group criteria, plus an additional 13% with hematologic improvement) and a longer time to acute leukemia transformation or death, in particular among those patients with an IPSS intermediate-2/high-risk score, or not previously treated. Overall survival was prolonged in patients responding to decitabine as compared to nonresponders (23.5 vs. 13.7 months). It is now approved by the FDA for use in MDS.

- **Decitabine 15 mg/m² as a 3-hour IV infusion every 8 hours for 3** consecutive days (9 total doses) every 6 weeks × 4 cycles; continue treatment as long as effective. Myelosuppression with cytopenic complications is an expected and frequent toxicity of decitabine, especially in the already cytopenic MDS patient. Other side effects include nausea, diarrhea, or constipation and cough. More convenient dosing schedules are being evaluated; the MD Anderson experience has reported overall clinical benefit in 76% of patients treated with a modified schedule of 20 mg/m² IV over 1 hour daily for 5 consecutive days every 4 weeks. It is not known if either DNA methyltransferase inhibitor is superior to the other.

   c. **Lenalidomide** is a thalidomide-related immunomodulator with greater potency. It has a wide range of biologic effects including suppression of angiogenesis, inhibition of inflammatory cytokines, potentiation of immune pathways, and other cellular ligand-induced responses. A landmark phase II study showed dramatic erythroid responses in erythropoietin-resistant patients. Major erythroid responses and cytogenetic responses occurred in 83% of patients with a 5q- deletion, but were not limited to this 5q- subset. Overall, 68% of patients with a low IPSS score, 50% with intermediate-1 IPSS, and over half of patients with normal cytogenetics, had erythroid responses. High-risk MDS patients had a much less frequent hematologic response (20%) but the refractory anemia with excess blasts (RAEB) patients responding also demonstrated decreased blast counts. It is approved by the FDA in patients with 5q- MDS.

- **Lenalidomide 10 mg orally daily** is continued so long as this dose is tolerated; the dose is reduced to a 21 out of 28-day schedule or 5-mg dosing if persistent or severe hematologic toxicity occurs. Marrow suppression with neutropenia and thrombocytopenia, the most frequent toxicity, is dose dependent and requires dose interruption in over half the number of patients. Other systemic side effects include low grade pruritus, diarrhea, rash, and fatigue.

   Thalidomide remains an option in treating MDS, but now with the availability of the more potent and potentially less toxic lenalidomide, it will likely find minimal use.

4. **Allogeneic stem cell transplantation.** This remains the only curative therapy but is limited to younger patients and preferably with a matched related donor. Treatment-related mortality and chronic morbidity remain very high. Given that the older age-group with MDS, less than 10% of patients are considered transplant candidates. It should always be considered in younger patients in IPSS high-risk or

intermediate-2-risk category with suitable sibling donors. Transplant studies show disease-free survival ranges from 29% to 40%, nonrelapse mortality of 37% to 50%, and relapse even with a sibling donor of 23% to 48%. Reduced-intensity conditioning transplants appear to carry promise for use in an older population but are still fraught with significantly high mortalities. The use of autologous SCT (high-dose chemotherapy with stem cell rescue) is limited to transformed or transforming acute leukemia.

5. Intensive chemotherapy. There is no clear consensus regarding the role of intensive chemotherapy in MDS. Its use is typically restricted to patients in IPSS intermediate- and high-risk groups. Induction chemotherapy utilizing acute leukemia–type regimens (e.g., **anthracycline/ cytosine arabinoside**) can induce CRs in 50% to 60% of MDS patients, but remissions tend to be brief and outcomes correlate strongly with karyotype associated chemoresistance mechanisms. **Topotecan**, a topoisomerase I inhibitor, has been postulated to have selectively favorable effectiveness in MDS, but its role is not well established as responses are brief and myelotoxicity is very high. The role of intensive chemotherapy in treating MDS is limited to overtly transformed acute leukemia or bridging selected patients to an allogeneic transplant. In hopes of minimizing toxicity, low-dose chemotherapy has been utilized, most notably with **cytarabine** at doses of 5 to 20 mg/m² daily, as a q12 hour SC injection, continued for 10 to 20 days. Hematologic responses are seen in 20% to 30% of patients, but without any significant survival benefit, and serious marrow suppression may result. **Melphalan** given at a dose of 2 mg PO daily, continued until progressive disease, toxicity, or response is seen, has been recently reported to give 40% response rate with minimal side effects, though patients with hypercellular marrow (the majority of MDS) or complex cytogenetic abnormalities do poorly. The effectiveness, tolerance, and availability of azacytidine, decitabine, and lenalidomide have now largely supplanted the use of low-dose chemotherapies in MDS.

6. Antithymocyte globulin (ATG). The immunosuppressive effects of ATG can be quite effective achieving transfusion independence along with other cytopenia responses in one third of a select subset of MDS patients, namely those who are younger, with hypocellular marrow, normal cytogenetics, shorter duration of transfusion dependency, and those who are HLA DR-15 positive.

- **ATG** 40 mg/kg/day × 4 days (common toxicities include infusion reactions, serum sickness (co-administration of prednisone may alleviate this), and immunosuppression).

Other immunosuppressive agents have been tried with mixed success. Prednisone is occasionally helpful in improving cytopenias (~10% response rate overall), particularly in those patients with evidence of hemolysis. **Cyclosporine** has shown high response rates in limited studies, utilizing 5 to 6 mg/kg/day initially, then monitored with dose adjustments to maintain serum levels of 100 to 300 ng/mL.

7. **Other agents** have shown some limited hematologic benefit in MDS. However, now with the availability of azacytidine, decitabine, and lenalidomide, and with a very narrow therapeutic index for either amifostine or arsenic trioxide, their use should be rare except in a clinical trial. **Pyridoxine** 100 to 200 mg daily is a reasonable trial in patients with increased ringed sideroblasts; however, benefit is infrequent. Developmental therapies targeting angiogenesis, apoptosis, cytokine, farnesyl transferase, tyrosine kinase, and histone deacetylase or other DNA methyltransferase epigenetic pathways, alone and in combination, are being evaluated in clinical trials.

8. **Supportive care**

   a. **Anemia.** RBC transfusions will become needed in most MDS patients to maintain quality of life. Hemoglobin goal (usually more than 9 g/dL) must be individualized on the basis of symptom, need, and improvement. Leukocyte-depleted packed RBCs should be used in all patients, with cytomegalovirus (CMV) negative blood if the patient is CMV negative, and irradiated blood products in potential SCT candidates.

   b. **Iron overload and chelation therapy.** Secondary hemochromatosis with cardiac, hepatic, endocrine, and hematopoietic dysfunction can develop after 20 to 30 units of red cell transfusion. Chelation therapy can improve visceral and marrow function, and should be a strong consideration in patients with an ongoing transfusion need who are expected to survive several years, as well as in patients with overt iron overload-related visceral dysfunction. Monitoring of ferritin levels should begin at a 20- to 30-unit transfusion threshold, with the institution of a chelating agent when the ferritin is more than 2,500 µg/L. The treatment goal is to lower ferritin to less than 1,000 µg/L.

   - **Desferrioxamine (Desferal)** 1 to 2 g by overnight (8–12 hours) SC infusion 5 to 7 nights/week; or
   - **Deferasirox (Exjade)** 20 mg/kg oral daily dispersed in water or orange/apple juice taken on an empty stomach. Toxicities are similar to desferrioxamine with nausea/vomiting, diarrhea, pyrexia, and abdominal pain but also with potential increased serum creatinine. The availability of this more convenient oral chelator will likely greatly improve this aspect of supportive care in MDS.

   c. **Infections.** Neutropenia and neutrophil dysfunction contribute to a high risk of bacterial infections in MDS. Antibiotics remain the mainstay of management, but prophylactic antibiotics are of unknown benefit. G-CSF can raise the neutrophil count in 90% of MDS patients, and its short-term use may be appropriate in infected, severely neutropenic patients; indications for long-term use of G-CSF are limited.

d. Bleeding. Symptomatic thrombocytopenia requires platelet transfusion support. Single-donor platelets delay alloimmunization, but this will eventually develop in most (30% to 70%) patients, limiting subsequent platelet transfusion increments. There is no absolute thrombocytopenia transfusion threshold, but platelet counts below 10,000 carry a spontaneous central nervous system hemorrhage risk. Two additional adjuncts to thrombocytopenic bleeding control are given:

- **Aminocaproic acid** 4 g IV over 1 hour, followed by 1 g/hour continuous infusion; or orally in a similar dosing schedule; or by a more convenient 2- to 4-g schedule orally every 4 to 6 hours. Tachyphylaxis and loss of antifibrinolytic stabilization will often occur after 48 consecutive hours of therapy.
- **Interleukin-11/oprelvekin** is a thrombopoietic cytokine that has increased platelet counts after chemotherapy. A low-dose regimen of 10 μg/kg/day can raise platelet counts in selected patients with bone marrow failure.

SUGGESTED READINGS

Myeloproliferative Diseases

Barosi G, Hoffman R. Idiopathic myelofibrosis. *Semin Hematol* 2005;42:248–258.

Harrison CN. Platelets and thrombosis in myeloproliferative diseases. *Hematology (American Society of Hematology Program)* 2005:409–415.

Harrison CN, Campbell PJ, Buck G, et al. Hydroxyurea compared with anagrelide in high-risk essential thrombocythemia. *N Engl J Med* 2005;353:33–45.

Kralovics R, Passamonti F, Buser AS, et al. A gain of function mutation of *JAK 2* in myeloproliferative disorders. *N Engl J Med* 2005;352:1779–1790.

Landolfi R, Marchioli R, Kutti J, et al. Efficacy and safety of low-dose aspirin in polycythemia vera. *N Engl J Med* 2004;350:114–124.

Marchioli R, Finazzi G, Landolfi R, et al. Vascular and neoplastic risk in a large cohort of patients with polycythemia vera. *J Clin Oncol* 2005;23:2224–2232.

Myelodysplastic Syndromes

Greenberg PL. Myelodysplastic syndromes: iron overload consequences and current chelating therapies. *J Natl Compr Canc Netw* 2006;4:91–96.

Greenberg PL, Baer MR, Bennett JM, et al. Myelodysplastic syndromes: clinical practice guidelines in oncology. *J Natl Compr Canc Netw* 2006;4:58–77.

Greenberg P, Cox C, Le Beau NM, et al. International scoring system for evaluating prognosis in myelodysplastic syndromes. *Blood* 1997;89:2079–2088.

Jadersten M, Montgomery SM, Dybedal I, et al. Long-term outcome of treatment of anemia in MDS with erythropoietin and G-CSF. *Blood* 2005;106:803–811.

Kantarjian H, Issa J-P, Rosenfield C, et al. Decitabine improves patient outcomes in myelodysplastic syndromes. *Cancer* 2006;106: 1794–1803.

Kantarjian H, O'Brien S, Giles F, et al. Decitabine low-dose schedule (100 mg/m2/course) in myelodysplastic syndrome (MDS): comparison of 3 different dose schedules. *Blood* 2005;106:2522a.

Kurzrock R, Cortes J, Thomas DA, et al. Pilot study of low-dose interleukin-11 in patients with bone marrow failure. *J Clin Oncol* 2001;19:4165–4172.

List A, Kurtin S, Roe DJ, et al. Efficacy of lenalidomide in myelodysplastic syndromes. *N Engl J Med* 2005;352:549–557.

Silverman LR, Demakos EP, Peterson BL, et al. Randomized controlled trial of azacytidine in patients with the myelodysplastic syndrome: a Study of the Cancer and Leukemia Group B. *J Clin Oncol* 2002;20:2429–2440.

Vardiman JW, Harris NL, Brunning RD. The World Health Organization (WHO) classification of the myeloid neoplasms. *Blood* 2002;100:2292–2302.

CHAPTER 22

Hodgkin's Lymphoma

Richard S. Stein and David S. Morgan

Hodgkin's lymphoma ([HL], Hodgkin's disease, HD) is a lymphoproliferative malignancy that accounts for approximately 1% of cancers in the United States. HL almost always presents as solitary or generalized lymphadenopathy, and as documented by clinical observation and by data collected during staging laparotomy, HL generally spreads in a contiguous manner. Most patients present with disease limited to lymph nodes or to lymph nodes and the spleen. The average age at presentation is 32 years with a bimodal incidence curve: one peak occurs at age 25, the other at age 55.

Patients with limited disease can be cured by radiation therapy; patients with advanced disease can be cured by combination chemotherapy. One of the major issues in HL therapy over the last two decades is where to draw the line between limited and advanced disease. Over time, the trend has been to consider chemotherapy for lesser stages of disease.

While HL is highly curable at presentation, patients with relapse following initial treatment may be cured by salvage therapy. Salvage chemotherapy may produce cures in patients initially treated with radiation therapy. Readministration of standard-dose chemotherapy or, more commonly, the administration of high-dose chemotherapy in conjunction with autologous stem cell transplantation may produce cures in patients initially treated with combination chemotherapy. Nevertheless, the potential for cure should not lead clinicians and patients to lose sight of the fact that HL is a malignancy and that approximately 20% to 25% of patients initially diagnosed with HL eventually die of the disease.

The success in the salvage therapy of HL makes it difficult to offer definitive recommendations regarding initial treatment. For most malignancies, disease-free survival is a valuable surrogate marker for overall survival. However, for HL, the success of salvage therapy means that the treatment options that are associated with superior disease-free survival may not necessarily produce superior overall survival when the results of salvage therapy are considered. Additionally, when therapies have significant long-term consequences such as secondary malignancies associated with larger radiation therapy fields or acute leukemia associated with combined-modality therapy, disease-free survival may overestimate the value of a specific therapy. Nevertheless, for each stage of HL, a number of rational therapeutic options exist.

I. Diagnosis and pathology. Diagnosis of HL requires biopsy of an involved node and review of the material by a hematopathologist. Lymph node biopsy is recommended for any patient with lymphadenopathy greater than 1 cm in diameter and persisting for more than 4 weeks. HL and other types of lymphoma may be suspected when the nodes are freely movable and rubbery rather than stony hard. However, these clinical features are not specific for HL or for lymphoma. Whenever the diagnosis of HL is made in a patient presenting at an extranodal site or at a nodal site below the diaphragm, the diagnosis should be subjected to greater than usual scrutiny.

HL has generally been subclassified into one of four subtypes: lymphocyte-predominant subtype (~5% of cases), nodular sclerosis subtype (~70% of cases), mixed cellularity subtype (~20% of cases), and lymphocyte-depleted subtype (<5% of cases). With the demonstration that lymphocyte-predominant HL is a B-cell neoplasm that is positive for CD20 and negative for CD30, the recent World Health Organization (WHO) classification of HL divides HL into two groups. The first group is nodular lymphocyte-predominant HL; the second group is "classical" Hodgkin's lymphoma, which includes nodular sclerosis HL, lymphocyte-rich classical HL, mixed cellularity HL, and lymphocyte depletion HL. Stage covaries with histology as patients with lymphocyte-depleted HL usually present with stage III or IV disease (retroperitoneal disease and/or bone marrow involvement). The average patient with mixed cellularity HL usually presents at a more advanced stage than the average patient with the nodular sclerosis subtype of HL. The presentation with cervical, supraclavicular, and mediastinal adenopathy in a young adult is classical for the nodular sclerosis type of HL. Because of this association of stage with histologic subtype, it is generally true that patients with the nodular sclerosis subtype of HL do better than patients with mixed cellularity HL, who, in turn, do better than patients with lymphocyte-depleted HL. However, whenever one stratifies patients by stage of disease, the impact of histopathology on prognosis is minimal.

II. Staging. In determining therapy for the patient with HL, the critical variable is the stage of the patient. Accurate staging also provides a baseline so that the completeness of a response can be determined when therapy has been completed.

  A. Cotswold staging system. The Cotswold modification of the Ann Arbor Staging System (Table 22.1) is used for patients with HL. Clinically, patients are placed in one of four stages and are further classified as to the absence "A" or presence "B" of symptoms. In addition, the subscript E (e.g., II_E) may be used to denote involvement of an extralymphatic site primarily or, more commonly, by direct extension, such as a large mediastinal mass extending into the lung. Stage III HL is often subdivided into stages III_1 and III_2 based on the extent of intra-abdominal disease.

  B. Staging tests. Staging must be performed with consideration of therapeutic options, and not just to complete a checklist. When performing staging tests, one should remember that HL tends to spread in a contiguous manner. Considering that the thoracic duct makes the left supraclavicular area and the abdomen contiguous sites, it is not surprising that abdominal disease is found in 40% of patients with left supraclavicular presentations and in only 8% of patients with right

Table 22.1. Cotswold modification of the ann arbor staging system for hodgkin's lymphoma

Stage	Description
Stage I	Involvement of a single lymph node region
Stage II	Involvement of two or more lymph node regions on the same side of the diaphragm
Stage III_1	Involvement of lymph node regions on both sides of the diaphragm Abdominal disease is limited to the upper abdomen, i.e., spleen, splenic hilar, celiac, and/or porta hepatis nodes
Stage III_2	Involvement of lymph node regions on both sides of the diaphragm Abdominal disease includes para-aortic, mesenteric, iliac, or inguinal nodes, with or without disease in the upper abdomen
Stage IV	Diffuse or disseminated involvement of one or more extralymphatic tissues or organs, with or without associated lymph node involvement
A	No symptoms
B	Fever, drenching sweats, weight loss
X	Bulky disease with greater than one-third widening of the mediastinum
E	Involvement of a single extranodal site contiguous to a nodal site

supraclavicular presentations. Procedures used in the staging of HL are as follows:

1. **History taking.** As with any patient, the staging of the patient with HL begins with history and physical examination. Special attention should be given to symptoms such as bone pain that might signal a specific extranodal site of disease. The symptoms that are considered "B symptoms" are fever, night sweats, and weight loss greater than 10% of body weight. Fever in HL can have any pattern. The pattern of days of high fever separated by days without fever, so-called "Pel-Ebstein fever," has been associated with HL for over a century but is quite rare in modern times when the diagnosis is usually made early in the course of disease and effective therapy is initiated. Pain at the site of HL in association with alcohol ingestion is a rare finding but may give hints as to the visceral sites of involvement.

2. **Complete physical examination.** Attention must be paid to all lymph node regions and the spleen. Splenomegaly is seen at presentation in approximately 10% of patients with HL and does not necessarily indicate splenic involvement by HL.

3. **Laboratory tests.** Complete blood counts, erythrocyte sedimentation rate, serum alkaline phosphatase, and tests of liver and kidney function should be obtained. Hepatic

enzymes may be elevated "nonspecifically" in patients with HL and do not necessarily indicate hepatic involvement by HL.

4. Chest x-ray and computed tomography (CT) scans. A chest x-ray and CT scans of the chest, abdomen, and pelvis are routinely obtained in patients with HL.

5. Positron emission tomography (PET) scan. PET scans have been shown to be highly reliable in detecting relapse and persistent disease and therefore should be obtained at baseline to document that tumor is PET positive. The PET scan is especially helpful when the posttreatment CT scan shows a residual mass that could be either scar or tumor.

6. Bone marrow biopsy. The test is rarely positive except in patients who are found to have at least stage III disease by other tests. However, because of the potential use of autologous bone marrow transplantation (ABMT) or stem cell transplantation as salvage therapy, a bone marrow biopsy is a reasonable baseline study in all patients with HL. Alternatively, if chemotherapy is planned and if blood counts are normal, the test may be omitted until the time that stem cell transplantation is considered.

7. Staging laparotomy. Staging laparotomy is the most accurate means of determining the extent of abdominal involvement with HL but is of historical interest only as staging laparotomy is rarely performed. Instead, most clinicians are willing to make clinical decisions on the basis of radiologic staging and to compensate for uncertain clinical staging by administering chemotherapy.

III. Therapy of Hodgkin's lymphoma

    A. General considerations. Therapy of HL must be considered on a stage-by-stage basis. The incidence of various stages of HL is presented in Table 22.2, which also presents an estimated cure rate for each stage. Historically, limited stages of HL (stages IA and IIA) have been treated with radiation therapy, while advanced stages (IIIB, IVA, and IVB) are generally treated with combination chemotherapy. For intermediate stages (IIB, IIIA), the tendency of most oncologists is to treat these patients with combination chemotherapy. Despite the success in the treatment of HL, decisions regarding the optimal choice of therapy for all stages of HL have become more complex.

    Late complications of radiation therapy for HL include breast cancer, lung cancer, hypothyroidism, thyroid cancer, coronary artery disease, and valvular heart disease. While the incidence of each of these complications is fairly low, the cumulative risk of all of these complications may be as much as 15% at 15 years following treatment. It is therefore reasonable to consider chemotherapy or chemotherapy plus involved field radiation therapy as an approach to limited-stage HL. Unfortunately, there are no data showing that the overall survival of patients with limited-stage HL can be improved with this alteration of therapy and studies designed to illustrate the superiority of this approach may require 15 to 20 years of observation to prove the point. Thus, after decades of "knowing" that radiation therapy was the optimal approach

Table 22.2.   Hodgkin's lymphoma: incidence of stages and results of therapy

Stage	Relative Incidence (%)	Potential Cure Rate (%)
IA	10	95
IIA	35	85
IB, IIB	13	70
III$_1$A	12	85
III$_2$A	8	65
IIIB	12	60
IVA, IVB	10	60

to limited-stage HL, there is now uncertainty as to whether this is the case.

While chemotherapy has clearly been established as the optimal therapy for advanced-stage disease, clinical trials have not resolved the question as to which regimen represents optimal treatment. Regardless of which chemotherapy regimen is chosen, standard regimens should not be altered arbitrarily as dose reductions may decrease the possibility of cure. Although most patients receive six cycles of chemotherapy, the data actually support the policy of administering a minimum of six cycles, with therapy being given until a complete remission (CR) has been achieved and then administered for an additional two cycles. While the tumor lysis syndrome has not been reported in HL, it is prudent to administer allopurinol during the first cycle of chemotherapy or during the first 2 weeks of radiation therapy.

B. Radiation therapy. Studies conducted in the 1960s established that the optimal dose for local control is 36 to 40 Gy given over 3.5 to 4.0 weeks. Standard radiation therapy ports are illustrated in Fig. 22.1.

With modern equipment, adequate radiation can be administered to involved areas while shielding adjacent tissues. As a result, radiation pneumonitis and radiation pericarditis occur only rarely. Because of the common occurrence of hypothyroidism and the less common occurrence of thyroid cancer in patients who receive radiation to the thyroid gland, thyroid-stimulating hormone (TSH) levels should be monitored yearly in these patients starting at 8 to 10 years following administration of radiation therapy. Patients with elevated levels of TSH, even if clinically euthyroid, should be placed on thyroid hormone replacement to limit stimulation of the irradiated thyroid gland by elevated levels of TSH. While radiation therapy alone has not been associated with an increased risk of acute leukemia, the use of radiation therapy in conjunction with combination chemotherapy has been associated with a risk of acute nonlymphocytic leukemia as high as 7% to 10% in the decade following therapy.

Women receiving radiation therapy for HL are at higher risk of developing breast cancer, and the younger the woman

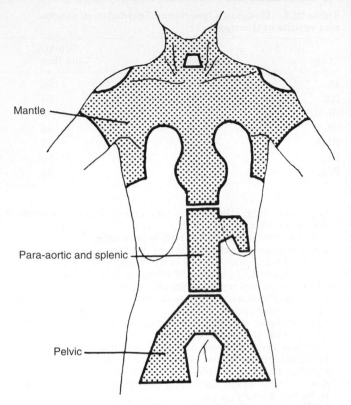

Mantle

Para-aortic and splenic

Pelvic

Figure 22.1.   Standard radiation ports used for the treatment of Hodgkin's lymphoma. For disease presenting above the diaphragm, the mantle plus para-aortic and splenic ports would be regarded as extended-field radiation therapy. The use of all three ports would be considered total nodal irradiation. (Reprinted by permission from Salzman JR, Kaplan HS. Effect of prior splenectomy on hematologic tolerance during total lymphoid radiotherapy of patients with Hodgkin's disease. *Cancer* **1972;27:472.)**

is at the time radiation therapy is administered, the higher the risk. Women who receive radiation therapy for HL should receive yearly mammograms starting 8 years following the completion of therapy.

C. Treatment by stage of disease

1. Stages IA and IIA. Patients with stage IA disease are most commonly treated with mantle irradiation when the disease occurs above the diaphragm (as it does in 90% of cases) or with pelvic radiation therapy when the disease presents in an inguinal node. Patients with stage IIA disease presenting above the diaphragm are most commonly treated with mantle plus para-aortic–splenic radiation therapy. While the use of more extensive radiation fields has been associated with a significantly lower rate of relapse, overall survival has not been shown to be significantly improved by the use of more extensive radiation ports. Additionally, the increased incidence of late malignancies with extended-field radiation therapy suggests that results that are superior at 10 years may not necessarily be superior at 15 or 20 years.

Alternatively, clinicians may treat patients with stage IA or IIA disease with chemotherapy such as ABVD plus involved field radiation therapy. While the addition of chemotherapy to radiotherapy in limited-stage disease has been shown to decrease the rate of relapse, as with the use of more extensive radiation therapy fields, this approach has not been associated with superior overall survival. This is due in large part to the fact that patients who relapse after radiation therapy alone may be salvaged by chemotherapy.

In attempts to limit long-term toxicity, investigators at Stanford have studied the use of involved field radiation in conjunction with a combination chemotherapy regimen that is less toxic than usually employed, specifically, vinblastine, bleomycin, and methotrexate (VBM). Early results have been encouraging, but long-term follow-up will be needed to determine if late complications are significantly decreased by this approach. At this time, the following treatment options can be justified for patients with stage IA or IIA disease:

- Involved field radiation therapy (for stage IA only),
- Extended field radiation therapy,
- Involved field radiation therapy with combination chemotherapy, and even
- Combination chemotherapy alone.

2. Stage II$_X$ disease with bulky mediastinal mass. Patients with bulky mediastinal masses (disease diameter greater than 10 cm or greater than one third of the chest diameter) present a special problem. When these patients, who are generally at stage II$_X$, are treated with radiotherapy alone, the risk of relapse approaches 50%. Combination chemotherapy with radiation therapy is most commonly employed in these patients. However, it is not clear that radiation therapy is necessary for all patients. Clearly, disease-free survival is superior when combined-modality therapy is given. However, as stated previously, disease-free survival is not a surrogate for long-term cure in Hodgkin's lymphoma. Combined-modality therapy is associated with an increased risk of acute leukemia, as high as 7% to 10% in the decade following therapy, and the addition of radiation therapy to chemotherapy creates a long-term risk of lung cancer and breast cancer. Therefore, the necessity of a combined-modality approach for all Stage II$_X$ patients is not established.

One approach is to treat the stage II$_X$ patients with combination chemotherapy and to give low-dose radiation therapy (20 Gy) only to patients who have residual disease on the basis of the PET scan obtained on completion of chemotherapy. When this is done, radiation is administered only to the area of residual disease. Unfortunately, whereas short-term results are encouraging, there are no long-term follow-up data to confirm that excellent clinical results can be achieved using PET scans to select patients who will not receive radiation therapy in this clinical situation.

3. Stages IB and IIB. In view of the limited number of patients with these stages of disease, available data do not allow firm treatment recommendations to be made. These patients are most commonly treated with extended field radiation therapy or radiation therapy in conjunction with combination chemotherapy such as MOPP, ABVD, or MOPP/ABV (Table 22.3). A discussion of the relative merits of the chemotherapy options for advanced-stage HL is found in the discussion of stage IIIB, IVA, and IVB disease.

4. Stage IIIA. Therapy for stage IIIA disease has become less controversial in the last 10 to 15 years, although consensus regarding the optimal therapy for these patients has not been achieved. Therapeutic options include total nodal radiation therapy alone, combination chemotherapy alone, or combined-modality therapy, that is, radiation therapy plus chemotherapy.

With the demonstration that combined-modality therapy was associated with a high risk of acute leukemia, this therapy fell out of favor. Additionally, studies in the early 1980s established that total nodal radiation therapy without chemotherapy was adequate only for patients with limited-stage III disease, that is, III_1 disease. For patients with III_2 disease, the use of radiation therapy alone was associated with a significant increase in mortality due to unacceptably high relapse rates and the inability of these patients to tolerate salvage chemotherapy at the time of relapse. If one decides to use different approaches to stage III_1 and stage III_2 disease, a staging laparotomy is necessary to definitively stage these patients. Since staging laparotomy is, essentially, never performed, the simplest approach to clinical stage III disease is to treat all stage III patients with combination chemotherapy.

5. Stages IIIB, IVA, and IVB. Combination chemotherapy is the standard approach to these stages of HL, although there remains some controversy as to which chemotherapy approach is optimal.

D. Chemotherapy. In 1970, the demonstration by investigators at the National Cancer Institute (NCI) that MOPP (mechlorethamine, Oncovin [vincristine], procarbazine, and prednisone) chemotherapy could cure advanced HL was one of the major milestones of the modern chemotherapy era as it was the first demonstration that a previously incurable advanced disease could be cured by combination chemotherapy. This has provided the rationale for the use of combination chemotherapy in medical oncology. However, more recent studies have indicated that the classic MOPP regimen is probably not the optimal regimen for patients with advanced HL.

1. Dose and duration of therapy. Arguments regarding selection of the "best" regimen should not obscure the following principles:

- Drugs should be administered in accordance with prescribed doses and schedules and not modified for toxicities

Table 22.3.   Chemotherapy regimens used in the treatment of Hodgkin's lymphoma

Regimen	Drugs and Dosages
MOPP	Mechlorethamine 6 mg/m^2 IV on days 1 and 8
	Vincristine (Oncovin) 1.4 mg/m^2 IV on days 1 and 8 (not to exceed 2.5 mg)
	Procarbazine 100 mg/m^2 PO on days 1–14
	Prednisone 40 mg/m^2 PO on days 1–14, cycles 1 and 4 only
	Repeat cycle every 28 days.
ABVD	Doxorubicin (Adriamycin) 25 mg/m^2 IV on days 1 and 15
	Vinblastine 6 mg/m^2 IV on days 1 and 15
	Bleomycin 10 U/m^2 IV on days 1 and 15
	Dacarbazine 375 mg/m^2 IV on days 1 and 15
	Repeat cycle every 28 days
MOPP/ABV	Mechlorethamine 6 mg/m^2 IV on day 1
	Vincristine (Oncovin) 1.4 mg/m^2 IV on day 1 (not to exceed 2.5 mg)
	Procarbazine 100 mg/m^2 PO on days 1–7
	Prednisone 40 mg/m^2 PO on days 1–14
	Doxorubicin (Adriamycin) 25 mg/m^2 IV on day 8
	Vinblastine 6 mg/m^2 IV on day 8
	Bleomycin 10 U/m^2 IV on day 8
	Repeat cycle every 28 days
VBM	Vinblastine 6 mg/m^2 IV on days 1 and 8
	Bleomycin 10 U/m^2 IV on days 1 and 8
	Methotrexate 30 mg/m^2 IV on days 1 and 8
	Repeat cycle every 28 days
Stanford V	Vinblastine 6 mg/m^2 IV weeks 1, 3, 5, 7, 9, and 11
	Doxorubicin 25 mg/m^2 IV weeks 1, 3, 5, 7, 9, and 11
	Vincristine 1.4 mg/m^2 IV (not to exceed 2 mg) weeks 2, 4, 6, 8, 10, and 12
	Bleomycin 5 U/m^2 IV weeks 2, 4, 6, 8, 10, and 12
	Mechlorethamine 6 mg/m^2 IV weeks 1, 5, and 9
	Etoposide 60 mg/m^2 IV daily × 2 weeks 3, 7, and 11
	Prednisone 40 mg/m^2 PO every other day on weeks 1–10, with tapering weeks 11 and 12 (No repeat)

such as nausea and vomiting (which should be controlled symptomatically).

- Full doses should be given when cytopenias are due to bone marrow involvement with HL.
- Vincristine should be decreased only in the presence of ileus, motor weakness, or numbness involving the whole fingers, not just the fingertips.
- Patients should be treated for a minimum of six cycles, but also until a CR is documented, and then for another two cycles. If tests are equivocal, it is better to treat with additional cycles rather than to prematurely discontinue therapy.

2. Classical MOPP therapy. When MOPP was initially administered, 81% of patients achieved a CR. Of these patients, 66% (representing 53% of the total series) remained in CR for 5 years, and an identical percentage remained in CR for 10 years. Thus, while late relapses have been seen on occasion, 5-year disease-free survival probably represents cure for most patients. Since salvage therapy can cure patients who are not cured by initial chemotherapy, the figure of 53% represents a minimal estimate for the cure of advanced HL.

3. Alternatives to MOPP induction therapy. Many efforts have been made to develop combination regimens that are more effective and less toxic than the standard MOPP regimen. Some regimens represent minimal modifications of MOPP, but the regimen that has attracted the most interest is ABVD (doxorubicin [Adriamycin], bleomycin, vinblastine, dacarbazine), a regimen composed of agents not cross-resistant to MOPP. In a large randomized trial, ABVD was shown to be superior to MOPP with respect to remission rates and survival.

Chemotherapy regimens have been created with alternate cycles of MOPP and ABVD or to use a hybrid of MOPP/ABV, in which all drugs are given during each cycle. With use of the MOPP/ABV hybrid, a CR rate of 84% has been achieved. This CR rate was elevated to 97% by administration of radiation therapy to areas of residual adenopathy. At a median follow-up approaching 4 years, 90% of complete responders remained free of disease for a projected disease-free survival of 88%.

In a randomized trial that compared hybrid MOPP/ABV with sequential MOPP and ABVD, the hybrid regimen was found to be superior to the sequential regimen. The MOPP/ABV hybrid produced CRs in 83% of patients with a failure-free survival rate of 64%. However, because of the increased incidence of myelodysplasia associated with MOPP/ABV, ABVD has become the regimen of choice among MOPP, MOPP/ABV, and ABVD.

Although some investigators have combined chemotherapy with radiation therapy for the treatment of advanced disease, there is no evidence that the standard use of this approach can improve results enough to compensate for the leukemogenic risk of that practice. In selected patients with bulky disease, however, it is reasonable to consider supplementing combination chemotherapy with local radiation therapy to sites of bulky disease.

Also, as high-intensity therapy in conjunction with stem cell transplantation has been shown to be effective salvage therapy of HL, more intense induction regimens have been studied in HL. Favorable results have been reported by German investigators using BEACOPP and by investigators at Stanford using Stanford V. Doses of the latter regimen are included in Table 22.3. However, it has not been established that long-term results using these regimens are superior to those achieved with ABVD.

4. Salvage therapy. Salvage therapy may produce cures in patients with HL who have a relapse following initial therapy. However, the chance of curing a patient with relapsed HL is greater if the relapse is nodal than if the relapse is visceral. Additionally, the chance of cure is greater when the initial stage of disease was limited than when the initial stage was advanced.

For patients with limited nodal relapses following radiation therapy, additional radiation therapy may be considered. If the recurrence represents a marginal miss at the edge of a radiation field, this may be feasible. However, if the recurrence is within a treatment field, further irradiation of the area is usually contraindicated and chemotherapy is needed. Furthermore, as fewer patients are treated with radiotherapy alone, this option is rarely clinically relevant.

For patients who have a relapse following chemotherapy, the variable that best predicts the chance of cure is the disease-free interval. Among patients initially treated with MOPP therapy, patients whose first CR lasted less than 1 year had a second CR rate of 29%, and only 14% of these second remissions lasted more than 4 years. Among patients whose first CR lasted more than 1 year, 93% achieved a second CR, and 45% of second CRs were projected to last more than 20 years. While the drugs used to obtain the first CR may be successful as salvage therapy, the general trend is to use drugs to which the patient has not been exposed. Thus, for patients treated with MOPP, the ABVD combination is the most commonly used salvage therapy. As ABVD has become a standard therapy, the regimens generally considered as salvage are MOPP, ICE, and ESHAP (Table 22.4).

However, rather than rely on salvage chemotherapy alone, the more common approach to salvage therapy is to follow a few cycles of salvage chemotherapy with high-dose chemotherapy in conjunction with ABMT or peripheral blood stem cell transplantation (PBSCT).

High-dose therapy in conjunction with ABMT or PBSCT is based on the rationale that bone marrow toxicity limits the dosages of the drugs that are most effective in HL. When autologous marrow or stem cells are stored and reinfused following chemotherapy, drug doses can be escalated to levels that would ordinarily be fatal in the absence of stem cell reinfusion. A number of standard preparative regimens

Table 22.4.   Salvage regimens in the treatment of Hodgkin's lymphoma

Regimen	Drugs and Dosages
ICE pre–stem cell transplant	Ifosfamide 5,000 mg/m^2 IV on day 2 over 24 h
	Mesna same dose as Ifosfamide, continuously with ifosfamide, with an additional dose after ifosfamide
	VP—16, 100 mg/m^2 IV day 1, 2, and 3
	Carboplatin AUC = 5, maximum 800 mg day 2
ICE in heavily pretreated patients	Ifosfamide 1000 mg/m^2 IV day 1 and day 2 (t = 0 to t = 1 h)
	Mesna 333 mg/m^2 IV 30 min before ifosfamide and 4 and 8 h after each dose of ifosfamide
	VP-16, 150 mg/m^2 IV b.i.d. day 1 and day 2
	Carboplatin 200 mg/m^2 IV day 1 and day 2
ESHAP	VP-16, 60 mg/m^2 IV daily, day 1–4
	Methylprednisolone 500 mg IV daily, day 1–4
	Cisplatin 25 mg/m^2 IV daily by continuous infusion over 24 h, day 1–4
	ARA-C 2,000 mg/m^2 IV on day 5

exist for use in conjunction with ABMT and PBSCT, and these regimens are presented in Table 22.5.

Controlled trials comparing preparative regimens for autologous transplantation have not been conducted, and in view of the heterogeneity of relapsed patients with respect to prior therapy, sensitivity to therapy, site of relapse, and disease-free interval, it is impossible to compare regimens across studies. Nevertheless, as improvements in supportive care, such as the use of granulocyte colony-stimulating factor ([G-CSF]; filgrastim) or granulocyte–macrophage colony-stimulating factor ([GM-CSF]; sargramostim), have lowered treatment-related mortality to approximately 5%, it appears that long-term disease-free survival may occur in approximately 50% of patients treated with ABMT or PBSCT. Patients who achieved long disease-free intervals with standard treatment seem to have the best chance for long-term disease-free survival and some studies have suggested that good performance status and persistent sensitivity to standard chemotherapy may predict an excellent response to autologous transplantation.

Table 22.5.   Regimens used preparatory to autologous transplantation in Hodgkin's lymphoma

Regimen	Drugs and Dosages
CBV	Cyclophosphamide 1,800 mg/m^2 IV on days -7, -6, -5, -4
	BCNU 600 mg/m^2 IV on day -3
	Etoposide (VP-16) 800 mg/m^2 IV on days -7, -6, -5
CBV	Cyclophosphamide 1,500 mg/m^2 IV on days -5, -4, -3, -2
	BCNU 300 mg/m^2 IV on day -5
	Etoposide (VP-16) 300 mg/m^2 IV on days -5, -4, -3
BEAM	BCNU 300 mg/m^2 IV on day -6
	Etoposide (VP-16) 100–200 mg/m^2 IV on days -5, -4, -3, -2
	Cytosine arabinoside 200–400 mg/m^2 IV on days -5, -4, -3, -2
	Melphalan 140 mg/m^2 IV on day -1

Day 0 is the day of reinfusion of progenitor cells. Therefore, day -5 would be 5 days before reinfusion.

E. Treatment of symptoms. Fever, and occasionally pruritus, may be disabling for some patients with HL. The basic approach to these problems is to treat the disease. However, if disease is drug resistant, that approach may be an oversimplification. Indomethacin 25 to 50 mg PO t.i.d. may be helpful in these patients. Anecdotal experience also supports the use of other nonsteroidal anti-inflammatory agents in these patients.

IV. Follow-up. HL patients who achieve a CR and who later relapse usually do so at a site of previous disease. Our policy for follow-up is to see the patient every 2 months for the first year, every 3 months for the second year, every 4 months during the third year, every 6 months during the fourth year, and every year thereafter. There is no standard panel of tests for routine follow-up but our practice is to obtain CT scans or a whole body PET/CT every 6 months for 1 to 2 years, then every year for 3 to 4 years. If such tests suggest that disease has recurred, it is advisable to obtain pathologic confirmation before initiating salvage therapy.

Because of the risk of acute leukemia following therapy, we obtain complete blood counts at the time of each visit for patients who have received combination chemotherapy. Monitoring for hypothyroidism was discussed in Section III.B. While elevated sedimentation rates and lactic dehydrogenase (LDH) levels may provide hints of relapse, we have not routinely used these tests for follow-up monitoring in our practice. Since women who receive radiation therapy above the diaphragm are at increased risk of breast cancer, we recommend yearly mammograms in these patients starting at age 40 or at 8 years following the completion of radiation therapy.

SUGGESTED READINGS

Andrieu JM, Ifrah N, Payen C, et al. Increased risk of secondary leukemia after extended field radiation combined with MOPP chemotherapy for Hodgkin's disease. *J Clin Oncol* 1990;8:1148– 1154.

Canellos GP, Anderson JR, Propert KJ, et al. Chemotherapy of advanced Hodgkin's disease with MOPP, ABVD, or MOPP alternating with ABVD. *N Engl J Med* 1992;327:1478–1484.

Crnkovich MJ, Leopold K, Hoppe RT, et al. Stage I to IIB Hodgkin's disease: the combined experience at Stanford University and the Joint Center for Radiation Therapy. *J Clin Oncol* 1987;5:1041– 1049.

DeVita VT Jr, Serpick AA, Carbone PP. Combination chemotherapy in the treatment of advanced Hodgkin's disease. *Ann Intern Med* 1970;73:881–895.

DeWit M, Baumann D, Beyer W, et al. Whole body positron emission tomography (PET) for diagnosis of residual mass in patients with lymphoma. *Ann Oncol* 1997;8(Suppl 1):57–60.

Diehl V, Franklin J, Hasenclever D, et al. BEACOPP, a new dose-escalated and accelerated regimen, is at least as effective as COPP/ABVD in patients with advanced stage Hodgkin's lymphoma: interim report from a trial of the German Hodgkin's Lymphoma Study Group. *J Clin Oncol* 1998;16:3810–3821.

Glick JH, Young ML, Harrington D, et al. MOPP/ABV hybrid chemotherapy for advanced Hodgkin's disease significantly improves failure-free and overall survival: the 8-year results of the intergroup trial. *J Clin Oncol* 1998;16:19–26.

Hancock SL, Cox RS, McDougall IR. Thyroid diseases after treatment of Hodgkin's disease. *N Engl J Med* 1991;325:599–605.

Horning SJ, Hoppe R, Hancock SL, et al. Vinblastine, bleomycin, and methotrexate. An effective regimen in favorable Hodgkin's disease. *J Clin Oncol* 1988;6:1822–1831.

Horning SJ, Williams J, Bartlett NL, et al. Assessment of the Stanford V regimen and consolidative radiotherapy for bulky and advanced Hodgkin's disease: Eastern Cooperative Oncology Group pilot study E1492. *J Clin Oncol* 2000;18:972–980.

Klimo P, Connors JM. An update on the Vancouver experience in the management of advanced Hodgkin's disease treated with MOPP/ABV hybrid regimen. *Semin Hematol* 1988;25(Suppl 2): 34–40.

Lister TA, Crowther D. Staging for Hodgkin's disease. *Semin Oncol* 1990;17:696.

Longo DL, Duffey PL, Young RC, et al. Conventional-dose salvage combination chemotherapy in patients relapsing with Hodgkin's disease after combination chemotherapy: the low probability of cure. *J Clin Oncol* 1992;10:210–218.

Mauch P, Larson D, Osteen R, et al. Prognostic factors for positive surgical staging in patients with Hodgkin's disease. *J Clin Oncol* 1990;8:257–265.

Mauch P, Tarbell N, Weinstein H, et al. Stage IA and IIA supra-diaphragmatic Hodgkin's disease: prognostic factors in surgically staged patients treated with mantle and paraaortic irradiation. *J Clin Oncol* 1988;6:1576–1583.

Salzman JR, Kaplan HS. Effect of prior splenectomy on hematologic tolerance during total lymphoid radiotherapy of patients with Hodgkin's disease. *Cancer* 1972;27:472.

Specht L, Gray RG, Clarke MJ, et al. Influence of more extensive radiotherapy and adjuvant chemotherapy on long-term outcome of early stage Hodgkin's disease: a meta-analysis of 23 randomized trials involving 3,888 patients. International Hodgkin's Disease Collaborative Group. *J Clin Oncol* 1998;16:830–848.

Stein S, Golomb HM, Wiernik PH, et al. Anatomic substages of stage IIIA Hodgkin's disease. *Cancer Treat Rep* 1982;66:733–741.

Vose JM, Bierman PJ, Armitage JO. Hodgkin's disease: the role of bone marrow transplantation. *Semin Oncol* 1990;17:749–757.

CHAPTER 23

Non–Hodgkin's Lymphoma

Richard S. Stein and John P. Greer

I.   Epidemiology. There is a worldwide epidemic of non–Hodgkin's lymphoma (NHL) with more than 60,000 cases diagnosed in the United States each year. Part of the increase is related to the development of NHL in patients with the human immunodeficiency virus (HIV). However, additional factors contributing to the NHL epidemic are listed in Table 23.1. The incidence of lymphomas is age related, with a steady increase in incidence from childhood through age 80; the median age of patients at the time of diagnosis of NHL is between 60 and 65 years. Lymphomas are the fifth most common cancer in the United States and they represent 4% of all cancers.

Extranodal presentations occur in 15% to 25% of adult cases in the United States with higher figures observed in Europe and the Far East. As the incidence of NHL has increased, there has been a disproportionate increase in cases with disease arising at extranodal sites as compared to that in nodal sites, in cases with a diffuse histologic pattern as compared to a follicular pattern, and in cases with an intermediate- to high-grade pattern as compared to low-grade disease. NHL of the brain has risen four times as rapidly as that in other extranodal sites, partly due to the association with HIV. However, the rise in central nervous system (CNS) lymphoma has also occurred in immunocompetent hosts as well. Familial aggregation of NHL plays a small role in the epidemic even though there is a twofold to fourfold increased risk for NHL in close relatives of patients with lymphoma or other hematopoietic neoplasms.

In addition to the association with HIV, other viruses have specific clinical associations with NHL. Chronic hepatitis C infection is often present in patients with type II cryoglobulin and many of these patients have an underlying indolent B-cell lymphoma. Helicobacter pylori infection in the stomach has been associated with gastric and duodenal ulcers, and it has been associated with gastric lymphoma, specifically, a low-grade B-cell lymphoma of mucosa-associated lymphoid tissue (MALToma).

The mechanism of developing lymphoma has best been studied in the lymphomas occurring in immunodeficiency states. These disorders can be divided into congenital (or primary) immunodeficiencies and acquired (or secondary) immunodeficiencies (Table 23.2). Common components to all these disorders are defects in immunoregulation, particularly in T-cell immunity, resulting in decreased cytokines and uncontrolled B-cell growth in lymphoid tissue, often in association with the Epstein-Barr virus (EBV) genome. Additionally, chronic inflammation, immune hyperactivity, and immunosuppression are elements of autoimmune disorders that predispose patients to lymphoma. With two exceptions, nearly all lymphomas that occur in association with immune suppression are B-cell lymphomas; ataxia

Table 23.1. Epidemiologic factors associated with an increased risk of non–Hodgkin's lymphoma

Immunosuppression

Infectious agents

 Epstein-Barr virus

 Human T-cell lymphotropic virus type I

 Helicobacter pylori

 Hepatitis C virus

 Human herpesvirus 8 (Kaposi's sarcoma)

 Human herpesvirus 6

 Human T-cell lymphotropic virus type II

Male gender

Increasing age

Family history of non–Hodgkin's lymphoma

Earlier cancer history

Drug history

 Immunosuppressive agents

 Phenytoin

 Methotrexate

 Tumor necrosis factor inhibitors

Occupational history

 Exposure to herbicides, pesticides, wood dust, epoxy glue, solvents

 Jobs in farming, forestry, painting, carpentry, tanning

---

telangiectasia is associated with T-cell lymphoma and as many as one tenth of the lymphomas that occur in organ transplant patients are of T-cell origin. Additionally, T-cell lymphomas have an increased incidence in patients with nontropical sprue, angioimmunoblastic lymphadenopathy, and lymphomatoid papulosis.

II. Pathologic classification of lymphoma. NHL is composed of a diverse group of malignancies in which the cell of origin is a lymphocyte. If the site of origin is the bone marrow, the disorder may be classified as a form of lymphocytic leukemia, but when disease is present in both nodes and marrow, the distinction between leukemia and lymphoma is somewhat arbitrary. The disorders included in NHL differ in many basic characteristics. At the time of presentation, some types of lymphoma such as small cleaved cell lymphoma (alternatively regarded as grade I follicular lymphoma) are almost always disseminated and the bone marrow is usually involved by lymphoma. By contrast, patients with large B-cell lymphoma present with disease limited to one or two lymph node areas in approximately one third of cases; in this histologic type of lymphoma, bone marrow involvement is seen at presentation less than 20% of the time.

Some types of lymphoma, primarily those lymphomas with a follicular pattern under the microscope, have a slow indolent course. Patients with small cleaved cell lymphoma, the most common follicular lymphoma, may initially do well with no treatment or with minimal therapy. Median survival for these patients is

Table 23.2.   Pre-lymphomatous conditions

Congenital	Acquired
Ataxia telangectasia	Immunodeficiency
Wiskott-Aldrich syndrome	Organ transplants
Severe combined immunodeficiency	Acquired immunodeficiency syndrome
Common variable immunodeficiency	Autoimmune disorders
Hyper immunoglobulin M	Sjogren syndrome
X-linked hypogammaglobulinemia	Hashimoto's thyroiditis
X-linked lymphoproliferative syndrome	Rheumatoid arthritis
Autoimmune lymphoproliferative syndrome	Inflammatory bowel disease
	Castleman disease
	Hodgkin's disease
	Predisposition to T-cell lymphoma
	Nontropical sprue
	Angioimmunoblastic lymphadenopathy
	Lymphomatoid papulosis

between 8 and 12 *years,* with patients experiencing a series of responses and relapses before the disease becomes refractory to further therapy and terminates fatally. In contrast, other types of lymphoma such as diffuse large B-cell lymphomas are fatal in 4 to 12 *months* in the absence of therapy but may be cured by combination chemotherapy in 40% to 50% of cases. For over 80% of patients with NHL, including the types previously discussed, the cell of origin is a B lymphocyte; for less than 15% of cases, the cell of origin is a T lymphocyte.

In view of this clinical diversity, accurate classification of NHL is essential for scientific and clinical purposes. Ideally, a classification system should identify types of NHL that are scientifically and clinically meaningful. A classification system should define entities that are relatively homogeneous from a clinical, morphologic, immunologic, and genetic point of view. One would also want a classification system that was associated with concordance among pathologists regarding the classification of individual cases. Unfortunately, such an ideal classification system does not exist. Nevertheless, a clinical consideration of NHL must start with a discussion of the classification of lymphoma.

Problems related to the pathologic classification of NHL can best be appreciated from a historical perspective. In the 1960s, Rappaport proposed a classification of NHL that divided the disorders on the basis of whether the predominant cell was small, large, or a mixture of small and large cells. Lymphomas were also categorized as nodular or diffuse. Studies conducted using this system demonstrated that nodular lymphomas composed of small lymphocytes were generally indolent disorders, whereas the so-called "histiocytic" lymphoma was curable with combination chemotherapy. However, the **Rappaport system** predated the understanding that lymphocytes were B cells or T cells and that the nodules of nodular lymphoma are composed of the same cells found in germinal follicles. Additionally, studies eventually established that the so-called "histiocytic lymphoma" was actually composed of many disorders, most of which were B-cell disorders and a minority of which were T-cell disorders. These findings established the need for better terminology and for a more scientific classification system.

In the 1970s, the Lukes-Collins classification in the United States and the Kiel classification developed by Lennert in Europe, subdivided lymphoma into B-cell and T-cell disorders. As flow cytometry and studies of surface markers were in their infancy, such systems were difficult to use and it was not clear that the entities being discussed were meaningful entities that could be identified reliably. In this setting, the National Cancer Institute assembled a working panel of hematopathologists who created the **New Working Formulation.** This classification considered many of the concepts of immunologically oriented systems. However, instead of defining entities on the basis of their "immunologic cell of origin," the New Working Formulation defined broad categories of lymphoma on the basis of general clinical prognosis. Specifically, the New Working Formulation defined low-grade lymphoma, intermediate-grade lymphoma, and high-grade lymphoma. The idea of this classification was to use the pathologic appearance of the lymphoma to tell the clinician how the lymphoma needed to be treated.

In the New Working Formulation, **low-grade lymphomas** are indolent lymphomas such as chronic lymphocytic leukemia (also known as *small B-cell lymphoma*) and follicular (nodular) small cleaved cell lymphoma. In asymptomatic patients, even in patients with widespread disease, watchful waiting (i.e., no initial treatment) may be appropriate management. These disorders are associated with a high response rate to single-agent or combination chemotherapy, but after a prolonged clinical course (8 to 12+ years), these diseases are usually fatal.

Intermediate-grade lymphomas were defined by the New Working Formulation as more aggressive lymphomas, associated with a fatal course within months to less than 2 years in the age of single-agent chemotherapy but curable 40% to 50% of the time in the era of combination chemotherapy. This category includes diffuse large cell lymphoma as well as diffuse forms of small cleaved cell lymphoma. Although most intermediate-grade lymphomas are B-cell lymphomas, this category also includes some T-cell lymphomas such as anaplastic large cell lymphoma (ALCL).

High-grade lymphomas as defined by the New Working Formulation are those lymphomas associated with a very high growth fraction and a rapidly lethal clinical course in the absence of effective therapy. This category includes Burkitt's and Burkitt's-like NHL. At the time the New Working Formulation was designed, the complete remission rate in patients with high-grade lymphoma was only 20%. However, in the intervening years, as cure rates in "intermediate-grade NHL" maintained a plateau of 40% to 50%, complete response rates in "high-grade lymphoma" rose from the 20% range to the 40% to 50% range with the use of more aggressive chemotherapy. Nevertheless, while response rates for intermediate- and high-grade lymphoma have come together, this distinction is still relevant as high-grade lymphomas will not show such response if treated with standard CHOP therapy, a regimen that is acceptable for intermediate-grade NHL.

On the basis of the assumption that the scientific study of lymphomas requires the delineation of scientifically meaningful entities, the **REAL (Revised European–American Classification of Lymphoid Neoplasms) classification system** was developed to delineate the entities that hematopathologists, immunologists, and molecular biologists had defined in the last 15 years. It has since been adopted and modified by the World Health Organization (WHO) as the REAL/WHO classification system.

The **REAL/WHO classification system** (Table 23.3) has the advantage of recognizing lymphomas that can be defined at the pathologic and molecular level but that are obscured by the use of the New Working Formulation. Entities such as mantle cell lymphoma, with its specific t(11;14) translocation, and ALCL are recognized as distinct entities in this system. However, in the REAL classification system (see Table 23.3), the largest entity, diffuse large B-cell disease (31% of cases), is likely a heterogeneous disease, and the division of follicular lymphoma (22% of cases) into three grades does not clarify the classification of those entities. Thus, the REAL/WHO classification may have the advantage of delineating uncommon lymphomas, while neglecting the lymphomas most commonly encountered in clinical practice. Only time will tell if this approach leads to a more scientific clinical analysis of lymphoma.

III.   Staging of lymphoma. The Cotswold modification of the Ann Arbor classification is generally used for patients with NHL as well as for patients with Hodgkin's lymphoma (HL). Despite the widespread use of this model, the clinical applicability of the four-stage model to NHL is uncertain. For practical purposes, many clinicians believe that there may be only two stages of NHL: limited disease (stage I) and advanced disease (stages II, III, and IV). In contrast to HL, it has been established that radiation therapy has no role in the curative treatment of stage II NHL. In fact, in the case of intermediate-grade lymphoma, for stage I disease, radiation therapy alone has been supplanted by chemotherapy plus radiation therapy as the treatment of choice. Additionally, in contrast to HL, which arises at an extranodal site in less than 1% of cases, approximately 10% to 20% of NHLs have an extranodal presentation.

Perhaps as important as the staging of lymphoma in general is the **International Prognostic Index** (IPI) for use in patients with "intermediate-grade lymphoma." This prognostic index (Table 23.4) predicts the probability of cure in intermediate-grade NHL on the basis of the age, stage, performance status, number of extranodal sites of disease, and lactate dehydrogenase (LDH) level. For patients of all ages, 5-year survival was 73% for low-risk patients, 51% for low intermediate-risk patients, 43% for high-/intermediate-risk patients, and 26% for high-risk patients. For patients under the age of 60, an age-adjusted prognostic system was developed (see Table 23.4). For

Table 23.3.   Revised European–American Classification of Lymphoid Neoplasms/World Health Organization classification of lymphoid neoplasms

B-cell lymphomas

Precursor B-cell neoplasms

   Precursor B lymphoblastic

Mature (peripheral) B-cell neoplasms

   Small lymphocytic lymphoma/(chronic lymphocytic leukemia) (7%)

   B-cell prolymphocytic leukemia

   Lymphoplasmacytic (1.2%)

   Splenic marginal zone B-cell lymphoma

   Hairy cell leukemia

   Plasma cell myeloma/plasmacytoma

   Extranodal marginal zone B-cell lymphoma of mucosa-associated lymphoid tissue (MALT) type (8%)

   Nodal marginal zone B-cell lymphoma with or without monocytoid B cell

   Mantle cell (6%)

   Follicle center, follicular (22.1%)

      Grade I (10%)

      Grade II (6%)

      Grade III (6%)

   Diffuse large B cell (31%)

   Mediastinal large B cell (2.4%)

   Primary effusion lymphoma

   Burkitt's lymphoma/Burkitt's cell leukemia (<1%)

T- and NK-cell lymphomas

Precursor T-cell neoplasms

   Precursor T-lymphoblastic lymphoma/leukemia precursor T cell

   Acute lymphoblastic leukemia (1.7%)

Mature (peripheral) T-cell neoplasms

   T-cell prolymphocytic leukemia

   T-cell granular lymphocyte leukemia

   Aggressive NK-cell leukemia

   Adult T-cell lymphoma/leukemia (human T-cell lymphotropic virus type I positive) (1%)

   Extranodal NK-/T-cell lymphoma nasal type (1.4%)

   Enteropathy-type T-cell lymphoma (<1%)

   Hepatosplenic $\gamma\delta$ T-cell lymphoma (<1%)

   Subcutaneous panniculitis-like T-cell lymphoma

   Mycosis fungoides/Sézary syndrome (<1%)

   Anaplastic large cell lymphoma T cell/null cell, primary cutaneous type

   Peripheral T cell, not otherwise specified (7%)

   Angioimmunoblastic T-cell lymphoma (1.2%)

   Anaplastic large cell lymphoma T cell/null cell, primary systemic type

Percentages represent the data presented after an international review of cases of NHL. Entities that represent ≥5% of cases are in boldface.

Table 23.4.   International Prognostic Index for non–Hodgkin's lymphoma

Variable	0 points	1 point
All patients[a]		
Age (years)	≤60	>60
Stage	I or II	III or IV
No. of extranodal sites	≤1	>1
Performance status	0 or 1	≥2
LDH	Normal	Elevated
Patients aged <60 years[b]		
Stage	I or II	III or IV
Performance status	0 or 1	≥2
LDH	Normal	Elevated

LDH, lactate dehydrogenase.
[a]Low risk, 0 or 1; low intermediate risk, 2; high intermediate risk, 3; high risk, 4 or 5.
[b]Low risk, 0; low intermediate risk, 1; high intermediate risk, 2; high risk, 3.

patients younger than 60, 5-year survival was 83% for low-risk patients, 69% for low-/intermediate-risk patients, 46% for high-/intermediate-risk patients, but only 32% for high-risk patients.

The evaluation of the patient with NHL begins with history and physical examination. When performing the physical examination, special care must be given to examining the Waldeyer's ring, epitrochlear nodes, femoral nodes, and popliteal nodes—sites that are almost never involved in HL but that may be involved in a small percentage of cases of NHL. The bone marrow biopsy is generally regarded as a key diagnostic procedure in the staging of NHL, owing to the high incidence of involvement, especially in small cleaved cell lymphoma (follicular lymphoma grade I). However, in follicular lymphoma grade I, the presence or absence of marrow involvement generally does not affect therapy as asymptomatic patients are treated with "watchful waiting" or single-agent chemotherapy regardless of marrow involvement. Thus, the clinical necessity of marrow biopsy is uncertain. In other histologic types of NHL, the test is important as a baseline test because of prognosis and the possible use of autologous bone marrow or stem cell transplantation at the time of relapse. Nevertheless, if a patient with NHL is going to be treated with chemotherapy, omitting the baseline bone marrow evaluation clearly does not compromise care.

Baseline computed tomography (CT) scans are an essential part of the staging of patients with NHL as much to establish a baseline for evaluating the response to treatment as for determining the actual extent of disease. In HL, involved nodes are often small and may be missed by CT scanning. However, in NHL, retroperitoneal masses, if present, are often large and easily detected by CT scans. In addition, whereas mesenteric nodes are rarely involved in HL, they are involved in most cases of nodular NHL and can be detected by CT scan.

With the advent of positron emission tomography (PET) scans, gallium scans have essentially become obsolete in the staging of lymphoma. Although PET scans may be negative in sites involved by low-grade lymphoma, they are generally positive in other histologic types of NHL. Additionally, studies have suggested that PET scans may be extremely well suited to evaluating residual masses detected by CT scanning as PET scans may reliably separate scar from active disease. In a recent study of patients with HL and NHL, 75 patients were studied with PET scans and CT scans following treatment; biopsies were obtained of areas that were suspicious for persistent or recurrent lymphoma. With a follow-up of 14 months, PET scans were far superior to CT scans in predicting relapse. If the PET scan is going to be used upon completion of therapy in a patient with a residual mass, it is rational to get a baseline PET scan to document that the tumor is PET positive. The optimal interval between posttreatment PET scans has not been determined.

Peripheral blood counts are an insensitive measure of bone marrow involvement. Most patients with small cleaved cell lymphoma (follicular lymphoma grade I) have focal marrow involvement, and almost all of these patients have normal peripheral blood counts. Abnormal blood counts may suggest marrow infiltration by lymphoma but may also occur when the spleen is infiltrated by lymphoma and extensively enlarged. As most patients with NHL will receive chemotherapy, evaluation of the blood counts is a basic part of staging of NHL. Serum LDH is an important prognostic indicator and is one of the variables considered in the IPI. Other molecular markers such as *bcl-2, bcl-6, p53, ALK* (anaplastic lymphoma kinase) in ALCL, and *cyclin D-1* in mantle cell lymphoma as well as markers for multidrug resistance are under active investigation as prognostic indicators but are not part of standard staging systems.

IV.   Radiation therapy of non–Hodgkin's lymphoma. Because most patients with NHL have disseminated disease, radiation therapy plays a limited role in NHL. However, the value of radiation therapy should not be overlooked. With most histologic types of follicular lymphoma, doses of 44 Gy can achieve control of local disease. Because disease occurs outside of treatment fields, such as in the bone marrow, radiation therapy is rarely curative. However, when patients with follicular lymphoma have large masses, local radiation therapy may be the most effective means of palliation. A dose–response curve for radiation therapy of large cell lymphoma is less well established, although radiation therapy may play a role in palliating patients with large cell lymphoma who have become refractory to chemotherapy.

Although 30% of patients with large cell lymphoma have stage I or II disease, the role of radiation therapy, as the sole treatment in these patients, has not been supported by clinical studies. Radiation therapy has been associated with cure rates exceeding 80% in stage I large cell lymphoma *only* when patients have been staged by laparotomy. Rather than subjecting these patients to a laparotomy, the usual approach is to treat clinical stage I and II intermediate-grade NHL patients with either six cycles of a chemotherapy regimen such as CHOP-Rituxan or three cycles of CHOP-Rituxan in conjunction with involved-field radiation therapy. In a randomized clinical trial, combined-modality therapy (chemotherapy plus radiotherapy) was associated with a projected 5-year progression-free survival of 77% as compared with a projected 5-year progression-free survival of 64% in patients receiving chemotherapy alone. However, with further follow-up, the survival curves have become almost overlapping, putting in doubt the superior value of combined-modality therapy in limited-stage patients.

V.   Therapy of low-grade NHL. As follicular small cleaved cell lymphoma (follicular lymphoma grade I) represents most cases of low-grade lymphoma, the following discussion relates to the management of that disease entity. Although the terms *follicular small cleaved cell lymphoma* and *low-grade lymphoma* are used somewhat interchangeably in the medical literature, it must be recognized that other disorders are included in the category "low-grade lymphoma," including small B-cell lymphoma (the nodal counterpart of chronic lymphocytic leukemia) and nodal marginal zone lymphoma. Most studies of low-grade lymphoma involve patient populations in which follicular small cleaved cell lymphomas are a majority, but not the totality, of the cases.

Follicular small cleaved cell lymphomas are associated with widespread disease at presentation. Bone marrow involvement is the most easily demonstrated site of advanced disease as it is found in 55% to 65% of cases on routine bone marrow biopsy. In patients whose bone marrow is negative by light microscopy, sensitive molecular techniques have often shown bone marrow involvement. This suggests that the true incidence of bone marrow involvement is at least 90% and may actually be close to 100%.

A.   Watchful waiting. Despite the advanced stage of disease at presentation, median survival in most series of patients with low-grade NHL ranges from 5 to 12 years. Patients are often "treated" initially with "watchful waiting," a strategy of watching the patient until the tumor burden is substantial or until symptoms develop. This is, in essence, the strategy used in chronic lymphocytic leukemia, when patients with elevated white blood cell counts and moderate adenopathy are simply observed until the disease becomes more advanced, as indicated by the development of anemia and/or thrombocytopenia. Often, patients can be followed for years without treatment. In a randomized trial, overall survival was similar for patients initially receiving aggressive combination chemotherapy as compared with those receiving no initial treatment. Although aggressive therapy led to patients spending more time in complete remission, the occurrence of myelodysplasia in the aggressively treated group prevented such therapy from achieving a therapeutic advantage.

B.   Chemotherapy. Alternatively, patients may be treated with single-agent chlorambucil, single-agent fludarabine, antibody therapy (such as rituximab), combination chemotherapy, or a combination of chemotherapy and rituximab.

- **Chlorambucil** is generally employed at a dose of 2 to 4 mg PO daily or 30 to 60 mg PO every 2 weeks.
- **Fludarabine** is generally administered at a dose of 25 mg/m^2 IV daily for 5 days every 4 weeks.

Combination chemotherapy regimens have produced complete remissions in up to 80% of patients. However, such remissions are not durable, and the administration of combination chemotherapy may be associated with myelotoxicity, nausea, vomiting, and neurotoxicity. In general, clinicians tend to avoid anthracyclines as part of initial chemotherapy in these patients. As therapy is palliative, in view of the age of the patients, the toxicity of anthracyclines may be disproportionate to the relative benefit of using a regimen such as CVP (see Table 23.5 for a description of individual regimens). Although combination chemotherapy is associated with higher response rates, it must be recognized that aggressive therapy has not been proved to produce superior overall survival in these patients.

For patients who relapse following initial therapy, several options are available. If initial therapy has been low-dose chlorambucil, a regimen such as CHOP, CNOP, or FND (see Table 23.5) would be reasonable. These regimens can be administered with or without the inclusion of rituximab. Another alternative for patients relapsing after initial treatment, or failing to respond to initial therapy, is the use of one of the salvage regimens designed for use in intermediate-grade lymphoma, that is, a regimen such as DHAP, ESHAP, MINT, or ICE (Table 23.6). As low-grade lymphomas are associated with prolonged survival despite multiple recurrences, there is no single clinical algorithm to be applied to all patients. Palliative treatments should be individualized on the basis of extent of disease, clinical pace of disease, and age of the patient.

C. Antibody therapy. Rituximab is an antibody to CD20, an antigen generally found on B lymphocytes. A dose of 375 mg/m^2/week × 4 to 8 weeks has become a popular choice for the therapy of low-grade lymphoma as the drug is effective in approximately half of the patients treated and has

Table 23.5. Initial combination chemotherapy regimens for non–Hodgkin's lymphoma

CVP[a]

  Cyclophosphamide 400–600 mg/m^2 IV on day 1
  Vincristine (Oncovin) 1.4 mg/m^2 IV on day 1 (maximum 2 mg)
  Prednisone 100 mg PO on days 1–5
   Repeat every 21 days

CHOP

  Cyclophosphamide 750 mg/m^2 IV on day 1
  Doxorubicin (Adriamycin) 50 mg/m^2 IV on day 1
  Vincristine (Oncovin) 1.4 mg/m^2 IV on day 1 (maximum 2 mg)
  Prednisone 100 mg PO on days 1–5
   Repeat every 21 days

FND

  Fludarabine 25 mg/m^2 IV on days 1–3
  Mitoxantrone (Novantrone) 10 mg/m^2 IV on day 1
  Dexamethasone 20 mg/m^2 PO on days 1–5
   Repeat every 21–28 days

[a]Primarily used in low-grade lymphoma.

Table 23.6. Combination chemotherapy regimens useful as salvage regimens in non–Hodgkin's lymphoma

ESHAP

Etoposide 60 mg/m^2 IV on days 1–4

Methylprednisolone 500 mg IV on days 1–4

Cytarabine 2 g/m^2 over 2 h on day 5[a]

Cisplatin 25 mg/m^2/d continuous infusion on days 1–4

Repeat every 28 days

DHAP

Dexamethasone 40 mg PO or IV on days 1–4

Cytarabine 2 g/m^2 IV over 2 h every 12 h for two doses on day 2[a]

Cisplatin 100 mg/m^2 continuous infusion over 24 h, day 1

Repeat every 3–4 weeks

MINT

Ifosfamide 1.3 g/m^2 IV over 1 h on days 1, 2, 3

Mesna 1.3 g/m^2 IV with ifosfamide on days 1, 2, 3

Mesna 1.3 g/m^2 IV over 1 h, 6 h after ifosfamide

Mitoxantrone 8 mg/m^2 IV on day 1 only

Paclitaxel (Taxol) 27.5 mg/m^2/day IV by continuous infusion × 4 days

Repeat every 3–4 weeks

ICE (one of several regimens with these three agents)

Ifosfamide 1,000 mg/m^2 IV over 1 h (h 0–1) on days 1 and 2

Etoposide (VP-16) 150 mg/m^2 IV b.i.d. (h 1–11 and 12–24) on days 1 and 2

Carboplatin 200 mg/m^2 IV (h 11–12) on days 1 and 2

Mesna 333 mg/m^2 IV 30 min before ifosfamide and 4 and 8 h after each dose of ifosfamide

Repeat every 3–4 weeks

[a]If age is >70 years, reduce to 1 g/m^2.

minimal toxicity. Although maintenance rituximab therapy can increase disease-free survival, there is no proof that such maintenance therapy produces better long-term results than can be obtained by simply waiting to use rituximab until the patient experiences a relapse.

Iodine-131 labeled tositumomab (Bexxar) and yttrium-90-labeled ibritumomab tiuxetan (Zevalin) have entered the clinical arena in the last 5 years. Both these radioimmuno-conjugates employ antibodies to CD20. However, the presence of radioactivity means that the drugs can be effective not only in cells that are CD20 positive but in nearby cells that lack CD20. Because of potential marrow toxicity, such therapy has been employed only when marrow involvement by tumor is less than 25%. Using Bexxar, response rates of 47% to 68%, with complete responses of 20% to 38% have been reported in patients relapsing after chemotherapy or refractory to rituximab; 30% of patients experienced long remissions (1–10 years). When used as initial therapy, Bexxar produced an overall response rate of 95% with 75% complete responses. By life-table estimate, 77% of patients with a complete remission are disease free at 5 years. However, considering that low-grade lymphoma is considered an incurable disease in which aggressive combination chemotherapy has not been shown to improve overall survival, the role of radioimmunoconjugates as initial therapy of low-grade lymphoma has yet to be established.

D. High-dose chemotherapy with stem cell transplantation. Another approach to low-grade NHL involves the use of very high dose chemotherapy, with or without total-body radiation therapy, in conjunction with autologous bone marrow or stem cell transplantation. This approach is limited by the fact that the bone marrow and presumably the peripheral blood are frequently involved in low-grade lymphoma. Even when genetic markers such as *bcl-2* are used to confirm successful purging of tumor cells, lymphoma may not be completely removed from the reinfused stem cell product. Autologous transplantation has produced long-term disease-free survival in patients whose disease remains sensitive to chemotherapy at the time of transplantation. However, as with other therapies for low-grade lymphoma, there is no evidence that these results represent cures. Additionally, the optimal timing of such therapy (after one, two, or three chemotherapy regimens), the optimal preparative regimen (with or without total-body irradiation), and the value of purging are issues that have not been resolved. The best results have been obtained in patients with sensitive disease who have received minimal therapy. However, as lead-time and selection bias confound these observations, autologous transplantation has not been established as part of standard therapy for low-grade lymphoma. Although allogeneic transplantation eliminates the risk of reinfusing tumor cells, it is associated with intrinsic risks such as graft-versus-host disease. Clinical results using allogeneic transplantation in this disorder have been highly variable, and the role of allogeneic transplantation in low-grade lymphoma (with either full intensity or reduced intensity preparative regimens) requires further evaluation. Nevertheless, it appears that allogeneic transplantation is the one approach to low-grade lymphoma that has a potential to achieve cure.

VI.   Therapy of intermediate-grade NHL. The most common intermediate-grade lymphoma is large B-cell lymphoma. Also included in this category are diffuse mixed cell lymphomas, diffuse small cleaved cell lymphoma, mantle cell lymphoma, immunoblastic lymphoma of B-cell origin, T-cell rich B-cell lymphoma, ALCL (generally a T-cell disease), and peripheral T-cell lymphoma. Although recommendations can be made for intermediate-grade lymphomas as if they were a single entity, one must recognize that some of the entities behave in a distinct manner. Specifically, although it is said that intermediate-grade lymphomas have a response rate between 70% and 80% and a cure rate between 40% and 50%, patients with peripheral T-cell lymphoma have a slightly lower response rate and are rarely cured (with the exception of ALK-positive ALCL and the small minority of peripheral T-cell lymphoma patients with low IPI). Additionally, patients with mantle cell lymphoma have a high

Table 26.2.   Treatment guidelines for Kaposi's sarcoma[a]

Disease Status of KS	HIV Disease Status	Treatment Options
Minimal cutaneous disease	CD4 count <200/μL; prior OI; B symptoms	Local therapy
	CD4 count $\geq$200/μL; no prior OI; no B symptoms	Interferon and antivirals or local therapy
Isolated, cosmetically disturbing disease	Any	Local therapy
Extensive cutaneous disease	CD4 count <200/μL; prior OI; B symptoms	Chemotherapy
	CD4 count $\geq$200/μL; no prior OI; no B symptoms	Interferon and antivirals or chemotherapy
Localized bulky or painful disease	Any	Radiation therapy or chemotherapy
Tumor-associated edema	Any	Chemotherapy
Symptomatic visceral disease	Any	Chemotherapy

HIV, human immunodeficiency virus; KS, Kaposi's sarcoma; OI, opportunistic infection.

[a] Best antiviral therapy is always a component of KS therapy.

Adapted with permission from Susan Krown SE. Highly active antiretroviral therapy in AIDS-associated Kaposi's sarcoma: implications for the design of therapeutic trials in patients with advanced, symptomatic Kaposi's sarcoma. *J Clin Oncol* 2004;22:399–402.

patients typically slough the oral mucosa in 24 to 48 hours, for which narcotic analgesics should be empirically provided. Intralesional IFN-α is occasionally effective even in patients who have failed systemic IFN. Topical alitretinoin has been approved for the local therapy of KS. The 0.1% retinoic acid gel is applied initially twice a day with escalation to three or four daily doses as tolerated. Overall

Table 26.3.   Intralesional chemotherapy for Kaposi's sarcoma

Chemotherapy Regimen[a]	Dosage
Vinblastine (0.2 mg/mL)	0.1 mL/0.5 cm of surface area of lesion (maximum 4 mL)
Interferon-α	3–5 $\times$ 10^6 U three times/week for 4 weeks

[a] Appropriate local anesthesia should be given before injection.

response rate but almost always have a relapse and die within a few years of diagnosis.

The clinical progress in treating intermediate-grade lymphoma not only represents one of the major success stories of modern oncology, but also represents a major caution regarding the problems associated with overinterpreting uncontrolled clinical observations. In the 1960s, patients with these lymphomas were routinely treated with single-agent therapy, usually chlorambucil. The median survival was 6 months; the 2-year survival rate was only 5% to 10%; cures were rare. In the early 1970s, parallel to the observation that MOPP (nitrogen mustard, Oncovin, procarbazine, and prednisone) could cure HL, workers at the National Cancer Institute reported that COPP (a regimen that substituted cyclophosphamide for nitrogen mustard) could produce complete remissions in 41% of patients with "histiocytic lymphoma" and long-term disease-free survival in 35%. This result was confirmed and slightly improved with investigators who used the CHOP regimen, a regimen that substituted doxorubicin (hydroxydaunorubicin, Adriamycin) for procarbazine.

The studies with COPP and CHOP established the basic principles regarding the chemotherapy of intermediate-grade lymphoma. First, the studies established that some patients within this group of lymphomas are curable with combination chemotherapy, although, with further data collection, we have come to realize that some subsets of patients, such as those with peripheral T-cell lymphoma, may be less curable than other subsets of intermediate-grade lymphoma. Second, the studies demonstrated that depending on how a complete remission is defined, from 60% to 80% of complete remissions represent cures. Many patients with lymphoma have residual masses upon completion of therapy. These residual masses may represent "scar" or may represent persistent disease. If the term *complete remission* is used only for patients who have no progression of residual masses for 3 months following completion of therapy, up to 80% of complete remissions may represent cures. Third, although complete remissions do not necessarily represent cures, complete remissions that persist for 2 years represent cures almost 95% of the time; that is, relapses after 2 years of remission are uncommon, although they do occur.

In the decade following the publication of the results of the CHOP regimen, a number of more intense combination chemotherapy regimens were studied in uncontrolled, single-institution, phase II studies. These regimens, shown in Table 23.7, suggested that long-term complete remission might be achieved in up to 75% of patients as compared with the 40% to 45% range observed with CHOP. However, even before randomized trials were conducted, there were several reasons to suspect that the improvement might be less than was suggested by uncontrolled phase II studies. First, as regimens became more dose intense, older patients, who generally do worse than younger patients, were selectively excluded on the grounds that they would be unable to tolerate the more intense therapy. The median age in the early CHOP study was 58 years; the median age in the MACOP-B study was 44 years. Second, with the demonstration that stage II disease was not routinely curable with radiation therapy, stage II patients became eligible for new

Table 23.7.   Combination chemotherapy regimens used as primary treatment of intermediate-grade lymphoma

CHOP[a]

Cyclophosphamide 750 mg/m^2 IV on day 1

Doxorubicin (Adriamycin) 50 mg/m^2 IV on day 1

Vincristine (Oncovin) 1.4 mg/m^2 IV on day 1 (maximum 2 mg)

Prednisone 100 mg PO on days 1–5

   Repeat every 21 days

CHOP plus rituximab[a]

Rituximab 375 mg/m^2 IV on day 1

Cyclophosphamide 750 mg/m^2 IV on day 3

Doxorubicin (Adriamycin) 50 mg/m^2 IV on day 3

Vincristine (Oncovin) 1.4 mg/m^2 IV on day 3 (maximum 2 mg)

Prednisone 100 mg PO on days 3–7

   Repeat every 21 days

BACOP

Bleomycin 5 U/m^2 IV on days 15 and 22

Doxorubicin (Adriamycin) 25 mg/m^2 IV on days 1 and 8

Cyclophosphamide 650 mg/m^2 IV on days 1 and 8

Vincristine (Oncovin) 1.4 mg/m^2 IV on days 1 and 8 (maximum 2 mg)

Prednisone 60 mg/m^2 PO on days 15–28

   Repeat every 28 days

m-BACOD

Methotrexate 200 mg/m^2 IV on days 1 and 8

Leucovorin 10 mg/m^2 PO q6h for 8 doses, start 24 h after methotrexate

Bleomycin 4 U/m^2 IV on day 1

Doxorubicin (Adriamycin) 45 mg/m^2 IV on day 1

Cyclophosphamide 600 mg/m^2 IV on day 1

Vincristine (Oncovin) 1 mg/m^2 IV on day 1 (maximum 2 mg)

Dexamethasone 6 mg/m^2 PO on days 1–5

   Repeat every 21 days

MACOP-B

Methotrexate 400 mg/m^2 IV weeks 2, 6, 10; one-fourth of dose as IV bolus, then three-fourths of dose over 4 h

Leucovorin 15 mg/m^2 PO q6h for 6 doses, start 24 h after each methotrexate dose

Doxorubicin (Adriamycin) 50 mg/m^2 IV in weeks 1, 3, 5, 7, 9, 11

Cyclophosphamide 350 mg/m^2 IV in weeks 1, 3, 5, 7, 9, 11

Vincristine (Oncovin) 1.4 mg/m^2 IV (maximum 2 mg), in weeks 2, 4, 6, 8, 10, 12

Bleomycin 10 U/m^2 IV in weeks 2, 4, 6, 8, 10, 12

Prednisone 75 mg/day PO for 12 weeks, taper to zero during weeks 10–12

[a]CHOP and CHOP-rituximab are considered the standard regimens.

chemotherapy regimens. By contrast, the early CHOP study contained only stage III and IV patients. As patients with lesser stages of disease would be expected to do better, including them in studies of newer regimens would favorably bias the results achieved with those regimens.

The key study regarding the role of chemotherapy in intermediate-grade lymphoma was the Intergroup Study, which randomly assigned patients with intermediate-grade lymphoma to CHOP, m-BACOD, MACOP-B, and ProMACE-CYtaBOM. Contrary to the expectations of clinicians who felt that these regimens were clearly better than CHOP, there were no significant differences among the regimens with respect to survival or disease-free survival. For all regimens, actuarial survival was between 40% and 45%.

A. Initial chemotherapy. Thus, until recently, CHOP remained the standard-of-care chemotherapy regimen for patients with intermediate-grade lymphoma. Randomized clinical trials have found higher remission rates to be associated with addition of rituximab to CHOP chemotherapy and **CHOP-rituximab has become a standard approach for treating these patients**. A population study has been reported from the Canadian province of British Columbia looking at all patients treated between 1999 and 2002; approximately half the number of patients were treated before rituximab became part of standard therapy and the other half were treated with rituximab as part of the initial combination regimen. Two-year progression-free survival increased significantly from 51% to 69% with the addition of rituximab; 2-year overall survival increased significantly from 52% to 78%.

B. Secondary chemotherapy. The fact that only 40% to 45% of patients with intermediate-grade lymphoma are cured with standard combination chemotherapy (at least before rituximab) means that most patients eventually become candidates for second-line treatment. Salvage chemotherapy regimens (see Table 23.6) can produce responses in 50% to 60% of patients, with 20% to 30% of patients achieving complete remission. However, cures with salvage chemotherapy are uncommon and occur in approximately 5% of patients.

C. High-dose chemotherapy with stem cell transplantation. As salvage chemotherapy rarely produces a cure, the standard approach to patients with relapsed or refractory intermediate-grade lymphoma has been to initiate salvage chemotherapy and to proceed to autologous stem cell transplantation in patients who respond to salvage therapy. The optimal preparative regimen for autologous transplantation has not been determined. Although some studies have suggested that results are equivalent whether total-body irradiation is included in the preparative regimen or not, even this point has not been firmly established.

1. Salvage chemotherapy and autologous transplantation. In a randomized clinical trial, patients with intermediate-grade lymphoma who were responding to salvage chemotherapy were randomized to continue on salvage chemotherapy or to switch over to high-dose therapy in conjunction with stem cell transplantation. **Five-year event-free survival was significantly**

higher in the group that switched to autologous transplantation (46%) as compared with 5-year event-free survival in the patients who continued on salvage chemotherapy (12%) (*p* = 0.001). Survival was also significantly better in the patients who switched to autologous transplantation as compared to survival in patients who continued to receive conventional salvage chemotherapy (53% vs. 32%, respectively; *p* < 0.05).

2. Autologous therapy as consolidation chemotherapy. With autologous transplantation being shown to be effective as salvage treatment in intermediate-grade NHL, a logical issue to pursue is whether such therapy might be effective for consolidation of complete remission. However, results using high-dose therapy as part of initial therapy have not consistently shown a clinical benefit and the role of this approach needs to be clarified by further clinical trials. Although this approach has the potential for increasing cures, it obviously subjects patients who can be cured by standard chemotherapy to unnecessary risks.

D. Advanced age and comorbid disease. The incidence of lymphoma increases with age. Thus, a common clinical problem involves the selection of appropriate therapy for a patient with intermediate-grade NHL over the age of 70 or older than 60 with significant comorbid disease. Clearly, older patients should not be denied a chance of cure on the basis of age alone, and elderly patients with good performance status and well-controlled comorbid disease are good candidates for curative therapy. Despite considerable efforts to design less intensive, better-tolerated therapies for older patients, there is no firm evidence that any of these regimens is equivalent to CHOP. The best strategy, therefore, is to attempt to administer CHOP plus rituxan therapy and use growth factors such as granulocyte colony-stimulating factor (G-CSF) or granulocyte–macrophage colony-stimulating factor (GM-CSF) starting with cycle 1 to limit marrow toxicity.

VII. Therapy of high-grade NHL. The most commonly seen high-grade lymphomas are Burkitt's and Burkitt's-like lymphoma, lymphoblastic lymphoma, and peripheral T-cell lymphomas (excluding anaplastic large cell lymphoma [ALCL], which has a prognosis similar to other intermediate-grade lymphomas). Because these diseases have different clinical manifestations, it is most reasonable to consider them separately.

A. Burkitt's lymphoma and Burkitt's-like lymphoma. These diseases have similar morphologic features and a similar prognosis. They are both B-cell lymphomas of small noncleaved cells, and both have been associated with a t(8;14) translocation. In the United States, Burkitt's lymphoma tends to occur in younger patients and to be associated with a higher incidence of gastrointestinal disease and a lower incidence of bone marrow involvement. Both diseases are relatively resistant to standard chemotherapy regimens such as CHOP as that therapy is generally associated with a median survival between 6 and 10 months. More intense therapy such as the high-intensity brief-duration regimen, the hyper-CVAD regimen, and the CODOX-M/IVAC regimen presented in Table 23.8 have been associated with long-term disease-free survival in

Table 23.8.   Therapy for high-grade lymphoma

High-intensity brief-duration therapy

Cyclophosphamide 1,500 mg/m^2 IV on days 1, 2, and 29

Etoposide 300 mg/m^2 IV on days 1, 2, and 3

Etoposide 100 mg/m^2 IV on days 29, 30, and 31; Cisplatin 30 mg/m^2
   IV on days 1, 2, 3, 29, 30, and 31

Doxorubicin 45 mg/m^2 IV on days 29 and 30

Prednisone 60 mg/m^2 PO on days 1–7 and on days 29–35

Vincristine 1.4 mg/m^2 IV on days 8, 22, 36, and 50 (capped at 2 mg)

Bleomycin 10 U/m^2 IV on days 8, 22, 36, and 50

Methotrexate 200 mg/m^2 IV on days 15, and 43

Leucovorin rescue 15 mg/m^2 IV or PO every 6 h for six doses,
   starting 24 h after methotrexate

Hyper-CVAD[a]

Cycles 1, 3, 5, and 7

   Cyclophosphamide 300 mg/m^2 IV over 2 h, every 12 h, for six
      doses

   Mesna 600 mg/m^2 IV daily, on days 1–3, starting 1 h before
      cyclophosphamide and completed 12 h after the last
      cyclophosphamide dose

   Vincristine 2 mg IV on days 4 and 11

   Doxorubicin 50 mg/m^2 IV over 2 h on day 4

   Dexamethasone 40 mg/day IV or PO on days 1–4 and 11–14

Cycles 2, 4, 6, and 8

   Methotrexate 1 g/m^2 IV over 24 h on day 1, *and*

   Leucovorin 50 mg IV to start 12 h after methotrexate, then
      15 mg IV every 6 h until serum methotrexate $<1 \times 10^{-8}$
      M, and

   Cytarabine 3 g/m^2 IV infusion over 1 h every 12 h × 4 doses on
      days 2 and 3 (reduce cytarabine dose to 1 g/m^2 for
      patients older than 60 years)

CODOX-M/IVAC

Cycles 1 and 3

   Cyclophosphamide 800 mg/m^2 IV on day 1

   Vincristine 1.5 mg/m^2 (maximum 2 mg) IV on days 1 and 8

   Doxorubicin 40 mg/m^2 IV on day 1

   Cytosine arabinoside 70 mg intrathecal on days 1 and 3

   Cyclophosphamide 200 mg/m^2 IV on days 2, 3, 4, and 5

   Methotrexate 1200 mg/m^2 IV over one h followed by 240 mg/m^2
      hourly for 23 h starting on day 10

   Leucovorin 192 mg/m^2 IV at h 36 of methotrexate therapy

   Leucovorin 12 mg/m^2 IV every 6 h until methotrextae level is
      $<5 \times 10^{-8}$ M

   G-CSF 5 mg/kg SC daily starting on day 13

   Methotrexate 12 mg intrathecal on day 15

   Leucovorin 15 mg PO 24 h after methotrexate

(continued)

Table 23.8.   (Continued)

Cycles 2 and 4

Etoposide 60 mg/m^2 IV over 1 h, daily, on days 1–5

Ifosfamide 1500 mg/m^2 IV over 1 h daily, on days 1–5

Mesna 360 mg/m^2 IV with ifosfamide, then every 3 h for seven additional doses each 24 h

Cytosine arabinoside 2 g/m^2 IV, over 3 h, every 12 h, for four total doses on day 1 and day 2

Methotrexate 12 mg intrathecal on day 5

Leucovorin 15 mg PO 24 h after methotrexate

G-CSF 5 μg/kg SC daily starting on day 7

G-CSF, granulocyte colony-stimulating factor.
[a]Filgrastim (G-CSF) should be administered starting on day 4 and again on day 32, and continued until granulocyte recovery occurs.

almost 50% of patients, but these results are dependent on stage. Patients with disease involving the CNS or bone marrow or with marked elevation of LDH levels have an especially poor prognosis. Salvage therapy with or without stem cell transplantation is less effective in high-grade lymphoma as compared with intermediate-grade lymphoma, especially when high-dose therapy is used as initial treatment. The role of stem cell transplantation in routine consolidation following initial high-dose therapy has not been established by clinical trials.

B. Lymphoblastic lymphoma. Lymphoblastic lymphoma is usually a T-cell malignancy that can be regarded as a variant of T-cell acute lymphoblastic leukemia (ALL). This disorder commonly presents with a mediastinal mass and bone marrow involvement. ALL-type therapy is most commonly employed to treat lymphoblastic lymphoma (see Chapter 19). However, excellent results have been reported with a regimen devised at Stanford University, which includes a CHOP-like induction, CNS prophylaxis, and consolidation that includes methotrexate and 6-mercaptopurine. In the initial report of this regimen, patients with marrow involvement, CNS involvement, and elevated LDH levels had a 5-year survival of only 19%, whereas patients without these features had a 5-year survival of 94%. Unfortunately, further studies of other regimens have not established that marrow involvement, CNS involvement, and LDH are the sole reliable prognostic factors in lymphoblastic lymphoma. As with Burkitt's lymphoma, high-dose therapy followed by stem cell transplantation as consolidation is a rational approach but one which has not been proven by randomized clinical trials.

C. Peripheral T-cell lymphomas. For many years, controversy has existed over whether the T-cell lymphomas included in intermediate-grade lymphoma have a prognosis that is the same as or worse than that of the B-cell lymphomas that make up most intermediate-grade lymphomas. Over the last several years, clinical pathologic studies have shed some light on this important issue. First, the entity of T-cell–rich B-cell lymphomas has been identified. These lymphomas are

B-cell lymphomas and have a prognosis similar to that of other B-cell lymphomas. However, as most cells in the lymphoma are nonmalignant T cells, these lymphomas may have been included in studies of T-cell lymphoma, falsely improving the prognosis. Second, the category of T-cell lymphomas includes ALCL, a group of lymphomas that have a prognosis similar to that of B-cell lymphomas. Once these lymphomas are excluded, the remaining T-cell lymphomas have a prognosis that is worse than that of B-cell intermediate-grade lymphomas, and as a result, the category of peripheral T-cell lymphomas may be considered as high-grade lymphomas, although this is not accepted by all investigators and clinicians.

Peripheral T-cell lymphomas are a heterogeneous group of lymphomas that constitute approximately 5% to 7% of adult NHLs (see Table 23.3). CHOP therapy is generally associated with long-term survival in 0% to 20% of patients with these disorders. With the exception of infrequent cases of peripheral T-cell lymphoma with low IPI, which do relatively well with CHOP, no optimal therapy for these patients has been defined, and the most rational course seems to be the use of one of the regimens employed for Burkitt's or Burkitt's-like lymphoma (see Table 23.8), or to employ a strategy that includes early transplantation. Active single agents that are under investigation for future inclusion in combination chemotherapy regimens for T-cell lymphomas include nucleoside analogues (gemcitabine, pentostatin), histone deacetylators (depsipeptide), and monoclonal antibodies (denileukin diftitox and alemtuzumab).

VIII. Therapy of other lymphomas. The classification of NHL into low grade, intermediate grade, and high grade is an oversimplification of this complex group of disorders. While a consideration of every entity is beyond the scope of this chapter, a number of subtypes of lymphoma have specific features that are worth noting.

A. Mantle cell lymphomas are composed of small B lymphocytes. The cell of origin is the mantle zone cell, which surrounds the lymphoid follicle and not the follicular center cell of follicular lymphoma. These lymphomas have a diffuse pattern, are generally CD5 positive and CD23 negative, are positive for cyclin D-1, and are associated with a t(11;14) chromosomal translocation. These lymphomas used to be included in low-grade lymphoma and were often regarded as diffuse forms of small cleaved cell follicular lymphoma. However, in contrast to small cleaved cell lymphoma, median survival in this type of lymphoma is between 3 and 4 years. Although responses are seen with CHOP, relapses are the rule rather than the exception, and cure is rarely, if ever, seen. The high incidence of marrow involvement limits the use of autologous stem cell transplantation, and early encouraging results using this approach as consolidation or salvage therapy have not been confirmed. This has led some investigators to advocate aggressive chemotherapy followed by allogeneic transplantation as consolidation therapy in this group of lymphomas. However, further data will be necessary to establish the role of that approach in mantle cell lymphoma.

B. Maltomas are *m*ucosa-*a*ssociated *l*ymphoid *t*umors, which are low-grade B-cell lymphomas that can occur at a number of sites including conjunctiva, thyroid, salivary gland, and gastrointestinal tract. Maltomas tend to be localized and are associated with a better survival than other low-grade lymphomas. Maltomas of the stomach have been associated with infection by *Helicobacter pylori,* and cures have been achieved with eradication of *H. pylori* by the use of antibiotics. This suggests that certain lymphomas may require continued antigenic stimulation in order to persist.

C. Anaplastic large cell lymphomas (ALCLs) are usually T-cell lymphomas, though null cell forms of ALCL exist. The lymphomas can be associated with a t(2;5) translocation and are generally CD30 positive. However, CD30 is not pathognomonic for ALCL as it may also be seen in HL, other B-cell and T-cell lymphomas, embryonal carcinoma, and seminoma. ALK-positive ALCL is commonly seen in young patients, usually is disseminated with nodal and extranodal sites (skin, bone), and has a prognosis similar to large B-cell lymphoma. ALK-negative ALCL involving lymph nodes is more resistant to chemotherapy. Additionally, there is a primary cutaneous form of ALK-negative ALCL, which is associated with a more indolent prognosis than node-based ALCL. The fact that ALCL limited to the skin is generally negative for t(2;5), i.e., ALK negative, suggests that these different forms of ALCL may have different etiologies.

IX. Special considerations

A. Central nervous system (CNS) prophylaxis. Involvement of the CNS by NHL is almost exclusively limited to small noncleaved cell lymphoma (Burkitt's and Burkitt's-like) and lymphoblastic lymphoma. As marrow involvement has been present in most cases with CNS involvement, a rational policy is to give intrathecal methotrexate and cranial irradiation to patients with these high-grade lymphomas and bone marrow involvement. Whether patients with intermediate-grade lymphoma and bone marrow involvement should receive CNS prophylaxis is not known. However, as testicular and nasopharyngeal involvement with intermediate-grade lymphoma is associated with an increased risk of CNS disease, such patients are rational candidates for CNS prophylaxis. As low-grade lymphomas do not involve the CNS unless transformation to intermediate-grade lymphoma has occurred, CNS prophylaxis is not needed for low-grade lymphoma despite the high incidence of bone marrow disease in these patients.

B. Lymphomas in patients with human immunodeficiency virus (HIV) infection. (Also see Chapter 26.) Among patients with HIV infection, 3% to 6% develop lymphoma. Lymphoma is an acquired immune deficiency syndrome (AIDS)–defining illness, and it is estimated that approximately one-fourth of new cases of NHL occur in patients with HIV. The lymphomas are generally intermediate-grade lymphoma (diffuse large B-cell lymphoma) and high-grade lymphoma (small noncleaved cell lymphoma). Over the last 15 years, there has been a histopathologic shift, and large B-cell lymphoma is now the most common lymphoma seen in these patients. Additionally, with the use of highly active antiretroviral therapy (HAART), the incidence of primary CNS lymphoma has decreased.

With the introduction of HAART, the incidence of AIDS-related lymphoma (ARL) decreased and the prognosis for patients with ARL has improved. Before HAART, median survival of patients with HIV who developed ARL was 5 months to 8 months for systemic disease and 2 months for patients with CNS lymphoma. For patients with systemic ARL in the era of HAART, median survival approaches 20 months. In view of the poor prognosis of these patients and their underlying immunosuppression, chemotherapy regimens characterized by dose reductions (such as half-dose or three-fourths–dose CHOP) have been investigated in patients with ARL. These regimens do not improve clinical results and standard dose regimens for lymphoma are recommended in patients with ARL. One *caveat* to this recommendation is that rituximab appears to augment the response to CHOP in patients without HIV infection, whereas in patients with HIV infection, the immunosuppression caused by rituximab appears to balance out an antitumor effect. As a result, **the role of rituximab in therapy of ARL is not established and requires further investigation.**

Patients with NHL and HIV infection should be evaluated for the presence of CNS disease including the presence of meningeal disease. If symptomatic CNS disease is present, therapy is indicated with an aim of improving quality, if not quantity, of life.

C. Extranodal lymphomas. NHLs arise at extranodal sites in approximately 10% to 20% of cases. In the past, these patients were often treated with radiation therapy alone. However, with extensive evidence that chemotherapy with or without radiation therapy can produce excellent results in patients with stage I lymphomas, these patients are rarely treated with radiation therapy alone. Certain extranodal sites present special considerations for which specific comments are needed.

  1. Stomach. The most common site for extranodal lymphoma is the stomach. Approximately one half of all gastric lymphomas are maltomas, and the next most common histology is large B-cell lymphoma (intermediate-grade lymphoma). Approximately two-thirds of gastric maltomas respond to antibiotic therapy for *H. pylori*. For gastric lymphomas not related to *H. pylori*, therapy is dependent upon histology and stage and may include chemotherapy, rituximab, and/or radiation therapy; chemotherapy is the treatment modality of choice. In the past, surgery was part of the standard therapy for gastric lymphomas owing to the risk of perforation during therapy. However, with most tumors diagnosed by endoscopic biopsy, surgery is rarely a part of the management of this disease.

  2. Primary central nervous system (CNS) lymphoma is commonly seen in patients with HIV but is also observed without HIV infection as a predisposition. All patients presenting with primary CNS lymphoma should be evaluated for possible HIV infection. In patients without HIV infection, the most common histologic types of lymphoma are large B-cell lymphoma and immunoblastic lymphoma.

Treatment with radiation therapy alone is generally associated with a median survival of less than 1 year and radiotherapy is no longer the treatment modality of choice for patients with primary CNS lymphoma. Recent trials employing chemotherapy, specifically high-dose methotrexate, as an alternative to radiation have produced superior results, with a median survival between 3 and 5 years. Although combined-modality therapy produces the best results, in patients over the age of 60, combined-modality therapy (chemotherapy plus radiotherapy) has been associated with clinical deterioration due to brain necrosis. Accordingly, an alternative approach is to give chemotherapy alone and reserve radiotherapy until the time of disease progression.

3. Testicular lymphomas represent the most common testicular tumor seen in elderly men, with large B-cell lymphoma being the most common histologic type. Therapy consists of orchiectomy, chemotherapy, and irradiation of the contralateral testis. Additionally, as testicular lymphoma is associated with CNS disease, prophylactic treatment of the CNS is indicated.

4. Nasopharyngeal lymphomas are more commonly seen in Asia than in the United States. In the United States, the most common type of NHL is large B-cell lymphoma. In contrast, the most common histologic type of NHL in Asia is angiocentric lymphoma of T-cell or natural killer (NK) cell origin. Formerly among the disorders included in the category lethal midline granuloma, this highly lethal lymphoma is often treated with radiation therapy and chemotherapy as well as with CNS prophylaxis. However, despite aggressive therapy, survival of greater than 1 year is uncommon.

5. Cutaneous lymphomas include a wide variety of diseases of both B-cell and T-cell origin. The most common cutaneous lymphoma is cutaneous or cerebriform T-cell lymphoma (CTCL), also known as *mycosis fungoides*. When there is generalized erythroderma and involvement of the peripheral blood, the syndrome is known as *Sézary syndrome*. Prognosis in CTCL depends on stage of disease, and special staging systems for CTCL exist (Table 23.9). Clinical Stage IA disease is so indolent that it does not impact on normal life expectancy, while prognosis worsens with more advanced stage of disease. The disease may exist as plaques in the skin for many years before progressing to involve skin tumors, adenopathy, or visceral disease. Often, this clinical progression occurs in association with a pathologic transformation to a large cell lymphoma. If disease is limited to the skin, topical therapy such as topical nitrogen mustard, electron beam radiotherapy, or psoralen in conjunction with ultraviolet radiation may be employed. Combination chemotherapy as employed for intermediate-grade lymphoma may be used for tumor stage of disease or for disease involving nodes or viscera. Unfortunately, such therapy may lead to simultaneous necrosis of skin tumors as well as the development of neutropenia, leading to fatal sepsis. Other approaches to this disease include the use of denileukin diftitox, an antibody to CD25, and bexarotene, a

Table 23.9.   Staging system for cutaneous T-cell lymphoma

Stage I : limited or generalized plaques without adenopathy or histologic involvement of lymph nodes

Stage II : limited or generalized plaques with adenopathy, or cutaneous tumors without adenopathy; without histologic involvement of lymph nodes or viscera

Stage III : generalized erythroderma, with or without adenopathy; without histologic involvement of lymph nodes or viscera

Stage IV : histologic involvement of lymph nodes or viscera with any skin lesions; with or without adenopathy

---

novel retinoid X receptor (RXR)–selective retinoid, or rexinoid. Use of the latter agent is commonly associated with a syndrome of central hypothyroidism as well as abnormal lipid metabolism and patients must be monitored for these complications.

X.   Posttransplant lymphomas. Following organ transplantation and the associated immunosuppression, the most common tumors are skin cancer and NHL. Extranodal sites of disease including the CNS and gastrointestinal tract are commonly observed, and the histologic appearance is that of an intermediate- or high-grade lymphoma. Many of these tumors are associated with Epstein-Barr virus (EBV), and if disease is limited in extent, one can employ therapy designed to increase the host response to EBV, such as withdrawing or decreasing immunosuppression, administering interferon, or giving lymphocytes from individuals who have had EBV infection. Such therapy is most effective in limited disease and in patients in whom the lymphocytes are polyclonal. Surgery or radiotherapy can be effective in localized disease. For more advanced disease and for disease in which the lymphocytes are monoclonal, chemotherapy is necessary, although rituximab has also been shown to be effective in this setting. Unfortunately, response rates are lower for transplant-associated lymphomas than for *de novo* lymphomas, and long-term survival is seen in less than 20% of patients.

SUGGESTED READINGS

Abrey L, Yahalom J, DeAngelis LM. Treatment for primary CNS lymphoma: the next step. *J Clin Oncol* 2000;18:3144–3150.

Banks PM, Chan J, Cleary ML, et al. Mantle cell lymphoma: a proposal for unification of morphologic, immunologic, and molecular data. *Am J Surg Pathol* 1992;16:637–640.

Coleman CN, Picozzi VJ, Cox RS, et al. Treatment of lymphoblastic lymphoma in adults. *J Clin Oncol* 1986;4:1628–1637.

Czuczman MS, Grillo-Lopez AJ, White CA, et al. Treatment of patients with low grade B-cell lymphoma with the combination of chimeric anti CD20 monoclonal antibody and CHOP. *J Clin Oncol* 1999;17:268–276.

Fisher RI, Gaynor ER, Dahlberg S, et al. Comparison of a standard regimen (CHOP) with three intensive chemotherapy regimens for advanced non-Hodgkin's lymphoma. *N Engl J Med* 1993;328:1002–1006.

Greer JP, Kinney MC, Collins RD, et al. Clinical features of 31 patients with Ki-1 anaplastic large-cell lymphoma. *J Clin Oncol* 1991;9:539–547.

Haioun C, Lepage E, Gisselbrecht C, et al. Comparison of autologous bone marrow transplantation with sequential chemotherapy for intermediate-grade and high grade non-Hodgkin's's lymphoma in first complete remission; a study of 464 patients. *J Clin Oncol* 1994;12:2543–2551.

Haioun C, Lepage E, Gisselbrecht C, et al. Benefit of autologous bone marrow transplantation over sequential chemotherapy in poor-risk aggressive non-Hodgkin's lymphoma: updated results of the prospective study LNH87–2. *J Clin Oncol* 1997;15:1131–1137.

Harris NL, Jaffe ES, Stein H, et al. A revised European–American classification of malignant lymphoid neoplasms: a proposal from the International Lymphoma Study Group. *Blood* 1994;84:1361–1392.

International Non-Hodgkin's Lymphoma Prognostic Factors Project. A predictive model for aggressive non-Hodgkin's lymphoma. *N Engl J Med* 1993;329:987–994.

Kaminski MS, Tuck M, Estes J, et al. 131-I-Tositmomab therapy as initial treatment for follicular lymphoma. *N Engl J Med* 2005;352:441–449.

Levine AM, Seneviratne L, Espina BM, et al. Evolving characteristics of AIDS related lymphoma. *Blood* 2000;96:4084–4090.

Maloney D, Grillo-Lopez A, White C, et al. IDEC-C2B8 (Rituxan AB) anti-CD20 monoclonal antibody therapy in patients with relapsed low grade non-Hodgkin's lymphoma. *Blood* 1997;90:2188–2195.

McKelvey EM, Gottleib JA, Wilson HE, et al. Hydroxyldaunomycin (adriamycin) combination chemotherapy in malignant lymphoma. *Cancer* 1976;38:1484–1493.

McMaster ML, Greer JP, Greco FA, et al. Effective treatment of small non-cleaved cell lymphoma with high intensity, brief duration chemotherapy. *J Clin Oncol* 1991;9:941–946.

Miller TP, Dahlberg S, Cassady JR, et al. Chemotherapy alone compared with chemotherapy plus radiotherapy for localized intermediate and high-grade non-Hodgkin's lymphoma. *N Engl J Med* 1998;339:21–26.

Non-Hodgkin's Lymphoma Pathologic Classification Project. National cancer sponsored study of classification of non-Hodgkin's lymphomas: summary and description of a working formulation. *Cancer* 1982;49:2112–2135.

Sehn LH, Donaldson J, Chhanabhai M, et al. Introduction of combined CHOP plus rituximab therapy dramatically improved outcome of diffuse large B-cell lymphoma in British Columbia. *J Clin Oncol* 2005;23:5027–5033.

Thomas DA, Cortes J, O'Brien S, et al. Hyper-CVAD program in Burkitt's type adult acute lymphoblastic lymphoma. *J Clin Oncol* 1999;17:2461–2470.

Young RC, Longo DL, Glatstein E, et al. The treatment of indolent lymphomas: watchful waiting v aggressive combined modality treatment. *Semin Hematol* 1988;25(Suppl 2):11–16.

Zinzani PL, Fanti S, Battista G, et al. Predictive role of positron emission tomography (PET) in the outcome of lymphoma patients. *Br J Cancer* 2004;91:850–854.

CHAPTER 24

Multiple Myeloma, Other Plasma Cell Disorders, and Primary Amyloidosis

Rachid Baz and Mohamad A. Hussein

I. Introduction

A. Types of plasma cell dyscrasias. Plasma cell dyscrasias represent a heterogeneous group of conditions characterized by an increased number of plasma cells and/or by the production of a monoclonal protein (M-protein). The following plasma cell dyscrasias will be discussed in this chapter: monoclonal gammopathy of undetermined significance (MGUS), multiple myeloma (MM), Waldenström's macroglobulinemia (WM), amyloidosis, and solitary plasmacytomas. Light-chain deposition disease, heavy-chain diseases, immunoglobulin (Ig) D multiple myeloma, nonsecretory multiple myeloma, osteosclerotic myeloma or peripheral neuropathy, organomegaly, endocrinopathy, monoclonal gammopathy, skin changes (POEMS) syndrome and primary plasma cell leukemia are beyond the scope of this text.

B. Monoclonal protein (M-protein). A monoclonal protein is detected in the serum and/or urine of most patients with plasma cell dyscrasias. The so-called M-protein is thought to be a measure of plasma cell burden although a correlation is not always evident. A notable discordance between the M-protein and disease burden could be noted in heavily pretreated patients where the malignant cells might have de-differentiated and become less secretory or nonsecretory. This is often accompanied by an increase in the serum lactate dehydrogenase (LDH) level. Exception aside, most plasma cell dyscrasias are best followed by serial measurements of the M-protein and parameters of end organ dysfunction. Current standard criteria rely on changes in the M-protein for determining response and progression after treatment. The basic Ig unit comprises two identical heavy chains (IgG, A, M, D or E) and two identical light chains (κ or λ). The serum protein electrophoresis used to quantify the monoclonal component of the globulin however fails to do so when the concentration of the latter is low because of lack of secretion or secondary to excretion in the urine. If there is a high clinical suspicion for the presence of a M-protein despite a negative electrophoresis, an immunoelectrophoresis should be performed in the serum and the urine as up to 15% of patients could show a negative serum immune fixation with positive urine. The urinary light-chain excretion (ULC, expressed in grams per 24 h) is used to follow the urinary M-protein. This is calculated from the 24 hours urine protein and the percentage contribution of light chain to proteinuria on the urine protein electrophoresis. It is critical to assess the percentage contribution of the light chain to the proteinuria especially in patients with other comorbidities such as hypertension and diabetes mellitus where the patient could present with a M-protein with the proteinuria consisting mainly of albumin secondary to other medical processes. Newer assays for serum free light chain are becoming increasingly available and often result in the detection of increased free light chain in the serum of many patients with nonsecretory MM (negative immune fixation of the serum and urine) and AL (primary or immunoglobulin light chain amyloid) amyloidosis. The latter assay does not demonstrate monoclonality of the light chain but relies on the ratio of κ to λ light chain to infer an excess of one of the light chains. Although some investigators have correlated changes in the free light chain induced by therapy with outcomes, the precise role of these markers beyond their contribution to the diagnosis remains unclear. Infections, autoimmune disorders, and poor renal function make interpretation of the free light-chain assay difficult.

II. Monoclonal gammopathy of undetermined significance (MGUS). This condition is usually characterized by a low M-protein (less than 3 g/dL), the absence of bone lesions, less than 10% plasma cells on the bone marrow biopsy, and the absence of attributable end organ damage such as anemia, hypercalcemia, and renal dysfunction. The prevalence of MGUS increases with age and has been described in as many as 3% of people older than 70 years. The rate of progression from MGUS to MM or other lymphoproliferative disorders varies on the basis of several factors, the most notable of which is the level of the serum M-protein. A high serum M-protein ($\geq$1.5 gm/dL), a higher bone marrow plasma cell burden, and possibly an abnormal κ to λ ratio on free light-chain analysis identify patients at higher risk of progression to MM. Patients with lower-risk MGUS may be followed up on a yearly or biannual basis, whereas patients with higher risk of progression are eligible for enrollment in prevention clinical trial and will probably benefit from closer follow-up. In a small number of patients, MGUS could be associated with peripheral neuropathy. Most patients with MGUS and peripheral neuropathy in association with an IgM M-protein have anti-myelin-associated glycoprotein (MAG) antibodies. This group of patients responds favorably to therapy with single agent rituximab.

III. Multiple myeloma (MM)

   A. General considerations and aims of therapy

      1. Diagnosis. MM is a clonal B-cell tumor of slowly proliferating plasma cells within the bone marrow. Table 24.1 illustrates diagnostic criteria required for a diagnosis of MM. The Durie and Salmon staging system was initially used for the staging of patients with MM (it is illustrated in Table 24.2). Its use has fallen out of favor because of difficulties inherent in its use. One such staging system developed by the Southwest Oncology Group (SWOG) is illustrated in Table 24.3. It relies on the serum β_2-microglobulin and on serum albumin. It was found to accurately prognosticate patient outcomes.

      With increased awareness, an increasing number of patients are being diagnosed with monoclonal gammopathy. A significant percentage of those patients are noted as an

Table 24.1.   Diagnostic criteria of multiple myeloma

Major criteria	1—Plasmacytoma of tissue biopsy
	2—Bone marrow plasmacytosis (greater than 30% plasma cell)
	3—IgG >3.5 g/dL or IgA >2.0 g/dL or urine light-chain excretion >1.0 g/24 h
Minor criteria	1—Bone marrow plasmacytosis (greater than 10% but less than 30% plasma cells)
	2—M-protein present in lower concentration as noted in major criteria
	3–Lytic bone lesions
	4—Hypogammaglobulinemia (IgM <50 mg/dL, IgA <100 mg/dL, or IgG <600 mg/dL)

The diagnosis of multiple myeloma is made in the following cases: any 2 major criteria; major criterion 1 and minor criteria 2, 3, or 4; major criterion 3 and minor criterion 1 or 3; minor criteria 1, 2, and 3, and minor criteria 1, 2, 4.

Table 24.2.   Durie-Salmon staging system

Stage	Criteria
I	All of the following:
	1. Hemoglobin >10 g/dL
	2. Serum calcium value normal ($\leq$12 mg/dL)
	3. On radiograph, normal bone structure or solitary bone plasmacytoma only
	4. Low M component production rates
	a. IgG value <5 g/dL
	b. IgA value <3 g/dL
	c. Urine light-chain M component on electrophoresis <4 g/24 h
II	Fitting neither stage I nor stage III
III	One or more of the following:
	1. Hemoglobin <8.5 g/dL
	2. Serum calcium value >12 mg/dL
	3. Advanced lytic bone lesions
	4. High M component production rates
	a. IgG value >7 g/dL
	b. IgA value >5 g/dL
	c. Urine light-chain M component on electrophoresis >12 g/24 h

Designation A and B are based on serum creatinine (A: serum creatinine <2.0, B: serum creatinine >2.0).
Ig, immunoglobulin.
Durie BG, Salmon SE. A clinical staging system for multiple myeloma.
Correlation of measured myeloma cell mass with presenting clinical features, response to treatment, and survival. *Cancer* 1975;36:842.

Table 24.3. Southwest Oncology Group (SWOG) staging system for multiple myeloma

β_2-Microglobulin (mg/L)	Albumin (g/dL)	SWOG Stage	Percent of Patients (%)	Median Survival (months)
<2.5	Any	I	14	55
≥2.5 and <5.5	Any	II	43	40
≥5.5	≥3.0	III	32	24
≥5.5	<3.0	IV	11	16

incidental finding and the decision to monitor or actively treat has become difficult with the old nomenclature.

a. End organ damage. The international multiple myeloma working group recently presented **the concept of multiple myeloma with active or inactive disease** based on the presence or absence of end organ damage respectively.

b. Criteria defining end organ damage are anemia, thrombocytopenia, renal failure, hypocalcaemia, severe osteoporosis or lytic bony disease, or any organ abnormality *that is attributed to the plasma cell dyscrasia*.

c. Patients without end organ damage should be monitored carefully as early intervention does not affect the outcome of the disease. Patients with inactive MM should be considered for clinical trials.

d. Even though MGUS is considered a premalignant condition, patients who meet the MGUS criteria and demonstrate end organ damage must be classified as having active MM and should receive active therapy.

2. Epidemiology. The annual incidence of MM is 4 per 100,000 population, with a peak incidence between the sixth and seventh decade of life. Patients of African-American descent have an incidence of MGUS and MM approaching twice the incidence for whites in the United States. Several agents have been strongly associated with the development of MM, ionizing radiation being the most described risk factor. Nickel, agricultural chemicals, petroleum products and other aromatic hydrocarbons, benzene and silicon have been considered potential risk factors as well.

3. Goals of therapy. Despite recent advances in the treatment of MM, the disease remains incurable. Accordingly, therapy is aimed at improving symptoms, preventing complications of the disease, thereby improving quality of life and survival. These goals could be achieved with different approaches: one aim is to transform the disease into a chronic process by using frequent low morbidity therapies, whereas the other approach attempts to eradicate the disease with intensive therapy. Currently, it is unclear which treatment methodology is superior; however, there is evidence that certain subgroups of patients might benefit from one or the other approach. With these uncertainties and because standard first-line therapy is not defined, patients with MM, regardless of age, stage of disease, or number of previous therapy must be considered for clinical trial enrollment.

In addition to the management of the malignant plasma cell clone, particular attention must be made to end organ dysfunction including skeletal health, prevention of infections, thrombotic, neuronal, and renal complications. Accordingly, response to therapy is based on changes to the M-protein concentration and the percentage of plasma cells in the bone marrow, and monitoring end organs for further change from baseline has been the tradition. The cooperative oncology groups in the United States and Europe have adopted different cutoffs to define response. Table 24.4 illustrates the response criteria adopted by the European Group for Blood and Marrow Transplantation.

4. Prognostic factors. Severe anemia, hypercalcemia, advanced lytic lesions, and very high M-protein are all associated with a high tumor burden and a poor survival and are the basis of the Durie and Salmon staging system. Renal failure, although not clearly correlated with disease burden, is associated with worse outcomes. Other established clinical poor prognostic factors include the following: advanced age, poor performance status at presentation, high serum LDH level, and lower platelet counts, bone marrow with greater than 50% plasma cells, greater than 2% bone marrow plasmablasts, high plasma cell labeling index, elevated serum β_2-microglobulin, and low serum albumin levels. The latter two are the basis for the SWOG staging system. The identification of cytogenetic prognostic factors using metaphase karyotyping relies on cellular growth, which is difficult as the MM plasma cells have a low proliferative rate, and therefore such information is available only in 20% to 40% of the patients. The presence of abnormalities with this method however is meaningful as it indicates a high proliferative index i.e., aggressive disease. Genomic prognostic factors include the deletion of chromosome 13, translocation of the Ig heavy chain (t(4,14), t(14,16)), and loss of 17p13. The t(11,14) on the other hand is not though to portend a worse outcome. Recently, interphase fluorescence *in situ* hybridization (FISH) has been used to detect specific cytogenetic abnormalities. Even though FISH analysis is more sensitive at detecting certain abnormalities such as chromosome 13, this might not be clinically meaningful without other additional poor prognosticators. Non–hyperdiploid karyotypes are frequently associated with Ig heavy chain rearrangements and worse clinical outcomes.

B. Initial treatment

1. General measures. Patients with a new diagnosis of MM occasionally have associated complications that require immediate attention, such as hypercalcemia, renal failure, severe cytopenias and spinal cord compression. These complications should be promptly identified and managed either simultaneously or before the start of therapy. Alternatively, asymptomatic patients and those

Table 24.4.   Criteria for response by the European Group for Blood and Marrow Transplantation (EBMT), Southwest Oncology Group (SWOG) and Eastern Cooperative Oncology Groups (ECOG)

	EBMT	SWOG	ECOG
Complete remission (CR)	Disappearance of all evidence of serum and urine M components on electrophoresis and by immunofixation studies for 6 weeks	≥75% decrease in calculated tumor mass and ≥ 90% decrease in Bence Jones proteinuria to <0.2 g in 24 h	Disappearance of all evidence of serum and urine M components on electrophoresis and by immunofixation and in the bone marrow
Partial remission (PR)	A >50% reduction in the serum paraprotein, and if present, a >90% reduction in the urine light-chain excretion for 6 weeks	50%–74% decrease in calculated tumor mass and 50–90% decrease in Bence Jones proteinuria	50% decrease in serum M-protein and 24 h urine light-chain excretion. Bence Jones proteinuria must decrease to <10% of baseline
Minimal remission (MR)	A 25%–49% reduction in serum paraprotein and a 50%–89% reduction in urine light-chain excretion for 6 weeks	Not defined	Not defined
Plateau phase (P) or stable disease (SD)	A stable serum and urine paraprotein (within 25%) maintained for at least 3 months	Does not meet criteria for progression or response	Does not meet criteria for progression or response

with smoldering MM may be followed without specific therapy until clear evidence of progression. Ambulation and hydration should be maintained throughout the initial therapy. Avoidance of nonsteroid anti-inflammatory drugs (NSAIDs), aminoglycosides, and intravenous contrast agent is important for renal health. If radiologic procedures involving the use of intravenous contrast agents are to be considered, appropriate hydration and the use of N-acetyl cysteine should be considered. The use bisphosphonates (either pamidronate or zoledronic acid) is recommended for nearly every myeloma patient with normal renal function, particularly in those with bony disease (see Section III.C.5.). We recommend holding the initiation of the bisphosphonates in the first cycle of therapy to help decrease renal complications from the use of these agents.

2. Systemic therapy for the newly diagnosed patient (see Sections III.B.3. for specific regimens). Although a plethora of therapeutic options for the treatment of newly diagnosed MM patients are available, there is no standard first-line therapy. **In this text, we will define non–high-dose therapy as traditional therapy and high-dose therapy with stem cell rescue as intensive**. The precise role of novel therapeutic agents (such as bortezomib, lenalidomide, and thalidomide) in the management of newly diagnosed MM remains unclear and is the subject of ongoing clinical trials. As therapy for MM does not result in cures, treatment recommendations are often individualized and are based on a patient's comorbidities, performance status, and preference, as well as on disease characteristics. For example, if high-dose therapy is considered during the course of therapy, avoidance of agents (e.g., melphalan and other alkylating agents) that impair stem cell collection is important. In the patient with significant symptoms from the disease, the choice of highly active first-line therapy that results in rapid responses is reasonable. Similarly, in patients with renal dysfunction at presentation, the choice of agents with a safe renal profile is recommended.

Patients with poor prognostic factors at presentation (chromosome 13 deletion by metaphase cytogenetics or t(4,14), high β_2-microglobulin, or increased plasma cell labeling index) fare poorly with all traditional therapy. Accordingly, these patients are best managed by enrollment to clinical trials. Alternatively, it is intuitive though unproved that intensive therapy (combination induction therapy followed by high-dose therapy) would result in improved outcomes.

For patients in whom high-dose therapy is not considered in first remission, therapy with thalidomide and dexamethasone, dexamethasone alone, or the combination of chemotherapy and thalidomide results in a higher response rate than melphalan and prednisone (MP) at the cost of increased toxicities. Overall survival benefit has not been demonstrated but avoidance of MP is reasonable to preserve bone marrow function. Although the duration of therapy remains unclear, we recommend treatment to best response or one to two cycles beyond best response. Chemotherapeutic regimens are described in the subsequent text.

Although most patients older than 70 years remain excellent candidates for aggressive induction therapy, those with significant comorbidities and decreased performance status are often better able to tolerate the combination of an alkylating agent (melphalan or cyclophosphamide) and prednisone. It remains a reasonable line of therapy in this patient group as it is well tolerated and results in responses in approximately 50% of patients. Modifications to this regimen have been described and patients with a good performance status benefit from the addition of thalidomide to first-line therapy with melphalan and corticosteroids. Alternative regimens in this patient population include the use of cyclophosphamide with prednisone as cumulative doses of this agent are not stem cell toxic.

3. Traditional chemotherapy recommendations. Although numerous additional chemotherapeutic regimens have been described, only commonly used agents in the treatment of MM are reviewed in the subsequent text.

　a. Dexamethasone. Dexamethasone is considered by many as the standard induction strategy in patients with MM.

- **Dexamethasone** is given at a dose of 40 mg PO on days 1 to 4, 9 to 12, and 17 to 20. Cycles are repeated every 28 days.

  Treatment is usually given for a minimum of 4 cycles or 2 cycles beyond best response. Significant toxicities include hyperglycemia, dyspepsia, fatigue, and muscle weakness. Additionally, patients often report agitation and insomnia with the use of this schedule of dexamethasone. Responses are observed in approximately 50% of patients and the median time to response is approximately 1 month.

　b. Thalidomide and dexamethasone. The addition of thalidomide to the earlier schedule of dexamethasone results in an increased response rates (~70%), at the cost of additional toxicity (in the form of thromboembolic events, rash, sedation, peripheral neuropathy, and constipation). Although thalidomide was started at 200 mg daily at bedtime on the pivotal clinical trial, our experience suggests improved patient tolerance with a more gradual start of thalidomide.

- We recommend initiating **thalidomide at 50 mg daily** at bedtime and increase the daily dose by 50 mg increments every week to a desired target dose not exceeding 400 mg daily or as dictated by patient tolerance. It should be noted however that there is no known minimal dose required for response where some (though rare) patients respond to dosages as low as 50 mg three times a week.
- In addition, after the second cycle of therapy, reduction of **dexamethasone to 40 mg on days 1 to 4** does result in improved patient tolerance.

- With the increased risks of thromboembolic events (~17% of patients receiving this combination), we recommend the use of **prophylactic low-dose aspirin (81 mg).** Other investigators have used different prophylactic strategies, which include low molecular weight heparin and therapeutic anticoagulation with warfarin.

c. DVd. The DVd regimen consists of the combination of an anthracycline, vincristine and dexamethasone, which is the backbone of the so-called VAD regimen. Intravenous chemotherapy is given on day 1 without the need for lengthy continuous infusions. This makes delivery easier in an outpatient setting. While efficacy is not compromised, tolerability is improved with this regimen.

- **The DVd regimen** consists of the following:
  — **Vincristine** 2 mg IVP on day 1, *and*
  — **Pegylated liposomal doxorubicin** 40 mg/m^2 IVPB on day 1, *and*
  — **Dexamethasone** 40 mg PO on days 1 to 4.
- Repeat cycles of DVd every 28 days for two cycles beyond best response and a minimum of four cycles.

Pegylated liposomal doxorubicin should be used with caution in patients with cardiac dysfunction and in patients with prior doxorubicin use (particularly those with higher cumulative doxorubicin doses). In addition, thalidomide can be combined with the DVd regimen (DVd-T) with the resultant overall response rate exceeding 90% and a rate of complete or near-complete response of approximately 30% to 40%. Caution must be used with the DVd-T regimen as toxicity is additive where prophylactic antibacterial (amoxicillin 250 mg PO b.i.d.), antiviral therapy (acyclovir 400 mg PO b.i.d.), low-dose aspirin (81 mg daily), and growth factor support should be given with this regimen.

d. Melphalan and prednisone (MP). Although more complex chemotherapy induction regimens have not clearly been proved to improve the overall survival as compared to MP, the use of this combination has fallen out of favor in younger patients because of concern over long-term bone marrow health and ability to collect stem cells. MP results in approximately 50% overall response rate in patients with newly diagnosed myeloma and a median time to progression of approximately 15 months. Although a number of different dosages and schedules for MP exist, we recommend the following:

- **Melphalan** 9 mg/m^2 PO on days 1 to 4, *and*
- **Prednisone** 100 mg PO on days 1 to 4.

For reliable absorption, melphalan should be taken on an empty stomach. Repeat cycle every 4 to 6 weeks depending on recovery of counts. MP is usually given for 6 to 9 cycles and treatment beyond 1 year does increase risks of myelodysplasia. Responses to MP tend to occur slower on average, making this a less attractive regimen in patients with significant symptoms. On the other hand, MP is well tolerated in myeloma patients with myelosuppression being the most significant adverse event.

e. Cyclophosphamide and prednisone (CP). CP is a forgotten alternative to melphalan and prednisone where cyclophosphamide does not need dose adjustments for renal failure, making it a useful agent in patients with a decreased performance status and/or comorbidities. It results in a response rate of approximately 50% and a progression-free survival of 12 to 15 months in treatment naïve patients. CP is given as follows:

- **Cyclophosphamide** 1,000 mg/m^2 IV on day 1, *and*
- **Prednisone** 100 mg PO on days 1 to 5

Cycles are repeated every 21 days.

CP is well tolerated and in distinction to MP does not result in significant compromise to stem cell reserve.

f. Bortezomib. Bortezomib is a proteasome inhibitor approved for relapsed or refractory MM. Although it is yet to have a defined role in newly diagnosed patients, combination therapy with dexamethasone, and with thalidomide and dexamethasone have shown promising results in this setting albeit at the cost of increasing toxicity. As a single agent in relapsed and refractory patients, it was shown to result in a response rate of approximately 30% to 40% and a median time to progression of 6 to 7 months, this was found to be superior to high-dose dexamethasone.

- **Bortezomib** is given at 1.3 mg/m^2 IVP on days 1, 4, 8 and 11 on a 21-day cycle.
- **Dexamethasone** 20 mg, on the day before and on the day of bortezomib, is often added after 2 cycles in patients with suboptimal responses. The addition of steroids however results in only a modest improvement in the response and/or the quality of the response.

Treatment is continued for a maximum of eight cycles. Grade 3 and 4 adverse events of bortezomib include the following: thrombocytopenia (30%), neutropenia (14%), anemia (10%), and neuropathy (8%). Neuropathy should be monitored carefully with special attention to autonomic neuropathy in the form of paralytic ileus and delayed peripheral neuropathy after the discontinuation of therapy. We do not recommend the use of this agent in newly diagnosed patients outside the context of a clinical trial.

g. Lenalidomide. Lenalidomide is an immunomodulatory drug with more potent tumor necrosis factor α (TNF-α) inhibition than thalidomide. In addition, lenalidomide has a different adverse event profile than thalidomide and does not usually cause significant sedation or neuropathy but does result in myelosuppression. Lenalidomide is currently approved in the United States for the treatment of myelodysplastic syndrome with 5q abnormalities but has significant activity in MM. In patients with relapsed or refractory MM, the combination of lenalidomide and dexamethasone resulted in responses in approximately 60% of patients with a progression-free survival of approximately 12 months. Similar combination in a small study of newly diagnosed patients resulted in response rates in more than 90% of patients. Lenalidomide and dexamethasone are given as follows:

- **Lenalidomide** 25 mg PO on days 1 to 21 of a 28-day cycle
- **Dexamethasone** 40 mg PO on days 1 to 4, 9 to 12, and 17 to 21

The optimal duration of therapy with lenalidomide is unclear and because clinical trials with this agent used continuing therapy, we recommend a similar approach in patients tolerating this agent well. After two cycles of therapy, consideration for decreasing the frequency of dexamethasone to 4 days must be given. Lenalidomide can also result in thromboembolic events and prophylaxis with low-dose aspirin daily is recommended. In addition, we have reported that the combination of lenalidomide with chemotherapy (specifically the DVd regimen) results in a high response rate (greater than 85%) and high complete and near-complete response rates (~30%). Lenalidomide is given at 10 mg for the first 21 days of the 28-day cycle with this combination. Similar to the DVd-T regimen, we recommend the use of prophylactic antimicrobials and growth factor support as in the preceding text. Until lenalidomide is approved for use in MM in the United States, we recommend that the use of this agent be restricted to clinical trials.

4. Treatment of patients with relapsed or refractory multiple myeloma (MM). Despite original responses to therapy, virtually all patients develop recurrent or refractory MM. In patients who experience a relapse more than 1 year after receiving chemotherapy, remission can frequently be obtained using the same regimen. Patients relapsing earlier will likely require an alternate treatment regimen. Patients with refractory myeloma have evidence of progressive disease while receiving active therapy despite possible original responses. This patient population has a worse outcome than patients with relapse do. Enrollment of patients with relapsed or refractory myeloma into clinical trial should be a first consideration in the choice of antineoplastic therapy. A number of novel therapeutic tools are emerging in the treatment of MM. These include the immunomodulatory drugs (lenalidomide and actimid), histone deacetylase inhibitors, mTOR (mammalian target of rapamycin) inhibitors, and RANK-L antibodies. Many of these will likely be approved first for the treatment of relapsed or refractory patients before gaining indication in newly diagnosed patients.

5. High-dose therapy with bone marrow or peripheral blood stem cell transplantation. (See also

Chapter 5.) The role of high-dose therapy and autologous stem cell transplantation for MM remains poorly defined. Initial reports of high-dose therapy generated significant enthusiasm for this approach, as it was associated with a survival advantage over standard therapy. Contemporary clinical trials comparing high-dose therapy to conventional therapy have failed to consistently confirm the results of initial trials, likely because of the improvement in standard therapy and the availability of novel active salvage therapies. Despite the lack of consistent overall survival advantage, high-dose therapy might be useful for a subgroup of patients that is yet to be defined. One such group are patients planning to receive a tandem transplant where the second transplant is administered in a timed manner following the first transplant (i.e., within 4 months of the first transplant). With the advent of novel agents, the role of high-dose therapy and its timing in MM therapeutic armamentarium will require revalidation.

For patients electing to proceed to high-dose therapy, available induction therapies include the use of dexamethasone alone, the combination of thalidomide and dexamethasone, or chemotherapy in the form of pegylated liposomal doxorubicin, vincristine, and dexamethasone (DVd) with and without the addition of thalidomide. Preliminary data suggest that patients achieving a more than 90% reduction of the M-protein might be the group benefiting most from a single high-dose therapy and stem cell support. If the patient and the treating physician are in agreement with this concept, the addition of thalidomide to the DVd regimen would be desirable to increase the number of high quality responders. It can be argued however that this group of patients will fare well regardless of therapy, and minimizing toxicity and therapy is a reasonable goal. Stem cells can be derived from the peripheral blood or the bone marrow. The former can be done with the use of granulocyte colony stimulating factor (G-CSF) with or without chemotherapy. Novel agents to facilitate stem cell collection are entering the clinical arena. Peripheral stem cell rescue results in faster engraftment as compared to bone marrow stem cell rescue and has accordingly supplanted the former in clinical use. High-dose therapy is usually in the form of melphalan given at 200 mg/m^2 for younger patients with intact renal function. Total-body radiation has mostly been abandoned in this setting in view of inferior results associated with its use. Although purging the graft of malignant cells seems intuitively useful, it has not been shown to improve outcomes and *in vivo* purging (with systemic therapy) remains the preferred modality. High-dose therapy with peripheral stem cell rescue has been carried out in an outpatient setting at some transplant centers, but remains an inpatient therapy for 2 to 3 weeks at most other centers.

French investigators reported promising results with a tandem transplant strategy. While awaiting confirmatory clinical trials, tandem transplants should be considered only as part of a clinical trial as long-term outcomes are not well defined and not all patients appear to benefit from a second course of high-dose therapy. Allogeneic transplantation remains experimental for patients with MM and is precluded by high transplant-related mortality. Reduced intensity conditioning regimen followed by allogeneic transplantation relies solely on graft-versus-myeloma effects. This approach remains experimental as well as long-term outcomes are unproved. Furthermore, only small subsets of patients with MM are candidates to receive such intensified therapy.

Advances in high-dose therapy will likely involve defining the role of vaccination and immunomodulatory drugs post–autologous stem cell transplantation, and supportive care improvement is needed to further increase the safety of this approach.

6. Duration of therapy and the role of maintenance therapy. Patients with stable M-protein for more than 6 months (the so-called "plateau phase") appear to have a favorable prognosis and should be monitored carefully at least every 3 months. No study has conclusively demonstrated benefit by continuing chemotherapy beyond 1 year in responding patients. Several investigators have noted earlier re-emergence of active myeloma after complete cessation of therapy, hence suggesting a benefit for maintenance therapy. A study by the SWOG has shown that maintenance therapy with prednisone given at 50 mg every other day improves overall and progression-free survival when compared to maintenance therapy with 10 mg of prednisone every other day. Although interferon maintenance resulted in a prolonged progression-free survival, overall survival was not increased and toxicity from interferon was notable. The use of thalidomide to maintain responses observed after induction chemotherapy that included this agent is common practice and has been associated with a survival benefit post–high-dose therapy. On the other hand, patients receiving continued thalidomide should be closely monitored for peripheral neuropathy and doses as low as 50 mg every other day are often all that patients are able to tolerate.

7. Role of radiotherapy. Although radiotherapy is sometimes curative in patients with solitary plasmacytomas, its use in patients with MM is palliative and adjunctive to the use of systemic therapy. Patients with symptomatic extraskeletal plasmacytomas, large lytic lesions threatening fracture of long bones, spinal cord or root compression by plasma cells and certain pathologic fractures are good candidates for radiotherapy. Conservative use of radiotherapy is wise as radiation of bone marrow can impair marrow reserves and render the patient less able to tolerate subsequent chemotherapy.

C. Complications of disease or therapy. Toxicity of each chemotherapeutic agent is described elsewhere. In addition, complications characteristic of MM are described here.

1. Hypercalcemia. Once a very frequent complication of MM, hypercalcemia is less often noted, likely as a result of more widespread use of bisphosphonate therapy for bone health. The pathophysiology of hypercalcemia in patients with MM is likely related to increased osteoclast activation as a result of binding of the latter to malignant plasma cells. Receptor activator of nuclear factor-κB (RANK) ligand produced by bone marrow stromal cells is the best-described cytokine mediating this effect. Antibodies to RANK ligand are entering the clinical arena and are currently being tested in clinical trials in patients with MM. Symptoms of hypercalcemia are often protean and overlap with adverse events of thalidomide, and a strong index of suspicion is required. Symptoms include anorexia, constipation and polyuria, and lethargy. Coma and death are the result of untreated hypercalcemia. Dehydration and potentially reversible renal dysfunction are frequently associated with hypercalcemia. Treatment of hypercalcemia involves aggressive saline hydration, use of loop diuretics once fluid overload occurs, use of corticosteroids (such as prednisone 60 mg for 7 days), and bisphosphonate therapy. Calcitonin is sometimes used but hemodialysis is reserved for refractory cases. When hypercalcemia occurs in previously untreated patients, prompt initiation of therapy for the MM in addition to the above usually results in effective, durable control.

   a. Bisphosphonates
      (1) Pamidronate 90 mg given as a 2-h IV infusion that can be repeated every 30 days **or**
      (2) Zoledronic acid 4 mg IV over 15 to 30 min in the absence of renal dysfunction.
   b. Calcitonin 100 to 300 U SC every 8 to 12 h for up to 2 to 3 days. Calcitonin is usually given with prednisone 60 mg PO daily to prolong its effectiveness.
   c. Hemodialysis is very effective but rarely needed.

2. Infections. (See also Chapter 28.) Patients with MM are at increased risk for infectious complications usually related to capsulated microorganisms. Deficiency of normal Igs, diminished bone marrow reserves, therapies for MM, and immobilization due to skeletal disease are important predisposing factors. Prompt evaluation of fever or other manifestations of infection and institution of empiric antimicrobial therapy are essential. The prophylactic and therapeutic use of growth factors (such as G-CSF) is often considered. Intravenous immunoglobulin (IVIG) is administered to patients with recurrent significant infectious complications.

3. Hyperviscosity. This is a rare manifestation of MM and is more commonly observed in patients with WM. It may present as central nervous system impairment (that is often subtle and noted as difficulty concentrating and headaches), and occasionally as congestive heart failure. Plasmapheresis is the treatment of symptomatic hyperviscosity; however, therapy should be combined with systemic therapy directed at the myeloma as benefits of plasmapheresis are short lived, owing to the fact that IgG and IgA are not confined to the vascular space.

4. Renal dysfunction. The possible causes of renal dysfunction in patients with MM include all of the following:

myeloma kidney or cast nephropathy, drugs such as nonsteroid anti-inflammatory drugs, bisphosphonates and intravenous contrast agents, hypercalcemia, hyperuricemia and urate nephropathy, amyloid deposition, pyelonephritis and other infections, hyperviscosity syndrome, plasma cell infiltration of both kidneys (rare), and renal tubular acidosis. In addition, MM patients are particularly susceptible to intravascular volume depletion and pre-renal azotemia. Adequate hydration, avoidance of possible culprit drugs when possible, high index of suspicion, and early identification of etiology will result in improved renal outcomes as most of the causes of renal dysfunction are reversible. Patients with MM with severe renal dysfunction in whom readily identifiable causes of renal dysfunction have been ruled out, may be assumed to have cast nephropathy without the need for a biopsy. Plasmapheresis in addition to institution of chemotherapy should be considered in such selected cases. Although plasmapheresis does not impact overall survival, it may result in improved dialysis-free survival. In patients with severe renal failure that has not improved with interventions mentioned earlier, hemodialysis should be considered if chemotherapy offers the potential for a prolonged remission.

5. Skeletal destruction. This remains a major cause of disability, pain, and immobilization for patients with MM. Adopting a multidisciplinary approach to the patient with bone disease cannot be overemphasized. Bisphosphonates are best given monthly in the first 1 to 2 years and less frequently thereafter. They have been shown to reduce the incidence of skeleton-related events. Pamidronate and zoledronic acid have both been associated with the development of osteonecrosis of the jaw. A dentist experienced in the management of this complication should promptly evaluate patients with symptoms referable to the jaw or teeth. In addition, bisphosphonates should be held for 1 month before and 2 months after any dental procedure or after confirmation of the total healing after the procedure. Radiation therapy is often used to palliate painful lytic lesions. Surgical intervention is used for prevention of impending fractures of weight-bearing bones, and the treatment of compression fractures causing pain and loss of height (kyphoplasty).

6. Anemia. Anemia is frequently observed in patients with MM. MM and its treatment are etiologic in most patients. In addition, a subset of patients was found to have vitamin B_{12} and folate deficiency and treatment with erythropoietic agents is thought to result in decreases in iron stores. Thus, monitoring of vitamin B_{12}, folate, and iron levels is recommended. The use of recombinant human erythropoietin yields results in approximately 80% of patients with anemia.

7. Leukemia. Acute myeloid leukemia (AML) develops in approximately 4% of myeloma patients who have received alkylator-based chemotherapy (melphalan). Myelodysplasia is present at diagnosis in a subset of patients as both conditions occur in older age-groups. Leukemia in this setting appears to be caused by the interaction of a carcinogenic drug with a predisposed host. With the avoidance of long-term therapy with alkylating agents, the incidence of this complication is declining.

IV. **Waldenström's macroglobulinemia (WM) (lymphoplasmacytic lymphoma)**

A. **Diagnosis and presentation.** WM is a B-cell lymphoproliferative disorder characterized by the production of a monoclonal Ig of the IgM subtype and by intertrabecular bone marrow infiltration with a lymphoplasmacytic infiltrate. The second international workshop on WM has proposed the following diagnostic criteria: an IgM M-protein of any concentration and bone marrow infiltration with small lymphocytes exhibiting plasmacytoid differentiation and with a suggestive immunophenotype (expression of surface IgM, CD19, CD20, CD25, CD27, FMC7, and CD138 without the expression of CD5, CD10, CD23, and CD103).

- **Symptoms attributable to WM** are related to tumor infiltration or to the M-protein. The former results in constitutional symptoms (fevers, sweats, and weight loss), cytopenias (secondary to bone marrow involvement), lymphadenopathy, and hepatosplenomegaly. Symptoms related to M-protein include those related to hyperviscosity, cryoglobulinemia, cold agglutinin, neuropathy, and amyloidosis.

B. **General considerations and aims of therapy.** There is no cure for WM. **Treatment is palliative and aimed at reduction of symptoms and prevention of complication of the disease.** Increasing numbers of patients without signs or symptoms are being diagnosed with WM. Expectant observation is the recommended approach for patients with asymptomatic WM. The level of the M-protein should not be used as an indication for treatment. The choice of the therapeutic option in symptomatic individual is guided by disease characteristics as well as possible patient characteristics. The available therapies include the following: oral alkylating agents, nucleoside analogs, rituximab monotherapy, combination of chemotherapy and rituximab, and autologous stem cell transplantation. Novel therapies include thalidomide, alemtuzumab, bortezomib, and sildenafil and are recommended only within the context of clinical trials. Limited randomized clinical trials have been conducted for WM, and treatment recommendations rely mostly on phase II studies. Patients with WM are monitored by repeated measurements of serum M-protein and serum viscosity when that is elevated, and/or by serial computed tomography (CT) scan. A complete response is defined as the disappearance of the M-protein, and by resolution of infiltration of lymph node and visceral organs confirmed on two separate evaluations 6 weeks apart. A partial response is defined as greater than 50% reduction in M-protein, and greater than 50% reduction in lymphadenopathy with the resolution of symptoms related to WM. Progressive disease is defined as a greater than 25% increase in the M-protein, worsening of cytopenias, organ infiltration, or disease-related symptoms. After the documentation of the best response, continued therapy is not clearly beneficial. The median survival of patients with WM has historically been 5 to 10 years, likely as a consequence of the older patient population and comorbidities.

C. Treatment

1. Cytopenias. Cytopenias in patients with WM are related to bone marrow involvement and occasionally to hypersplenism. Anemia in patients with WM is common and often responds to erythropoietic agents. Although transfusions are generally safe, it is generally done with caution in patients with hyperviscosity as red blood cells contribute to whole blood viscosity. Thrombocytopenia and leukopenia usually are indications to initiate treatment and improvement in these cytopenias is often regarded as evidence of response to therapy. Platelet transfusions are occasionally needed, especially after chemotherapy is given to the patient with baseline thrombocytopenia.

2. Hyperviscosity. Hyperviscosity syndrome readily responds to plasmapheresis. Plasmapheresis should not be regarded as a long-term treatment, and consolidation of that response with chemotherapy is ultimately needed to render the patient independent of that procedure.

3. Chemotherapy

a. Oral alkylating agents

- **Chlorambucil** 2 to 6 mg PO daily, *or*
- **Cyclophosphamide** 50 to 100 mg PO daily.

(**Prednisone** 40 to 60 mg PO on days 1 to 4 every 4 weeks is often added.)

Complete responses are rare with the use of alkylating agents, whereas partial responses approach 50% in some series. The time to response has been slow with alkylating agents. The use of alkylating agents should be considered in older patients in whom rapid control of the disease is not necessary.

b. Nucleoside analog

- **Fludarabine** 25 mg/m^2 IV on days 1 to 5.

Cycles are repeated every 28 days.

Although many patients are able to tolerate this regimen, older individual and patients with significant cytopenias at baseline are best treated by dose reduction in the early cycles. We recommend 2 to 3 days of the above dose of fludarabine in the first two cycles and would consider dose increases if the patient is able to tolerate therapy well and responses are suboptimal. Nucleoside analogs have been shown to result in a higher response rate than oral alkylators but a survival benefit has not been demonstrated. The time to response is shortened by the use of nucleoside analogs. We recommend the use of these agents in younger patients in whom autologous stem cell transplantation is not considered and who require a fast tumor control.

c. Rituximab

- **Rituximab** 375 mg/m^2 IV weekly for four doses, consider repeating for another four doses.

Rituximab is a monoclonal antibody targeting CD20 on B lymphocytes. Response rates range from 20% to

70% in the in newly diagnosed patients and approximately 30% in patients with relapse. Time to response to rituximab is in the order of 3 months. A flare reaction has been described in patients treated with rituximab and is characterized by a transient increase in the serum IgM of patients. A serum IgM lower than 5 g is predictive of response to this agent. We recommend the use of this agent in younger patients, with minimal symptoms of their disease and with a lower serum IgM level.

d. High-dose therapy and autologous stem cell transplantation. Autologous stem cell transplantation has resulted in high rates of responses (approaching 90%), and lasting responses (progression-free survival approaching 70 months) in small series of patients. The small number of patients, the nonrandomized nature of the studies, and the potential for treatment-related morbidity make it difficult to routinely recommend this approach in many patients. It should however be considered in younger patients after cytoreductive treatment with rituximab. Treatment with alkylating agents and nucleoside analog may impair the ability to collect stem cells and should be judiciously used in younger patients.

V. Amyloidosis. Only primary amyloidosis (AL amyloidosis) with or without associated plasma cell neoplasms is considered in this section. In these disorders, fragments of Ig light chain accumulate and deposit in the affected tissues. These deposits are characterized by a pathognomonic apple green birefringence on polarized microscopy. These deposit lead to organ dysfunction. AL amyloid characteristically infiltrates the tongue, heart, skin, ligaments, and muscle and occasionally the kidney, liver, and spleen. Diagnosis requires biopsy of the affected organ although occasionally a fat pat biopsy may obviate that need. In patients with documented lymphomas or plasma cell neoplasms, treatment is directed at the underlying neoplasm, but the decline in the amount of amyloid is often minimal. With primary amyloidosis without a demonstrable underlying neoplasm, treatment with alkylator-based therapy such as MP has been used historically and is of moderate benefits. The use of high-dose dexamethasone is often prescribed as well. High-dose therapy with stem cell rescue is considered in only a minority of patients as most patients are not eligible and procedure-related mortality remains high. Patients with cardiac amyloidosis have dismal outcomes, often measured in months, if they have concomitant heart failure. Novel effective therapies are needed and enrollment of patients to clinical trials should be considered early.

SUGGESTED READINGS

Attal M, Harousseau JL, Stoppa AM, et al. A prospective, randomized trial of autologous bone marrow transplantation and chemotherapy in multiple myeloma. Intergroupe Francais du Myelome. *N Engl J Med* 1996;335:91–97.

Barlogie B, Kyle RA, Anderson KC, et al. Standard chemotherapy compared with high-dose chemoradiotherapy for multiple myeloma: final results of phase III U.S. intergroup trial S9321. *J Clin Oncol* 2006;24:929–936.

Baz R, Li L, Kottke-Marchant K, et al. The role of aspirin in the prevention of thrombotic complications of thalidomide and anthracycline-based chemotherapy for multiple myeloma. *Mayo Clin Proc* 2005;80:1568–1574.

Berenson JR, Crowley JJ, Grogan TM, et al. Maintenance therapy with alternate-day prednisone improves survival in multiple myeloma patients. *Blood* 2002;99:3163–3168.

Bergsagel PL, Kuehl WM. Molecular pathogenesis and a consequent classification of multiple myeloma. *J Clin Oncol* 2005;23:6333–6338.

Blade J, Kyle RA. Nonsecretory myeloma, immunoglobulin D myeloma, and plasma cell leukemia. *Hematol Oncol Clin North Am* 1999;13:1259–1272.

Cavo M, Terragna C, Renzulli M, et al. Poor outcome with front-line autologous transplantation in t(4;14) multiple myeloma: low complete remission rate and short duration of remission. *J Clin Oncol* 2006;24:e4–e5.

Crawley C, Szydlo R, Lalancette M, et al. Outcomes of reduced-intensity transplantation for chronic myeloid leukemia: an analysis of prognostic factors from the Chronic Leukemia Working Party of the EBMT. *Blood* 2005;106:2969–2976.

Dhodapkar MV, Hussein MA, Rasmussen E, et al. Clinical efficacy of high-dose dexamethasone with maintenance dexamethasone/alpha interferon in patients with primary systemic amyloidosis: results of United States Intergroup Trial Southwest Oncology Group (SWOG) S9628. *Blood* 2004;104:3520–3526.

Dimopoulos MA, Kyle RA, Anagnostopoulos A, et al. Diagnosis and management of Waldenstrom's macroglobulinemia. *J Clin Oncol* 2005;23:1564–1577.

Durie BG, Salmon SE. A clinical staging system for multiple myeloma. Correlation of measured myeloma cell mass with presenting clinical features, response to treatment, and survival. *Cancer* 1975;36:842–854.

Fonseca R, Barlogie B, Bataille R, et al. Genetics and cytogenetics of multiple myeloma: a workshop report. *Cancer Res* 2004;64:1546–1558.

Frassica DA, Frassica FJ, Schray MF, et al. Solitary plasmacytoma of bone: mayo clinic experience. *Int J Radiat Oncol Biol Phys* 1989;16:43–48.

Greipp PR, San Miguel J, Durie BG, et al. International staging system for multiple myeloma. *J Clin Oncol* 2005;23:3412–3420.

Holland J, Trenkner DA, Wasserman TH, et al. Plasmacytoma. Treatment results and conversion to myeloma. *Cancer* 1992;69:1513–1517.

Jacobson JL, Hussein MA, Barlogie B, et al. A new staging system for multiple myeloma patients based on the Southwest Oncology Group (SWOG) experience. *Br J Haematol* 2003;122:441–450.

Owen RG, Treon SP, Al-Katib A, et al. Clinicopathological definition of Waldenstrom's macroglobulinemia: consensus panel recommendations from the Second International Workshop on Waldenstrom's Macroglobulinemia. *Semin Oncol* 2003;30:110–115.

Rajkumar SV, Blood E, Vesole D, et al. Phase III clinical trial of thalidomide plus dexamethasone compared with dexamethasone alone in newly diagnosed multiple myeloma: a clinical trial coordinated by the Eastern Cooperative Oncology Group. *J Clin Oncol* 2006;24:431–436.

Rajkumar SV, Hayman SR, Lacy MQ, et al. Combination therapy with lenalidomide plus dexamethasone (Rev/Dex) for newly diagnosed myeloma. *Blood* 2005;106:4050–4053.

Richardson PG, Sonneveld P, Schuster MW, et al. Bortezomib or high-dose dexamethasone for relapsed multiple myeloma. *N Engl J Med* 2005;352:2487–2498.

Rifkin RM, Gregory SA, Mohrbacher A, et al. Pegylated liposomal doxorubicin, vincristine, and dexamethasone provide significant reduction in toxicity compared with doxorubicin, vincristine, and dexamethasone in patients with newly diagnosed multiple myeloma: a Phase III multicenter randomized trial. *Cancer* 2006;106:848–858.

Rosen LS, Gordon D, Kaminski M, et al. Long-term efficacy and safety of zoledronic acid compared with pamidronate disodium in the treatment of skeletal complications in patients with advanced multiple myeloma or breast carcinoma: a randomized, double-blind, multicenter, comparative trial. *Cancer* 2003;98:1735–1744.

Segeren CM, Sonneveld P, van der Holt B, et al. Overall and event-free survival are not improved by the use of myeloablative therapy following intensified chemotherapy in previously untreated patients with multiple myeloma: a prospective randomized phase 3 study. *Blood* 2003;101:2144–2151.

Srkalovic G, Elson P, Trebisky B, et al. Use of melphalan, thalidomide, and dexamethasone in treatment of refractory and relapsed multiple myeloma. *Med Oncol* 2002;19:219–226.

Stewart AK, Fonseca R. Prognostic and therapeutic significance of myeloma genetics and gene expression profiling. *J Clin Oncol* 2005;23:6339–6344.

Treon SP, Gertz MA, Dimopoulos M, et al. Update on treatment recommendations from the Third International Workshop on Waldenstrom's macroglobulinemia. *Blood* 2006;107:3442–3446.

CHAPTER 25

Metastatic Cancer of Unknown Origin

James M. Leonardo

In approximately 5% to 10% of patients with newly diagnosed cancer (excluding nonmelanoma skin cancer), the primary site remains unknown despite a detailed pretreatment evaluation. Even after postmortem examination, a primary tumor is not found in up to half the number of these patients. However, the frequency of cancers with truly occult primary sites is decreasing, in part because of advances in technology to detect the primary site(s). The problem of metastatic cancer of unknown origin raises difficult questions for both diagnosis and treatment. Although the median survival time of patients with cancer of unknown origin has been reported to be 6 to 9 months, subgroups of patients have been defined who have a more favorable outlook with aggressive management. With current therapeutic modalities, the overall survival of these patients appears to be improving. A major responsibility of the clinician is to identify those patients with a characteristic presentation who might benefit from a specific strategy and to identify the increasingly large group of patients who might benefit from a trial of chemotherapy.

Tumors thought to be more amenable to treatment, and therefore to have a more favorable prognosis, include poorly differentiated cancers with midline distribution, squamous cell carcinoma (SCC) involving cervical lymph nodes, papillary adenocarcinoma of the peritoneal cavity in women, and adenocarcinoma involving only axillary lymph nodes in women. Conversely, adverse prognostic findings include adenocarcinoma metastatic to the liver or other organs, nonpapillary malignant ascites, and multiple metastases to brain, bones, or lungs.

I. **General considerations and aims of therapy**
   A. **Histology and presenting clinical manifestations.** Moderately differentiated adenocarcinoma and poorly differentiated carcinoma or adenocarcinoma respectively comprise up to 60% and 30% of all cancers of unknown origin. SCC and poorly differentiated cancers other than adenocarcinoma each account for approximately 5% of unknown primary tumors. Other histologies that may present as cancer of unknown origin include lymphomas, germ cell tumors, and neuroendocrine carcinomas. These histologies are particularly important to identify because they represent tumors that may be effectively managed with systemic chemotherapy. Nearly half of all patients with unknown primaries and more than half the number of those with adenocarcinoma present with hepatomegaly, abdominal mass, or other abdominal symptoms. Lymphadenopathy is the presenting clinical manifestation in 15% to 25% of patients. Lower cervical or supraclavicular lymph nodes usually contain adenocarcinoma or undifferentiated carcinoma,

and middle to high cervical adenopathy generally represents SCC. Between 10% and 20% of patients present with manifestations of bone, lung, or pleural involvement, whereas fewer than 10% present with evidence of central nervous system disease. Most of the latter group is eventually found to have either lung or gastrointestinal tract primaries.

Two presentations of advanced carcinoma of unknown primary site have been recognized as more treatable than others: poorly differentiated carcinoma or adenocarcinoma, especially with predominant sites of involvement in the mediastinum, retroperitoneum, lymph nodes, or lungs and adenocarcinoma in women predominantly involving the peritoneal surfaces. In these instances, platinum-based chemotherapy regimens designed for germ cell or ovarian cancers have produced many useful objective responses and occasional long-term disease-free survival.

B. Sites of origin. It is sometimes possible to predict the most likely primary sites from the histology and location of the metastatic lesion of unknown origin. Pancreas and lung are the most common ultimately determined sites of origin. Together they represent more than 40% of the adenocarcinomas of unknown origin in which the site can be ultimately determined. Colorectal, gastric, and hepatobiliary carcinoma each represent about another 10%.

In general, adenocarcinomas or undifferentiated carcinomas presenting with hepatic metastases or left supraclavicular adenopathy are eventually demonstrated to be of gastrointestinal origin. SCCs that present in the supraclavicular or low cervical lymph nodes are usually from lung primaries, whereas similar lesions of higher cervical nodes are more likely to have originated from occult primary lesions in the head and neck region.

The pattern of metastatic involvement associated with occult primary tumors may differ from that associated with overt primaries. For example, occult lung cancer rarely involves bone, a common site of metastasis from overt lung cancer; however, bone metastases appear to be more common in patients with gastrointestinal cancer who have occult primaries than in those who have overt primaries. Nonetheless, occult primaries can metastasize to any site and, in general, one should not rely on the pattern of metastatic spread to predict the site of origin.

C. Aims of diagnostic evaluation. The first objective in the management of a patient newly diagnosed with cancer of unknown origin is to plan the appropriate diagnostic evaluation. There are three chief aims of this evaluation:

   1. Identify a tumor in which cure or effective disease control is possible.

   2. Determine if the tumor is regionally confined or widely metastatic.

   3. Identify any complication for which immediate local therapy is indicated.

D. Goals of treatment. In patients with tumors for which effective systemic therapy is available and in patients with disease regionally confined to peripheral lymph nodes alone, the primary goal of treatment is prolongation of life through extended disease control; in some cases cure should be considered. These patients represent approximately 25% of those with occult primaries. For the remaining patients, the chance of prolonging life has been less likely, but with the advent of new cytotoxic agents and targeted drugs, prospects for this group are improving. Treatment should also address palliation of symptoms and preservation of the best possible quality of life.

II. Diagnostic evaluation

A. Initial work-up. The initial evaluation of a patient presenting with a metastatic tumor should include a complete history and physical examination including a pelvic and rectal examination. Routine laboratory studies (complete blood count [CBC], electrolytes, creatinine, blood urea nitrogen [BUN] and calcium, liver function tests) should also be done early on in the evaluation. The clinical scenario should dictate more specialized laboratory testing. It is wholly reasonable to measure a CA-125 in the setting of a woman with ascites, for example. Imaging studies should include a chest radiograph at minimum; additional studies such as mammography may be useful depending on the location of the metastases and symptoms. Computed tomography (CT) scanning is now being routinely used to evaluate patients with occult primary tumors and may be responsible for the decreased frequency of cancers that remain of truly unknown origin. The role of positron emission tomography (PET) scan is not clear, but some series have reported a usefulness of this modality for identifying the primary site, particularly when the presentation is in cervical lymph nodes. More invasive testing, such as endoscopy or colonoscopy, should be guided by the patient's symptoms.

B. Analysis of the biopsy specimen. If possible, the pathologist should receive fresh, unfixed material to allow electron microscopy, histochemistry, immunohistology, and hormone receptor studies to be done, if needed, after routine examination. Careful review of the biopsy material should be undertaken to attempt to classify the tumor conclusively as SCC, adenocarcinoma, or other identifiable histology. Up to 40% of cancers of unknown origin are undifferentiated or poorly differentiated tumors based on evaluation of hematoxylin and eosin–stained material. Electron microscopy, when available, may be useful for the further classification of these tumors through the identification of desmosomes and intercellular bridges (SCC); tight junctions, microvilli, and acinar spaces (adenocarcinoma); premelanosomes (amelanotic melanoma); neurosecretory granules (small cell or neuroendocrine carcinoma); and absence of junctions (lymphoma). Immunohistochemistry is an indispensable part of the evaluation of carcinoma of unknown primary site. The expression of cytokeratins, particularly CK7 and CK20, may be useful in narrowing down the origin of a tumor. Immunohistochemical studies on the tumor may be used to demonstrate the presence of prostate-specific antigen (PSA; prostate carcinoma), human chorionic gonadotropin (β-hCG; germ cell tumors), α-fetoprotein (germ cell tumors or hepatocellular carcinoma), or monoclonal immunoglobulin (lymphoma, plasmacytoma). Immunoglobulin or T-cell receptor gene rearrangements may be helpful in identifying tumors of lymphoid origin. Undifferentiated carcinomas or adenocarcinomas in women should be evaluated for estrogen and progesterone receptors. Mucin positivity is helpful in eliminating the possibility of renal cell carcinoma.

Clearly, the use of many of these specialized studies must be balanced against their cost. If judiciously applied, they can aid in the identification of some of the undifferentiated or poorly differentiated tumors of unknown origin and help focus their subsequent diagnostic evaluation and management.

C. Squamous cell carcinoma (SCC). One exception to the policy of seeking a definitive histologic diagnosis as the first step in evaluating a tumor of unknown origin is when the patient presents with a potentially resectable neck mass (other than supraclavicular adenopathy) and no other apparent lesion. In these patients, a head and neck primary should be sought by detailed head and neck examination, radiographs of the sinuses, and, if necessary, panendoscopy under general anesthesia to include laryngoscopy, bronchoscopy, esophagoscopy, and nasopharyngoscopy with blind biopsy of the base of the tongue, piriform sinuses, nasopharynx, and tonsillar fossae if no gross primary is found. A CT scan of the head and neck may also be of value. [18F]Fluorodeoxyglucose positron emission tomography (FDG-PET) scanning has also been utilized in this setting. If this work-up is not diagnostic, biopsy of the neck mass is undertaken. This order of evaluation is chosen so that if a resectable SCC of the head and neck is found, the neck mass can be removed as part of the curative procedure.

For SCCs with apparent involvement of only one lymph node group, the possibility of long-term survival exists if proper treatment is carried out. The diagnostic evaluation depends on the lymph node region involved. The most common lymph node presentation for SCCs of unknown origin is in the cervical or supraclavicular region. Cervical lymph node metastases above the supraclavicular region usually originate from head and neck primary lesions. The diagnostic approach to these lesions is discussed in the preceding paragraph. Because surgery, irradiation, or both, with curative intent, are employed if disease is localized to this region, distant metastases should be excluded with a bone scan, a chest radiograph, and, in some instances, a chest CT scan. SCC of supraclavicular lymph nodes is usually of lung or esophageal origin and seldom represents regionally confined disease. Evaluation is the same as that for disease that extends beyond regional lymph nodes.

SCC in axillary or inguinal lymph nodes is rarely associated with an occult primary. Regional skin and lung should be examined as possible primary sites with axillary disease, whereas the skin, anus, and genitalia should be carefully examined when the presentation is SCC in the inguinal nodes.

SCC with generalized lymphadenopathy or, more commonly, with disease that extends beyond the lymph nodes represents disease that cannot be satisfactorily controlled by present-day techniques. The search for the primary lesions should be done mainly by a chest radiograph and careful physical examination of the appropriate organs. Serum chemistries, including the calcium level, should be determined. Further diagnostic studies are needed only if indicated by signs, symptoms, or abnormalities on the initial studies.

D. Adenocarcinoma and poorly differentiated carcinoma. Women with adenocarcinoma or poorly differentiated carcinoma of unknown origin should undergo mammography, careful pelvic examination, and hormone receptor evaluation of the tumor. In men, serum acid phosphatase, PSA, β-hCG, and α-fetoprotein should be determined to help exclude prostate and germ cell tumors, respectively. An elevated CA 27.29 level would point toward a breast primary. All patients should have stools and urine examined for occult blood, and the serum should be tested for abnormalities in the liver chemistries, creatinine, and electrolytes. With disease apparently confined to axillary lymph nodes, mammography is particularly important in women and should be considered in men as well. If there is a strong suspicion of breast cancer and the mammogram is negative, magnetic resonance imaging (MRI) should be considered. Undifferentiated carcinoma found only in middle to high cervical lymph nodes should be evaluated in the same manner as described in Section II.C. for cervical node SCC.

Traditional contrast studies such as intravenous pyelogram, barium enema, and upper gastrointestinal series are not indicated unless specifically suggested by signs or symptoms (e.g., occult blood in the stool). Abdominal CT scan with intravenous contrast medium is a reasonable option in view of the frequency with which it detects carcinoma of the pancreas or hepatobiliary cancer in this setting.

E. Malignant melanoma. The finding of malignant melanoma confined to a single lymph node group and without a detectable primary lesion represents stage II disease and is associated with a 5-year survival rate of 30% after lymphadenectomy. Evaluation to exclude more extensive disease should include a history, physical examination (emphasizing skin and ophthalmoscopic examination), chest radiograph, liver chemistries, liver scan, and brain CT scan.

III. Treatment

A. General strategy. The importance of identifying tumors that may be treated effectively, such as lymphomas, germ cell tumors, trophoblastic tumors, and breast, prostate, ovarian, and neuroendocrine carcinomas, is readily apparent. Once identified, these lesions should be treated as described in the respective chapters. In patients whose primary lesion remains obscure, a therapeutic distinction must be made between those with disease confined to one lymph node region and those with more widespread disease or involvement of visceral organs. In the former, some may be treated with curative intent, whereas in the latter, the aims of treatment are palliative.

B. Squamous cell carcinoma (SCC). Patients with SCC confined to the cervical lymph nodes above the supraclavicular region should receive full-course radiotherapy to a field extending from the base of the skull to the clavicles. Alternatively, they may be treated with radical lymph node dissection followed by radiation therapy. In either case, the irradiation is designed to include any possible head and neck primary carcinoma. Survival of patients so treated is at least as good as that for patients with known head and neck primaries. More limited lymph node dissection or regional irradiation may also be indicated for SCC confined to unilateral involvement of the axillary or inguinal nodes.

More widespread SCCs of unknown origin are treated with a palliative intent. No treatment except for local radiotherapy to symptomatic lesions is the standard approach. In patients with symptomatic or progressive disease who desire chemotherapy, regimens designed mainly for head and neck (Chapter 6) or non–small cell lung cancer (Chapter 7) should be considered.

C. Adenocarcinoma and poorly differentiated carcinoma. In women, if these carcinomas are confined to the unilateral axillary lymph nodes, they should be considered as possible breast cancer and treated accordingly as stage II disease (see Chapter 10). A woman with adenocarcinoma or poorly differentiated carcinoma predominantly confined to the peritoneal surface should be considered for a platinum-based ovarian cancer regimen. Undifferentiated carcinoma confined to the middle or high cervical lymph nodes should be treated actively as SCC (see Section II.C.). Men with adenocarcinoma of unknown primary and a positive tumor or serum PSA should have a' trial of hormonal therapy.

Patients with more advanced adenocarcinoma or poorly differentiated carcinoma in which the evaluation previously described in Section II does not suggest breast, prostate, or other highly treatable primary or a primary site should be managed according to the histology. Platinum-based combination chemotherapy may be valuable in the treatment of poorly differentiated carcinoma and poorly differentiated adenocarcinoma. In patients with mediastinal or retroperitoneal tumors, the germ cell regimen of bleomycin, etoposide, and cisplatin (BEP) or EP (BEP without the bleomycin) has been studied in a series of 220 patients. This combination may produce more than a 60% objective response rate and more than a 20% complete response rate with up to a 13% long-term survival rate.

BEP

- **Cisplatin** 20 mg/m^2 IV over 30 minutes on days 1 to 5, *and*
- **Etoposide** 100 mg/m^2 IV on days 1 to 5, *and*
- **Bleomycin** 30 U IV push weekly on days 1, 8, and 15

Repeat cycle every 21 days regardless of blood cell counts for two (adjuvant therapy), three (good-risk patients), or four (intermediate or poor risk) cycles.

Patients with widespread adenocarcinoma that is well or moderately well differentiated may be responsive to systemic therapy. Combinations such as paclitaxel, carboplatin, and oral etoposide (PCE) or gemcitabine and carboplatin followed by paclitaxel yield objective responses in 25% to 45% of patients.

PCE

- **Paclitaxel** 200 mg/m^2 as a 1-hour IV infusion on day 1 and
- **Carboplatin** area under the curve (AUC) 6 IV over 30 to 60 minutes on day 1 and
- **Etoposide** 50 to 100 mg PO on alternate days for 1 to 10 days.

Gemcitabine and carboplatin

- **Carboplatin** AUC of 5 on day 1
- **Gemcitabine** 1,000 mg/m² IV on day 1 and 8

Repeat each cycle every 3 weeks.

Both regimens are worthy of consideration in patients with good performance status because occasional durable responses have occurred. Reports on both of these regimens are based on limited accrual phase II studies. Responding patients show improvement within two cycles, and chemotherapy should be stopped after two cycles if no improvement is seen. PCE is also effective in patients with poorly differentiated adenocarcinoma and poorly differentiated carcinoma, and may be considered as an alternative to BEP.

D. Malignant melanoma. For disease confined to a single lymph node group, radical lymph node dissection yields long-term survival in 30% of treated patients. Treatment of disseminated melanoma is discussed in Chapter 15.

E. Neuroendocrine carcinoma. Poorly differentiated neuroendocrine carcinoma may represent up to 13% of cases of poorly differentiated carcinoma or adenocarcinoma. The diagnosis is secured by recognition of neurosecretory granules on electron microscopy. Localized lesions are uncommon and should be treated with surgery or radiation therapy. Metastatic disease frequently responds to platinum-based chemotherapy such as etoposide plus cisplatin or newer regimens, such as irinotecan and cisplatin.

EP

- **Etoposide** 120 mg/m² IV on day 1 to 3 *or* 120 mg/m² PO b.i.d. on day 1 to 3 *and*
- **Cisplatin** 60 mg/m² IV on day 1

IP

- **Irinotecan** 60 mg/m² IV on days 1,8,15.
- **Cisplatin** 60 mg/m² IV on day 1.

IV. Future directions. Advances in our understanding of the molecular events leading to carcinogenesis and metastasis have led to the development of gene profiling for specific types of cancer. Retrospective studies of archival breast tumor specimens, for example, in which genetic profiles are identified and compared to the known treatment outcomes have led to prospective studies in which gene profiles are being used to guide specific therapy. It is not only conceivable, but also likely, that in the near future genetic profiling will be used routinely to characterize most tumors. This approach should identify the tissue of origin of most tumors, leading to a further decline in the apparent incidence of true occult primary tumors. More importantly, effective, targeted therapies that act at defined points in the cancer cell could then be chosen on the basis of the molecular characteristics of the tumor rather than on the basis of the purported tissue or organ of origin.

Acknowledgement. The author is indebted to Dr. Martin Oken who contributed to the previous editions of this chapter. Much of the content and text of this chapter represents Dr. Oken's work and has been included verbatim in this revision of the handbook.

SUGGESTED READINGS

Abbruzzese JL, Abbruzzese MC, Hess KR, et al. Unknown primary carcinoma: natural history and prognostic factors in 657 consecutive patients. *J Clin Oncol* 1994;12:1272–1284.

Altman E, Cadman E. An analysis of 1539 patients with cancer of unknown primary site. *Cancer* 1986;57:120–124.

Ettinger DS, Arnoletti JP, Gockerman JP, et al. Occult primary. *NCCN Pract Guidelines Oncol* V.I.2007. Available at http://www.NCCN.org/professionals/physician_gls/PDF/occult.pdf.

Greco FA, Burris HA III, Litchy S, et al. Gemcitabine, carboplatin, and paclitaxel for patients with carcinoma of unknown primary site: a Minnie Pearl Cancer Center Research Network Study. *J Clin Oncol* 2002;20:1651–1656.

Greco FA, Vaughn WK, Hainsworth JD. Advanced poorly differentiated carcinoma of unknown primary site: recognition of a treatable syndrome. *Ann Intern Med* 1986;104:547–556.

Hainsworth JD, Erland JB, Kalman LA, et al. Carcinoma of unknown primary site: treatment with one-hour paclitaxel, carboplatin, and extended schedule etoposide. *J Clin Oncol* 1997;15: 2385–2393.

Hainsworth JD, Greco FA. Treatment of patients with cancer of an unknown primary site. *N Engl J Med* 1993;329:257–263.

Hainsworth JD, Johnson DH, Greco FA. Poorly differentiated neuroendocrine carcinoma of unknown primary site: a newly recognized clinicopathologic entity. *Ann Intern Med* 1988;109:364–371.

Hainsworth JD, Johnson DH, Greco FA. Cisplatin-based combination chemotherapy in the treatment of poorly differentiated carcinoma and poorly differentiated adenocarcinoma of unknown primary site: results of a 12-year experience. *J Clin Oncol* 1992;10:912–922.

Hainsworth JD, Spigel DR, Raefsky EL, et al. Combination chemotherapy with gemcitabine and irinotecan in patients with previously treated carcinoma of an unknown primary site: a Minnie Pearl Cancer Research Network Phase II trial. *Cancer* 2005;104(9): 1992–1997.

Kolesnikov-Gauthier H, Levy E, Merlet P, et al. FDG PET in patients with cancer of an unknown primary. *Nucl Med Commun* 2005;26(12):1059–1066.

Lenzi R, Hess KR, Abbruzzese MC. Poorly differentiated carcinoma and poorly differentiated adenocarcinoma of unknown origin: favorable subsets of patients with unknown-primary carcinoma. *J Clin Oncol* 1997;15:2056–2066.

Moertel CG. Adenocarcinoma of unknown origin. *Ann Intern Med* 1979;91:646–647.

Neumann KH, Nystrom JS. Metastatic cancer of unknown origin: nonsquamous cell type. *Semin Oncol* 1982;9:427.

Stokkel MP, Terhoard CH, Hordij KFJ, et al. The detection of unknown primary tumors in patients with cervical metastases by dual-head positron emission tomography. *Oral Oncol* 1999;35:390–394.

Strnad CM, Grosh WW, Baxter J, et al. Peritoneal carcinomatosis of unknown primary site in women: a distinctive subset of adenocarcinoma. *Ann Intern Med* 1989;11:213–217.

Woods RL, Fox RM, Tattersall MH, et al. Metastatic adenocarcinomas of unknown primary site: a randomized study of two combination chemotherapy regimens. *N Engl J Med* 1980;303:87–89.

CHAPTER 26

Human Immunodeficiency Virus

Mary E. Cianfrocca

I. Introduction. Four malignancies are considered acquired immunodeficiency syndrome (AIDS)–defining illnesses: Kaposi's sarcoma (KS), primary central nervous system (CNS) lymphoma (PCNSL), non–Hodgkin's lymphoma (NHL), and cervical cancer. Although other malignancies appear to have an increased incidence in human immunodeficiency virus (HIV)–infected patients (e.g., squamous cell anal cancer and Hodgkin's disease), their precise relationship to HIV infection has not yet been established. The management of any cancer in an HIV-infected patient requires an integrated team approach. Treatment of the underlying HIV infection must be incorporated into the overall treatment plan, in addition to aggressive prophylaxis and treatment of opportunistic infections, maintenance of general health and nutrition, and psychosocial support.

II. Kaposi's sarcoma (KS)

A. Epidemiology. KS is one of the most common HIV-associated malignancies. The incidence of KS in both developed and developing countries rose steadily in the 1970s and 1980s, peaked around 1994, and declined dramatically since the introduction of highly active antiretroviral therapy (HAART). As an AIDS-defining illness, the incidence of KS has decreased from approximately 33% of patients in the early 1980s to 14% in the early 1990s to only 6.4% in 1998. In recent years, KS most often presents as a late, non–AIDS-defining manifestation of HIV infection. In developing counties, however, the incidence of KS remains high. In some parts of Africa, KS is the most common cancer in men, accounting for up to 50% of all cancers in men. There is significant evidence that points to the importance of human herpes virus type 8 (HHV-8) in the pathogenesis of KS. HHV-8 DNA is identified in more than 90% of KS biopsies. Serologic studies demonstrate detectable antibodies to HHV-8 in a high percentage of KS patients. Furthermore, antibodies to HHV-8 have been associated with the subsequent development of KS.

B. Presentation and detection. The natural history of KS is extremely variable. KS most often presents as a pink or brown–purple papule or plaque on the skin or mucous membranes. Lesions are frequently symmetric and follow Langer's lines. KS can present anywhere but has a predilection for the retroauricular areas, soles of the feet, extremities, genitalia, and face. In addition to their cosmetic unacceptability, KS lesions can cause significant morbidity and organ dysfunction. Dermal lymphatic involvement, most commonly involving the lower extremities, genitalia, and periorbital area, can cause painful and disfiguring lymphedema. The edema is often out of proportion to the visible skin involvement. Oral cavity lesions occur in approximately 45% of patients with cutaneous KS, and the oral cavity is the first site of disease in 15% of patients. Oral lesions can interfere with speech and eating. Gastrointestinal involvement, present in up to half the number of patients, is often asymptomatic but can cause pain, diarrhea, and bleeding. Pulmonary involvement is the most common life-threatening manifestation of KS. It may be difficult to differentiate from opportunistic infection because the chest radiograph may show a reticulonodular or nodular infiltrate, with or without pleural effusions. Bronchoscopy is useful to visualize the characteristic erythematous plaque-like bronchial lesions of KS. However, biopsy is rarely done because of the risk of bleeding from these highly vascular tumors. Thallium and gallium scans may be useful to differentiate KS from an opportunistic pulmonary infection.

C. Staging. KS is a multicentric tumor and hence does not easily fit the usual TNM categorization. Because the overall prognosis may be more closely related to the degree of underlying immune dysfunction than to sites of disease involvement, the AIDS Clinical Trials Group (ACTG) developed a staging system that reflects various prognostic factors (Table 26.1). Patients are defined as good or poor risk on the basis of tumor burden, sites of involvement, CD4 lymphocyte count, history of opportunistic infections, systemic symptoms, and performance status. In the pre-HAART era, a study validating the ACTG staging system identified tumor burden as a significant predictive factor only in patients with a CD4 count of at least 200 cells/μL. The presence of systemic symptoms was not a predictor of outcome, and a CD4 count of 150 cells/μL, rather than 200 cells/μL, was a better discriminator of outcome. In

Table 26.1. AIDS Clinical Trials Group staging for epidemic Kaposi's sarcoma[a]

	Relative Risk	
Disease status	Good risk (0) (all of the following)	Poor risk (1) (any of the following)
Tumor (T)	Confined to skin, minimal oral disease, or both	Edema; extensive oral ulcers; visceral and gastrointestinal disease
Immune status (I)[a]	CD4 count ≥ 150/μL	CD4 count < 150/μL
Systemic illness (S)	No prior opportunistic infection or thrush; no B symptoms	Prior opportunistic infection or thrush; B symptoms; performance status <70%; other HIV-related illness

B Symptoms, unexplained fever, weight loss >10%, night sweats, diarrhea >2 weeks.
[a] Modified by validation study.

the post-HAART era however, a reassessment of the ACTG staging system was recently reported. Multivariate analysis indicated that tumor burden and presence of HIV-related systemic disease but not CD4 count were predictive of survival. In particular, analysis of the interaction between tumor stage and systemic disease identified two main risk categories with T1S1 patients having a significantly worse survival as compared to all other groups (T1S0, T0S1, T0S0). Furthermore, within the T1 risk category, pulmonary involvement was associated with a significantly worse survival as compared with the other T1 sites.

The initial evaluation of a patient with KS should involve a careful physical examination, including a rectal examination with Hemoccult testing. The history should focus on the rate of progression of KS and lesion-associated symptoms (pain, edema, disfigurement), as well as the history of HIV treatment, HIV-related opportunistic infections, the rate of decline in CD4 lymphocyte counts, and viral load. Even though the lesions are characteristic, a biopsy should be done to exclude other cutaneous processes. A baseline chest radiograph is important to look for asymptomatic visceral disease. Computed tomography (CT) scans are not indicated unless the patient's symptoms suggest abdominal disease. Upper endoscopy and colonoscopy are not indicated in the absence of unexplained gastrointestinal bleeding or symptoms. Medications should be reviewed to ensure that patients are receiving appropriate HAART and prophylaxis for opportunistic infections as well as to identify potentially myelosuppressive drugs that may complicate the use of chemotherapeutic agents (e.g., trimethoprim–sulfamethoxazole, sulfadiazine, and zidovudine).

D. Treatment. Effective treatment of KS is dependent on clear communication between the doctor and patient with regard to the risks and benefits of the proposed therapy, its interaction with HIV treatment, and the patient's overall expectations. **KS is not a curable tumor.** The first decision to be made is whether to initiate therapy. Indications to initiate treatment for KS include prevention of disease progression, cosmesis, palliation of symptoms, and visceral disease. In general, local therapies are used for minimal, primarily cosmetically disturbing KS or for patients with severe multisystem compromise who may not tolerate systemic treatment. Systemic therapy is indicated for bulky, rapidly progressing, symptomatic, or life-threatening disease (Table 26.2). The determination of appropriate therapy is based on an evaluation of both tumor and immune status. Regardless of the extent of KS, effective HIV suppression tends to improve both the response to KS treatment and the durability of the response.

    1. Local therapy. Limited numbers of small lesions can be treated by radiotherapy, topical therapy, cryotherapy, or intralesional injection. Surgery is occasionally useful for an isolated pedunculated lesion. Cryotherapy with liquid nitrogen can lead to hypopigmentation, which may be cosmetically unacceptable to dark-skinned patients. Intralesional therapy with vinblastine or interferon (IFN) can be effective but is limited by the need for multiple injections (Table 26.3). After the injection of oral lesions,

response rates for individual lesions range from 27% to 49%. The main adverse effect is local skin irritation and local pain. There is no evidence of systemic absorption. Radiation therapy is effective for local control of KS. Depending on the dose and schedule, radiation therapy results in the most satisfying cosmetic result and longest duration of benefit of all the available local interventions.

2. Highly active antiretroviral therapy (HAART). Patients with HIV-associated KS should be treated with HAART whenever possible. HAART has been shown to prolong the time to treatment failure and improve survival in patients receiving chemotherapy for HIV-related KS. Furthermore, regression of KS after institution of HAART alone has been well-documented. At the present time, however, the evidence suggests that HAART-induced regression primarily occurs in patients with limited KS who were not previously treated with HAART.

3. Systemic therapy

    a. Biologic response modifiers. IFN-α is the best-studied biologic response modifier. A clear-cut dose–response relationship has not been established. Responses have been reported with doses ranging from 1×10^6 U/day to 36×10^6 U three times per week (Table 26.4 for recommended dosing). Immune function, as measured by CD4 lymphocyte counts, is the best predictor of response to IFN as a single agent. Patients with CD4 lymphocyte counts of more than 400 cells/μL have an overall response rate of 45%, whereas patients with CD4 lymphocyte counts of less than 100 cells/μL respond less than 10% of the time. Although it may take more than 8 weeks to respond, the responses are often durable, with a median response duration of 1 to 2 years. IFN is best prescribed in combination with antiretroviral agents. IFN plus azidothymidine (AZT) results in a response rate of greater than 40%, with responses seen even in patients with CD4 counts below 100 cells/μL. IFN has been evaluated in combination with protease inhibitor–based antiretroviral therapy

Table 26.4. Selected systemic treatment regimens for Kaposi's sarcoma

Regimens	Dosage
Biologic response modifier	
Interferon-α	$1–10 \times 10^6$ U/day SC
Chemotherapy	
Liposomal doxorubicin (Doxil)	20 mg/m² IV every 3 weeks
Liposomal daunorubicin (DaunoXome)	40 mg/m² IV every 2 weeks
Paclitaxel	100 mg/m² IV every 2 weeks, *or*
	135 mg/m² IV every 3 weeks

in a recent phase I trial. Dose-limiting toxicities were neutropenia and malaise and the maximum tolerated IFN dose was 5 million IU/day. Most practitioners begin with antiretroviral therapy and relatively low-dose IFN-α, 1 to 5 $\times$ 10^6 U SC daily.

b. Chemotherapy. Chemotherapy provides rapid palliation of KS-related symptoms for most patients (see Table 26.4). Liposomal anthracyclines (e.g., liposomal daunorubicin [DaunoXome], liposomal doxorubicin [Doxil]) are currently considered the chemotherapeutic agents of choice for advanced KS. Multiple randomized trials of bleomycin and vincristine, with or without doxorubicin (Adriamycin), compared with one of the liposomal anthracyclines have consistently demonstrated less toxicity and equal or better response rates and response durations with the liposomal anthracyclines. For second-line therapy, paclitaxel 100 mg/m^2 every 2 weeks or 135 mg/m^2 every 3 weeks has produced response rates of 50% to 70% associated with significant palliation of tumor-related symptoms. Doses of paclitaxel may need to be reduced for patients who are also receiving HAART with drugs metabolized by the same cytochrome P-450 pathway.

Patients often require growth factor support between cycles. Granulocyte colony-stimulating factor 5 μg/kg SC given on days 7 to 12 of a 14-day (or 21-day) treatment cycle is often sufficient to preserve adequate neutrophil counts to prevent infection and allow timely administration of therapy. An absolute neutrophil count of 750/μL is adequate to deliver therapy with liposomal anthracyclines.

The duration of treatment is variable. Treatment should be continued until the maximal response is obtained; however, intercurrent illness may interrupt therapy. Although lesions may progress after therapy is discontinued, an effective maintenance therapy has not yet been defined. Maximal viral suppression with highly active antiretroviral therapy (HAART) may suppress KS tumor regrowth after discontinuation of chemotherapy.

III. Non–Hodgkin's lymphoma (NHL)

A. Background. HIV-related lymphomas have increased as a percentage of first AIDS-defining illness since the increased use of HAART. Studies to determine if the use of HAART has led to a decrease in the overall incidence of HIV-related lymphomas have been inconclusive. HIV-associated NHLs are high-grade B-cell lymphomas similar to those seen in other immunocompromised patients. In comparison to NHL in the general population, HIV-associated NHLs are more likely to have advanced disease with bone marrow involvement and leptomeningeal disease and B symptoms. Primary CNS lymphoma accounts for less than 15% of the new AIDS-associated NHL, occurs in patients with severe immunodeficiency, and is universally associated with Epstein-Barr virus (EBV).

B. Presentation and detection. The most common presentations for HIV-associated NHL are constitutional symptoms (fevers, night sweats, and weight loss) or an enlarging mass.

Extranodal presentations, although once common, have become less frequent since the introduction of HAART. Nodal presentations occur in 60% of patients, and the remainder present with extranodal disease, most commonly involving the gastrointestinal tract, bone marrow, and liver. Very unusual sites of NHL have been seen, including the ear lobe, heart, and bile ducts. Seventy-five percent of patients present with advanced disease (stage III or IV).

C. Staging. The Ann Arbor staging classification is commonly used to stage HIV-related NHL (see Chapter 23); however, the correlation between stage and prognosis is weaker with HIV-associated cases. In the pre-HAART era, treatment of patients with HIV-related NHL was frequently complicated by severe hematologic toxicity and increased infectious mortality. Complete remissions (CRs) were uncommon and median survival was less than 6 months. In a pre-HAART study, four important adverse prognostic factors were identified for HIV-associated NHL: CD4 lymphocyte counts of less than 100 cells/μL, age more than 35 years, stage III or IV, and use of IV drugs. The presence of three or four of these indicators was associated with a median survival of only 18 weeks as compared with 46 weeks for patients with one or none of these indicators. Similarly, in a retrospective review of 60 patients, two prognostic subgroups were identified on the basis of immune function, performance status, and bone marrow involvement (Table 26.5). Use of HAART, however, has been associated with improved tumor response and survival.

Table 26.5. Prognostic stratification for HIV-associated non–Hodgkin's lymphoma

From Levine	From Strauss
Good prognosis: median survival = 11.3 months No prior AIDS diagnosis, *and* Karnofsky performance status >70%, *and* No bone marrow involvement	Good prognosis: Presence of 0–1 indicators, median survival of 46 weeks.
Poor prognosis: median survival = 4.0 months Prior AIDS diagnosis, *or* Karnofsky performance status <70%, *or* Bone marrow involvement	Poor prognosis: Presence of 3–4 indicators, median survival of 18 weeks Prognostic factors: • Age <35 • CD4 <100 • Stage III or IV • Use of IV drugs

HIV, human immunodeficiency virus; AIDS, acquired immunodeficiency syndrome.
From Levine AM, Sullivan-Halley J, Pike MC, et al. Human immunodeficiency virus-related lymphoma: prognostic factors predictive of survival. *Cancer* 1991;68:2466–2472; and Strauss, with permission.

Complete staging evaluation should include CT scans of the head, chest, abdomen, and pelvis; bilateral bone marrow biopsies; and lumbar puncture with cerebrospinal fluid (CSF) sent for protein and cytologic evaluation. Before the availability of HAART, 40% of patients had CNS involvement; therefore, all patients should undergo CSF evaluation regardless of clinical stage. The incidence of CNS involvement at presentation in the HAART era is unknown but appears to be decreasing.

D. Treatment

1. General approach. The best therapy for HIV-associated NHL remains to be defined. As is the case for KS, aggressive treatment of the underlying HIV infection is an important component of treatment. Fortunately, many clinical trials are ongoing to improve our understanding and treatment of this disease. Therapy must be tailored to the overall condition of each individual patient.

2. Systemic therapy. Before the availability of HAART, patients with AIDS-related NHL had a high incidence of opportunistic infections, limited bone marrow reserve, and poor outcomes with dose-intensive treatment. Because of this, the ACTG compared standard m-BACOD (Table 26.6) with low-dose (50% doses of cyclophosphamide and doxorubicin) m-BACOD in patients with HIV-associated NHL. There was no difference in the complete response rate or median survival between the two groups, but the low-dose group had significantly less hematologic toxicity. This led to the recommendation of low-dose treatment, particularly for patients with CD4 counts less than 200 cells/μL.

In the HAART era, standard chemotherapy should be recommended for patients with well-controlled HIV infection. The optimal treatment recommendation for patients with poorly controlled HIV infection is unclear. French/Italian randomized studies have shown that for patients with good performance status and relatively preserved immune function, treatment with standard-dose CHOP is feasible and leads to a complete response (59%) and event-free survival rates (33% at 2 years) significantly higher than those obtained with low-dose CHOP.

On the basis of data suggesting that longer exposure of tumor cells to drugs may enhance drug efficacy, a 4-day infusional regimen of cyclophosphamide, etoposide, and doxorubicin (CDE) has been evaluated in HIV-associated NHL. Phase II studies demonstrated a CR rate (46%) similar to that obtained with standard regimens but with prolongation of the median time to progression to 17 months and a near doubling of the 1-year survival rate (48%). Randomized trials comparing infusional versus bolus chemotherapy are underway.

While HIV suppression is consistently associated with improved overall survival for patients with HIV-associated malignancies, it is not clear that HAART and NHL therapy must be delivered concurrently. A possible downside of chemotherapy plus HAART is the potential for enhanced toxicity. Protease inhibitors interfere with the excretion of drugs metabolized through hepatic cytochrome P-450,

Table 26.6. Selected chemotherapy regimens for HIV-associated non–Hodgkin's lymphoma

Low-dose m-BACOD

Bleomycin	4 mg/m^2 IV on day 1
Doxorubicin	25 mg/m^2 IV on day 1
Cyclophosphamide	300 mg/m^2 IV on day 1
Vincristine	1.4 mg/m^2 IV on day 1 (not to exceed 2 mg total)
Dexamethasone	3 mg/m^2 PO on days 1–5
Methotrexate	500 mg/m^2 IV on day 15
Leucovorin	25 mg PO every 6 h for four doses, on day 16 beginning exactly 24 h after methotrexate

CHOP

Cyclophosphamide	750 mg/m^2 IV on day 1
Doxorubicin	50 mg/m^2 IV on day 1
Vincristine	1.4 mg/m^2 IV on day 1, not to exceed 2 mg total
Prednisone	100 mg/m^2 PO on days 1–5

CDE chemotherapy

Cyclophosphamide	200 mg/m^2/24 h CIV on days 1–4
Doxorubicin	12.5 mg/m^2/24 h CIV on days 1–4
Etoposide	60 mg/m^2/24 h CIV on days 1–4

Infusional EPOCH regimen (repeated q3wk × 6cycles)

Etoposide	50 mg/m^2/day CIV × 4 days
Vincristine	0.4 mg/m^2/day CIV × 4 days
Doxorubicin	10 mg/m^2/day CIV × 4 days
Cyclophosphamide	187 mg/m^2 IV on day 5 for CD4+ count <100, *or*
	375 mg/m^2 IV on day 5 for CD4+ count ≥100
Prednisone	60 mg/m^2 PO on days 1–5
G-CSF	Starting on day 6

HIV, human immunodeficiency virus; G-CSF, granulocyte colony-stimulating factor; CIV, continuous IV infusion.

and indinavir, in particular, decreases cyclophosphamide clearance by 40%. Recommendations for dose modifications based on these pharmacologic interactions are not yet available. Saquinavir has been associated with significant mucositis in patients receiving myelosuppressive chemotherapy.

Little and colleagues treated patients with infusional EPOCH treatment (see Table 26.6) and withheld HAART until the completion of chemotherapy. The observed CR rate was 77% with an overall survival of 74%, after approximately 30 months median follow-up. The median survival has not yet been reached. Resumption of HAART after chemotherapy leads to rapid repopulation of CD4+ cells and suppression of HIV viral load within 3 months.

The role of rituximab in the treatment of HIV-related NHL is controversial. The AIDS Malignancy Consortium (AMC) conducted a phase III trial randomizing patients to standard-dose CHOP versus CHOP with rituximab. Although the CR rate was higher in the R-CHOP arm (57% vs. 47%), this did not reach statistical significance. Death due to lymphoma was also lower in the R-CHOP arm. There were more deaths from infection, however, in the R-CHOP arm (15% vs. 2%; $p = 0.027$). Interpretation of these results is complicated by the fact that more patients in the R-CHOP arm had a CD4 count of less than 50 cells/mm^3 and of the 15 patients on the R-CHOP arm who died of infection, 9 had a CD4 count less than 50 cells/mm^3. Since more than 60% of the infectious deaths overall occurred in patients with CD4 counts of less than 50 cells/mm^3, it raises the question of whether the higher infectious mortality on the R-CHOP arm was due to the severe immunosuppression of the patients on that arm. Furthermore, other trials have confirmed the high CR rate with rituximab-based chemotherapy without additional infectious complications. A current AMC trial is evaluating EPOCH with concurrent versus sequential rituximab.

For patients with well-controlled HIV infection, who are not eligible for a randomized clinical trial, standard-dose CHOP, infusional EPOCH, or infusional CDE plus or minus rituximab are reasonable therapeutic options (see Table 26.6). Careful observation for increased or unusual toxicities is essential. Growth factor support is frequently needed. Aggressive prophylaxis against opportunistic infections is important. Regardless of CD4 lymphocyte count, all patients should receive prophylaxis for *Pneumocystis carinii* pneumonia during the treatment of a high-grade lymphoma (Table 26.7).

3. Central nervous system (CNS) prophylaxis/treatment. CNS involvement at presentation occurs in 10% to 20% of patients with HIV-related NHL. The presence of EBV in the primary tumor is an independent predictor for CNS involvement either at diagnosis or during relapse. CNS prophylaxis is recommended for patients with small noncleaved cell tumors or epidural, bone marrow, paraspinal, paranasal sinus or testicular involvement. CNS prophylaxis should include four weekly treatments of either preservative-free methotrexate (12 mg) or

Table 26.7. Prophylaxis regimens for *Pneumocystis carinii* pneumonia

Trimethoprim–sulfamethoxazole (Bactrim DS) 1 tablet PO, Monday, Wednesday, Friday, *or*

Dapsone 100 mg PO daily[a]

[a]Exclude glucose-6-phosphatase deficiency by quantitative spectrophotometry in high-risk patients before initiating therapy.

cytosine arabinoside (50 mg). In patients with documented meningeal disease, intrathecal therapy should be given three times per week until the CSF clears, then weekly for 8 weeks and monthly for 10 months. An Ommaya reservoir should be placed to facilitate therapy.

4. Burkitt's lymphoma (BL). While survival of patients with HIV-associated diffuse large cell lymphoma has improved in the HAART era, survival of HIV-associated BL remains poor. At present, patients with HIV-associated BL are not treated differently than HIV-positive patients with diffuse large cell lymphoma. However, there is data supporting the use of more intensive chemotherapy regimens such as those used in HIV-negative patients in this population.

5. Follow-up. In this era of cost containment, repeat staging studies are often controversial. Despite this zeal to minimize testing, documentation of a complete response as early as clinically warranted is important to minimize the duration of therapy in this already-immunocompromised group of patients. Treatment should be continued for a minimum of four cycles or for two cycles after attainment of complete response.

6. Salvage therapy. Some patients who have a relapse after initial treatment have been successfully treated with an alternative NHL regimen. Suitable patients should be considered for high-dose chemotherapy with autologous stem cell transplantation.

IV. Primary central nervous system lymphoma (PCNSL)

A. Background. The incidence of PCNSL has declined since the introduction of HAART. Unlike systemic HIV-associated NHL, which can occur at earlier stages of HIV infection, PCNSL typically occurs in profoundly immunocompromised patients with CD4 lymphocyte count less than 50 cells/μL. The Epstein-Barr virus (EBV) genome is identified in virtually all investigated cases of HIV-associated PCNSL. This supports the belief that EBV may have a direct etiologic role in the development of this disease.

B. Presentation and detection. The diagnosis of PCNSL is often difficult to make. Most patients present with a focal neurologic deficit. CT scan or magnetic resonance imaging (MRI) of the head typically shows single or multiple contrast-enhancing masses with surrounding edema. These lesions are often in a periventricular location and may be difficult to distinguish from those of toxoplasmosis. CSF cytology is rarely diagnostic, and stereotactic biopsy is often recommended to establish a tissue diagnosis. Because 95% of HIV-positive patients with toxoplasmosis have serologic evidence of *Toxoplasma* sp. infection, the *Toxoplasma* titer can be useful to determine a course of action.

- If the *Toxoplasma* titer is negative, stereotactic biopsy should be considered.
- If the *Toxoplasma* titer is positive and the patient is either clinically unstable or the clinician feels uncomfortable without a tissue diagnosis; based on the clinical scenario, stereotactic biopsy should be considered.

- If, however, the *Toxoplasma* titer is positive and the patient is clinically stable, a 1- to 2-week trial of empiric therapy for a presumptive diagnosis of toxoplasmosis may be appropriate. If there is no evidence of clinical or radiologic improvement or if there is evidence of clinical decompensation, stereotactic biopsy should be considered.

This approach requires close and frequent monitoring for signs of neurologic deterioration or progression. A newer alternative to the above is the use of EBV polymerase chain reaction (PCR) in the spinal fluid as a diagnostic clue. The presence of EBV by PCR in the CSF is a sensitive and highly specific (80% and 100%, respectively, in a recent study) marker for primary PCNSL. Therefore, in the context of either a suggestive MRI or CT of the brain and a positive thallium scan, EBV-detection in the CSF may be considered highly suggestive of PCNSL in the absence of a tissue diagnosis.

C. Treatment. Whole-brain radiation therapy is the standard therapy. Temporary control and improvement of neurologic deficits occur in 70% of patients. A range of radiation doses (2,000 to 6,000 cGy) has been used. In one retrospective review, survival was found to be a function of performance status, not the total radiation dose administered. **Median survival with radiation is only 2 to 5 months.** Recent data suggests that the addition of HAART to radiation therapy improves survival. Furthermore, tumor regression with HAART alone has been reported. The role of chemotherapy or chemoradiation for HIV-related PCNSL is not well established. Treatment with combined-modality therapy (CHOP plus radiation therapy) based on the experience in non–HIV-related PCNSLs was evaluated and did not demonstrate superior results to radiation therapy alone. High-dose methotrexate, with or without intrathecal chemotherapy, has been reported to lead to prolongation of median survival to as much as 40 months; however, studies done to date have been very small. Small clinical trials evaluating preradiation chemotherapy with CHOD/BVAM (cyclophosphamide, doxorubicin, vincristine, and dexamethasone alternated with BCNU, vincristine, ara-C, and methotrexate) have reported prolonged survival but with significant toxicity including dementia and leukoencephalopathy.

V. Cervical cancer

A. Background. It was not until 1993 that cervical cancer became an AIDS-defining illness. As in non–HIV-infected women, the development of cervical squamous carcinoma has been directly linked to prior infection with human papilloma virus (HPV). Although both HIV and HPV are sexually transmitted diseases, other immunosuppressed populations also have an increased incidence of HPV infection, suggesting that immune competence is a deterrent to the development of HPV coinfection. The presence of HPV, especially types 16, 18, and 31, is correlated with a higher incidence of cervical intraepithelial neoplasia (CIN).

B. Presentation and detection. Presentation is similar to that of non–HIV-related cervical cancer, except that the disease is often more aggressive in HIV-infected patients and advanced disease is more common. Routine Papanicolaou's

(Pap) smears may not be sensitive enough to detect this aggressive neoplasm. It has been recommended that colposcopy, not Pap smears, be the standard for following up HIV-infected women at high risk of CIN. Because CIN may progress at a faster rate in HIV-infected women, annual screening may not detect "curable" disease. Women with rapidly progressing CIN should probably be tested for HIV. The effect of HAART on CIN has been examined and the findings have been mixed, with some studies showing no effect and others suggesting modest regression (12.5% regression in one study).

C. Staging. The International Federation of Gynecology and Obstetrics (FIGO) staging system, used for non–HIV-infected patients, is used in this population as well (see Chapter 11). Stage for stage, however, the prognosis appears worse in HIV-infected women owing to their compromised immune function.

D. Treatment. In a small study, women with CD4 lymphocyte counts of less than 500 cells/μL did significantly worse than women with intact immune function. Until these results are confirmed in larger trials, HIV-positive women with invasive cervical cancer should be treated in the same manner as women without HIV infection.

VI. Other malignancies. Hodgkin's lymphoma, testicular carcinoma, and anal cancers are also seen frequently in HIV-infected patients. Anecdotally, these malignancies appear more aggressive than their usual counterpart in immunocompetent patients, but no large trial has yet confirmed either increased virulence or increased incidence. It is interesting to speculate that EBV may play a role in the development of Hodgkin's disease. The role of HPV in the development of anal cancers has been well described. We recommend treatment of these malignancies with standard therapy. However, close attention should be paid to the prophylaxis and treatment of opportunistic pathogens as well as to the appropriate use of antiretroviral agents.

SUGGESTED READINGS

Adieh-Greant L, Li R, Levine AM, et al. Highly active antiretroviral therapy and cervical squamous intraepithelial neoplasia lesions in human immunodeficiency virus-positive women. *J Natl Cancer Inst* 2004;96:1070–1076.

Bower M, Fox P, Fife K, et al. Highly active antiretroviral therapy prolongs time to treatment failure in Kaposi's Sarcoma. *AIDS* 1999;13:2105–2111.

Boue F, Gabarre J, Gisselbrecht C, et al. CHOP chemotherapy plus rituximab in HIV patients with high grade lymphoma-results of an ANRS trial. *Blood* 2002;100:470a. (Abstract 1824).

Bundow D, Aboulafia DM. Potential drug interaction with paclitaxel and highly active antiretroviral therapy in two patients with AIDS-associated Kaposi's sarcoma. *Am J Clin Oncol* 2004;27:81–84.

Cingolani A, De Luca A, Larocca LM, et al. Minimally invasive diagnosis of acquired immunodeficiency syndrome-related primary central nervous system lymphoma. *J Natl Cancer Inst* 1998;90:364–369.

Cingolani A, Gastaldi R, Fassone L, et al. Epstein-Barr virus infection is predictive of CNS involvement in systemic AIDS-related non-Hodgkin's lymphomas. *J Clin Oncol* 2000;18:3325–3330.

Formenti SC, Gill PS, Lean E, et al. Primary central nervous system lymphoma in AIDS: results of radiation therapy. *Cancer* 1989;63:1101–1107.

Gill PS, Wernz J, Scadden DT, et al. Randomized phase II trial of liposomal daunorubicin (DaunoXome) versus doxorubicin, bleomycin, vincristine (ABV) in AIDS-related Kaposi's sarcoma. *J Clin Oncol* 1996;14:2353–2364.

Gill PS, Tulpule A, Espina BM, et al. Paclitaxel is safe and effective in the treatment of advanced AIDS-related Kaposi's sarcoma. *J Clin Oncol* 1999;17:1876–1883.

Heard I, Schmitz V, Costagliola D, et al. Early regression of cervical lesions in HIV-seropositive women receiving highly active antiretroviral therapy. *AIDS* 1998;12:1459–1464.

Hoffman C, Tabrizian S, Wolf E, et al. Survival of AIDS patients with primary central nervous system lymphoma is dramatically improved by HAART-induced immune recovery. *AIDS* 2001;15:2119–2127.

Holkova B, Takeshita K, Cheng DM, et al. Effect of highly active antiretroviral therapy on survival in patients with HIV-associated Kaposi's sarcoma treated with chemotherapy. *J Clin Oncol* 2001;19:3848–3851.

International Collaboration on HIV and Cancer. Highly active antiretroviral therapy and incidence of cancer in human-immunodeficiency virus-infected adults. *J Natl Cancer Inst* 2000; 92:1823–1830.

Kaplan LD, Lee JY, Ambinder RF, et al. Rituximab does not improve clinical outcome in a randomized phase 3 trial of CHOP with or without rituximab in patients with HIV-associated non-Hodgkins lymphoma: AIDS-Malignancies Consortium Trial 010. *Blood* 2005;106:1538–1543.

Knowles DM. Etiology and pathogenesis of AIDS-related non-Hodgkin's lymphoma. *Hematol Oncol Clin North Am* 1996;10:1081–1109.

Krishnan A, Molina A, Zaia J, et al. Durable remission with autologous stem cell transplantation for high-risk HIV-associated lymphomas. *Blood* 2005;105:874–878.

Krown SE. Highly active antiretroviral therapy in AIDS-associated Kaposi's sarcoma: implications for the design of therapeutic trials in patients with advanced, symptomatic Kaposi's sarcoma. *J Clin Oncol* 2004;22:399–402.

Krown SE, Lee JL, Lin L, et al. Interferon-α2b with protease inhibitor-based antiretroviral therapy in patients with AIDS-associated Kaposi Sarcoma: an AIDS Malignancy Consortium Phase I Trial. *J Acquir Immune Defic Syndr* 2006;41:149–153.

Lebbe C, Blum L, Pellet C, et al. Clinical and biological impact of antiretroviral therapy with protease inhibitors on HIV related Kaposi's sarcoma. *AIDS* 1998;12:F45–F49.

Levine AM, Sullivan-Halley J, Pike MC, et al. Human immunodeficiency virus-related lymphoma: prognostic factors predictive of survival. *Cancer* 1991;68:2466–2472.

Levine AM, Wernz JC, Kaplan L, et al. Low-dose chemotherapy with central nervous system prophylaxis and zidovudine maintenance in AIDS-related lymphoma. *JAMA* 1991;266:84–88.

Lim ST, Karim R, Nathwani BN, et al. AIDS-related Burkitt's lymphoma versus diffuse large-cell lymphoma in the pre-highly active antiretroviral therapy (HAART) and HAART eras: Significant differences in survival with standard chemotherapy. *J Clin Oncol* 2005;23:4430–4438.

Maiman M, Fruchter RG, Guy L, et al. Human immunodeficiency virus infection and invasive cervical carcinoma. *Cancer* 1993;71: 402–406.

McGowan JP, Shah S. Long-term remission of AIDS-related primary central nervous system lymphoma associated with highly active antiretroviral therapy. *AIDS* 1998;12:952–954.

Miles SA. Pathogenesis of AIDS-related Kaposi's sarcoma: evidence of a viral etiology. *Hematol Oncol Clin North Am* 1996;10:1011–1021.

Minkoff H, Ahdieh L, Massad LS, et al. The effect of highly active antiretroviral therapy on cervical cytologic changes associated with oncogenic HPV among HIV-infected women. *AIDS* 2001; 15:2157–2164.

Nasti G, Talamini R, Antinori A, et al. AIDS-related Kaposi's Sarcoma evaluation of potential new prognostic factors and assessment of the AIDS Clinical Trial Group Staging System in the HAART era—the Italian Cooperative Group on AIDS and tumors and the Italian cohort of patients naïve from antiretrovirals. *J Clin Oncol* 2003;21:2876–2882.

Newell ME, Hoy JF, Cooper SG, et al. Human immunodeficiency virus-related primary central nervous system lymphoma: factors influencing survival in 111 patients. *Cancer* 2004;100:2627–2636.

Saville MW, Lietzau J, Pluda JM, et al. Treatment of HIV-associated Kaposi's sarcoma with paclitaxel. *Lancet* 1995;346:26–28.

Schafer A, Friedmann W, Mielke M, et al. The increased frequency of cervical dysplasia–neoplasia in women infected with the human immunodeficiency virus is related to the degree of immunosuppression. *Am J Obstet Gynecol* 1991;164:593–599.

Sparano JA, Wiernik PH, Strack M, et al. Infusional cyclophosphamide, doxorubicin and etoposide in HIV-1 and HTLV-1-related non-Hodgkin's lymphoma: a highly active regimen. *Blood* 1993;81: 2810–2815.

Spina M, Sparano JA, Jaeger U, et al. Rituximab and chemotherapy is highly effective in patients with CD-20-positive non-Hodgkin's lymphoma and HIV infection. *AIDS* 2003;1:137–138.

Stelzer KJ, Griffin TW. A randomized prospective trial of radiation therapy for AIDS-associated Kaposi's sarcoma. *Int J Radiat Oncol Biol Phys* 1993;27:1057–1061.

Straus DJ, Huang J, Testa MA, et al. Prognostic factors in the treatment of human immunodeficiency virus-associated non-Hodgkin's lymphoma: analysis of AIDS Clinical Trials Group protocol 142—low-dose versus standard-dose m-BACOD plus granulocyte-macrophage colony-stimulating factor. *J Clin Oncol* 1998;6:3601–3606.

Wang ES, Straus DJ, Teruya-Feldstein J, et al. Intensive chemotherapy with cyclophosphamide, doxorubicin, high-dose methotrexate/ifosfamide, etoposide and high-dose cytarabine (CODOX-M/IVAC) for human immunodeficiency virus-associated Burkitt lymphoma. *Cancer* 2003;6:1196–1205.

SECTION IV

Selected Aspects of Supportive Care of Patients with Cancer

CHAPTER 27

Side Effects of Cancer Chemotherapy

Janelle M. Tipton

Systemic cancer chemotherapy agents play a valuable role in cancer treatment; however, there are undesirable effects both to normal replicating and quiescent cells. Rapidly dividing normal cells that are vulnerable to damage include cells of the bone marrow, hair follicles, and mucous membranes, and reproductive system. Other toxicities may occur that are unrelated to cell growth and are particular to individual agents. The side effects of cancer chemotherapy agents may be acute, self-limited, and mild or can be chronic, permanent, and potentially life threatening in nature. Many advances have been made in the last 10 to 15 years in the management of side effects of chemotherapy. Although much progress has been made, the management of side effects continues to be of utmost importance for the tolerability of therapy and effect on overall quality of life. The implementation of evidence-based interventions has received increased emphasis and is critical in making appropriate clinical decisions for the management of side effects.

I. **Acute reactions**
   A. **Extravasation.** Extravasation is defined as the leakage or infiltration of drug into the subcutaneous tissues. *Vesicant* drugs that extravasate are capable of causing tissue necrosis or sloughing. *Irritant* drugs cause inflammation or pain at the site of extravasation. Common vesicant and irritant agents and potential antidotes are listed in Table 27.1.
      1. **Risk factors for peripheral extravasation** include small, fragile veins, venipuncture technique, site of venipuncture, drug administration technique, presence of superior vena cava syndrome, peripheral neuropathy, limited vein selection due to lymph node dissection, and concurrent use of medications that may cause somnolence, altered mental status, excessive movements, vomiting, and coughing.

Table 27.1.   Common vesicant and irritant drugs and potential antidotes

Chemotherapy Agent	Pharmacologic Antidote	Nonpharmacologic Antidote	Method of Administration
Mechlorethamine HCl	Sodium thiosulfate	None	Prepare 1/6 M solution: if 10% Na thiosulfate solution, mix 4 mL with 6 mL sterile water for injection. Through existing IV line, inject 2 mL for every 1 mL extravasated. Inject SC if needle is removed.
Cisplatin	Sodium thiosulfate	None	For large extravasations only (>20 mL) of cisplatin solution with 0.5 mg/mL). Use 2 mL of 10% sodium thiosulfate solution for each 100 mg cisplatin. Administer as with mechlorethamine.
Doxorubicin Daunorubicin Epirubicin Idarubicin Mitoxantrone	None	Topical cooling	Apply cold pad with circulating ice water, ice pack, or cryogel pack for 15–20 min at least 4 times/day for first 24–48 h. Some studies suggest benefit with 99% dimethyl sulfoxide (DMSO) 1–2 mL applied to site every 6 h.
Vincristine Vinblastine Vinorelbine	Hyaluronidase 150 units/1 mL SC	Warm compresses	Apply heat for 15–20 min at least 4 times/day for first 24–48 h. Hyaluronidase is instilled as multiple SC injections around extravasated area, using a small gauge needle (25 g).
Etoposide	None	Warm compresses	Treatment necessary only if large amount of concentrated solution extravasates. Treat as vincristine or vinblastine extravasations.
Oxaliplatin	Case reports of use of anti-inflammatory drugs and high-dose dexamethasone.	Case reports of topical cooling, but may make neuropathy worse.	
Paclitaxel (Taxol)	None	Topical cooling	Apply ice pack for 15–20 min at least 4 times/day for first 24 h

2. The **incidence of extravasation** for vesicant chemotherapy is recorded as 1% to 6% in the literature for peripheral chemotherapy. Extravasation may also occur with central venous catheters. Potential causes for central venous catheter extravasation include backflow secondary to fibrin sheath or thrombosis in the central venous catheter, needle dislodgement from a venous access port, central venous catheter damage, breakage, or separation, and displacement or migration of the catheter from the vein.

3. **Common signs and symptoms of extravasation** are pain or burning at the IV site, redness, swelling, inability to obtain a blood return, and change in the quality of the infusion. Any of these complaints or observations should be considered a symptom of extravasation until proved otherwise.

4. **Procedures to manage peripheral extravasation** are imperative to have in place, including guidelines or orders for extravasation management of vesicant and irritant agents before administration. If an extravasation is suspected, the following actions should be taken:

1. Stop administration of the chemotherapy agent.
2. Leave the needle/catheter in place and immobilize the extremity.
3. Attempt to aspirate any residual drug in the tubing, needle, or suspected extravasation site.
4. Notify the physician.
5. Administer the appropriate antidote, as shown in Table 27.1. This may include instillation of a drug antidote or application of heat or cold to the site. Of note, hyaluronidase was not commercially available from 2001 to late 2004. It is now available as Amphadase (hyaluronidase injection, Amphastar Pharmaceuticals, Rancho Cucamonga, CA).
6. Provide the patient and/or caregiver with instructions, including the need to elevate the site for 48 hours and the continuation of antidote measures as appropriate.
7. Discuss the need for further intervention with the physician, and photograph if indicated.
8. Document extravasation occurrence according to institutional guidelines.
9. Continued monitoring of extravasation site at 24 hours, 1 week, 2 weeks, and additionally as guideline recommends. Secondary complications such as infection and pain may occur. Follow-up photographs at these periods, if possible, are helpful in monitoring extent of injury and progress in healing.

5. **Procedures for central extravasation** are also critically important to follow, as extravasation of chemotherapeutic agents in the upper torso or neck area is difficult to manage and may result in extensive defects, requiring reconstructive surgery. Extreme caution should be taken by nurses administering chemotherapy by this route. Procedures followed in central extravasation are similar to peripheral extravasation. Assessment of lack of blood return, patient reports in changes of sensation, pain, burning, or swelling at the central venous catheter site or chest warrant immediate discontinuation of chemotherapy. Prompt administration of the appropriate antidote is recommended, but if the extravasation has been extensive, the actions may not prevent damage. Collaboration with the physician regarding the need for further studies to identify the cause of the extravasation will be necessary as well as other decisions for future plans for venous access.

B. Hypersensitivity and anaphylaxis. Specific drugs with the potential for hypersensitivity with or without an anaphylactic response should be administered under constant supervision of a competent and experienced nurse and with a physician readily available, preferably during the daytime. Important preassessment data to be documented include the patient's allergy history, though this information may not predict an allergic reaction to chemotherapy. Other risk factors include previous exposure to the agent and failure to administer effective prophylactic medications. Drugs with the highest risk of immediate hypersensitivity reactions are asparaginase, murine monoclonal antibodies (e.g., ibritumomab tiuxetan), the taxanes (paclitaxel and docetaxel), and platinum compounds (cisplatin, carboplatin, oxaliplatin). Drugs with a low to moderate risk include the anthracyclines, bleomycin, IV melphalan, etoposide, and humanized (e.g., trastuzumab) or chimeric (e.g., rituximab) monoclonal antibodies. Test doses or skin tests may be performed if there is an increased suspicion for hypersensitivity. In specific occasions, this is generally done with carboplatin, bleomycin and asparaginase. A skin testing protocol for carboplatin skin testing is shown in Table 27.2.

1. Type 1 hypersensitivity reactions are the most common chemotherapy-induced type of reactions. These reactions characteristically occur within 1 hour of receiving the drug; however, with paclitaxel, the hypersensitivity reactions often occur within the first 10 minutes of the start of the infusion. Common manifestations of a type 1 reaction

Table 27.2. Sample carboplatin skin testing protocol

1. All patients receiving their sixth and each subsequent doses of carboplatin will have skin test dosing.
2. Patients receive an intradermal injection of 0.02 mL of an undiluted aliquot from the carboplatin preparation planned for subsequent infusion. This dose is then diluted in 50 mL of 0.9% normal saline.
3. Following the intradermal injection, the injection site is examined at 5, 15, and 30 min.
4. A positive skin test is a wheal of ≥ 5 mm in diameter, with surrounding redness. A strongly positive skin test was one with ≥ 1 cm in diameter. If a patient develops a positive skin test, the physician is notified.
5. If the skin test is negative, the patient is then pretreated for the carboplatin with antiemetics, dexamethasone, diphenhydramine, and famotidine. Thirty minutes after the premedications are given, the carboplatin is given.

include urticaria, respiratory distress, bronchospasm, hypotension, angioedema, flushing, chest and back pain, and anxiety. With appropriate premedication, the incidence of the hypersensitivity reactions has markedly decreased with paclitaxel. Commonly used premedications include dexamethasone, diphenhydramine, and an H_2-histamine antagonist such as cimetidine, ranitidine, or famotidine. Emergency equipment should be immediately accessible, including oxygen, an Ambu respiratory assist bag, and suction equipment. The following parenteral drugs should also be stocked in the treatment area: epinephrine 1:1,000 or 1:10,000 solution, diphenhydramine 25 to 50 mg, methylprednisolone 125 mg, and dexamethasone 20 mg. The development of a clinical guideline for hypersensitivity reactions, with or without true anaphylaxis, may be helpful in preparing for a potential reaction, reducing delays in response time to a reaction, and standardizing the management of a reaction with standing orders. Table 27.3 provides a sample preprinted/standing order for the management of hypersensitivity and anaphylactic reactions.

2. Retreatment and rechallenge of patients who have experienced paclitaxel-associated hypersensitivity reactions are supported in the literature. If rechallenge is considered, paclitaxel should be administered in the appropriate setting where immediate emergency situations may be handled. The decision to reinstitute paclitaxel should be based on the clinical importance of using the drug in

Table 27.3. Sample standing orders for hypersensitivity reactions to chemotherapy agents

1. Have the following medications available:
   a. Diphenhydramine (Benadryl) 50 mg IV
   b. Methylprednisolone (Solu-Medrol) 125 mg IV or equivalent hydrocortisone
   c. Epinephrine (1:10,000) 10 mL single-dose vial (or 1 mL of 1:1,000, 1-mg vial)
2. If signs/symptoms of hypersensitivity occur (such as urticaria [hives], respiratory distress, bronchospasm, hypotension, angioedema, flushing, chest/back pain, anxiety), stop infusion of chemotherapy/biotherapy agent.
3. Maintain IV access with IVF normal saline at 200 mL/h until blood pressure stabilizes.
4. Administer oxygen at 2–4 L/min and measure pulse oximetry.
5. Administer methylprednisolone 125 mg IVP.
6. Administer diphenhydramine (Benadryl) 50 mg IVP.
7. Monitor blood pressure, pulse, and oxygen saturation continuously.
8. Notify physician immediately for further orders.
9. If symptoms do not resolve or if they worsen, administer epinephrine as directed by physician.
10. Initiate a code if airway patency is not maintained or cardiopulmonary arrest occurs.

IVF, intravenous fluid.

the particular disease setting. Patients have been success-fully retreated within hours to days of the initial paclitaxel reactions at full doses.

   a. Reinstitution of paclitaxel after experiencing a hypersensitivity reaction includes immediate discontin-uation of the paclitaxel infusion at the onset of symptoms and rapid administration of additional diphenhydramine and methylprednisolone. Following stabilization of the patient and waiting approximately for 30 minutes, the paclitaxel infusion is reinitiated, with initial infusion rates of 10% to 25% of the total infusion rate. If toler-ated, the rate can be gradually increased over the next several hours. Nursing care would also include vital signs every 5 minutes or continuous observation for the first 15 minutes, then every 15 minutes through the first hour, then hourly until the infusion is completed. An alternative is to pretreat the patient for 24 hours with dexamethasone 10 mg three times orally and to restart the infusion at the rate indicated earlier on the second day.

   b. Desensitization approaches. Rechallenge after a severe hypersensitivity reaction of the second episode of hypersensitivity reaction to paclitaxel and carboplatin are documented in the literature; however, planning for the "desensitization" is necessary. Regimens including dexamethasone 20 mg orally at 36 and 12 hours before chemotherapy and on the morning of chemotherapy have been studied. A full 30 minutes before the chemotherapy, other IV premedications such as dexamethasone 20 mg, diphenhydramine 50 mg, and H_2-histamine antagonist are given. For paclitaxel, the desensitization procedure continues with the administration of a test dose of 2 mg in 100 mL of normal saline over 30 minutes. If there is no reaction, 10 mg in 100 mL of normal saline is given over 30 minutes, followed by the remaining full dose in 500 mL of normal saline over 3 hours if still no reaction. If a reaction is experienced, the usual diphenhydramine and methylprednisolone medications are given.

II. Nausea and vomiting. Patients who are about to be-gin chemotherapy are often concerned and apprehensive about nausea and vomiting. Nausea and vomiting can be distressing enough to the patient to cause extreme physiologic and psy-chological discomfort, culminating in withdrawal from therapy. With the advent of more effective antiemetic regimens in the last 15 years, many improvements in the prevention and control of nausea and vomiting have led to a better quality of life for patients receiving chemotherapy. The goal of therapy is to pre-vent the three phases of nausea and vomiting: that which occurs before treatment is administered (anticipatory), that which fol-lows within the first 24 hours after treatment (acute), and that which occurs more than 24 hours after treatment (delayed). It is also important to assess nausea and vomiting separately because they are different events and may have different causes. Factors related to the chemotherapy that can affect the likelihood and severity of symptoms include the specific agents used, the doses of the drugs, and the schedule and route of administration. Other patient characteristics that may effect emesis include history of poor emetic control, history of alcoholism, age, gender, and history of motion sickness.

A. Emetic potential of the drug. To plan an effective approach to control nausea and vomiting, the chemotherapeutic agents are grouped according to their emetic potential (Table 27.4). This type of categorization is helpful in making decisions regarding possible antiemetics to be used and how aggressive the antiemetic regimen should be for patients receiving chemotherapy for the first time or in subsequent treatments. It is important to select appropriate antiemetics from the various antiemetic classes, and not to undertreat the patient for nausea and vomiting in the initial chemotherapy cycle. Failure to control nausea and/or vomiting may result in a conditioned response and subsequent anticipatory nausea and vomiting.

B. Antiemetic drugs. Agents that have been effective in preventing and treating nausea and vomiting (Table 27.5) come from various pharmacologic classes. They work by different mechanisms that may relate to the pathophysiologic processes causing nausea and vomiting. For many years, the mainstays of antiemetic therapy have been agents that block dopamine receptors. These agents have been somewhat effective but have limited value for highly emetogenic agents and, in escalating doses, have caused problematic side effects. Within the last 15 years, it was discovered that agents that block predominately the serotonin (5-hydroxytryptamine) subtype 3 (5-HT3) receptors, rather than the dopamine receptors, have greater efficacy in the prevention of nausea and vomiting. More recent research indicates that the tachykinins, including a peptide called *substance P*, play an important role in emesis. Substance P binds to the neurokinin type 1 (NK-1) receptor. Thus, the NK-1-receptor antagonists are now validated in their role in inhibiting nausea and vomiting with moderately and highly emetogenic chemotherapy. Oral NK-1-receptor antagonists are thought to improve acute nausea and vomiting associated with chemotherapy when combined with standard regimens (i.e., dexamethasone and 5-HT3 receptor antagonists) and to have additional effect during the period of delayed nausea and vomiting, alone or in combination with dexamethasone.

C. Combination antiemetic therapy. Several antiemetic regimens are effective, but their design should be based on two general principles:

- Combinations of antiemetics are more effective than single agents. It is common to use two or more antiemetics to prevent or manage nausea and vomiting.
- Preemptive treatment and scheduled administration are more effective than reactive therapy to prevent nausea and vomiting early in therapy and to manage potential delayed nausea and vomiting in the days following treatment.

Table 27.6 shows examples of antiemetic regimens that may be used when the chemotherapy has a high, moderate, and low emetic potential.

D. Nonpharmacologic interventions. Patients who are likely to experience or who have experienced anticipatory

Table 27.4. Emetogenic potential for commonly used chemotherapeutic agents[a]

Highly Emetogenic Agents (≥75% Potential for Nausea, Vomiting, or Both)	Moderately Emetogenic Agents (50%–75% Potential for Nausea, Vomiting, or Both)	Mildly Emetogenic Agents (25%–50% Potential for Nausea, Vomiting, or Both)
Carmustine	Carboplatin	Asparaginase
Cisplatin (>40 mg/m^2)	Cisplatin (<40 mg/m^2)	Bleomycin
Cyclophosphamide (>1 g/m^2)	Cyclophosphamide (200 mg/m^2 to 1 g/m^2)	Busulfan
		Capecitabine
	Cytarabine	Bevacizumab
Cytarabine (>1 g/m^2)	(200 mg/m^2 to 1 g/m^2)	Bortezomib (Velcade)
Dacarbazine (days 1 and 2)	Daunorubicin	Cetuximab
	Doxorubicin (<60 mg/m^2)	Cladribine
Dactinomycin	Etoposide	Cyclophosphamide (<200 mg/m^2)
Doxorubicin (>60 mg/m^2)	Gemcitabine	
Epirubicin	Idarubicin	Cytarabine (<200 mg/m^2)
Ifosfamide (>1.2 g/m^2)	Ifosfamide (<1.2 g/m^2)	Docetaxel
Mechlorethamine	Irinotecan	Fludarabine
Methotrexate (>1 g/m^2)		

Mitomycin (>15 mg/m²)	Methotrexate (50 mg/m² to 1 g/m²)	Fluorouracil
Oxaliplatin	Mitomycin (<15 mg/m²)	Hydroxyurea
Streptozocin	Mitoxantrone	Imatinib
	Procarbazine	Liposomal doxorubicin
	Topotecan	Melphalan
	Vinorelbine	Methotrexate (<50 mg/m2)
		Paclitaxel
		Pemetrexed
		Rituximab
		Temozolomide
		Thioguanine or mercaptopurine (6-MP)
		Vinblastine
		Thiotepa
		Trastuzumab
		Vinblastine
		Vincristine

[a]High-dose therapy requiring progenitor cell support is not included in this table.

Table 27.5. Agents used for chemotherapy-induced nausea and vomiting

Agent	Route of Administration	Dose	Comments
Phenothiazines			
Prochlorperazine (Compazine)	PO PO (sustained release) IM or IV PR	10 mg every 4–6 h 15–30 mg every 12 h 2–10 mg every 4–6 h 25 mg every 12 h	Some EPS; potential for postural hypotension when given IV
Thiethylperazine (Torecan)	PO, IM, or PR	10 mg every 6–8 h	Some EPS
Trimethobenzamide (Tigan)	PO IM or PR	250 mg every 4–6 h 200 mg every 4–6 h	Some EPS
Butyrophenones			
Haloperidol (Haldol)	IM, PO, or IV	2–5 mg every 2–4 h	Some EPS
Droperidol (Inapsine)	IV or IM	0.5–2.5 mg every 4 h	Causes sedation, cardiac arrhythmias, EPS, hypotension. Not recommended.
Substituted benzamide			
Metoclopramide (Reglan)	PO or IV	10–40 mg q.i.d. to 1- to 2-mg/kg dose at 2-h intervals	EPS common in higher doses that should be given with diphenhydramine; EPS worse with younger patients; may have diarrhea in higher doses

	Route	Dose	Comments
Benzodiazepines			
Lorazepam (Ativan)	PO, SL, or IV	1–2 mg every 4–6 h; 0.5–2 mg every 4–6 h	Causes sedation, amnesia, and confusion
Corticosteroids			
Dexamethasone (Decadron)	IV	4–20 mg (10–20 mg × 1), otherwise every 4–6 h	Potential for agitation, delirium
	PO	4–8 mg every 4 h	
Serotonin (5-HT$_3$) antagonists			
Ondansetron (Zofran)	IV	8–32 mg × 1; 0.15 mg/kg, every 4 h × 3	For highly emetogenic chemotherapy; lower doses effective for less emetogenic regimens
	PO	8 mg b.i.d.	
Granisetron (Kytril)	IV	1 mg × 1	Similar to ondansetron
	PO	1–2 mg × 1	
Dolasetron (Anzemet)	IV or PO	100 mg before chemotherapy	Similar to above
Palonosetron (Aloxi)	IV	0.25 mg IV (single dose only)	
Cannabinoids			
Dronabinol (Marinol)	PO	2.5–10 mg every 4–6 h	Causes sedation, may be habit forming, a controlled substance
NK-1 Receptor Antagonists			
Aprepitant (Emend)	PO	Tri-pack: 125 mg 30 min before chemotherapy day 1, then 80 mg daily on days 2 and 3	

EPS, extrapyramidal symptoms.

Table 27.6. Examples of antiemetic regimens for prevention and management of chemotherapy-induced nausea and vomiting

Level 1: patients receiving a mildly emetogenic agent

Dexamethasone 8–10 mg PO/IV before chemotherapy

With or without

Prochlorperazine 10 mg PO before chemotherapy, then 10 mg PO every 4–6 h p.r.n., *or*

Lorazepam 1 mg PO every 4–6 h p.r.n., *or both*

Level 2: patients receiving a moderately emetogenic agent or patients receiving a mildly emetogenic agent who have failed to respond to or are intolerant of at least two level 1 regimens

Aprepitant 125 mg PO before chemotherapy day 1, then 80 mg PO daily on days 2 and 3, *and*

Palonosetron[a] 0.25 mg IV before chemotherapy, *and*

Dexamethasone 10–12 mg IV/PO before chemotherapy, then 8 mg PO daily on days 2–4

With or without

Lorazepam 1 mg PO or IV before q4–6 h p.r.n., *or*

Prochlorperazine 10 mg PO q4–6 h p.r.n., *or both*

Level 3: patients receiving a highly emetogenic agent or patients receiving two or more moderately emetogenic agents or patients who have failed a level 2 regimen

Aprepitant 125 mg PO before chemotherapy on day 1, then 80 mg PO daily on days 2 and 3, *and*

Palonosetron[b] 0.25 mg IV before chemotherapy, *and*

Dexamethasone 10–12 mg PO/IV before chemotherapy, then 8 mg PO on days 2–4, *and*

Lorazepam 1 mg PO or IV before chemotherapy, then q4–6 h p.r.n.

In addition, for delayed nausea and vomiting:

Metoclopramide 40 mg PO q6 h × 4 days, *with*

Dexamethasone 4 mg PO q6 h × 3 days, then 4 mg PO q12 h × 1 day (if not given already with Aprepitant)

Give antiemetics 20–30 min before chemotherapy when using the IV route and 1 h before chemotherapy when using the PO route. Given in this manner, oral medication is usually as effective as the same medication IV, and the cost is considerably less.

---

[a]Alternatives (5-HT$_3$): ondansetron 10 mg IV × 1 before chemotherapy, *or* dolasetron 100 mg PO or IV, or granisetron 1 mg PO or IV before chemotherapy.

[b]Alternatives (5-HT$_3$ antagonists): ondansetron 32 mg IV before chemotherapy; dolasetron 100 mg PO or IV, or granisetron 1 mg PO or IV before chemotherapy.

nausea and vomiting related to chemotherapy may benefit from the use of nonpharmacologic interventions in addition to the pharmacologic agents taken. The use of acupuncture, acupressure, guided imagery, music therapy, and progressive muscle relaxation are often effective in preventing nausea and vomiting. Many of these are forms of distraction that assist patients in maintaining a feeling of control over their treatment effects. Massage therapy, hypnosis, exercise, and acustimulation with wristband devices have insufficient data, and further studies are needed to support their use as interventions. With increasing attention to complementary therapies, it is hoped that more clinical studies will determine their value in patient care. Patients who are able to have little or no nausea and vomiting with their first chemotherapy treatment often assert that positive thinking is helpful as well. Patients may also prepare for their chemotherapy treatments by eating foods that do not have offensive odors or spicy taste. Clear liquids, foods served at room temperature, soda crackers, and carbonated beverages are sometimes good suggestions. Following chemotherapy, smaller, more frequent meals are less likely to promote the development of nausea and vomiting.

E. Herbal remedies: ginger. There have long been anecdotally based recommendations for the use of ginger to help prevent and minimize chemotherapy-induced nausea and vomiting. Few randomized controlled trials have been done to evaluate ginger as an intervention in this patient population. Although early studies show safety and little toxicity, it is difficult to recommend the use of ginger because of the lack of evidence, particularly with respect to dosages and schedules.

III. Other short-term complications related to cancer chemotherapy

A. Stomatitis and other oral complications. The oral mucosa is vulnerable to the effects of chemotherapy and radiotherapy because of its rapid growth and cell turnover rate. Radiotherapy also interferes with the production of saliva and may increase oral complications because of a consequent reduction in the protective effect of the saliva. It is crucial to manage oral complications effectively because patients may experience considerable discomfort or develop secondary infections from the disruption of the oral mucosa. The likelihood of the development of stomatitis from a drug is dependent on the agent, the dose, and the schedule of administration. Continuous rather than intermittent administration is more likely to cause stomatitis with the antimetabolites.

1. Specific chemotherapy agents that may cause stomatitis include the following:

Antimetabolites: methotrexate, fluorouracil (particularly continuous infusion), capecitabine, cytarabine, irinotecan

Antitumor antibiotics: doxorubicin, idarubicin, dactinomycin, mitomycin, bleomycin

Plant alkaloids: vincristine, vinblastine, vinorelbine

Taxanes: docetaxel, paclitaxel

Alkylating agents: high doses of busulfan, cyclophosphamide

Biologic agents: interleukins, lymphokine-activated killer cell therapy

2. Prevention and early detection. If oral complications are anticipated, it is important to implement a good oral hygiene program before the initiation of therapy. Dental consultation is recommended in specific groups of patients, including those undergoing bone marrow transplant and those with leukemia or head and neck malignancies. Maintaining good nutrition and dental hygiene is also a primary preventive measure. Normal saline is the preferred mouth rinse. Alternative rinsing agents such as sodium bicarbonate or nonalcoholic mouthwashes, if preferred by patients, may be used. **Chlorhexidine and hydrogen peroxide mouth rinses should *not* be used.** For patients receiving bolus fluorouracil, it is recommended that patients perform oral cryotherapy. This involves holding ice chips in the mouth starting 5 minutes before the bolus of fluorouracil and for 30 minutes after the administration of the drug. This intervention is effective for bolus administration only, and should not be done when oxaliplatin is also given because of the potential for increase in acute neurotoxicity. Systematic oral assessments should be integrated into the physical examination at regular intervals. Special attention should be given to the tongue, the gingiva, the buccal mucosa, the soft palate, and the lips. It is also important to assess the patient for soreness, functional ability to swallow, and any effects on eating.

3. Management of oral complications. Although the primary goal is prevention, once oral complications develop, the focus of care should shift to the continuation of good oral hygiene and treatment of symptoms. Agents used for oral care are categorized according to function: cleansing agents, lubricating agents, analgesic agents, and preventive agents. Table 27.7 lists several commonly used agents. Commercial mouthwashes and lemon glycerin swabs are not recommended for use because of their irritating and drying effects. If painful ulcerations do develop, topical relief may be best obtained by using single agent topical analgesics such as UlcerEase (Med-Derm Pharmaceuticals, Johnson City, TN) or lidocaine. Compounded analgesic mouth rinses such as "magic mouthwash" consisting of various components such as lidocaine, diphenhydramine, antacids, and/or sodium bicarbonate do not have established data to recommend in practice. Systemic pain control measures such as oral or parenteral narcotics should be implemented if topical analgesics are ineffective.

4. Xerostomia that follows radiation therapy to the mouth area may require treatment with artificial saliva. It may also be benefited by the administration of pilocarpine 5 to 10 mg PO t.i.d. before meals. Before the initiation of radiation therapy to the head and neck area, dental consultation is necessary to evaluate oral hygiene, the state of repair of the teeth, and the health of the gums. Amifostine shows promise as a protective agent for xerostomia and is used concurrently with radiation to the head and neck.

5. Secondary oral infections should be treated promptly and as accurately as possible. Fungal infections may be treated with nystatin suspension, clotrimazole troches, or

Table 27.7.   Agents for oral care

Agent	Indications and Comments
Cleansing agents	
Normal saline solution (preferred) (1/2 tsp salt in 8 oz of water)	Economical, nondamaging
Sodium bicarbonate	Nonirritating, debriding
Lubricating agents	
Saliva substitutes (mucin-based preferred)	Decreases dryness
Water- or oil-based lubricants	Useful emollient; oil-based lubricants should not be used in mouth because of danger of aspiration
Analgesic agents	
a. *Healing and coating agents*	
Vitamin E	Protection to mucosa, healing properties
	Effectiveness not yet established
Allopurinol	May decrease intensity of mucositis with fluorouracil
Gelclair bioadherent oral gel	
L-Glutamine	May decrease mucositis intensity
b. *Topical anesthetics*	
Lidocaine viscous	Transient pain relief, absorbed systemically
Diclonine hydrochloride	Transient pain relief
Benzocaine	Transient pain relief
Zilactin	Burns on application
Capsaicin	Active ingredient in chili peppers; given in candy vehicle will decrease pain
Morphine	
c. *Systemic analgesics*	
Nonsteroidal anti-inflammatory drugs	Take before meals and as needed
Narcotic analgesics	
Prevention agents—hematologic growth factors	
Filgrastim, Sargramostim	Less severe mucositis experienced by patients receiving growth factors
Keratinocyte growth factors (Palifermin)	Approved for patients with hematologic malignancies receiving stem cell transplant

oral fluconazole. Viral infections may be reactivated after chemotherapy and are commonly treated with oral or IV acyclovir. The benefit of prophylactic use of antiviral agents or antifungal agents is not well established. However, in patients with a known history of cold sores or positive herpes simplex virus titers, it may be advantageous to administer prophylactic acyclovir.

Patients with dentures may be encouraged to remove them during the period after chemotherapy when they are at risk for infection, except at mealtime. In addition, the dentures should be cleansed before use. Although removal of the dentures may be detrimental to the patient's self-esteem, irritation of the dentures may lead to inflammation, ulceration, and secondary infection.

B. Alopecia. Chemotherapy-induced hair loss is not necessarily a serious physiologic complication, but psychologically, it can be one of the most devastating side effects. Partial or total hair loss can contribute to a perceived negative body image owing to the emphasis placed on the hair and overall appearance in society. The hair loss from chemotherapy, which often occurs 2 to 3 weeks after chemotherapy, is usually temporary. Hair growth begins in approximately 1 to 2 months after the treatment is completed, but it may be approximately 4 to 5 months before the patient will feel comfortable not wearing a wig. The new hair may have a different texture or color from its pretreatment characteristics. In addition to scalp hair loss, it is important to remind patients of the hair loss that may occur in other areas such as the eyebrows, eyelashes, axilla, pubis, and other fine hair.

   1. Specific chemotherapy agents with a high potential of causing alopecia include doxorubicin, cyclophosphamide, ifosfamide, vincristine, and paclitaxel. Other drugs capable of causing alopecia include bleomycin, dactinomycin, daunorubicin, etoposide, vinblastine, methotrexate, and mitoxantrone. The extent of alopecia depends on the mechanism of the drug, the dose, the serum half-life, the infusion technique (bolus vs. continuous infusion), and the use of combinations of drugs.

   2. Nursing interventions start with informing and preparing the patient for the possibility of alopecia. It is helpful to encourage purchasing wigs and other head wear before the alopecia occurs so that the hair color and style may be used in selecting a wig as well as allowing time for adjustment. It is important to encourage discussion of feelings regarding the hair loss for both men and women and to recognize their concerns and fears. The American Cancer Society's program "Look Good, Feel Better" is helpful in providing guidance about wigs, makeup, and skin care. Scalp hypothermia has been used in the past as an attempt to restrict the circulation to the scalp, with the goal of minimizing alopecia. Because of the concern for scalp metastases and sanctuary sites, scalp hypothermia is no longer recommended.

C. Diarrhea. Among the many causes of diarrhea in patients with cancer are chemotherapy, radiotherapy, the cancer itself, medications, supplemental feeding, and anxiety. Osmotic diarrhea refers to that caused by chemotherapy agents, where the actively dividing epithelial cells of the gastrointestinal tract are destroyed. Unabsorbable substances draw water into the intestinal lumen by osmosis, resulting in increased stool volume and weight. Secretory diarrhea may result from infectious causes (e.g., *Clostridium difficile* or other enterocolitis-causing bacteria), with or without concurrent neutropenia. The opportunistic infection may intensify the inflammatory reaction in the gut, causing excessive intestinal mucosal secretion of electrolytes and fluids from the bacterial toxins. Prolonged diarrhea can lead to discomfort, severe electrolyte imbalances and dehydration, altered social life, and poor quality of life. In the past, little attention has been paid to the prompt evaluation and management of diarrhea, but with increasing use of agents such as irinotecan, the observation of severe and potentially life-threatening problems has heightened awareness of this side effect. The elderly, in particular, may be at increased risk for treatment-related diarrhea and may require close monitoring.

1. Chemotherapy and biologic agents may contribute to the development of diarrhea and most commonly include the antimetabolites such as fluorouracil, capecitabine, methotrexate, cytarabine, and irinotecan. In addition, agents such as dactinomycin, floxuridine, hydroxyurea, idarubicin, the nitrosoureas, and paclitaxel cause diarrhea relatively frequently. When diarrhea from fluorouracil, floxuridine, or irinotecan is present while on therapy, it is a sign of toxicity that must be monitored closely and that could escalate to severe levels at which the drug might need to be held or discontinued. With the increased use of biologic agents, diarrhea has been noted with interferon-α and interleukin-2. High-dose chemotherapy regimens used in stem cell transplantation may also be associated with severe diarrhea and may be caused by acute graft-versus-host disease.

2. Assessment of a patient experiencing diarrhea should begin with a baseline history of usual elimination patterns, pattern of symptoms, and concurrent medications. The duration of the diarrhea and frequency of stool passage should be noted with reference to a stool diary if indicated. Physical examination may disclose abdominal tenderness, signs of dehydration, and disruption in perianal or peristomal skin integrity. Laboratory data may be obtained to assess serum chemistries, complete blood count, and stool samples for *Clostridium difficile* toxin and other enteropathic bacteria.

3. Management of treatment-related diarrhea is often symptomatic and requires little or no alteration in cancer therapy. Agents that decrease bowel motility should not be used for longer than 24 hours unless significant infections have been excluded. In the absence of obvious inflammation and infection, it is appropriate to treat most patients with nonspecific treatment for diarrhea, including opioids (loperamide, diphenoxylate, and codeine), anticholinergics (atropine, scopolamine), or both. More recently, it has been recognized that octreotide is often effective in

Table 27.8. Pharmacologic management strategies for diarrhea

Agent	Comments
Kaolin pectin (Kaopectate)	30–60 mL PO after each loose stool
Loperamide (Imodium)	2 capsules (4 mg) PO 4 h initially, then add 1 capsule (2 mg) after each loose stool; should not exceed 16 capsules daily
Diphenoxylate hydrochloride, atropine sulfate (Lomotil)	1–2 tablets PO 4 h; should not exceed 8 tablets daily; there may be anticholinergic effects due to atropine
Atropine	May give 0.25-1 mg IV before irinotecan, or IV/SQ for cholinergic symptoms
Paregoric	1 tsp PO 4 times/day; may alternate with Lomotil
Octreotide	May be useful for fluorouracil induced diarrhea; starting dose: 0.05–0.1 mg SC t.i.d; may be increased to 1.8 mg/day in refractory diarrhea
	Sandostatin LAR Depot is indicated for carcinoid and VIPomas. It is a slow-release drug that is dosed at 20–30 mg every 4 weeks.

controlling chemotherapy-related diarrhea and diarrhea associated with the carcinoid syndrome. Table 27.8 lists common agents used to treat diarrhea. Nonpharmacologic measures that may also assist in the prevention and management of diarrhea are a low-residue diet and increased fluids. If the diarrhea is severe, IV hydration is necessary to prevent serious hypovolemia, electrolyte disturbances, and shock. In patients who experience severe irinotecan-associated diarrhea, antibiotic therapy such as ciprofloxacin is recommended because of a high incidence of infectious contribution to the gastrointestinal problems, including functional ileus, which may be associated.

D. Constipation. In patients whose cancer has resulted in debility or immobility or in those who require narcotic analgesics, constipation can be a particular problem. Constipation may also develop in patients who have received neurotoxic chemotherapy agents including the vinca alkaloids, etoposide, and cisplatin, each of which may cause autonomic dysfunction. Decreased bowel motility due to intra-abdominal disease, hypercalcemia, dehydration, and antiemetic use can also contribute to constipation. Chronic constipation in patients with cancer is a problem that is more easily prevented than treated. A diet high in bulk fiber, fresh fruits and vegetables, and adequate fluid intake may help to minimize constipation. Patients started on narcotic analgesics should also begin a bowel regimen, first with mild stool softeners and bulk laxatives and then proceeding to stimulants or osmotic laxatives if the milder regimen is not effective. A bowel regimen example for a patient at risk for constipation is as follows:

1. Docusate sodium 100 mg b.i.d. alone or with casanthranol (Peri-Colace), 1 capsule b.i.d.
2. If no bowel movement, add:
   a. Senna at bedtime (dose varies with the preparation), *or*
   b. Milk of magnesia 30 mL at bedtime
3. If no bowel movement with the above, the following may be added:
   a. Bisacodyl one to three tablets or one 10-mg suppository, at bedtime, *or*
   b. Lactulose one to four tablespoons daily
4. Other more aggressive alternatives, if there is no impaction, include the following:
   a. Fleet enema
   b. Magnesium citrate 1 bottle
   c. Tap-water enema

E. Altered nutritional status. Patients with cancer often experience progressive loss of appetite and sometimes severe malnutrition during the course of the disease and treatment. Malnutrition may result from a side effect of the therapy or a direct effect of the cancer (e.g., gut obstruction or hepatic or brain metastases). The resulting effects of malnutrition are a poorer response to therapy, increased incidence of infections, and an overall worsening of patient well-being. Many times, one of the presenting signs that lead to the diagnosis of cancer is weight loss; therefore, the patient is most likely experiencing some alteration already in nutritional status. Malnutrition is reported to occur in 50% to 80% of patients with advanced disease. Nutritional management of the patient with cancer involves early intervention using a supportive health care team.

1. **Effects of chemotherapy and radiation therapy on nutrition.** Chemotherapy has a major effect on nutritional status because of the direct insult on the gastrointestinal tract. Among the gastrointestinal effects are anorexia, nausea, vomiting, taste alterations, stomatitis, esophagitis, colitis, constipation, and diarrhea. Not only are the effects physiologic in nature, but also the added psychologic impact of the disease and therapy can result in anxiety and depression, which can contribute to the lack of interest in food.

2. **Nutritional assessment.** Early in the patient's treatment, a thorough nutritional assessment should be completed by the health care team. The assessment should include diet history, nutrient intake, anthropometric measurements (height, weight, and skin-fold thickness and midarm circumference, if possible), laboratory tests for

anemia and serum albumin, and an evaluation of activity and functional status. A serum pre-albumin is a very sensitive indicator of changes in nutritional status. A level of <15 mg/dL is indicative of protein depletion. A good nutritional assessment may help identify patients who are already at risk of malnutrition or those who may be prone to developing problems during the course of the illness and treatment.

3. Nutritional intervention. Nutritional intervention should be considered during the initial and ongoing assessments. Situations that warrant nutritional intervention include involuntary weight loss (more than 10% within the last 6 months, especially when combined with weakness and fatigue), history of recent physiologic stress, serum albumin below 3.2 g/dL, or severe immunocompromise. Nurses, dietitians, and even family members can identify problems and may be the first to act to promote weight gain. Various approaches that help increase weight are changes in diet; symptomatic treatment of nausea and vomiting, stomatitis, and other gastrointestinal effects of chemotherapy, and supplemental nutrition.

    a. Nutritional supplements. Several nutritional supplements are commercially available for oral use. One benefit of nutritional supplements is that they are a concentrated form of nutrition for protein and calories. Some of the disadvantages are the unappealing taste and the high cost to the consumer. Some patients and their families are able to develop some creative high-protein and high-calorie supplements using household items with some suggestions from the health care team.

    b. Tube feedings. Enteral nutrition through a nasogastric or gastrostomy tube may be an alternative if oral intake is not possible. Enteral feedings are the recommended route if the gastrointestinal tract is functional. Advantages of enteral feeding include lower cost and fewer complications than with parenteral feedings and maintenance of normal gastrointestinal function. Some care and maintenance are involved with feeding tubes, and patients and their families need to be given information regarding available options for feeding.

    c. Total parenteral nutrition (TPN). Parenteral nutrition should be considered in patients who do not have a functioning gastrointestinal tract or in those for whom supplemental nutrition is anticipated for a short period of time. Patients who receive TPN usually require the insertion of a central venous catheter, which may result in other iatrogenic complications such as pneumothorax, vein thrombosis, and catheter-related infections. In many situations, TPN used in the patient with cancer increases morbidity, especially from infection, without improving survival. Thus, TPN has considerable economic, ethical, and medical consequences that must be evaluated in conjunction with the patient's overall prognosis.

4. Pharmacologic interventions. A recent area of interest is pharmacologic appetite stimulation. One of the agents currently used is megestrol acetate oral suspension

800 mg/day (20 mL/day). Agents such as megestrol acetate have documented evidence in promoting increased weight gain in some patients and at least a decreased weight loss in others. Dronabinol (Marinol) is also an agent that may stimulate appetite.

F. Neurotoxicity. The incidence of neurotoxicity associated with chemotherapy is increasing, potentially because of the greater use of high-dose chemotherapy and newer drugs causing neurotoxicity used in combination. In many cases, early detection and treatment of neurotoxicity (i.e., reduction of drug dose or discontinuation) allow for the reversal of symptoms. The neurotoxic symptoms may manifest as altered level of consciousness or coma, cerebellar dysfunction, ototoxicity, or peripheral neuropathy, which may be temporary but can cause significant changes in functional ability that persist as a long-term effect. It is also important to assess renal function because poor renal function may reduce clearance of the chemotherapy agent, leading to increased neurotoxicity.

1. Chemotherapy and biologic agents with known potential for neurotoxicity include high-dose cytarabine, high-dose methotrexate, vincristine, vinblastine, vinorelbine, ifosfamide, cisplatin, carboplatin, oxaliplatin, paclitaxel, docetaxel, procarbazine, bortezomib, thalidomide, interleukin 2, and the interferons.

2. Prevention and early detection of neurotoxicity is key to prevention of permanent neurologic damage. Assessment of symptoms of neurotoxicity should be documented on a routine basis. In certain treatment regimens, altering the drug sequence can markedly decrease the symptoms.

3. Management of peripheral neurotoxicity is being studied, with the goal of slowing, halting, and reversing the neuropathy. One agent that has shown some activity with mixed results is the cytoprotectant amifostine. Pyroxidine or vitamin B_6 may also be used, 100 mg b.i.d., in an attempt to minimize peripheral neuropathy. Glutamine has been shown to reduce peripheral neuropathy associated with paclitaxel. If pain becomes a major concern, anticonvulsants (gabapentin or carbamazepine) or tricyclic antidepressants (amitriptyline) may also be used. The drug pregabalin (Lyrica), similar to gabapentin, has shown promise in postherpetic neuralgia and in diabetic neuropathy, and has increasing attention in chemotherapy-induced neuropathy. Dosages of 75 mg b.i.d. have been effective, with improvements observed within 1 week of starting pregabalin. Whether there is any advantage over gabapentin is not clear. Topical analgesics and opioids may also be effective. Conventional nondrug interventions with some report of effectiveness include exercise, physical therapy, massage, and transcutaneuous electric nerve stimulation (TENS).

G. Palmar–plantar erythrodysesthesia or hand–foot syndrome. Palmar–plantar erythrodysesthesia (PPE) is not a new side effect due to cancer chemotherapy. It has been seen with continuous-infusion fluorouracil in the past but has captured attention recently because of a high incidence with some newer chemotherapeutic drugs such as capecitabine and liposomal doxorubicin. PPE is a toxic drug reaction that begins as a cutaneous eruption of the integument on the palms of the hands and plantar surfaces of the feet. It has been postulated that PPE occurs because of drug extravasation in the micro-capillaries of the hands and feet due to local everyday trauma or by drug concentration and accumulation in sweat glands found in the palms and soles with resultant tissue damage. PPE is time exposure dependent and occurs with protracted, chronic exposure over long periods (i.e., >3 to 4 weeks).

Prevention or minimization of PPE has been observed through regional cooling during the infusion of pegylated liposomal doxorubicin by having patients keep ice packs around the wrists and ankles, and consume iced liquids. These interventions were continued for 24 hours after completion of the chemotherapy. In this study, regional cooling decreased the frequency and severity of PPE in 94% of the patients in the intervention group. Although this is a single study, the minimal cost, relatively simple procedure, and well-tolerated intervention may be helpful.

1. **Chemotherapeutic agents** with a known potential for the development for PPE include fluorouracil (primarily with continuous infusions), capecitabine, doxorubicin, and liposome-encapsulated doxorubicin.

2. **Clinical findings** of PPE include tingling, numbness, pain, dryness, erythema, swelling, rash, blister formation, and pruritus of the hands and feet. Clinical knowledge of the potential for PPE and early assessment is imperative for adjustments of dose or withholding of therapy. Table 27.9 shows a staging scale that can be utilized to evaluate functional and clinical criteria for dose modification.

3. **Management of PPE** and symptomatic treatment result from prompt identification of symptoms. At the first sign of PPE, the drug should be stopped, or the interval between doses should be increased, or the drug dose should be reduced. If identified at grade 2 toxicity, symptoms typically improve within a few days of stopping the drug. If

Table 27.9. Hand–foot syndrome (palmar–plantar erythrodysesthesia) grading scale

Grade 1	Grade 2	Grade 3	Grade 4
Painless erythema, or welling, numbness, dysesthesia/paresthesia, and tingling that do not disrupt activities of daily living	Painful erythema with swelling that affects activities of daily living, blisters or ulcerations <2 cm	Moist desquamation, ulceration, blistering, and severe pain, interference with normal daily activities, cannot wear regular clothing	Diffuse or local process causing infectious complications, a bed-ridden state or hospitalization

Based on National Cancer Institute of Canada CTG Expanded Common Toxicity Criteria.

untreated, grade 2 side effects may quickly progress to grade 3 or 4, requiring more intense medical concern and intervention. Depending on the drug used, recommendations are available for dose modifications. Education on preventative measures should be given to patients before beginning the drug where PPE is likely. Patients should be counseled to avoid tight-fitting shoes and rings or repetitive rubbing pressure to the hands or feet. Other precautionary measures include avoiding excessive pressure and heat on the skin for 3 to 5 days after treatment, avoidance of hot baths, showers, or hot tubs (hot water for 24 hours before and 72 hours after treatment), and friction-causing activities such as exercise for 3 to 5 days after treatment. Patients should also be advised to use emollients such as Bag Balm (Dairy Association Co., Lyndonville, VT), Udderly Smooth (Redex Industries, Salem, OH), or other petroleum- or lanolin-containing creams liberally and frequently. Patients should also be instructed to notify their health care providers at the first signs or symptoms of PPE. If the grade of toxicity worsens, supportive care related to analgesia and prevention of infection is important. Other anecdotal interventions include topical steroids and oral premedication with steroids, application of a nicotine patch, and oral administration of pyridoxine. Further studies need to be done to evaluate which interventions are helpful for PPE and do not exacerbate the skin toxicity.

SUGGESTED READINGS

Armstrong T, Almadrones L, Gilbert MR. Chemotherapy-induced peripheral neuropathy. *Oncol Nurs Forum* 2005;32:305–311.

Cawley MM, Benson LM. Current trends in managing oral mucositis. *Clin J Oncol Nurs* 2005;9:584–592.

Eilers J. Nursing interventions and supportive care for the prevention and treatment of oral mucositis associated with cancer treatment. *Oncol Nurs Forum* 2004;31:13–23.

Ezzo J, Vickers A, Richardson MA, et al. Acupuncture-point stimulation for chemotherapy-induced nausea and vomiting. *J Clin Oncol* 2005;23:7188–7198.

Gobel BH. Chemotherapy-induced hypersensitivity reactions. *Oncol Nurs Forum* 2005;32:1027–1035.

Kostler WJ, Hejna M, Wenzel C, et al. Oral mucositis complicating chemotherapy and/or radiotherapy: one option for prevention and treatment. *CA Cancer J Clin* 2001;51:290–315.

Markman M, Kennedy A, Webster K, et al. Paclitaxel-associated hypersensitivity reactions: experience of the gynecologic oncology program of the Cleveland Clinic Cancer Center. *J Clin Oncol* 2000; 18:102–105.

Markman M, Zanotti K, Peterson G, et al. Expanded experience with and intradermal skin test to predict for the presence or absence of carboplatin hypersensitivity. *J Clin Oncol* 2003;21:4611–4614.

Molpus KL, Anderson LB, Craig CL, et al. The effect of regional cooling on toxicity associated with intravenous infusion of pegylated liposomal doxorubicin in recurrent ovarian carcinoma. *Gynecol Oncol* 2004;93:513–516.

National Comprehensive Cancer Network (NCCN). *Antiemesis practice guidelines in oncology.* Version 2. www.nccn.org. 2006.

Polovich M, White JM, Kelleher LO, eds. *Chemotherapy and bio-therapy guidelines and recommendations for practice*, 2nd ed. Pittsburgh: Oncology Nursing Society, 2005.

Schulmeister L. Managing extravasations. *Clin J Oncol Nurs* 2005;9: 472–475.

Sliesoraitis S, Chikhale PJ. Carboplatin hypersensitivity. *Int J Gynecol Cancer* 2005;15:13–18.

Stricker CT, Sullivan J. Evidence-based oncology oral care clinical practice guidelines: development, implementation, and evaluation. *Clin J Oncol Nurs* 2003;7:222–227.

Warr DG, Hesketh PJ, Gralla RJ, et al. Efficacy and tolerability of aprepitant for the prevention of chemotherapy-induced nausea and vomiting in patients with breast cancer after moderately emetogenic chemotherapy. *J Clin Oncol* 2005;23:2822–2830.

Zanotti KM, Rybicki LA, Kennedy AW, et al. Carboplatin skin testing: a skin-testing protocol for predicting hypersensitivity to carboplatin chemotherapy. *J Clin Oncol* 2001;19:3126–3129.

CHAPTER 28

Infections: Etiology, Treatment, and Prevention

Joan M. Duggan

Infections in patients with cancer that are commonly seen by the practicing oncologist can be associated with significant morbidity and mortality. For example, infection occurs in more than 50% of patients undergoing aggressive chemotherapy for acute leukemia. The keys to successful management of infection in the oncology patient are an understanding of the risk factors for infection and the commonly associated etiologic agents, institution of a thorough and prompt diagnostic work-up guided by the most likely etiology, and early institution of appropriate antibiotic therapy. In general, most bacterial and fungal infections seen in oncology patients develop from the patient's own endogenous flora, especially in the presence of neutropenia.

I. **Etiology of infections in patients with cancer**
   A. **General considerations.** Patients with cancer are immunocompromised hosts for a variety of reasons. The underlying malignancy may damage the immune system directly or indirectly, or the treatments for the malignancy may result in neutropenia or other alterations in white blood cell (WBC) function (e.g., decreased cell-mediated immunity). Clinical changes accompanying cancer and its treatment, such as protein malnutrition or mucositis, may change immune system function as well. It is important to understand the major etiologic agents associated with the wide variety of immune system defects seen in patients with cancer for proper diagnosis and treatment. Common organisms that are associated with each of the etiologic categories are shown in Table 28.1.
   B. **Neutropenia.** Neutropenia is generally defined as a neutrophil count of less than 500 neutrophils/μL or less than 1,000 μL total WBCs. Patients with neutropenia develop infections most commonly from endogenous bacteria and fungi in the gastrointestinal (GI) tract or from indwelling intravascular access devices.
   C. **Altered cellular immunity.** Prolonged steroid use, purine analogs (such as fludarabine), protein malnutrition, and hematopoietic stem cell transplant (HSCT) are some of the factors that can decrease cell-mediated immunity (CMI). In addition, certain malignancies such as Hodgkin's lymphoma have intrinsic abnormalities in CMI. Risk of infections from microbes controlled by CMI may increase when the CD4 cell count ("T-helper cell") falls below 200 cells/μL. These organisms are usually opportunistic pathogens. However, because CD4 cell function may be abnormal at higher counts in oncology patients, opportunistic infections can also occur at higher CD4 cell counts. Intact CMI is required for fully functional humoral immunity as well.

Table 28.1.   Etiology of infection in patients with cancer

Immune System Deficit	Chemotherapeutic Agent	Gram-Positive Bacteria	Gram-Negative Bacteria	Fungi	Others
Neutropenia	***Neutropenia ≤ 4 weeks*** Carboplatin, alemtuzumab, alkylating agents, cytarabine, Daunorubicin, Doxorubicin, Etoposide, Fluorouracil, Ifosfamide, methotrexate, Rituximab, vinblastine ***Neutropenia ≥ 4 weeks*** Busulfan, Carmustine, lomustine, mitomycin, purine analogs, Cladribine	*Staphylococcus* species *(S. aureus, S. epidermidis)* *Streptococcus* (including *S. pneumoniae, S. pyogenes, viridans streptococcus), Enterococcus faecalis* and *E. faecium,* Diphtheroids	*Pseudomonas* species, Enteric gram-negative rods (e.g., *Escherichia coli, Klebsiella)*	*Candida* species *(C. albicans* and *C. glabrata, C. krusei,* and *C. lusitaniae), Aspergillus, Fusarium* species, *Trichosporon*	—
Decreased cell-mediated immunity (especially CD4 cell count <200/cells/mm³)	Alemtuzumab, corticosteroids, purine analogs	*S. pneumoniae, Listeria monocytogenes*	*Neisseria meningitidis, Salmonella* species	*Candida, Aspergillus,* endemic mycosis (e.g., *Histoplasmosis, Coccidioidomycosis), Pneumocystis jiroveci, Cryptococcus neoformans*	Mycobacterium (e.g., *M. tuberculosis, M. avium* complex), HSV, VZV, CMV, *Toxoplasmosis*

Decreased humoral immunity or functional asplenia	Alkylating agents, corticosteroids, methotrexate rituximab	*S. pneumoniae, Haemophilum influenza, S. aureus*	*E. coli, N. meningitidis, C. canimorsus*	—	Malaria, Ehrlichiosis, Babesiosis
Nosocomial infections					
Indwelling line infections		*S. epidermidis, S. aureus, Enterococcus*	Gram-negative rods (e.g., *Pseudomonas, Klebsiella, E. coli*)	*Candida* species	—
Urinary tract infections		*S. Epidermidis* (with Foley), *Enterococcus*	*E. coli, Klebsiella, Proteus, Pseudomonas, Providencia*	*Candida* species (with Foley)	—
Diarrhea		*Clostridium difficile*	—	—	—
Surgical site infections (superficial)		*S. aureus, S. epidermidis*	—	—	—

D. Altered humoral immunity. Decreased ability to produce opsonizing antibodies can occur through decreased cell-mediated immune system function, use of alkylating agents or from malignancies such as multiple myeloma or chronic lymphocytic leukemia. Common etiologic agents and organisms in patients with altered humoral immunity as shown in Table 28.1.

E. Asplenia. Splenectomy or functional asplenia can increase the risk for infections with encapsulated organisms, especially *Streptococcus pneumoniae*. Postsplenectomy sepsis can also occur from dog bites with *Capnocytophaga canimorsus*. Reports of severe infection in asplenic patients have also been described with malaria, babesiosis and ehrlichiosis.

F. Nosocomial infections. Infections acquired after 48 hours in the hospital are defined as *nosocomial infections*. Some of the more common causes of nosocomial infections and associated etiologic agents are listed below.

   1. Indwelling lines. Long-term venous access catheters can become infected through a variety of mechanisms.

   2. Urinary tract catheter. Any bladder instrumentation increases the risk of urinary tract infections (UTIs) (including intermittent catheterization, indwelling Foley catheters, and suprapubic catheters).

   3. *Clostridium difficile*. Risk factors for *C. difficile* colitis include prior use of antibiotics, GI surgery, proton pump inhibitors, tube feedings or hyperalimentation, and exposure to *C. difficile* in the hospital environment (e.g., infected roommate).

   4. Postoperative infections. Surgical site infections can occur at the incision or in the deep tissue/organs involved in surgery. The majority are acquired at the time of surgery. For cases not involving an enteric or mucosal surface, the most common pathogens are *S. aureus* and *Staphylococcus epidermidis*. Infections involving viscus or mucosal surfaces are usually polymicrobic, and similar to the microbes normally found in the surrounding area.

   5. Obstruction/necrosis of tissues secondary to the underlying malignancy. Patients with tracheobronchial obstruction are predisposed to infections with oral bacterial flora, such as anaerobes and gram-negative rods. Malignancies with secondary GI obstruction predispose patients to infection with anaerobes, gram-negative rods and gram-positive cocci such as enterococcus. Genitourinary (GU) tract obstruction can result in infection with gram-negative rods, especially unusual or more resistant bacteria.

G. Other sources of infection

   1. Travel. Most infections associated with travel are respiratory tract infections or GI tract infections. The majority will present within the first month of return from travel. Infections that may be acquired from remote travel and reactivated in the immunocompromised patient with cancer include tuberculosis, endemic fungal infections such as *Histoplasmosis*, or parasitic infections such as strongyloidiasis.

2. Exposure to community-acquired pathogens. Susceptible patients with cancer are at increased risk of infection when exposed to commonly occurring community pathogens such as influenza, pneumococcus, and varicella zoster virus (VZV).

3. Reactivation of previously latent or asymptomatic infections. Decreased function of the cell-mediated immune system can cause reactivation of previously controlled pathogens. Herpes Simplex virus (HSV) infection and VZV infections (shingles) are common reactivation infections in oncology patients. These viruses can disseminate as well. Other common pathogens that can reactivate with serious systemic infections after clinical latency include cytomegaloviruses infection and tuberculosis.

II. Diagnosis of infections in patients with cancer

A. General overview. Any patient who has cancer and develops fever or other signs and symptoms of infection (such as hypotension, tachypnea, tachycardia, organ system dysfunction, hypothermia, and/or clinical deterioration) requires urgent evaluation and prompt institution of empiric antibiotic therapy directed at the most likely clinical pathogens. Clinicians should have a low threshold for starting broad-spectrum antimicrobial therapy and should not withhold therapy while waiting for the results of diagnostic tests such as blood cultures. The general work-up and therapy should focus on the most likely infectious sources and pathogens for a given clinical scenario. Therefore, the work-up and initial therapy of a patient with fever, cough, and a bronchial obstruction due to lung cancer would be significantly different from that of a patient with febrile neutropenia and an indwelling venous access catheter.

B. Clinical history. The clinical history should be thorough and directed toward discovering underlying risk factors for infection, likely alterations in immune system function, and localizing complaints or changes in clinic status. It is important to note that severe infections in immunocompromised hosts may present with very subtle changes. For example, pneumonia in a neutropenic patient may present with only mild shortness of breath or cough initially. In addition, infections in any organ system can present with nonspecific symptoms such as fever or malaise. All new changes in clinical history should be thoroughly investigated.

1. Cancer treatment. In addition to knowing the type and extent of malignancy, it is important to know the treatment history as this will impact the presentation and etiology of infection in the patient with cancer.

a. Chemotherapeutic agents. Many commonly used chemotherapeutic drugs are cytotoxic, resulting in significant lymphopenia and/or neutropenia. The duration, severity and type of myelosuppression can be related to the type of chemotherapeutic agent, the amount of drug exposure, and the underlying degree of bone marrow involvement (see Table 28.1).

(1) CD4/CD8 suppression (cellular immune system suppression). The following chemotherapeutic agents may result in prolonged suppression of the T-helper/suppressor arm of the immune system:

- Alemtuzumab—median duration of neutropenia is 28 days.
- Corticosteroids—significant T-cell function suppression can be seen with dose of equal to or more than 15 mg prednisone/day for equal to or more than 1 month.
- Purine analogs (cladribine, fludarabine, and pentostatin) may result in CD4 cell count suppression of equal to or more than 200 for several years after therapy.

(2) Suppressed B-cell function (altered humoral immunity). The following chemotherapeutic agents may cause suppression of antibody production by B cells:

- Alkylating agents (cyclophosphamide, chlorambucil, melphalan)
- Corticosteroids—use of greater than 40 mg/day may decrease antibody production
- Methotrexate
- Rituximab

   2. Type of malignancy
   a. Solid tumors. These malignancies can cause significant obstruction in affected tissues, leading to infection behind the obstruction. Postobstructive pneumonias are common in patients with bronchogenic carcinomas, for example. Tissue necrosis secondary to malignancy may also create an area of potential sequestrum, which can become infected during an episode of bacteremia or from translocation of bacteria from a normally nonsterile area to a sterile area. Finally, some solid tumors may mimic an infectious etiology without any microbial involvement, such as the presence of fever and malaise in a patient with renal cell carcinoma.
   b. Hematologic malignancies. Leukemias and lymphomas result in significant compromise of immune system function through a variety of mechanisms.
C. Clinical evaluation. The clinical examination should be thorough with special emphasis on areas of symptomatology. Like the clinical history, the review of systems and clinical examination can present with subtle or atypical findings in the presence of severe infection. Special attention should be directed to the following areas and potential infectious etiologies.
   1. Review of systems/symptoms of infection
   a. Head, eyes, ears, nose, and throat (HEENT)—changes in vision, ear or sinus tenderness, oral lesions, changes in dentition.
   b. Lungs—cough, shortness of breath, pleuritic chest pain.
   c. Abdomen—difficulty swallowing, abdominal pain, rectal pain, discomfort or pruritus, or bleeding, diarrhea, nausea or vomiting.
   d. Skin—any new skin lesions or skin changes.

e. GU system—urinary frequency, dysuria, urinary urgency, GU discharge, flank tenderness, decreased urination.

f. Central nervous system (CNS)—altered mental status, new onset focal deficits.

g. Catheter sites—redness, tenderness at the insertion site including that along the subcutaneous tract of the catheter.

2. Signs of infection—signs of infection in patients with malignancy and altered immune system function may be subtle or atypical. In general, a thorough clinical examination focusing on changes or alteration in function is essential. Special attention should be directed to the areas listed in Table 28.2 and the associated potential etiologic agents.

a. HEENT

(1) Retina. Hemorrhages, necrosis of the retina, yellow lesions next to scarred retina ("headlight in fog"), white, infiltrative lesions on the retina, chorioretinitis with retinal detachment, or fulminant endophthalmitis are all signs of serious infection.

(2) Sinuses. Sinus tenderness, orbital cellulitis, or edema can indicate bacterial or fungal infection of the sinuses. Black material in the sinuses may indicate mucormycosis.

(3) Oropharynx and dentition. Special attention should be paid to the oral cavity during clinical examination, as this area can give important clues to a wide variety of microbiology infections. Bacterial infections, especially anaerobic infections, may present with reddened gums, loosened teeth, pain or discomfort in the teeth or gums, or referred pain to the sinus area in addition to frank abscess formation. The presence of a draining sinus tract may be significant for *Actinomycosis*. Ulcerations can be caused by a variety of infectious agents, including viruses, fungi, and tuberculosis. Viral ulcerations are generally shallow and painful, and may have extensive oropharyngeal involvement in the patient with cancer. The viruses that usually cause ulcerations are the herpes viruses and coxsackie viruses (herpangina). Fungal infections such as *Histoplasmosis* may present with painful, deep ulcers with heaped up edges. *Candida* can present with characteristic white plaques on the buccal mucosa (thrush) or less commonly, erythema of the mucosal surfaces or angular cheilitis.

b. Cardiovascular system. The presence of new murmurs or suspected line infections should prompt an evaluation for endocarditis. The most common cause of endocarditis in this population is *S. aureus*. Pericarditis and pericardial tamponade are uncommon, but should be suspected in patients with chest pain, shortness of breath, fever and/or pericardial rub. A variety of infectious agents can cause pericarditis, including common agents such as *S. aureus, S. pneumoniae* and coxsackie

Table 28.2.   Potential etiologic agents of infection and associated signs and symptoms

Clinical Change	Potential Etiologic Agent
HEENT	
Changes in vision	
Retinal hemorrhage	*Staphylococcus aureus* (endocarditis), CMV
Retinal necrosis	HSV, VZV
Retinal exudate with scarring	*Toxoplasmosis*
Chorioretinitis, white infiltrate retinol lesions, or endophthalmitis	*Candida* species
Sinus tenderness	
Black discharge or orbital cellulitis/edema	Mucormycosis (zygomycosis)
Oropharynx	
Painful, bleeding gums	Anaerobes
Ulcerations	
Shallow, painful	HSV, coxsackievirus
Deep, painful	*Histoplasmosis*
Erythema or white plaques	*Candida*
Cardiovascular	
Murmur or line infection	*Staphylococcus epidermidis, S. aureus*
Chest pain/SOB/fever/rub/ pericarditis	*S. aureus, Streptococcus pneumonia,* coxsackievirus, *Candida, Aspergillus*
Pulmonary	
Consolidation	*S. pneumoniae, Legionella sp., Haemophilus influenza*
Diffuse interstitial pattern/patchy alveolar infiltrate	CMV, PCP, *Mycoplasma,* other viruses (e.g., influenza, adenovirus)
Postobstructive	
Neutropenic	Anaerobes + Gram-negative rods *S. aureus, Pseudomonas, Candida, Aspergillus*
Abdomen	
Pain, nausea/vomiting— suspect typhilitis	Polymicrobic; gram-positive cocci, gram-negative rods, anaerobes
Rectal discomfort—suspect rectal abscess	Polymicrobic; gram-positive cocci, gram-negative rods, anaerobes
Diarrhea	*C. difficile*
Skin	
Petechia/purpura	Coxsackievirus, echovirus, CMV, *Neisseria meningitidis, Haemophilus* species, *Rickettsia* species, *S. aureus, S. pneumoniae, C. canimorsus, Listeria monocytogenes*

Table 28.2. *(Continued)*

Clinical Change	Potential Etiologic Agent
Macules/papules	*Pseudomonas* and other gram-negative rods, *S. aureus, Rickettsia* species, *Candida, Aspergillus,* other endemic, mycosis, viral infections (multiple), mycobacterium
Vesicles/bullae	VZV, HSV
Vesicles/bullae—suspect ecthyma gangrenosus	*Pseudomonas* species, *Vibrio vulnificus* and other gram-negative rods, *S. aureus, Mucormycosis, Aspergillus, Candida*
Lines	
Pain, swelling, erythema	*S. epidermidis, S. aureus, Candida*, gram-negative rods (e.g., *Pseudomonas*)

CMV, cytomegalovirus; HSV, herpes simplex virus; VZV, varicella zoster virus; PCP, *Pneumocystis Jiroveci (carinii)* pneumonia

viruses and uncommon agents such as *Candida* species and *Aspergillus* in patients with cancer with prolonged neutropenia and antibiotic therapy.

c. Lungs. Signs of consolidation and/or pleural effusion may indicate the presence of pneumonia (including postobstructive pneumonia). In neutropenic hosts, pneumonia may present with minimal changes on examination. Also, atypical pulmonary infections such as *Pneumocystis jiroveci* pneumonia (formerly *Pneumocystic carinii* pneumonia/PCP), can present initially with minimal or no changes on pulmonary examination.

d. Abdomen. Peritonitis may present with minimal findings of pain, rebound, or rigidity and can be somewhat benign initially, especially in neutropenic hosts with neutropenic enterocolitis (typhilitis) or patients on medications such as narcotics or steroids. Perirectal abscesses can be present with minimal discomfort or pruritus and on physical examination, may reveal only minimal erythema, tenderness, or swelling.

e. Skin. All areas of skin including perineal area, soles and palms should be thoroughly examined for new lesions. The pattern of skin involvement and type of lesions are important. Some of the following skin changes can signal disseminated infection with the following microbes.

(1) Petechia and purpura. Both viral and bacterial infections may present with scattered petechiae or purpura. *Neisseria meningitidis* is the most common bacterial agent causing petechiae, especially in asplenic patients.

(2) Macules and papules. A wide variety of gram-negative bacteria (including *Pseudomonas* and *Enterobacteriaceae*) may present with papules or macules, as can *S. aureus* and atypical bacteria such as Rickettsial species. Disseminated fungal infections (including *Candida, Cryptococcus, Histoplasma, Coccidioides and Fusarium*) will most commonly present with maculopapular, umbilicated, or nodular skin lesions. Common viral illnesses (and childhood viral illnesses such as adenovirus, rubella, or rubeola) may present with maculopapular eruptions as well. Mycobacterial infections such as *Mycobacterium haemophilum* may present with nodules.

(3) Vesicles and bullae. Classic herpes virus infections, such as varicella or herpes simplex may have vesicles in localized areas (dermatomal or mucocutaneous) or extensive cutaneous dissemination with other organ system involvement such as lungs or CNS. Two bacterial infections that may present with rapidly evolving vesicles or bullae (ecthyma gangrenosum) in immunocompromised hosts are *Vibrio vulnificus* and *Pseudomonas* species. Lesions can initially present as macules with or without vesicles, but quickly evolve into hemorrhagic bullae. These bullae later slough, revealing a deep underlying ulceration with surrounding erythema. Other infectious causes of ecthyma gangrenosum include fungal infections (such as *Mucormycosis, Aspergillus* or *Candida*), *S. aureus* and a variety of gram-negative rods.

f. Lines/catheters. Infections in lines and catheters may present with minimal erythema, tenderness, and swelling.

D. Microbiologic evaluation. Any patient with cancer with suspected infection should have a complete microbiologic evaluation of blood, urine and sputum at a minimum. Other specimens should be obtained depending on the patient's presentation (e.g., stool, skin biopsy, cerebrospinal fluid). Diagnostic studies such as blood cultures may need to be repeated periodically to document adequate response to therapy or identify the etiology of infection.

1. Blood cultures. Blood cultures are the single most important microbiologic test ordered and should be obtained in all patients with fever or suspected infection. In patients without longer-term indwelling intravenous access, all cultures should be drawn through separate peripheral venopuncture sites. Initially two to three sets of blood cultures are drawn at least 10 minutes apart and may be repeated in 48 to 72 hours, or sooner if the patient is clinically unstable. Ideally, 10 mL of blood should be drawn in each bottle. Blood cultures should be drawn in aerobic and anaerobic bottles with enriched media, to encourage growth of bacteria in the presence of antibiotics. Fungal blood culture bottles may be used if fungal infections such as *Coccidioides* or *Aspergillus* are suspected. However, most commercially available blood culture systems are able to detect *Candida* species in the blood. Therapy should not be delayed pending results of blood cultures, but ideally antibiotics should be started after the blood cultures are obtained, provided the cultures are obtained in an urgent manner.

  a. Catheter-related infections. In patients with longer-term percutaneous indwelling central catheters (PICCs), subcutaneously implanted catheters, and other central catheters, blood cultures are often obtained from both peripheral sites and from the catheters. Unfortunately, positive blood cultures from catheters for organisms such as *S. epidermidis, Bacillus* species or diphtheroids may represent either true infection or contamination and are difficult to interpret without removal of the catheter and culture of the tip.

2. Sputum. Expectorated sputum should be obtained for Gram stain, culture, and sensitivity. If patients cannot produce a sputum sample and a pulmonary source of infection is suspected, bronchoscopy with or without transbronchial biopsy may be indicated. When bronchoscopy is performed on an immunocompromised host, the following studies are usually obtained on lavage and biopsy specimens: routine Gram stain, culture, sensitivity, fungal stains and culture, acid-fast bacillus stains and cultures, modified acid-fast stains (for *Nocardia*), viral culture, silver stain (for Pneumocystis), and histopathology.

3. Urine. Urine should be sent for Gram stain, culture and urinalysis. If the patient is unable to produce a clean-catch urine specimen, urine should be obtained by catheterization. Leukocytes may be absent in urinalysis in a neutropenic host.

4. Stool. If patients have loose stools, initial specimens at the time of admission should be sent for routine culture (often this includes *Salmonella, Shigella, Campylobacter, Yersinia* and *Escherichia coli* 0157.H7), *C. difficile* toxin, ova and parasites, *Giardia* antigen, and cryptosporidium antigen. Except for *C. difficile* toxin, these tests have a low yield in patients who have been hospitalized for more than 3 days and then develop diarrhea. The exception to this is reactivation of a parasitic cause of diarrhea (such as *Strongyloides*).

5. Cerebrospinal fluid. Lumbar punctures are not indicated in the routine evaluation of patients with fever unless a meningeal source is suspected (e.g., significant headache, focal deficits, altered mental status, or nuchal rigidity). A relative contraindication to lumbar puncture is thrombocytopenia (<50,000) or coagulopathy. When cerebrospinal fluid is obtained, it should be sent at a minimum for cell count with differential, glucose, protein, routine culture and Gram stain, and cryptococcal antigen. Other tests such as acid-fast bacillus smear and cultures and fungal smear and cultures should be ordered if clinically warranted.

6. Other microbiologic tests. Other microbiologic tests that can be clinically useful include the following:

Cytomegalovirus (CMV) polymerase chain reaction (PCR) of blood.

Legionella urine antigen (>93% sensitive in detecting *Legionella pneumophila* serogroup).

Histoplasmosis urinary antigen.
HSV PCR of cerebrospinal fluid.
Semiquantitative cultures of catheter tips.

E. Radiology
   1. Chest x-rays. All patients with malignancy and suspected infection should have a baseline chest radiograph
   (including a lateral view if possible).
   2. Computer tomography (CT). CT scans should be ordered on an individualized basis. Patients with pulmonary
   complaints should undergo a CT scan of the chest if the
   chest x-ray (CXR) is noncontributory. Patients with abdominal complaints should have a CT of the abdomen and
   pelvis.
   3. Magnetic resonance imaging (MRI). MRI scans are
   especially useful in evaluating the brain and spine, hepatobiliary system and pancreas, soft tissue and bone.
   4. Ultrasound. Ultrasounds are noninvasive or minimally invasive tests without the need for IV contrast. All
   patients with suspected endocarditis should receive a TEE
   (transesophageal echocardiogram) unless contraindicated.
   Ultrasonography is especially useful in imaging the liver,
   biliary tree and gallbladder, pancreas, and kidneys.
   5. Other radiological tests. Other imaging studies such
   as gallium scans or tagged WBC scans are relatively nonspecific and rarely used. Positron emission tomography
   (PET) scans detect differential glucose metabolism of normal and abnormal tissues, but cannot differentiate between
   infection or underlying malignancy.
F. Other tests. All patients with cancer with suspected infection should have a complete blood count with differential
   and basic chemistry profile including electrolytes, blood urea
   nitrogen, creatinine, and liver function tests in order to assess
   possible multiple organ system involvement and presence of
   neutropenia.
G. Invasive diagnostic procedures. Bronchoscopy should
   be performed, preferably with biopsy in all patients with pneumonia without etiology, pneumonia with failure to improve
   with empiric therapy, or suspected pulmonary site of infection
   with a negative CXR or CT scan (especially in neutropenic
   patients). Liver biopsy and bone marrow biopsies are rarely
   required, but may be indicated when a thorough fever work-up
   is negative in a patient with an inadequate response to empiric
   therapy. In addition to routine Gram stains and cultures, bone
   marrow aspirates and liver biopsies are often sent for acid-
   fast bacillus smears and cultures, fungal smears and cultures,
   viral cultures, and histopathology for stains such as Warthin-
   Starry. Consultation with the clinical microbiology laboratory
   and pathology laboratory is important before obtaining these
   specimens.
III. Treatment
   A. General overview. Fever or suspected infection in a patient with cancer requires urgent evaluation and initiation of
   treatment. In certain populations (neutropenia, asplenia), it
   constitutes a medical emergency. Antibiotic therapy should
   never be withheld while the work-up for a fever source is
   in progress, but empiric therapy against the most likely

pathogens should be promptly instituted. If possible, however, blood cultures should be drawn before antibiotics are begun if this does not result in a treatment delay. Empiric therapy in febrile neutropenic and non-neutropenic hosts with suspected infection is reviewed as well as directed therapy against specific pathogens. Commonly used dosages of antimicrobials are listed in Table 28.3.

B. Febrile neutropenia. An excellent guideline for the management of a patient with febrile neutropenia has been published by the Infectious Diseases Society of America (IDSA, last updated in 2002).

    1. Febrile neutropenia is usually defined as fever (two episodes of temperatures >100.4°F or one episode of temperature >101°F) in a patient with a neutrophil count of less than 500 cells/µL or WBC count less than 1,000 cells/µL with neutrophils predicted to be less than 500 cells/µL. Most fevers in neutropenic patients stem from bacteria and fungi that are normal colonizers of the skin and alimentary canal. Mucosal damage with secondary bacterial and fungal translocation is thought to be an important initial step in the pathogenesis of febrile neutropenia.

    2. Microbiology. The most common organisms causing fever in neutropenic hosts are gram-positive cocci such as *Staphylococcus* species (*S. aureus* and *S. epidermidis*), *Streptococcus, Enterococcus, Pseudomonas* and other gram-negative rods (such as *Enterobacter* and *Proteus* species), and anaerobes (such as *Bacteroides* and *Clostridium* species). Fungi such as *Candida* species occasionally can cause primary infections, but usually occur as secondary infections ("super infections").

    3. Empiric antibiotic therapy. All neutropenic patients with fever without localizing source or suspected infection in the absence of fever should receive urgent empiric antibiotic therapy to cover gram-positive organisms such as *Staphylococcus* species and *Streptococcus* species and gram-negative rods such as *Pseudomonas*. Antifungal antibiotics are not usually included in the initial empiric antibiotic regimen unless a fungal infection is suspected (i.e., use of hyperalimentation).

        a. Monotherapy. Use of a single broad-spectrum antimicrobial such as a third- or fourth-generation cephalosporin or a carbapenem has been shown in multiple clinic trials to be as effective as multidrug treatment regimens for febrile neutropenia. Treatment options for empiric therapy include the following:

- Ceftazidime
- Cefepime
- Carbapenems (imipenem–cilastatin or meropenem)
- Piperacillin–tazobactam
- For patients with severe penicillin allergies, no monotherapy regimens are available and multidrug regimens are required.

        b. Two-drug therapy. Multidrug therapy does not offer any specific clinical advantages over monotherapy

Table 28.3. Dosages of commonly used antibiotics in oncology patients

Antibacterials	Renal Adjustment Required for Cr Cl <50	Comments
Vancomycin 1 g IV q12 h	Yes	Monitor peak and trough Nephrotoxicity increased with aminoglycosides
Piperacillin–tazobactam 3.375 g IV q6 h	Yes	Piperacillin needs aminoglycosides for synergy with *Pseudomonas* infections.
Ampicillin–clavulanate 875 mg PO q12 h	Yes	Diarrhea common
Imipenem–cilastatin 0.5 g IV q6 h	Yes	Seizures can occur if dose not reduced for renal insufficiency
Meropenem 1 g IV q8 h	Yes	Approved for meningitis in patients ≥3 months of age
Aztreonam 2 mg IV q8 h	Yes	Can use in patients with β-lactam allergy
Ciprofloxacin 400 mg IV q12 h	Yes	Avoid in children <16 years old
Ceftriaxone 2 g IV q2 h	No	High doses can result in sludge in gallbladder—no *Pseudomonas* or enterococcal coverage.
Cefepime 2 g IV q8 h	Yes	Covers *Pseudomonas*, not *Enterococcus*
Ceftazidime 2 g IV q8 h	Yes	Covers *Pseudomonas*, not *Enterococcus*
Trimethoprim–culfamethiazole 1 DS PO q12 h	Yes	Can increase creatinine/PCP doses—5 mg/kg q8 h IV based on a trimethoprim component.
Metronidazole 500 mg PO q6 h	No	Dose adjustment with dialysis—avoid alcohol.
Linezolid 600 mg PO or IV q12 h	No	Anemia, thrombocytopenia, leukopenia common—monitor CBC weekly if treatment >2 weeks.
Daptomycin 4 mg/kg IV q.d.	Yes	Not effective in pneumonia
Quinupristin/ dalfopristin 7.5 mg/kg IV q8 h	Yes	Infuse through central line

Table 28.3. (*Continued*)

Antibacterials	Renal Adjustment Required for Cr Cl <50	Comments
Gentamicin—dosing varies based on clinical scenarios	Yes	Nephrotoxicity/ototoxicity common—monitor peak and trough.
		Use ideal body weight or adjusted body weight with obesity.
Antifungals		
Amphotericin B up to 1.5 mg/kg/day	No, unless due to drug itself	Nephrotoxicity (increased with radiographic contrast, cisplatinum, other nephrotoxic agents)
Fluconazole 200–400 mg IV q.d.	Yes	Drug–drug interactions common
Voriconazole 400 mg PO q12 h on day 1, then 200 mg PO q12 h if >40 kg	No	Avoid IV if Cr Cl <50
Caspofungin 70 mg IV on day 1, then 50 mg IV q.d.	No	Decrease dose with liver dysfunction
Antivirals		
Ganciclovir 5 mg/kg IV q12 h	Yes	Neutropenia, thrombocytopenia
Valganciclovir 900 mg PO q12 h	Yes	Prodrug of ganciclovir—oral form only
Foscarnet 60 mg/kg IV q8 h	Yes	Significant renal toxicity
Acyclovir 10–12 mg/kg IV q8 h	Yes	Not active against CMV. Seizures can occur if dose is not adjusted for renal insufficiency.

Cr Cl, creatinine clearance.

in recent clinical trials using carbapenems or antipseudomonal cephalosporins. However, the addition of an aminoglycoside (gentamicin, tobramycin, amikacin) can be used for potential synergistic effects against gram-negative rods.

c. Severe penicillin allergy. There are no published clinical trials evaluating the treatment of febrile neutropenia in patients with a severe penicillin or β-lactam allergy. A fluoroquinolone with antipseudomonal activity such as ciprofloxin combined with aztreonam and vancomycin should provide effective coverage against the most likely pathogens.

d. Vancomycin. Vancomycin should be included in the initial antibiotic regimen of febrile neutropenia if any of the following additional clinical situations are noted:

- Suspected catheter infection
- Cellulitis or mucositis
- Known colonization or previous infection with a β-lactam–resistant gram-positive organism or methicillin-resistant *Staphylococcus aureus* (MRSA)
- Blood cultures with gram-positive organisms
- Sepsis, hypotension or signs of cardiovascular or endovascular infection (e.g., new murmur, petechia)
- Significant institutional presence of β-lactam–resistant gram-positive organisms
- Use of quinolones as antibiotic prophylaxis before the onset of fever

4. **Duration of antimicrobial therapy**
   a. In patients in whom a source of infection is found, standard therapy should be continued for the standard duration (i.e., treat Group A streptococcal pharyngitis with penicillin for 10 days).
   b. In patients in whom no specific infection is found, antimicrobial therapy can generally be discontinued when the neutrophil count is more than 500 cells/mm³ and the patient is afebrile for more than 48 hours and without signs of infections.
   c. In patients who become afebrile within 3 to 5 days but remain neutropenic, no specific treatment strategy is well defined. Options include the following:

   - Continue empiric antimicrobial therapy for 5 to 7 afebrile days.
   - Continue empiric antimicrobial therapy during the period of neutropenia.

5. **Continued fever in neutropenic patients on empiric therapy without a source.** Patients with febrile neutropenia should undergo a thorough history and physical examination daily looking for a source of infection, including a review of all labs, microbiology data, and radiologic studies. If a source of fever is found, antimicrobial therapy should be adjusted accordingly for most likely etiologic organisms.
   a. If no source of fever is found after 5 days and a change of antibiotic therapy is not indicated on the basis of the results of the work-up, an empiric antifungal agent should be added.
   b. Options include amphotericin B compounds, voriconazole, or caspofungin. Both caspofungin and voriconazole have been shown to be as effective as liposomal amphotericin B. Fluconazole is generally not recommended for empiric antifungal therapy, as it does not cover *Aspergillus* or *Candida* species such as *Candida krusei* or *Candida glabrata*.

C. **Empiric therapy in non-neutropenic patients.** Patients with infection and neutrophil count greater than 1,000 cells/μL may present with fever or infection from a known or unknown source. As with febrile neutropenia, urgent evaluation and initiation of prompt empiric therapy is indicated.

1. **Patients with altered cell-mediated immunity (CMI).** Patients with altered cellular immunity due to treatment or underlying diseases (such as non–Hodgkin's lymphoma in a patient with acquired immune deficiency syndrome [AIDS]) may present with fever without a known source.

   a. **Microbiology.** In addition to routine bacterial pathogens such as *S. pneumoniae* or *S. aureus*, patients with altered CMI are at risk for infection with atypical organisms such as PCP, *Mycobacterium, Nocardia, Listeria*, viral infections such as CMV and fungal infections such as *Cryptococcus*.

   b. **Treatment.** In patients with altered cell-mediated immunity, diagnostic work-up of fever before initiating treatment is important if the patient is clinically stable. Work-up before antimicrobial therapy should include at a minimum blood cultures, acid-fast bacillus blood cultures, viral cultures, urinalysis and culture, CXR, or CT scan of chest and abdomen. Urgent infectious diseases consultation is recommended for the clinically unstable patient with suspected infection and altered CMI.

2. **Patients with altered humoral immunity and/or splenectomy.** Patients with hypogammaglobulinemia or agammaglobulinemia may lack opsonizing antibodies to encapsulated bacteria.

   a. **Microbiology.** Encapsulated bacteria such as *S. pneumoniae, Haemophilus influenza, N. meningitidis, C. canimorsus*, and encapsulated strains of other bacteria such as *S. aureus* and *E. coli* are potential pathogens.

   b. **Treatment.** Antibiotic therapy in patients with asplenia and/or altered humoral immunity must be instituted immediately as a delay in treatment may lead to death. No clinical trials have been performed in this patient population, but treatment is aimed at covering the major pathogens. An appropriate empiric antibiotic regimen would be vancomycin and a third-generation cephalosporin such as ceftriaxone. In patients with severe penicillin allergy, a fluoroquinolone such as levofloxacin could be substituted for ceftriaxone. In patients with documented or suspected bacteremia, the duration of therapy is at least 14 days.

3. **Nosocomial infections.** Nosocomial infections are generally defined as infections occurring in a health care setting 48 hours after admission. These infections are often multidrug resistant, resulting in severely limited treatment options. They can be associated with high morbidity and mortality.

   a. **Lungs.** Hospital-acquired pneumonia is commonly polymicrobic with resistant gram-negative rods (such as *Pseudomonas, Klebsiella* and *Acinetobacter* species) and gram-positive cocci (such as methicillin-resistant

Staphylococcus aureus [MRSA]). In hospitalized patients, the oropharynx becomes colonized with microbes from the hospital environment within 48 hours. Microaspiration of oropharyngeal bacteria is the main cause of pneumonia. Empiric antimicrobial therapy should be directed against common multidrug resistant organisms such as *Pseudomonas* species or MRSA. Examples of an initial empiric regimen for nosocomial pneumonia would be as follows:

(1) Antipseudomonal β-lactam (cefepime or ceftazidime) or

(2) Carbapenem (imipenem-cilastatin, meropenem) or

(3) Piperacillin–tazobactam + antipseudomonal fluoroquinolone (levofloxacin or ciprofloxacin) + vancomycin or linezolid.

Duration of therapy is probably 3 weeks in immunocompromised hosts.

b. Lines. Intravascular catheter-related infections are common nosocomial infections and can occur in central venous catheters (CVC) (tunneled and nontunneled), arterial catheters, and implantable devices. They are a major cause of morbidity and mortality, and may result in significant complications such as endocarditis or distant metastasis or infection. The most common organisms involved in line infections are *Staphylococcus* species (*S. epidermidis*, *S. aureus*), gram-negative rods, and *Candida* species. Treatment of catheter-related infections requires removal of the catheter if possible, in addition to systemic antibiotics.

(1) Empiric antibiotic therapy in patients with a nontunneled CVC. In patients with a suspected indwelling line infection with an easily removable venous access catheter (i.e., PICC line and severe infection), the line should be removed and inserted at a new site if possible. Semiquantitative cultures of the catheter tip should be performed. Empiric antibiotic therapy with vancomycin and an antipseudomonal penicillin or cephalosporin (such as piperacillin or cefepime) is indicated. If the patient has been receiving hyperalimentation through the line, empiric therapy against *Candida* species with amphotericin B or caspofungin may be also needed. Owing to the increasing incidence of resistant *Candida* species, fluconazole should not be used empirically for suspected fungemia. If associated septic thrombophlebitis is present, surgical excision or drainage of the vein is generally required.

When the organism has been identified through blood cultures or by the presence of more than 100 colony-forming units (CFU)/mL from quantitative culture of the catheter tip, directed therapy can begin. If *S. aureus* is present on blood cultures, a TEE should be performed to rule out infective endocarditis. If there is no evidence of endocarditis, 2 weeks of antistaphylococcal therapy guided by sensitivity data can be used. Otherwise, 4 to 6 weeks is indicated. Infection with distant colonization (such as osteomyelitis) may require more than 6 weeks. In patients with positive fungal cultures, an ophthalmologic examination to rule out endophthalmitis is indicated. Blood cultures need to be repeated until they are negative and antifungal therapy is continued for 2 weeks after documented clearance of the fungemia. Infection with gram-negative rods is generally treated for 2 weeks as well. In patients with coagulase-negative staphylococcus (*S. epidermidis*), treatment may be indicated for 5 to 7 days after catheter removal.

If the catheter is not removed in nonvirulent infections such as *S. epidermidis* line infections, an attempt can be made to clear the catheter infection using intraluminal ("antibiotic lock therapy") intravenous antibiotics. A common antibiotic regimen for antibiotic lock therapy for *S. epidermidis* is vancomycin at 1 to 5 mg/mL instilled into the catheter lumen (s) to fill all lumens completely for more than 12 hours/day for 2 weeks in combination with intravenous antibiotics. A wide range of study results using antibiotic lock therapy to clear *S. epidermidis* line infections have been published with success rates of 18% to 100%, but in general successful clearance of infection is usually less than 50%.

(2) Empiric antibiotic therapy in patients with a tunneled CVC. In patients in whom the CVC cannot be easily removed, it is important (if possible) to determine if the catheter is the actual source of infection. Insertion site infections, tunnel infections, clinically unstable patients with possible line infection, evidence of metastatic disease or infection with *Candida* species, gram-negative rods, or *S. aureus* require catheter removal and treatment as previously mentioned. Salvage therapy of the line with systemic antibiotic therapy and antibiotic lock therapy can be attempted in selected stable patients with nonvirulent pathogens such as *S. epidermidis*, but clinical deterioration, continued bacteremia, or failure to improve requires catheter removal.

c. Foley catheter/urinary tract infections (UTIs). Complicated UTIs in hospitalized patients with or without Foley catheters are commonly caused by *E. coli* and *Enterococcus* species. Other microbes that can cause nosocomial infection of the urinary tract include *Pseudomonas* species, and other enterobacteriaceae bacteria/gram-negative rods (*Proteus, Klebsiella, Providencia*). *S. epidermidis* may cause catheter-associated UTIs. The presence of *S. aureus* in the urine should prompt a search for bacteremia and metastatic staphylococcal infection. Treatment involves removal of the Foley catheter and correction of any associated obstructions or renal-related problems (e.g., azotemia) if possible. Empiric therapy for complicated UTIs could include quinolones with good urinary concentration such as ciprofloxacin or levofloxacin, extended spectrum β-lactams such as ticarcillin–clavulanate or piperacillin–tazobactam, or carbapenems such as imipenem–cilastatin or meropenem. Antibiotic resistance in commonly occurring gram-negative rods (such as *E. coli*) to trimethoprim–sulfamethoxazole (TMP–SMZ) is equal to or more than 20% in most areas, making this a poor choice for empiric therapy in immunocompromised hosts. Ampicillin plus gentamicin has been the traditional therapy for complicated UTIs but newer agents available carry less toxicity risks than gentamicin and are generally preferred.

Duration of therapy is usually 2 weeks but patients should be improving and afebrile within 72 hours. Patients who remain febrile or who are initially clinically unstable should undergo ultrasound or CT to rule out perinephric abscess or obstruction.

d. **Diarrhea**

(1) **The major nosocomial pathogen causing diarrhea is *C. difficile*.** Recently, an epidemic strain of binary toxin producing *C. difficile* associated with an aggressive form of colitis has been described. In addition, hospitalized patients with neutropenia and diarrhea may also develop neutropenic enterocolitis (typhlitis). Typhlitis is probably caused by mucosal disruption and enteric bacterial invasion of the mucosa during neutropenia. Clostridial organisms (e.g., as *Clostridium septicum*), *Pseudomonas*, anaerobes, and occasionally *Candida* are commonly occurring pathogens. Fungemia and/or bacteremia can be associated with typhilitis as well. Work-up of a hospitalized patient with diarrhea and/or neutropenia should include *C. difficile* toxin assay and CT of the abdomen. For diarrhea developing in the hospital, unless reactivation of a parasitic illness is suspected (e.g., *Strongyloides*), ova and parasite examination of stool has a relatively low yield.

(2) **Empiric therapy of suspected *C. difficile* colitis** is metronidazole 500 mg orally three times a day or 250 mg orally four times a day. Metronidazole is preferred initially over vancomycin. Both are equally effective but use of vancomycin may lead to vancomycin-resistant enterococcus (VRE).

(3) **In patients with suspected typhlitis** broad-spectrum antibiotic therapy with good anaerobic coverage is indicated, such as imipenem–cilastatin, meropenem or piperacillin–tazobactam. If *C. difficile* colitis has not been excluded, oral metronidazole should be added as well. In patients with continued fever or clinical deterioration an antifungal agent such as caspofungin should be added. Initial surgical consultation is recommended for patients with suspected typhlitis, because perforation or clinical deterioration may require urgent laparotomy and resection of involved bowel.

Table 28.4. Directed therapy against specific pathogens

Organism	Antibiotics
Staphylococcus aureus	
Methicillin sensitive	Nafcillin, cefazolin, ceftriaxone
Methicillin resistant	Vancomycin, linezolid, daptomycin, quinupristin−dalfopristin
Staphylococcus epidermidis	Vancomycin, linezolid, daptomycin, quinupristin−dalfopristin
Enterococcus	Vancomycin, linezolid, daptomycin, quinupristin−dalfopristin, penicillin/amoxicillin + aminoglycoside
Pseudomonas	Cefepime, piperacillin, imipenem or meropenem, ciprofloxacin, aztreonam + aminoglycoside
Candida	
C. albicans	Fluconazole, amphotericin B, voriconazole, caspofungin
C. glabrata	Amphotericin B, caspofungin, voriconazole
C. krusei	Amphotericin B, caspofungin, voriconazole
Aspergillus	Voriconazole, amphotericin B, caspofungin
Pneumocystis jiroveci (formerly *carinii*)	Trimethoprim−sulfamethoxazole, pentamidine, atovaquone
Cytomegalovirus	Ganciclovir, valganciclovir, foscarnet, cidofovir

D. Directed therapy against specific pathogens. Before the results of sensitivity testing, empiric therapy against specific or suspected pathogens needs to be chosen on the basis of the most likely sensitivity results. Microbial sensitivities are influenced by a number of factors, including earlier antibiotic exposure, clinical scenario of infection and institutional and community resistance patterns (Table 28.4).

1. **Staphylococcus aureus.** As previously mentioned, risk factors for methicillin-resistant *S. aureus* (MRSA) infection include catheter infections, cellulitis, mucositis, previous colonization with resistant organisms, sepsis or possible endovascular infections, earlier use of quinolones, or significant institutional presence of MRSA. Good treatment options for MRSA include vancomycin, linezolid, daptomycin, and quinupristin−dalfopristin. For methicillin-sensitive *Staphylococcus aureus* (MSSA), good treatment options include β-lactam antibiotics such as nafcillin, cefazolin or ceftriaxone, β-lactam/β-lactamase inhibitor combinations such as piperacillin−tazobactam

or vancomycin, if allergic to β-lactams. Bacteriostatic antibiotics such as TMP–SMZ, clindamycin, fluoroquinolones, or doxycycline should generally not be used as first-line therapy in patients with severe *S. aureus* infections.

2. *Staphylococcus epidermidis.* Coagulase-negative Staphylococci are often resistant to β-lactams (>80%). When these infections are suspected (often line-associated) good initial antibiotic choices include vancomycin, linezolid, daptomycin, or quinupristin–dalfopristin.

3. *Enterococcus.* Treatment of enterococcal endocarditis or other severe enterococcal infection generally requires synergy with a β-lactam (penicillin or amoxicillin) or glycopeptide (such as vancomycin) in combination with an aminoglycoside at synergistic doses. Cephalosporins have no activity against *Enterococcus.* Linezolid is bacteriostatic against vancomycin-resistant enterococcus (VRE), but has been used successfully in cases of severe enterococcal infection as monotherapy. Other antibiotics with activity against enterococcus include daptomycin and quinupristin–dalfopristin (active against *Enterococcus faecium*, but not *Enterococcus faecalis*). Nitrofurantoins, quinolones such as ciprofloxacin, and doxycycline also have some enterococcal activity, but should be used only for UTIs after data are available on sensitivity.

4. *Pseudomonas aeruginosa.* Serious *Pseudomonas* infections (e.g., bacteremia, ecthyma gangrenosum) often require synergistic combinations of antipseudomonal β-lactams (such as piperacillin or cefepime) and an aminoglycoside. Other treatment options include monotherapy with an antipseudomonal β-lactam, imipenem or meropenem, ciprofloxacin or aztreonam. Resistance can occur with treatment, resulting in treatment failure.

5. *Candida* species. *Candida albicans* is usually sensitive to fluconazole, amphotericin B, caspofungin, and voriconazole. *C. glabrata* and *C. krusei* have decreased sensitivities to fluconazole (85% and 5% sensitive, respectively) but are usually sensitive to amphotericin B, caspofungin, and voriconazole. Two other commonly seen *Candida* species (*Candida parapsilosis* and *Candida tropicalis*) are usually sensitive to fluconazole, amphotericin B, voriconazole, and caspofungin, but have decreased sensitivity to itraconazole.

6. *Aspergillus.* *Aspergillus* species (*Aspergillus fumigatus, Aspergillus flavus, Aspergillus terreus* and *Aspergillus niger*) are resistant to fluconazole. Voriconazole is more effective than amphotericin B in one large study of invasive aspergillosis in immunocompromised hosts. In addition to amphotericin B and voriconazole, caspofungin has activity in invasive aspergillosis. Combination therapy with caspofungin and voriconazole has been successfully used in patients with invasive aspergillosis, but large-scale randomized studies are lacking.

7. *Pneumocystis jiroveci* **pneumonia (PCP).** TMP–SMZ at high doses (5 mg/kg IV q8 h) is the primary treatment for PCP. If the Pao_2 is less than 70 mm/kg, prednisone

40 mg orally q12 hours is added for 5 days, then 20 mg daily for 11 days. Other commonly used treatment choices for PCP include pentamidine (intravenous) or atovaquone (oral).

8. **Cytomegalovirus (CMV).** CMV can cause a variety of end-organ diseases. CMV pneumonia is generally treated with high-dose ganciclovir (2.5 mg/kg IV q8 h) with intravenous immunoglobulin (IVIG). CMV retinitis can be treated with oral valganciclovir or intravenous ganciclovir. Other antivirals with CMV activity include foscarnet and cidofovir.

IV. **Infections in hematopoietic stem cell transplant recipients (HSCT).** The management of HSCT patients with infection is extremely complex and depends on a number of variables—type of transplantation, latent infections in the recipient, timing of humoral and cellular reconstitution, development of graft-versus-host disease, conditioning regimen, and time after transplantation. Several excellent reviews of infection in HSCT recipients are available and are listed in the references.

A. **Evaluation of infection based on temporal approach.** One classic approach to the evaluation of infection in bone marrow transplant patients is to divide the transplant immunodeficiencies and pathogen susceptibilities into three separate periods—pre-engraftment, early postengraftment, and late postengraftment. Engraftment is defined as the time when a patient can sustain an absolute neutrophil count (ANC) greater than 500 cells/μL and platelet count of more than 20,000 μL for three or more consecutive days without transfusion.

1. **Pre-engraftment** (Phase I: generally first month after transplant). Pathogens likely to cause infection in the pre-engraftment period include the following:
   a. **Viral.** HSV, seasonal respiratory and enteric viruses
   b. **Bacteria.** *S. epidermidis, S. aureus*, vidians streptococcus, *Pseudomonas* species, Enterobacteriaceae and other gram-negative rods
   c. **Fungus.** *Candida* species, *Aspergillus*

2. **Early postengraftment** (Phase II: generally first 30 to 100 days after transplant)
   a. **Other human herpes viruses such as Epstein-Barr virus** (EBV), seasonal respiratory and enteric viruses
   b. **Bacterial.** *Listeria monocytogenes, Legionella* species, *S. epidermidis, Streptococcus* species, *S. aureus*
   c. **Fungus.** *Aspergillus* and other molds (e.g., *Pseudallescheria boydii*), *P. jiroveci*
   d. **Parasites.** *Toxoplasma gondii, Strongyloides stercoralis*

3. **Late postengraftment** (Phase III: generally more than 100 days after transplant).
   a. **Viral.** VZV, EBV, and other human herpes viruses (e.g., CMV, HHV-8), hepatitis B, hepatitis C, seasonal respiratory and enteric viruses
   b. **Bacteria.** Encapsulated bacteria such as *S. pneumonia, H. influenza, N. meningitidis*
   c. **Fungi.** *P. jiroveci, Aspergillus,* and other molds
   d. **Parasitic.** *T. gondii*

V.   Prophylaxis of infection in patients with cancer. Given
the high rate of infection in oncology patients and the associated
morbidity and mortality, multiple studies have evaluated preventive strategies for fungal, bacterial, and viral infections in
different oncology populations.

A.   Prophylaxis of infection in non-HSCT patients

1.   Antibacterial prophylaxis. Multiple randomized placebo controlled studies of antibiotic prophylaxis in afebrile
neutropenic patients have been performed over the last
30 years with differing results. Many studies have shown
reductions in febrile illnesses using antibiotic prophylaxis
during afebrile neutropenia, but significant side effects
have been noted. These include fungal superinfection and
development of resistant organisms. The most widely studied prophylactic antibiotics have been oral nonabsorbable
antibiotics for selective GI decontamination (e.g., aminoglycosides, oral vancomycin) and systemically absorbed antibiotics such as trimethoprim–sulfamethoxazole (TMP–SMZ)
and fluoroquinolones. Oral nonabsorbable antibiotics for
prophylaxis in afebrile neutropenic patients with cancer
are not recommended on the basis of previous studies, but
controversy exists regarding the use of TMP–SMZ and
quinolones.

a.   TMP–SMZ. Studies on use of TMP–SMZ for the
most part have shown some decrease in infection rates
in afebrile neutropenia with little effect on overall mortality. The development of resistant organisms and
potential bone marrow suppression has been important disadvantages in the routine prophylactic use of
TMP–SMZ. The current 2002 IDSA guidelines for use
of antimicrobial agents in neutropenic patients with
cancer recommend prophylactic use of TMP–SMZ only
for PCP in patients at risk.

b.   Fluoroquinolones. Oral quinolones have been studied extensively for prophylaxis in afebrile neutropenic
patients with mixed results. Use of agents such as
ciprofloxacin in randomized trials has shown a decrease
in gram-negative rod infections, but an increase in infections with resistant organisms and gram-positive cocci.
The current 2002 IDSA guidelines for use of antimicrobial agents in neutropenic patients with cancer recommends against prophylactic use of quinolones in afebrile
neutropenia. However, a recent meta-analysis of antibiotic prophylaxis in neutropenia patients showed potential reduction in mortality with fluoroquinolone use.
There are no adequate large-scale trials yet on the use of
newer quinolones with improved gram positive-coverage
(such as moxifloxacin). For now, use of quinolones for
routine antibiotic prophylaxis in afebrile neutropenia is
not recommended.

2.   Antifungal prophylaxis. The 2002 IDSA guidelines
for antimicrobial prophylaxis in neutropenic patients recommends against routine use of itraconazole or fluconazole
for antifungal prophylaxis. Several studies have shown a
decrease in fungal infections and associated mortalities in

patients receiving fluconazole or itraconazole prophylaxis, but this is outweighed by possible development of antifungal resistance. Additional studies are in progress for specific oncologic populations, such as AML.

3. **Antiviral prophylaxis.** Antiviral prophylaxis is not recommended for afebrile neutropenic patients.

B. **Prophylaxis of infection in hematopoietic stem cell transplant (HSCT).** The American Society for Blood and Marrow Transplantation and the IDSA recommend prophylaxis for encapsulated bacteria, *Pneumocystis*, HSV and VZV seropositive patients, (with prophylactic or preemptive therapy for CMV), and antifungal prophylaxis for patients on chronic steroids and until engraftment. In addition, they recommend antibiotic prophylaxis for patients undergoing dental procedures as per the current American Heart Association guidelines for endocarditis prophylaxis.

1. **Bacterial prophylaxis.** There are no recommendations for use of specific antibiotics for bacterial prophylaxis in HSCT patients. Physicians who use single antibiotics for prophylaxis of encapsulated organisms after transplant should choose agents on the basis of factors such as local antimicrobial resistance patterns. IVIG can be used in patients with severe hypogammaglobinemia during the early postengraftment phase.

2. **Fungal prophylaxis.** Fluconazole 400 mg orally per day until engraftment.

3. **Pneumocystis** jiroveci prophylaxis (PCP prophylaxis) and toxoplasmosis prophylaxis. One TMP–SMZ double strength tablet daily or three times per week. Prophylaxis for PCP should begin before transplantation.

4. **Viral prophylaxis.** Multiple strategies (prophylaxis or preemptive) exist to decrease the incidence of CMV infection and reactivation in HSCT patients. One strategy is the use of intravenous ganciclovir 5 g/kg IV q12 h for 1 week, then 5 days/week till day 100 post-transplant in seropositive patients at risk. Prophylaxis against HSV reactivation is recommended for HSV seropositive transplant recipients. Acyclovir (200 mg orally three times per day) can be given at the start of conditioning until engraftment or resolution of mucositis.

5. **Other prophylactic strategies**

   a. **Vaccination.** The following vaccines are commonly given 12 to 24 months after HSCT transplantation in adults: tetanus–diphtheria toxoid vaccine, hepatitis B series, 23-valent pneumococcal polysaccharide vaccine, influenza vaccine, and inactivated polio vaccine. Measles, mumps, and rubella (MMR) vaccine and varicella vaccine are contraindicated. No recommendation has yet been made on the use of meningococcal vaccine or the newly developed tetanus–diphtheria–acellular pertussis vaccine for adults due to limited data.

   b. **Infection control measures.** Strict attention to infection control measures should be practiced by HSCT patients, caregivers, and health care workers, especially strict attention to hand washing. Some unique aspects of infection control include the following:

(1) While in hospital, strict attention should be paid to air-flow and air filtration, possible exposure to construction in the hospital environment, and exposure to health care workers with seemingly minor infections such as adenovirus conjunctivitis.

(2) HSCT patients should avoid exposure to respiratory and enteric viruses (i.e., wear surgical mask during close contact with people with respiratory illness).

(3) Contact with sick pets should be minimized and excellent pet health should be maintained.

(4) Patients should avoid reptiles, chicks, ducklings, and exotic pets.

(5) Patients should avoid well water.

(6) Strict attention to food safety practices (e.g., use of separate cutting boards for raw chicken; cleaning of surfaces and knives after each use; and washing all produce) should be practiced by everyone involved in meal preparation for HSCT patients.

(7) Use of a low microbial diet (e.g., avoid sushi, salad dressings made with raw eggs) is recommended.

(8) Vaccination of family members and household contacts should be done as per current Advisory Committee on Immunization Practices (ACIP) guidelines. Currently, family members and household contacts should receive all age-appropriate vaccinations and influenza and hepatitis A, MMR and varicella vaccination if indicated. Oral polio vaccine should be avoided. Updated information about vaccines can be accessed at www.cdc.gov/nip.

SUGGESTED READINGS

Centers for Disease Control and Prevention. Recommended adult immunization schedule–United States, October 2005-September 2006. *MMWR Morb Mortal Wkly Rep* 2005;54(48):Q1–Q4.

Dykewicz CA, Kaplan JE, Jaffe HW, et al. Guidelines for preventing opportunistic infections among cell transplant recipients. *MMWR Morb Mortal Wkly Rep* 2000;49(RR10):1–128.

Gafter-Gvili A, Fraser A, Paul M, et al. Meta-analysis: antibiotic prophylaxis reduces mortality in neutropenic patients. *Ann Intern Med* 2005;142(12 Pt 1):979–995.

Hall K, Farr B. Diagnosis and management of long-term central venous catheter infections. *J Vasc Interv Radiol* 2004;15(4):327–334.

Helbig JH, Uldum SA, Bernander S, et al. Clinical utility of urinary antigen detection for diagnosis of community-acquired, travel-associated and nosocomial legionnaires' disease. *J Clin Microbiol* 2003;41(2):838–840.

Hughes WT, Armstrong D, Bodey GP, et al. Guidelines for the use of antimicrobial agents in neutropenic patients with cancer. *Clin Infect Dis* 2002;34:730–751.

McDonald LC, Killgore GE, Thompson A, et al. An epidemic, toxin gene-variant strain of clostridium difficile. *N Engl J Med* 2005;353:2442–2449.

Mermel L, Farr B, Sherertz RJ, et al. Guidelines for the management of intravascular catheter-related infections. *Clin Infect Dis* 2001;32:1249–1272.

Pappas PG, Rex JH, Sobel JD, et al. Guidelines for treatment of candidiasis. *Clin Infect Dis* 2004;38:161–189.

Rizzo JD, Wingard JR, Tichelli A, et al. Recommended screening and preventive practices for long-term survivors after hematopoietic cell transplantation: joint recommendations of the European group for blood and marrow transplantation, the center for international blood and marrow transplant research, and the American society of blood and marrow transplantation. *Bone Marrow Transplant* 2006;37:249–261.

Rubin RH, Young LS. *Clinical approach to infections in the compromised host*. New York, NY: Kluwer Academic Plenum Publishers, 2002.

Sable Ca, Donowitz GR. Infections in bone marrow transplant recipients. *Clin Infect Dis* 1994;18:223.

Safdar N, Fine JP, Maki DG. Meta-analysis: methods for diagnosing intravascular device-related bloodstream infection. *Ann Intern Med* 2005;142(6):451–466.

Van Burik J, Weisdoft D. Infections in recipients of hematopoietic stem cell transplantation. In: *Principles and practices of infectious diseases*. Mandel GL, Bennett JE, Dolin R, eds. Philadelphia: Elsevier Churchill Livingstone, 2005.

Vetter E, Torgerson C, Feuker A, et al. Comparison of the BACTEC MYCO/F lytic bottle to the Isolator Tube, BACTEC Plus Aerobic F/Bottle, and BACTEC Anaerobic Lytic/10 Bottle and Comparison of the BACTEC Plus Aerobic F/Bottle to the Isolator Tube for Recovery of Bacteria, Mycobacteria and F. *J Clin Microbiol* 2001;39(12):4380–4386. ungi from Blood. Dec;

Walsh TJ, Pappas P, Winston DJ, et al. Voriconazole compared with liposomal amphotericin B for empirical antifungal therapy in patients with neutropenia and persistent fever. *N Engl J Med* 2002;346(4):225–234. Jan 24;

Walsh TJ, Teppler H, Donowitz GR, et al. Caspofungin versus liposomal amphotericin B for empirical antifungal therapy in patients with persistent fever and neutropenia. *N Engl J Med* 2004; 351(14):1391–1402. Sep 30;

CHAPTER 29

Transfusion Therapy, Bleeding, and Clotting

Mary R. Smith and NurJehan Quraishy

Disorders of the hemostatic mechanisms are common in patients with malignancy. Abnormalities associated with thromboembolic events cause significantly more morbidity and mortality than disorders leading to hemorrhage.

I. **Thromboembolism in cancer**

A. **Pathophysiology.** The thromboembolic risk associated with neoplasia reflects an imbalance between platelet number, platelet function, levels of coagulation factors, and generation of thromboplastins as compared with the levels of inhibitors of hemostasis and fibrinolytic activity. Thrombosis may be minor and localized or widespread and associated with multiple-organ damage. There may also be hemorrhage of varying degrees of severity in association with the thromboembolic events.

1. **Factors that may affect the risk of thromboembolism** vary widely from patient to patient and include the following:

- Specific type of tumor
- Nutritional status of the patient
- Type of chemotherapy
- Response to chemotherapy (e.g., tumor lysis syndrome)
- Liver and renal function
- Patient immobility and venous stasis

2. **Factors that can initiate thrombus formation** are common to many cancers:

- Circulating tumor cells adhere to the vascular endothelium and form a nidus for clot formation.
- Tumors may penetrate the vessel, destroying the endothelium and promoting clot formation.
- Neovascularization associated with many tumors may stimulate clotting.
- Arterial thrombosis associated with tumors may result from vasospasm.
- A systemic hypercoagulable state develops (e.g., decreased protein C).
- External compression of vessels by tumor masses impedes blood flow and leads to stasis and clot development.

3. **Platelet abnormalities associated with an increased risk of thromboembolism** include thrombocytosis and increased platelet adhesion and aggregation. Tumors may produce substances that cause increased platelet aggregation with subsequent release of platelet factor III and ensuing acceleration of coagulation.

B. Clinical syndromes. A variety of noteworthy clinical syndromes are associated with the "hypercoagulable state" of malignancy and its treatment.

 1. Disseminated intravascular coagulation (DIC). DIC is a syndrome with many signs, symptoms, and abnormal laboratory results (Table 29.1). As many as 90% of patients with metastatic neoplasms have some laboratory manifestation of DIC, but only a small fraction of these patients suffer morbidity from the coagulation process or subsequent depletion of coagulation factors and consequent bleeding due to DIC. The initiating factor for DIC is apparent in some situations but unknown in others. Among the common initiators of DIC are the following:

- Thromboplastic substances in granules from promyelocytes of acute promyelocytic leukemia (DIC may worsen with therapy). There is a significant concomitant fibrinolysis in many patients.
- Sialic acid from mucin produced by adenocarcinomas of the lung or gastrointestinal tract.
- Trypsin released from pancreatic cancer.
- Impaired fibrinolysis associated with hepatocellular carcinoma.
- DIC in any patient may be fostered by sepsis or other causes of the systemic inflammatory response syndrome (SIRS).

Table 29.1. Laboratory diagnosis of disseminated intravascular coagulation (DIC)

Laboratory Tests	Acute DIC	Chronic DIC
Screening		
PT, aPTT	Usually prolonged	Normal
Platelets	Usually decreased	Normal or slightly decreased
Fibrinogen	Usually decreased but may be normal[a]	Usually normal[a]
Confirmatory[b]		
Fibrin monomer	Positive	Positive
FDP	Strongly positive	Positive
D-Dimer	Positive	Positive
Thrombin time	Normal or abnormal	Usually normal
Factor assays	Decreased factors V and VIII	Normal factors V and VIII
Antithrombin III	May be reduced	Usually normal

PT, prothrombin time; aPTT, activated partial thromboplastin time; FDP, fibrinogen degradation products.

[a]Fibrinogen is usually elevated in advanced malignancy or acute leukemia that is not complicated by DIC. Therefore, a normal fibrinogen level may actually be decreased for the physiologic state of the patient.

[b]Changes indicated are confirmatory if present; the absence of the indicated findings in some of the confirmatory tests does not exclude the diagnosis.

2. Lupus anticoagulant in neoplastic disease. The lupus anticoagulant is an antiphospholipid antibody (immunoglobulin G or M). Antiphospholipid antibodies are reported to be associated with a number of malignant disorders including hairy cell leukemia, lymphoma, Waldenström's macroglobulinemia, and epithelial neoplasms. The lupus anticoagulant leads to a prolonged activated partial thromboplastin time (aPTT) but is paradoxically associated with an increased risk of thrombosis.

3. Trousseau's syndrome (tumor-associated thrombophlebitis). The possibility of neoplasia should be suspected in the following circumstances:

- An unexplained thromboembolic event occurs after the age of 40 years.
- Thromboses occur in unusual sites.
- The thromboses affect superficial as well as deep veins.
- The thromboses are migratory.
- The thromboses tend not to respond to the "usual" anticoagulant therapies.
- An unexplained thrombosis occurs more than once.

4. Thrombotic events that occur after surgery for tumors of the lung, ovary, pancreas, or stomach.

5. Nonbacterial thrombotic endocarditis may be found in association with carcinoma of the lung. These thrombi are formed from accumulations of platelets and fibrin. The mitral valve is the most frequent site of origin of these thrombi, which frequently embolize.

6. Thrombotic thrombocytopenic purpura (TTP) is a poorly understood syndrome characterized by thrombocytopenia, microangiopathic hemolytic anemia, fever, fluctuating neurologic signs and symptoms, and acute renal failure. TTP and the hemolytic–uremic syndrome (thrombocytopenia, hemolysis, and acute renal failure) have been associated with untreated malignancies as well as with a number of drugs used for treating malignant disease. The agent most often reported is mitomycin, but other drugs including bleomycin, cisplatin, cyclophosphamide, gemcitabine, and vinca alkaloids may also be associated with these syndromes. TTP may be difficult to diagnose in this setting because the chemotherapy suppresses platelet production, some agents may impair renal function, and many of the features of TTP are similar to those of DIC. Careful review of the peripheral blood smear is required to identify the changes in red blood cells (RBCs) that are associated with a microangiopathic hemolytic process.

There is growing evidence that damage to the endothelium is seen in association with TTP. For many patients with TTP, von Willebrand–cleaving protease levels are very low or absent, leading to the presence of unusual ultralarge multimers of von Willebrand factor (vWF). The von Willebrand–cleaving proteolytic activity is thought to be inhibited by an anti–vWF-cleaving protease immunoglobulin G.

The prognosis of patients with TTP is poor, and its therapy has been varied. Plasmapheresis and transfusion with fresh frozen plasma (FFP) appear to be the best modalities of therapy. Plasmapheresis and FFP infusion replace the von Willebrand–cleaving protease that is missing in patients with TTP. In patients who are nonresponders to plasmapheresis or plasma transfusion, immunoadsorption of the patient's plasma by staphylococcal protein A columns has been used.

Complications from platelet transfusions are not as common in TTP associated with malignancy and bone marrow transplantation as in other cases of TTP; therefore, platelet transfusion can be used especially if there is a threat of bleeding.

7. **Thromboembolism associated with chemotherapy**
   a. The use of **central arterial or venous catheters** has markedly facilitated the delivery of chemotherapy, but all such catheters are associated with a significant risk of vascular thrombosis. The empiric use of low doses of warfarin (1 mg/day) decreases the risk of thrombosis without inducing a hemorrhagic state. It is not necessary to monitor the prothrombin time (PT) with low-dose warfarin.

   b. Many **chemotherapy agents** cause significant chemical phlebitis. The most common offending agents are mechlorethamine (nitrogen mustard), anthracyclines, nitrosoureas, mitomycin, fluorouracil, dacarbazine, and epipodophyllotoxins.

   c. **L-Asparaginase** inhibits the synthesis of proteins, including coagulation factors. This inhibition may cause either hemorrhage or thrombosis. Patients with preexisting hemostatic disorders are at particular risk for complications when using L-asparaginase. L-Asparaginase also decreases antithrombin III (AT-III) activity.

   d. **Tamoxifen** has been associated with thromboembolic events. This effect may be magnified when tamoxifen is combined with chemotherapeutic agents.

   e. **Thalidomide** and **lenolidomid** are associated with a high frequency of thromboembolism, particularly when used in combination with high dose steroids in the treatment of multiple myeloma.

   f. **Estrogens** may increase the risk of thromboembolism. This is likely due, at least in part, to a decrease in protein S and an increase in coagulation factors.

   g. **Superior vena cava syndrome** is nearly always associated with thrombosis in the thoracic venous system cephalad to the site of obstruction and may lead to upper-extremity thrombosis.

C. **Principles of therapy for thrombosis associated with neoplasia**
   1. **Discrete vascular thrombosis**
      a. **General guidelines.** Therapy should be directed at controlling the neoplasm. As an anticoagulant, heparin is superior to warfarin in these patients. Warfarin and antiplatelet drugs have been used with varying degrees of success in some patients with thromboembolism associated with tumors. The use of heparin, warfarin, and antiplatelet agents alone or in combination may be associated with normalization of hemostatic parameters.

Despite this, patients with malignant disease are often resistant to anticoagulant therapy and may continue to have thrombotic events even while receiving what appears to be adequate anticoagulant therapy. Great care must be exercised in the use of both heparin and warfarin in patients with malignant disease because hemorrhage into areas of necrotic tumor can be hazardous. The use of anticoagulant therapy is generally contraindicated in patients with central nervous system metastases. Bulky disease is a relative contraindication, especially if central necrosis of the tumor is suspected and particularly if the lesion is in the mediastinum or pleural spaces.

The decision to treat thromboembolism occurring in a patient with malignancy may be difficult. One must carefully weigh the risks of therapy against expected benefits. The patient's life expectancy, concurrent therapy, and type of malignancy also influence the decision.

b. Heparin. Low doses of heparin (5,000 U given SC every 12 hours) can be used to protect patients with malignant disease from thromboembolism during perioperative periods. Heparin may be used as the initial or long-term therapy for thromboembolic events in patients with malignant disease. Heparin may be administered either IV or by the SC route. Generally, the IV route is preferred for initial therapy so that the anticoagulant effect begins at once and adjustment of doses can be easily achieved. An initial dose of 5,000 U (70 U/kg) of heparin is given as an IV bolus followed by 1,000 to 1,200 U (15 U/kg)/hour as a continuous infusion. One should check the aPTT 1 hour after the heparin bolus to ensure that the patient is heparinizable (i.e., not AT-III deficient), 6 hours after beginning therapy, and 6 hours after any change in the dose of heparin. Some patients with malignant disease may appear to be refractory to heparin; in all likelihood, this reflects low levels of AT-III, owing to poor production or increased consumption, both of which may occur in patients with malignant disease. (*Note*: infusion therapy with L-asparaginase has been associated with reduced levels of AT-III.) As long as the AT-III activity is above 50% of normal, it is usually possible to achieve the desired anticoagulant effect if adequate doses of heparin are given. If AT-III activity is less than 50% of normal, AT-III may be replaced using AT-III concentrates or FFP.

Heparin may be administered by the SC route for both acute and chronic management of thromboembolism associated with malignancy. Using the SC route may be less desirable when treating acute events because the onset of anticoagulant effect is somewhat slower (2–3 hours), and adjusting the therapeutic effect may be more difficult. SC heparin can be considered for chronic therapy, provided that the patient can manage the twice-daily injection and weekly monitoring of the aPTT. In a patient who has been receiving IV heparin, half the total dose of IV heparin received in the previous 24 hours should be given SC twice a day (e.g., 1,000 U/hour by IV infusion equals an SC dose of 12,000 U b.i.d.). For the patient being started on SC heparin, the initial dose is 7,500 to 10,000 U SC, b.i.d. The aPTT should be checked 6 hours after the third dose of heparin. Otherwise, the aPTT should be checked 6 hours after an SC dose of heparin. The goal for the aPTT should be similar to that of IV heparin, namely, 1.5 to 2 times the patient's baseline aPTT.

Low molecular weight (LMW) heparin(s) can be used for thromboembolism and for primary prevention. The selection of drug and its dosing schedule should be made by the treating physician. If monitoring of the drug is indicated owing to liver or kidney dysfunction in the patient, one must use anti-Xa levels as the aPTT is not indicative of the anticoagulant effect of LMW heparins.

c. Warfarin is often selected as the therapy of choice for the chronic management of thromboembolic events associated with malignant disease. The use of warfarin in this setting is of concern because patients with malignant disease are frequently taking multiple medications that can alter the patient's response to warfarin. An additional concern about the use of warfarin in patients with malignancy is the development of purpura fulminans. This complication may be due to lower-than-normal protein C levels in patients who had DIC before initiation of warfarin therapy. Warfarin should not be used if there is laboratory evidence of DIC.

Despite these caveats, warfarin is often used for the prevention and treatment of clotting problems in patients with cancer. For most patients, an international normalized ratio (INR) of 2 to 3 is required; for patients with mechanical prosthetic valves, recurrent systemic embolism, or lupus anticoagulant with thrombosis, an INR of 2.5 to 3.5 is necessary (Table 29.2). Table 29.3

Table 29.2.   Clinical indications and international normalized ratio (INR) goals: using the INR for anticoagulation monitoring

A. Clinical indications requiring an INR of 2.0–3.0

Prophylaxis of venous thrombosis (high-risk surgery)

Treatment of venous thrombosis

Treatment of pulmonary embolism

Prevention of systemic embolism

Tissue heart valves

Valvular heart disease

Atrial fibrillation

Recurrent systemic embolism

Cardiomyopathy

B. Clinical indications requiring an INR of 2.5–3.5

Mechanical prosthetic valves (high risk)

Acute myocardial infarction

Table 29.3.   Vitamin K₁ administration for patients on warfarin doses of vitamin K₁ to reduce INR in patients on warfarin

INR	Vitamin K₁ Dosage (slow IVP)[a]	Time Expected for Response to Vitamin K or to Repeat INR
>3.5 but <5	None, hold warfarin	24 h
≥5 but <9.0 (no significant bleeding)	Omit one or two doses, monitor closely and resume at a lower dose *or* Give 0.5–1.0 mg; may repeat dosage if INR is still high at 24 h	Reduction of INR expected at 8 h; therapeutic INR expected at 24–48 h
≥9.0 (no significant bleeding)	3–5 mg; may repeat dosage if INR is still high at 6–12 h	Reductions of INR expected at 6 h; repeat INR every 6–12 h
(significant bleeding)	Vitamin K 10 mg IV slowly and fresh frozen plasma or prothrombin complex if situation is urgent Hold warfarin	
(life-threatening bleeding)	Give prothrombin complex or recombinant factor VIIa	

[a] If patient is bleeding, a procedure is planned, or patient has just had a procedure, consider the use of fresh frozen plasma or prothrombin complex.
Modified from Ansell J, Hrish J, Poller L, et al. The pharmacology and management of oral vitamin K antagonists. *Chest* 2004;126:204S–233S

also gives the recommended vitamin K dose necessary to reduce the INR to therapeutic levels in patients who are taking warfarin and have INR values higher than 5. Care must be taken to balance the risks of bleeding in patients with elevated INRs—with or without thrombocytopenia—against the risks of clotting and thrombosis if the reversal of anticoagulation is too vigorous.

d. The use of platelet-inhibiting drugs such as aspirin, other nonsteroidal anti-inflammatory agents, and dipyridamole has met with varying degrees of success in the prevention of repeated thromboembolic events in patients with malignant disease. Care must be taken with the use of such drugs, especially in thrombocytopenic patients, because the risk of bleeding associated with thrombocytopenia is increased.

e. Fibrinolytic therapy. Systemic malignancy is a relative contraindication to fibrinolytic therapy.

f. Vascular interruption devices such as inferior vena caval filters may be used in patients who cannot tolerate anticoagulant therapy or who develop emboli while on adequate anticoagulant therapy.

2. Disseminated intravascular coagulation. Therapy for DIC includes the following:

- Correct shock urgently (if present).
- Treat the underlying disease process; when it is not possible to treat the underlying disease process it is unlikely that the complicating DIC can be successfully managed.
- Replace depleted blood components (e.g., platelets, cryoprecipitated antihemophilic factor [AHF] for fibrinogen and factor VIII, FFP for other factors) if clinically significant bleeding is present.
- Consider the use of heparin only in the following situations:
  — In patients with acute promyelocytic leukemia (see Chapter 19)
  — When there is clear evidence of ongoing end-organ damage due to microvascular thrombosis
  — If venous thrombosis occurs

The latter two complications of DIC are most likely to occur as a component of the SIRS, and the treatment of the underlying cause of the SIRS is necessary in addition to treatment with heparin. There is no evidence that chronic warfarin therapy is of value for treating the chronic DIC seen in some patients with neoplasia if thromboses are absent. Warfarin may predispose to the development of purpura fulminans in the presence of chronic DIC due to acquired protein C deficiency.

II. Bleeding in patients with cancer

A. Tumor invasion. It is well recognized that bleeding may be a warning sign of cancer. Bloody sputum may indicate carcinoma of the lung, blood in the urine may be a sign of carcinoma of the bladder or kidney, blood in the stool may be due to carcinoma of the alimentary tract, and postmenopausal vaginal bleeding may be caused by endometrial carcinoma. In each of these instances, bleeding can be directly related to the invasive properties of cancer and disruption of normal tissue integrity.

B. Hemostatic abnormalities. Often bleeding in patients with cancer is not due to the direct effects of the neoplasm but rather due to indirect effects of the cancer or its therapy on one of the components of the hemostatic system. Because of the special management problems caused by abnormalities in the hemostatic system in patients with cancer and the frequency with which these problems occur, it is important to consider the possible causes and corrective measures in detail.

1. Increased vascular fragility may be due to chronic corticosteroid therapy, chronic malnutrition, or "senile purpura." Bleeding is usually not severe, but bruising, particularly around IV sites, is common. Hemostatic therapy is not necessary.

2. Thrombocytopenia may occur for a variety of reasons. Some of the more common causes are as follows:

a. Chemotherapy and radiotherapy regularly cause depression of platelet production. Serial blood cell counts must be monitored while patients are being treated.

b. Bone marrow invasion or replacement causing thrombocytopenia is commonly seen only with leukemias or lymphomas but may occur in other cancers that invade the bone marrow.

c. Splenomegaly with splenic sequestration is most common with leukemia or lymphoma.

d. Folate deficiency with decreased platelet production is common in patients with cancer because of poor nutrition. Dietary history should provide the clues to the diagnosis.

e. Neoplasm-induced immune thrombocytopenic purpura. Patients with lymphoproliferative malignancies (e.g., chronic lymphocytic leukemia, Hodgkin's disease) often develop immune thrombocytopenic purpura (ITP). ITP may also be the presenting symptom of a nonhematologic malignancy. Usually, the ITP improves with prednisone 1 mg/kg/day followed by treatment of the malignancy.

f. Drug-induced immune thrombocytopenia. Many nonchemotherapy medications used to treat patients with malignancy can cause immune thrombocytopenia. Offending agents to consider are heparin, vancomycin, H_2-receptor antagonists, penicillins, cephalosporins, interferon, and sulfa-containing antibiotics, diuretics, and hypoglycemic agents.

g. Graft-versus-host disease developed after bone marrow transplantation may produce a chronic (often isolated) immune-mediated thrombocytopenia. The platelet count may respond to increased immunosuppression.

3. Abnormalities of platelet function must be suspected in patients who have a normal or near-normal platelet count but signs or symptoms of bleeding and a documented prolonged bleeding time. Most cases are secondary to drug effects including aspirin and other non-steroidal anti-inflammatory agents, antibiotics (e.g., ticarcillin), antidepressants (e.g., tricyclic drugs), tranquilizers, and alcohol. Consider any drug that the patient is taking as a possible offender until proved otherwise. The presence of fibrin degradation products is a common cause of platelet dysfunction in patients with malignancy who also have DIC. Platelet dysfunction may occur in patients with malignant paraproteinemias as a result of the coating of platelet surfaces by the immunoglobulin. When renal failure develops or is present in such patients, the platelet dysfunction is magnified.

4. Coagulation factor deficiencies may develop in patients with malignancy for several reasons:

- Acute (decompensated) DIC depletes most clotting factors but to variable degrees.
- Liver failure causes deficiency of all clotting factors except factor VIII.
- Malnutrition leads to deficiency of factors II, VII, IX, and X (the vitamin K–dependent factors).
- Fibrinolysis may be due to the release of urokinase in prostate cancer or secondary to DIC. This may produce

hypofibrinogenemia as well as fibrin split products, which act as circulating anticoagulants.

- Functionally abnormal clotting factors are occasionally seen. The most commonly diagnosed abnormality is dysfibrinogenemia.

5. Acquired circulating anticoagulants may develop in patients with a number of different tumors. Many of these anticoagulants are heparinoid in nature. The most common associations are with carcinoma of the lung and myeloma. Other anticoagulants act as antithrombins; in this case, the most common association is with carcinoma of the breast.

6. Chemotherapy and other drug-induced bleeding

Mithramycin, although rarely used now, may lead to platelet dysfunction and a reduction in multiple coagulation factors. Hemorrhage due to these effects may occur in up to half the number of patients treated with mithramycin.

Anthracyclines may be associated with primary fibrinolysis or fibrinogenolysis and hemorrhage.

Dactinomycin is a powerful vitamin K antagonist that causes defective synthesis of all vitamin K–dependent proteins (factors II, VII, IX, and X, protein C, and protein S).

Melphalan, cytarabine, doxorubicin, vincristine, and **vinblastine** are all associated with platelet dysfunction.

Mitomycin, daunorubicin, cytarabine, bleomycin, CDDP, methyl-CCNU, tamoxifen, deoxycoformycin, gemcitabine, atorvastatin, clopidogrel, ticlopidine, cyclosporine, sulfonamides, tacrolimus, sirolimus, "crack" cocaine, penicillin, rifampin, penicillamine, oral contraceptives, arsenic, quinine, and **iodine** are all associated with TTP.

III. Laboratory evaluation of hemostasis in patients with malignancy. About half of all patients with cancer and approximately 90% of those with metastases manifest abnormalities of one or more routine coagulation parameters (Table 29.4). These abnormalities may be minor early in the patient's disease, but as the disease progresses, the hemostatic abnormalities become more pronounced. Serial coagulation tests may offer the clinician a clue to response to therapy or recurrence of malignant disease. Serial evaluations of coagulation tests are of more value in patients with no symptoms of hemostatic disruption than is a single determination.

A. Screening tests for bleeding. The following tests provide an adequate screening battery: **platelet count, bleeding time or whole blood platelet function screening testing, aPTT, PT, thrombin time,** and **fibrinogen level.**

B. Interpretation of screening laboratory studies. Abnormal results of the screening tests reflect hematologic problems caused by blood vessels, platelets, or coagulation factors. The following list provides clues to the interpretation of the screening test results that help determine the most likely cause or causes of the patient's bleeding.

Table 29.4. Coagulation tests that may show an abnormality in patients with cancer without clinical bleeding or thrombosis

Test	Common Results in Patients with Malignancy
Antithrombin III	Decreased
β-Thromboglobulin	Increased
Cryofibrinogen	Present
D-Dimer	Increased
Factor VIII	Increased
Fibronectin	Decreased
Fibrin monomer (soluble)	Present
Fibrinogen	Increased
Fibrin(ogen) degradation products	Present
Fibrinopeptide A	Increased
Fibrinopeptide B	Increased
Plasmin	Increased
Plasminogen	Decreased
Platelet count	Increased or decreased
Platelet factor 4	Increased
Protein C	Decreased

1. **Platelet count**
   Normal: 150,000 to 450,000/μL.
   If **thrombocytopenia** is less than 100,000/μL, consider the following:

- Bone marrow failure
- Increased consumption of platelets
- Splenic pooling of platelets

   Thrombocytosis with a platelet count of more than 500,000/μL has the following characteristics:

- It is common in patients with neoplasms.
- It may be seen in association with iron deficiency (e.g., secondary to gut neoplasm).
- It usually poses no risk of arterial thrombosis unless the patient has a myeloproliferative disorder.

2. **Bleeding time.** This is a useful screening test if the platelet count is normal and platelet dysfunction is suspected.

- A normal bleeding time requires normal platelet number, normal platelet function, and normal function of the blood vessels and connective tissues.
- A prolonged bleeding time may be due to thrombocytopenia, abnormal platelet function, and, rarely, inadequate vessel function. The bleeding time may be spuriously prolonged in elderly people with "tissue-paper" skin.
- The following formula is a rough rule of thumb to be used to estimate what the bleeding time should be in

patients who have platelet counts between 10,000 and 100,000/μL. Although it was derived using the Mielke template, the principle should still hold for contemporary bleeding time devices: bleeding time (minutes) =30−([platelet count/μL]/4,000).

Whole blood platelet function screening is replacing bleeding time tests in many laboratories. This method of screening for platelet function abnormalities appears to be a better predictor for the risk of bleeding due to platelet function abnormalities than the bleeding time.

3. Prolonged prothrombin time. This is seen in the presence of the following:

- Deficiency of one or more of the following clotting factors: VII, X, V, II (prothrombin), or I (fibrinogen); oral anticoagulant therapy leads to a deficiency of factors II, VII, IX, and X
- Circulating anticoagulants against factor VII, X, V, or II
- Dysfibrinogenemia

4. Prolonged activated partial thromboplastin time

- Deficiency of any of the following clotting factors: XII, XI, IX, VIII, X, V, II, or I. Factor XII deficiency is not associated with bleeding. Fletcher and Fitzgerald factor deficiencies (both rare) may also prolong the aPTT.
- Circulating anticoagulants directed against the factors mentioned earlier or the lupus inhibitor.
- Anticoagulant therapy with heparin or oral anticoagulants.

5. Prolonged thrombin time. Prolongation of the thrombin time may be due to the following:

- Hypofibrinogenemia (fibrinogen <100 mg/dL)
- Some forms of dysfibrinogenemia
- Fibrin–fibrinogen split products
- Heparin therapy
- Paraproteins

If the thrombin time is prolonged, further studies to clarify the cause may be required.

6. Low fibrinogen level. When evaluating the results of a fibrinogen assay, one must be familiar with the assay method used. Many laboratories use immunologic assays, which measure both functionally normal and abnormal fibrinogens. If such an assay is in use, the thrombin time can be used to evaluate the functional integrity of the fibrinogen. A low functional fibrinogen level means that production is decreased, consumption is increased, or a dysfibrinogen is present. Fibrinogen is an acute-phase reactant and is often elevated with advanced malignancy. A fibrinogen level in the normal range may actually be relatively low for the patient's physiologic state and therefore may be a sign of DIC (see Table 29.1).

C. Laboratory findings in patients with disseminated intravascular coagulation. Acute DIC is often associated with significant hemorrhage, whereas chronic DIC may be asymptomatic or associated with thromboses. Screening and confirmatory laboratory tests are shown in Table 29.1.

D. Review of peripheral smear for schistocytes and decrease numbers of platelets if TTP suspected.

IV. **Treatment of hemorrhagic syndromes in patients with malignant disease**

A. **Transfusion therapy**

1. **General guidelines**

a. **Regard elective transfusion with allogeneic blood as an outcome to be avoided.** Consider the factors that will influence the use of blood products, including the following:

- Alternative forms of therapy that could control bleeding (e.g., topical measures or desmopressin).
- *How symptomatic is the patient?* Do not treat for an abnormal laboratory test in a symptom-free patient. For example, patients with chronic DIC may demonstrate prolongation of both the PT and the aPTT and mild to moderate thrombocytopenia. If there is no demonstrable bleeding, transfusion therapy is not necessary.

b. **Use the specific blood component needed by the patient.**

c. **Minimize complications** of transfusion by using the following:

- Only the amount and type of blood product indicated for the patient in the specific clinical setting
- Leukoreduced blood products, irradiated blood, or both, when indicated

2. **Blood component therapy**

a. **Platelet transfusions**

(1) **Available forms of platelets for transfusion.** Platelets may be ordered and transfused in various ways. Because most patients with an underlying malignancy have the potential for needing long-term platelet support, platelet products should be leukocyte reduced from the initiation of transfusion (see Section IV.A.3. in the subsequent text). In general, patients who need platelet support can be started with whole blood–derived platelets. Given the added expense and the limited number of platelet apheresis donors in many centers, single donor and human leukocyte antigen (HLA)–matched platelets should be reserved for patients who have become refractory to whole blood derived platelets (see Section IV.A.2.a. (4) in the subsequent text). There are no solid data to suggest that starting with platelet apheresis products decreases the incidence of alloimmunization. In fact, the Trial to Reduce Alloimmunization to Platelets Study Group study (1997) did not show any benefit in the use of platelet apheresis products over whole blood–derived platelets. Conversely, patients who are candidates for bone marrow transplantation should receive single-donor platelets (if available) from the initiation of platelet therapy. Many blood centers have geared up production of platelet apheresis, and this product may be more

readily available in some places than in others. Patients who are candidates for transplantation with bone marrow from an HLA-matched sibling should not receive apheresis products from the potential donor before the transplantation.

(a) **Whole blood–derived platelets (Random-donor platelets or platelet concentrates).** Four to 6 U (usually pooled in one bag) are considered an adequate dose for a 70-kg adult.

(b) **Platelets obtained by apheresis (single-donor platelets) and HLA-matched platelets obtained by apheresis.** These come as a single pack and represent the platelets obtained by apheresis from a single donor. One unit of platelets obtained by apheresis is equivalent to 4 to 6 U of platelet concentrate.

(2) **Check platelet count** 10 minutes to 1 hour, and then 24 hours after platelet transfusion to estimate survival of platelets in the patient. Each unit of platelet concentrate should increase the platelet count by approximately 7,000/μL. The expected 1-hour posttransfusion rise in platelets is 15,000 platelets/μL divided by the patient's body surface area in square meters for each unit of platelet concentrate (Therefore, for a person of 2 m^2, 6 U should produce a rise of 45,000/μL [6 × 15,000/2]).

(3) **Criteria for transfusing platelets**

(a) For patients with **reduced platelet production,** criteria for transfusion are shown in Table 29.5.

(b) **Increased platelet destruction.** Platelet transfusions are of limited benefit in patients with thrombocytopenia due to increased destruction as a result of either antibodies or consumption. If potentially life-threatening bleeding complicates thrombocytopenia due to increased destruction, platelet transfusions may be given; however, only small increments in the platelet count usually occur. γ-Globulin 1 g/kg IV daily × 2 days given before the platelet transfusions might improve the response.

(c) **Dysfunctional platelets.** One must stop any drugs known to cause platelet dysfunction. Although the use of platelet transfusions should be considered, pharmacologic methods of enhancing platelet function, such as desmopressin, should be used if possible (see Section IV.B.1.).

(4) **Refractoriness to platelet transfusions** rise of <5,000/μL after 5 to 6 U of platelet concentrates or 1 U of platelets obtained by apheresis on two separate occasions) is a common problem in multiply transfused patients. Alloimmunization is the most difficult form to treat and is therefore best prevented (see Section IV.A.3). Apparent refractoriness to platelets may be due to shortened platelet lifespan

Table 29.5. Guidelines for platelet transfusion in patients with reduced platelet production

Platelet Count	Recommendation
0–5,000/μL	Transfuse with platelets even if there is no evidence of bleeding
6,000–10,000/μL	Transfuse with platelets in the presence of the following:
	Fresh minor hemorrhage
	Temperature of 38°C or active infection
	Rapid decline in platelet count (>50%/day)
	Headache
	Significant gastrointestinal blood loss
	Recent chemotherapy that may be expected to cause severe stomatitis or gastrointestinal ulceration
	Presence of confluent petechiae (as opposed to scattered petechiae)
	Continuous bleeding from a wound or other sites
	Planned minor procedure such as a bone marrow biopsy
11,000–20,000/μL	Transfuse with platelets if there is more rapid bleeding or if more complicated procedures are anticipated
>20,000/μL	If major surgery is planned or when life-threatening bleeding occurs, the platelet count should be increased to at least 50,000/μL
	For intracranial surgery or opthalmic surgery, transfuse to a platelet count of at least 100,000/μL (bleeding time must be checked before surgery and must be normal)
	In fully anticoagulated patients, it is advisable to keep the platelet count at least at 50,000/ mL.

from fever, septicemia, DIC, splenomegaly, drugs, infections, or bleeding.

(a) Evaluation. Patients who become refractory to platelet transfusions should have a laboratory evaluation for alloimmunization. They should also be evaluated for infection and DIC. Further, all potentially offending medications should be stopped.

(b) Therapy. The therapeutic modalities for ITP (corticosteroids, IV globulin, danazol) are generally ineffective for platelet refractoriness due to alloimmunization. Two therapeutic options exist:

(i) Human leukocyte antigen (HLA)–matched platelets

(ii) Cross-matched platelets. Because platelets are available at most blood centers, if a blood center performs cross-matching, it is often easier to obtain cross-matched platelets since no specific donor qualification is required. This product is as effective as HLA-matched platelets in producing a platelet response in the alloimmunized patient. Either platelet concentrates or apheresed platelets can be cross-matched with the recipient. Nonreactive or, in extenuating circumstances, the least reactive platelets can then be selected for transfusion.

b. **Coagulation factor support**

(1) **Fresh frozen plasma** (FFP) contains all clotting factors (but not platelets) and should be used for multiple coagulation factor deficiencies. FFP requires 20 to 30 minutes to thaw and must be thawed at 37°C. Once thawed, FFP must be transfused within 5 days of thawing as long as it is maintained at 1°C to 6°C.

(2) **Plasma frozen within 24 hours of phlebotomy is often used interchangeably with FFP.**

(3) **Cryoprecipitated antihemophilic factor** is a source of factor VIII–vWF complex, fibrinogen, and factor XIII. Each bag of cryoprecipitated AHF contains approximately 50% of the factor VIII–vWF complex (minimum of 80 U) and 20% to 40% of the fibrinogen (minimum of 150 mg) harvested from 1 U of blood. Cryoprecipitated AHF is stored in a frozen state and has the advantage of concentrating the clotting factors in a small volume (10 to 15 mL/bag). It is used primarily in deficiencies of fibrinogen. The goal is to keep the fibrinogen level higher than 100 mg/dL. The usual dosage of cryoprecipitated AHF to correct hypofibrinogenemia is one bag of cryoprecipitated AHF for every 5 kg body weight. Because 50% is recovered after transfusion, this may raise the fibrinogen level only by approximately 50 mg/dL. Larger doses may be needed for severe hypofibrinogenemia or "flaming" DIC. The patient is evaluated to determine if the laboratory values have been corrected.

(4) **Factor IX concentrates** are available as factor IX complex concentrates, which contain factors II, VII, IX, and X, or as coagulation factor IX concentrates. The latter are highly purified factor IX concentrates with few or no other coagulation factors. Several precautions are worth noting regarding the factor IX concentrates:

(a) This concentrate is made from pooled plasma but is treated with viral attenuation processes such (i) dry or vapor heat in the case of factor IX complex concentrates (therefore the risk is significant) or (ii) solvent-detergent or monoclonal antibody in the case of coagulation factor IX concentrates. The dose depends on the preparation to be used. The goal is to bring the factor concentration to no more than 50% of normal.

(b) There is a small risk of DIC resulting from the use of factor IX complex concentrates. Patients with liver dysfunction and newborns are at increased risk. The coagulation factor concentrates are far less thrombogenic and should be used in cases at increased risk for venous thrombosis or DIC.

(c) Factor IX concentrates are stored in the lyophilized state. Do not shake when reconstituting.

3. **Leukocyte reduction.** Patients who have not previously received transfusions and who will need long-term blood product support should receive leukocyte-reduced ($<5 \times 10^6$ leukocytes/bag) blood products. Leukocyte reduction may prevent febrile transfusion reactions, prevent cytomegalovirus (CMV) infections, and delay alloimmunization. Controversy still exists as to whether tumor recurrence and infections are a result of immunomodulatory effects of blood transfusion and if they can be reduced by leukoreduction. Two methods of leukocyte reduction by filtration are currently available: bedside and prestorage.

a. Bedside filtration involves leukocyte reduction at the time of transfusion. Disadvantages include plugging of the filter, the presence of leukocyte breakdown products, bag breakage, and lack of consistency of products. Filters are available for RBCs and platelets.

b. AS-1 or AS-3 prestorage filtered red blood cells are RBCs that have been leukocyte reduced generally within 8 to 24 hours of collection. Advantages are fewer leukocyte breakdown products, ease of administration, and consistent quality (guaranteed less than 5×10^6 leukocytes/bag). Cost may be perceived as a disadvantage. However, this is offset by the expense of stocking filters, training of staff in the use of filters, and breakage. There is ongoing controversy as to whether leukocyte-reduced blood products should be provided to all patients, not just patients at risk.

4. **Cytomegalovirus-negative blood.** Only patients known to be anti-CMV negative with impaired immunity should be considered for the use of CMV-negative blood. This group includes children, for the most part. The use of CMV-negative blood seriously restricts the potential donor pool for these patients. Leukocyte-reduced blood products (less than 5.0×10^6/bag) are, in general, equivalent to CMV-negative screened products and both are considered "CMV-reduced risk" products.

White blood cell (WBC) depletion filters also remove CMV since it resides in the WBCs. Irradiation of blood products does not render them CMV-free. Frozen deglycerolized blood is considered free of CMV contamination.

5. **Irradiated blood products.** These prevent the development of graft-versus-host disease. Irradiated blood

products, in the case of patients with cancer or hematologic malignancies, are indicated in the following situations:

- Congenital immunodeficiency
- Bone marrow, peripheral blood stem cell, or umbilical cord stem cell transplantation
- Directed blood donations to blood relatives
- HLA-matched or cross-matched platelets
- Granulocyte transfusions
- High-dose chemotherapy with growth factor or stem cell rescue
- Hodgkin's lymphoma
- Leukemia and non–Hodgkin's lymphoma (relative indication)
- Fludarabine treatment

B. **Other forms of therapy**

1. **Desmopressin.** Desmopressin 0.3 μg/kg IV over 30 minutes every 12 to 24 hours for 2 to 4 days may be used to elevate factor VIII and vWF levels as well as to improve platelet function. Tachyphylaxis may occur if therapy is continued for longer periods. Intranasal desmopressin 0.25 mL b.i.d. using a solution containing 1.3 mg/mL has been given for minor bleeding episodes.

2. **Fibrin glue.** This is a topical biologic adhesive. Its effects imitate the final stages of coagulation. The glue consists of a solution of concentrated human fibrinogen, which is activated by the addition of bovine thrombin and calcium chloride. The resulting clot promotes hemostasis and tissue sealing. The clot is completely absorbed during the healing process. The best adhesive and hemostatic effect is obtained by applying the two solutions simultaneously to the open wound surface. Fibrin glue has been used primarily in surgical settings. It has been most effective when used for surface, low-pressure bleeding. There is a small risk of anaphylactic reaction because of the bovine origin of the thrombin.

3. **Antifibrinolytic agents.** ε-Aminocaproic acid (EACA) and tranexamic acid have been used to control bleeding associated with primary fibrinolysis as seen in patients with prostatic carcinoma and in a small number of patients with refractory thrombocytopenia. Great care must be taken in the use of these agents because of a possible increased risk of thrombosis. EACA may be used topically to control small-area, small-volume bleeding.

4. **Oprelvekin (interleukin-11).** Oprelvekin has recently been approved by the U.S. Food and Drug Administration for the treatment and prevention of chemotherapy-related thrombocytopenia. Oprelvekin is a thrombopoietic growth factor that directly stimulates the proliferation of hematopoietic stem cells and megakaryocyte progenitor cells as well as megakaryocyte maturation, resulting in increased platelet production. It may cause substantial fluid retention and should be used with caution in patients who have congestive heart failure (CHF), those with a history of CHF, and those being treated for CHF. One must also

be cautious in using this agent in patients who are receiving diuretic therapy or ifosfamide because sudden deaths have been reported as a result of severe hypokalemia. Oprelvekin should be used to prevent thrombocytopenia, which would be severe enough to require platelet transfusions. Therapy usually begins 6 to 24 hours after the completion of chemotherapy, and patients should be monitored for any signs or symptoms of allergic reactions or cardiac dysfunction.

SUGGESTED READINGS

Anand SS, Wells PS, Hunt D, et al. Does this patient have deep vein thrombosis? *JAMA* 1998;279:1094–1099.

Baker WF Jr. Thrombosis and hemostasis in cardiology: review of pathophysiology and clinical practice. II. Recommendations for anti-thrombotic therapy. *Clin Appl Thromb Hemost* 1998;4:143– 147.

Bauer KA, ten Cate H, Barzegar S, et al. Tumor necrosis factor infusions have a pro-coagulant effect on the hemostatic mechanism of humans. *Blood* 1989;74:165.

Bern MM, Lokich JJ, Wallach SR, et al. Very low doses of warfarin can prevent thrombosis in central venous catheters: a randomized prospective trial. *Ann Intern Med* 1990;112:423.

Beutler E. Platelet transfusions: the 20,000/µl trigger. *Blood* 1993; 81:1411–1413.

Brennan M. Fibrin glue. *Blood Rev* 1991;5:240.

College of American Pathologists Task Force. Practice parameter for the use of fresh-frozen plasma, cryoprecipitate, and platelets. *JAMA* 1994;271:777–781.

Dzik S. Leukodepletion blood filters: filter design and mechanisms of leukocyte removal. *Transfus Med Rev* 1993;7:65.

Dzik WH. Leukoreduced blood components, laboratory and clinical aspects. In: Rossi EC, Simon TL, Moss GS, et al., eds. *Principles of transfusion medicine*, 2nd ed. Baltimore: Williams & Wilkins, 1996:353–373.

Esparaz B, Kies M, Kwaan H. Thromboembolism in cancer. In: Kwaan HC, Samama MM, eds. *Clinical thrombosis*. Boca Raton: CRC Press, 1989:317–333.

Friedberg RC. Clinical and laboratory factors underlying refractoriness to platelet transfusions. *J Clin Apheresis* 1996;11:143– 148.

Gelb AB, Leavitt AD. Crossmatch compatible platelets improve corrected count increments in patients who are refractory to randomly selected patients. *Transfusion* 1997;37:624–630.

Ginsberg JS. Management of venous thromboembolism. *N Engl J Med* 1996;335:1816–1828.

Griffin MR, Stanson AW, Brown ML, et al. Deep venous thrombosis and pulmonary embolism: risk of subsequent malignant neoplasms. *Arch Intern Med* 1987;147:1907–1911.

Hillyer CD, Emmens RK, Zago-Novaretti M, et al. Methods for the reduction of transfusion transmitted cytomegalovirus infection: filtration versus the use of seronegative donor units. *Transfusion* 1994;34:929–934.

Hirsh J, Dalen JE, Deykin D, et al. Oral anticoagulants. Mechanism of action, clinical effectiveness, and optimal therapeutic range. *Chest* 1992;102(suppl):312.

Hull RD, Pineo GF. Prophylaxis of deep vein thrombosis and pulmonary embolism: current recommendations. *Clin Appl Thromb Hemost* 1998;4:96–104.

Humphries JE. Transfusion therapy in acquired coagulopathies. *Hematol Oncol Clin North Am* 1994;8:1181–1201.

Kunkel LA. Acquired circulating anticoagulants in malignancy. *Semin Thromb Hemost* 1992;18:416–423.

Lane TA. Leukocyte reduction of cellular blood component: effectiveness, benefits, quality control and costs. *Arch Pathol Lab Med* 1994;118:392–404.

Legler TJ, Fischer I, Dittman J, et al. Frequency and course of refractoriness in multiply transfused patients. *Ann Hematol* 1997;74:185–189.

Mannucci DM. Desmopressin: a non-traditional form of treatment for congenital and acquired bleeding disorders. *Blood* 1988;72:1449–1455.

McCarthy PM. Fibrin glue in cardiothoracic surgery. *Transfus Med Rev* 1993;7:173–179.

Murgo A. Thrombotic microangiopathy in the cancer patient including those induced by chemotherapy agents. *Semin Hematol* 1987;24:161–177.

O'Connell B, Lee EJ, Schiffer CA. The value of 10 min posttransfusion platelet counts. *Transfusion* 1988;28:66–67.

Pisciotto PT, Benson K, Hume H, et al. Prophylactic versus therapeutic platelet transfusion practices in hematology and/or oncology patients. *Transfusion* 1995;35:498–502.

Poon M. Cryoprecipitate: uses and alternatives. *Transfus Med Rev* 1993;7:180–192.

Przepiorka D, LeParc GF, Stovall MA, et al. Use of irradiated blood components: practice parameter. *Am J Clin Pathol* 1996;106:6–11.

Przepiorka D, LeParc GF, Werch J, et al. Prevention of transfusion associated CMV infection: practice parameter. *Am J Clin Pathol* 1996;106:163–169.

Schafer A. The hypercoagulable state. *Ann Intern Med* 1985;102:814–828.

Schiffer CA, Anderson KC, Bennett CL. Platelet transfusion for patients with cancer: clinical practice guidelines of the American Society of Clinical Oncology. *J Clin Oncol* 2001;19:1519–1538.

Slichter SJ. Algorithm for managing the platelet refractory patient. *J Clin Apheresis* 1997;2:4–9.

Sorenson HT, Mellemkjaer L, Steffensen FH, et al. The risk of the diagnosis of cancer after primary deep venous thrombosis or pulmonary embolism. *N Engl J Med* 1998;338:1169–1173.

Tefferi A, Silverstein MN, Hoagland HC. Primary thrombocythemia. *Semin Oncol* 1995;22:334–340.

Trial to Reduce Alloimmunization to Platelets Study Group. Leukocyte reduction and ultraviolet B irradiation of platelets to prevent alloimmunization and refractoriness to platelet transfusions. *N Engl J Med* 1997;337:1861–1869.

CHAPTER 30

Oncology Emergencies and Critical Care Issues—Anaphylaxis, Spinal Cord Compression, Cerebral Edema, Superior Vena Cava Syndrome, Hypercalcemia, Tumor Lysis Syndrome, and Respiratory Failure

Roland T. Skeel

Spinal cord compression, cerebral edema, superior vena cava syndrome (SVCS), anaphylaxis, respiratory failure, tumor lysis syndrome, and bone metastasis can be major causes of morbidity and, in some cases, potential mortality in patients with cancer. Because of the critical nature of these complications of cancer and its treatment, oncologists, oncology nurses, and other oncology health professionals must be prepared to recognize the signs and symptoms of these disorders promptly, so that appropriate therapy can be instituted without delay.

I. Spinal cord compression

A. Tumors. The most common tumors resulting in spinal cord compression are breast cancer, lung cancer, prostate cancer, and renal cancer, although it may also occur with sarcoma, multiple myeloma, and lymphoma. Purely intradural or epidural lesions are uncommon because more than three-fourths of cases arise from either metastasis to a vertebral body or other bony parts of the vertebra or, less commonly, direct extension from a paravertebral soft tissue mass. Seventy percent of the bone lesions are osteolytic, 10% osteoblastic, and 20% mixed. More than 85% of patients with metastases to the vertebra have lesions that involve more than one vertebral body.

B. Symptoms and signs. The most common early symptoms seen in patients with spinal cord compression are localized vertebral or radicular pain. These are not from the cord compression per se but rather from involvement of the vertebral structures and nerve roots at the level of the compression. Localized tenderness to pressure or percussion over the involved vertebrae is often found on physical examination. Because pain is seen initially in up to 90% of patients, localized back pain, radicular pain, or spinal tenderness in a patient with cancer should evoke the clinical suspicion of the physician and prompt further evaluation to determine whether the patient has potential or early cord compression. Muscle weakness, evidenced by subjective symptoms or objective physical findings, is present in 75% of patients by the time of diagnosis. The clinician must be aware that progression of this symptom can vary from a gradual increase in weakness over several days to a precipitous loss of function over several hours that may worsen rapidly to the point of paraplegia. If muscle weakness is present, it is incumbent on the physician to act urgently to obtain consultation with the neurosurgeon and the radiation oncologist. It is not appropriate to wait until the next morning! By the time there is muscle weakness, most patients also have sensory deficits below the level of the compression and often have changes in bladder and bowel sphincter function. When compression is diagnosed late or if treatment is not started emergently, only 25% of patients who are unable to walk when treatment is started will regain full ambulation.

C. Diagnosis. Magnetic resonance imaging (MRI) is the diagnostic modality of choice, although high-resolution computed tomography (CT) with myelography is an alternative. Plain radiographs and bone scans give evidence of metastases to vertebrae, but, in and of themselves, they are not diagnostic of spinal cord involvement.

When there is evidence of bony involvement of the spine on a plain radiograph, CT scan, or bone scan, our approach is to obtain an MRI for those patients who have subjective or objective evidence of weakness, radicular pain, paresthesia, or sphincter dysfunction because these patients are at the highest risk of spinal cord compression. Routine MRIs in patients who have completely asymptomatic bony spine metastases (without pain, tenderness, or neurologic findings on a comprehensive clinical examination) are not cost effective. In patients with only localized pain or tenderness to correspond with the bone scan or radiographic findings, the yield of additional tests is also low. Thus, the clinical determination of whether to obtain additional invasive or costly diagnostic tests is more difficult and requires a careful assessment of all clinical features of the patient. All patients with metastasis to the spine require close follow-up, and they and their families must be urged to report relevant symptoms immediately.

D. Treatment. As noted in the preceding text, immediate consultation with radiation oncology and neurosurgery is imperative. Because of potentially precipitous deterioration when neurologic deficits have developed, treatment should be started immediately.

   1. Corticosteroids. When a radiologic study identifies the level of cord compression or a neurologic deficit is detected on physical examination, dexamethasone should be started to reduce spinal cord edema. The recommended dose is 10 to 20 mg IV as a loading dose and then 4 to 6 mg PO or IV every 6 hours, to be continued through the initial weeks of radiation therapy. Some recommend higher doses up to 96 mg daily, but whether there is any real benefit is not established and toxicity of the steroids is clearly greater. At completion of radiotherapy, the dexamethasone therapy may be tapered.

   2. Radiotherapy
      a. Although the preferences of individual centers vary, we generally recommend the **immediate initiation**

of radiotherapy once cord compression is diagnosed. This is based on both randomized and nonrandomized studies showing no significant improvement in outcome for patients treated with surgery plus radiation as compared with those treated with radiation alone. Secondly, metastatic disease to the spine is often not totally resectable, so that follow-up radiation therapy is frequently required. Thirdly, because patients with evidence of spinal metastases frequently have either overt or microscopic evidence of metastases elsewhere that would likely grow during the postoperative recuperation period after surgery, the use of radiotherapy instead allows the initiation of some form of systemic therapy concurrently.

b. Dose and Schedule. Radiation therapy is most frequently given to a total dose of 40 to 45 Gy with daily dose fractions of 200 to 250 cGy. Alternatively, 400 cGy daily may be given initially for the first 3 days of therapy and then subsequently decreased to standard-dose levels for the completion of the radiation course. Short-course therapies with higher dose fractions have also been used. These appear to have similar functional outcome in patients with a short prognosis, but local control is maintained for a longer time when long course (standard) therapy is used. The longer course is thus recommended for patients with better prognosis from their overall disease. In selected cases, stereotactic radiosurgery, which is more commonly used in brain metastases, may be effective.

c. The clinical response to radiation is dependent not only on the degree of cord involvement and the duration of symptoms but also on the underlying cell type. In general, patients with severe deficits such as complete paraplegia or a long duration of neurologic deficit are unlikely to have returned to normal function. This underscores the need to diagnose and treat these patients rapidly. Lymphoma, myeloma, and other hematologic malignancies, along with breast and prostate cancers and small cell lung carcinoma, tend to be more responsive than adenocarcinomas of the gastrointestinal tract, non–small cell lung cancer, renal cancer, and others.

3. Surgery. Surgery still plays a crucial role for some patients. Traditional approaches include decompressive laminectomy for posterior lesions or anterior approaches for other lesions. Newer treatment options include minimally invasive vertebroplasty and kyphoplasty, which may effectively maintain function and reduce pain in appropriately selected patients and have a shorter recovery time than other procedures. Indications for surgery include worsening of neurologic signs or symptoms or the appearance of new neurologic findings during the course of radiation treatment, vertebral collapse at presentation, a question of spinal stability, and disease recurrence within an earlier radiation port. In select patients, the use of surgery to remove disease in the vertebral bodies followed by stabilization can result in dramatic improvement in pain and function.

II. Cerebral edema

A. Clinical evaluation

1. Neurologic signs and symptoms. Intracranial metastases commonly manifest as a variety of neurologic symptoms and signs, including headache, change in mentation, visual disturbances, cranial nerve deficits, focal motor or sensory abnormalities, difficulty with coordination, and seizures. In the more critical condition of brain stem herniation, there may be gradual to rapid loss of consciousness, neck stiffness, unilateral or bilateral pupillary abnormalities, ipsilateral hemiparesis, or respiratory dysfunction; the specific findings depend on whether there is uncal, central, or tonsillar herniation. Any new neurologic complaint from a patient with cancer should be viewed by members of the oncology team with a high index of suspicion that it represents metastasis, especially if metastasis to the brain is commonly associated with the patient's tumor type.

The history and physical examination provide the first clue to the presence of a metastatic lesion or associated cerebral edema. In general, a history of gradual progression of neurologic symptoms before the development of a significant deficit is more consistent with a metastatic lesion, whereas the absence of symptoms followed by the abrupt onset of a severe deficit is suggestive of a cerebrovascular event.

2. Radiologic studies. MRI is the imaging modality of choice because it has greater sensitivity than CT in detecting the presence of metastatic lesions, evaluating the posterior fossa, and determining the extent of cerebral edema. CT is substituted for MRI in many institutions because of availability, ease of administration, shorter test time and less cost. However, although CT is sufficient to detect the presence of cerebral edema in most patients, it is necessary to realize that CT fails to diagnose some lesions and may underestimate cerebral edema. If CT of the brain reveals no definite abnormality in the presence of persistent neurologic findings, MRI is the recommended next step. Delay of appropriate imaging studies (either CT or MRI) to examine plain skull radiographs or to obtain radionuclide studies in patients experiencing neurologic difficulties is not warranted.

Warning: In a patient with cancer who has focal neurologic signs or symptoms, headache, or alteration in consciousness, a lumbar puncture to evaluate for possible neoplastic meningeal spread should not be done until a CT scan or MRI shows no evidence of mass, midline shift, or increased intracranial pressure. To do the lumbar puncture without this assurance could precipitate brain stem herniation, which is often rapidly fatal.

B. Treatment

1. Symptomatic therapy. Once the presence of cerebral edema is established, dexamethasone 10 to 20 mg IV to load, followed by 6 mg IV or PO four times daily should be started. The rationale for the use of steroids centers around the etiology of cerebral edema. It appears that the invasion of malignant cells releases leukotrienes and other soluble mediators responsible for vasodilation, increased capillary permeability, and subsequent edema. Dexamethasone inhibits the conversion of arachidonic acid to leukotrienes, thereby decreasing vascular permeability. Additionally, steroids appear to have a direct stabilizing effect on brain capillaries. There is some evidence to suggest that patients who do not have lessening of cerebral edema with the dexamethasone dose just described may respond to higher doses (50 to 100 mg/day). Because of the risk of gastrointestinal bleeding and other side effects of doses higher than 32 mg/day, higher doses are usually not given for more than 48 to 72 hours.

Patients with severe cerebral edema leading to a life-threatening rise in intracranial pressure or brain stem herniation should also receive mannitol 50 to 100 g (in a 20% to 25% solution) infused IV over approximately 30 minutes. This may be repeated every 6 hours if needed, although serum electrolytes and urine output must be monitored closely. Patients with severe cerebral edema should be intubated to allow for mechanical hyperventilation to reduce the carbon dioxide pressure to 25 to 30 mm Hg in order to decrease intracranial pressure.

2. Therapy of the intracerebral tumor. Once the patient has been stabilized, appropriate therapy for the cause underlying the cerebral edema should be implemented. Radiation is the usual modality for most metastases, but surgery may be considered in addition for suitable candidates with easily accessible lesions; combined surgery and radiotherapy may result in a longer disease-free and total survival if there are only one or two metastatic lesions and the systemic disease is controlled. Stereotactic radiosurgery combined with whole brain radiation is an effective and equivalent alternative to surgery plus whole brain radiation, provided the lesions are not too large and limited in number.

3. Nonmalignant causes of cerebral edema, such as subdural hematoma in thrombocytopenic patients and brain abscess, toxoplasmosis, or other infections in immunocompromised patients, must always be considered.

III.   Superior vena cava syndrome (SVCS). The superior vena cava is a thin-walled vessel located to the right of the midline just anterior to the right main-stem bronchus. It is ultimately responsible for the venous drainage of the head, neck, and arms. Its location places it near lymph nodes that are commonly involved by malignant cells from primary lung tumors and from lymphomas. Lymph node distention or the presence of a mediastinal tumor mass may compress the adjacent superior vena cava, leading to superior vena cava syndrome (SVCS). Similarly, the presence of a thrombus due to a hypercoagulable state secondary to underlying malignancy or a thrombus developing around an indwelling central venous catheter may also lead to the development of this syndrome.

A. Symptoms and signs. Patients who develop SVCS commonly complain of dyspnea, orthopnea, paroxysmal nocturnal dyspnea, and facial, neck, and upper-extremity swelling. Associated symptoms may include cough, hoarseness, and chest or neck pain. Headache and mental status changes may also be seen. A patient's symptoms may be gradual and progressive, with only mild facial swelling being present early in the course of this disorder. These early changes may be so subtle that the patient is unaware of them. Alternatively, if a clot develops in the superior vena cava in association with narrowing of the vessel, the signs and symptoms may appear suddenly. Physical examination may reveal a spectrum of findings from facial edema to marked respiratory distress. Neck vein distention, facial edema or cyanosis, and tachypnea are commonly seen. Other potential physical findings include the presence of prominent collateral vessels on the thorax, upper-extremity edema, paralysis of the vocal cords, and mental status changes.

B. Radiologic evaluation. Patients may often be diagnosed by physical findings plus the presence of a mediastinal mass on chest radiographs. Although it was thought previously that the superior venacavogram was required to establish the diagnosis and delineate the extent of obstruction, current opinion now appears to favor the use of CT instead. CT permits a more detailed examination of surrounding anatomy, including adjacent lymphadenopathy; may differentiate between extrinsic compression and an intrinsic lesion (primary thrombus); poses less risk to the patient; aids in treatment planning for radiation therapy; and allows for possible percutaneous biopsy of a compressing mass.

SVCS may occur in patients with subclavian or internal jugular IV catheters. The injection of contrast material into these catheters is useful to determine the presence of a thrombus. However, a thrombus forms in the venous vasculature distal to the caval obstruction in most patients with SVCS secondary to external compression. Thus, a clot may be primary or secondary; determination of the cause and the appropriate treatment depends on both the clinical situation and the radiologic findings.

C. Tissue diagnosis. Although some patients present with such severe respiratory compromise as to require emergent treatment, most patients are clinically stable and may undergo biopsy for a tissue diagnosis if they are not previously known to have cancer. Tissue may be acquired through multiple methods including bronchoscopy, CT-guided biopsy, mediastinoscopy, mediastinotomy, and thoracoscopy. Thoracotomy is the most invasive option and is rarely needed. Because of increased venous pressure and dilated veins distal to the obstruction, extreme care must be taken to ensure adequate hemostasis after any biopsy procedure.

D. Treatment. Initially, patients with SVCS may be treated with oxygen for dyspnea, furosemide 20 to 40 mg IV to reduce edema, and dexamethasone 16 mg IV or PO daily in divided doses. The benefit of dexamethasone is not clear. In patients with lymphoma, there is probably a lympholytic effect with resultant decrease in tumor mass; in patients with most other tumors, the effect is probably limited to decreasing any local inflammatory reaction from the tumor and from subsequent initial radiotherapy.

1. **Neoplasms.** Therapy for SVCS ultimately involves radiation therapy for most tumors but possibly chemotherapy as a single modality for particularly sensitive tumor types such as small cell lung cancer, lymphomas, and germ cell cancers. Radiation therapy may be given in relatively high-dose fractions (e.g., 4 Gy) for several days, followed by a reversion to "standard doses" thereafter. Dexamethasone is continued for approximately 1 week after the start of radiation treatment.

2. **Thrombi.** SVCS secondary to vascular thrombi has been treated in the past with thrombolytic therapy, though this treatment is less commonly used now. It is particularly important to avoid thrombolytic therapy in patients with a tumor that might bleed, and when thrombi are secondary to external SVC pressure from neoplasms, thrombolytics are not needed. A newer highly effective treatment for the relief of signs and symptoms is percutaneous stent placement in the superior vena cava. Anticoagulation with heparin after thrombolytic therapy or stent placement is recommended, because clot formation is common, even when external pressure was the primary cause of the obstruction. Depending on the situation, therapeutic doses of warfarin may be indicated to prevent propagation of the clot (see Chapter 29).

IV. **Anaphylaxis**

A. **Causes.** Anaphylaxis, although infrequent, is one of the most catastrophic potential side effects of biologic and chemotherapy. Anaphylaxis is a hyperimmune reaction mediated by the release of immunoglobulin E. This emergency situation may arise in oncology patients who are exposed to serum products, bacterial products such as L-asparaginase, certain cytotoxic agents (such as paclitaxel [Taxol] or the Cremophor component of paclitaxel), antibiotics such as penicillin, iodine-based contrast material, latex, and monoclonal antibodies (which have murine components). However, virtually any drug can lead to a hyperimmune response resulting in anaphylaxis.

B. **Clinical manifestations.** Patients may display anxiety, dyspnea, and presyncopal symptoms. Urticaria, generalized itching, and evidence of bronchospasm and upper-airway angioedema may occur. Peripheral vasodilation may manifest as facial flushing or pallor, can result in significant hypotension, and may lead to syncope.

C. **Management.** Prompt recognition and treatment can be invaluable in blunting an adverse response and may prevent a reaction from becoming life threatening. Patients must be assessed rapidly to ensure that an open airway is present and maintained. Supplemental oxygen should be given for respiratory symptoms. Endotracheal intubation may be necessary. If severe laryngeal edema rather than bronchospasm is the cause of respiratory distress, tracheostomy or cricothyrotomy is necessary.

1. **Epinephrine** 0.3 to 0.5 mg (0.3 to 0.5 mL of 1:1,000 epinephrine or 3 to 5 mL of a 1:10,000 solution) IV is given every 10 minutes for severe reactions with laryngeal stridor, major bronchospasm, or severe hypotension, for

a maximum of three doses (1 mg) or until the episode resolves, whichever occurs first. For milder reactions, a dose of 0.2 to 0.3 mL of 1:1,000 epinephrine may be given SC and repeated every 15 minutes for two additional doses if needed. In the event of life-threatening anaphylaxis, 0.5 mg (5 mL of a 1:10,000 solution) should be given IV; this dose may be repeated once in 10 minutes if needed. Because of the cardiovascular stress associated with epinephrine, its use in relatively minor allergic reactions, such as pruritus alone, should be avoided. Alternatively, epinephrine may be administered through the endotracheal tube if IV access is unavailable.

2. Intravenous fluids (either normal saline or lactated Ringer's solution) may be given for hypotension. Hypotension unresponsive to these measures requires the use of vasopressors such as dopamine.

3. Albuterol or metaproterenol aerosol treatments can be used to treat bronchospasm.

4. Diphenhydramine 25 mg IV may be followed by a second dose, if necessary. Blood pressure must be monitored because hypotension can result.

5. Corticosteroids have a slow onset of action measured in hours. Although their administration may be reasonable for their later effects, they do not have a primary role in the acute management of this emergent condition. Hydrocortisone 100 to 500 mg IV or methylprednisolone 125 mg IV may be given for their later effects.

6. Cimetidine 300 mg IV or any other H_2-blocker may be given for urticaria; it has no significant role in acute, severe episodes, although it has a preventive role in averting reactions from paclitaxel along with dexamethasone and diphenhydramine.

V. **Respiratory failure**

A. **Causes.** Respiratory failure in patients with cancer may have many potential causes:

- Bacterial or other pneumonias, especially in patients who are neutropenic due to therapy
- Sepsis (and other causes of the systemic inflammatory response syndrome)
- Interstitial pulmonary spread of cancer
- Overwhelming parenchymal pulmonary metastases
- Radiation injury
- Lung damage from chemotherapy agents (such as bleomycin, mitomycin, high-dose cyclophosphamide, or methotrexate)
- Pulmonary edema secondary to cardiac damage from cytotoxic agents (such as doxorubicin), or capillary leak syndrome from biologic agents (such as IL-2)
- Retinoic acid syndrome from tretinoin (all-*trans*-retinoic acid) therapy of acute promyelocytic leukemia
- Pulmonary emboli, either multiple small or single large

B. **Management.** The management of severe respiratory failure requires intubation and mechanical ventilation, which is usually managed by pulmonologists or critical care specialists. However, because the prognosis of most patients with advanced solid tumors who develop respiratory failure is poor, careful consideration of a patient's entire medical situation must be made. Relevant factors include the patient's underlying medical illnesses, such as concurrent cardiopulmonary disease, and their particular tumor type and potential for response to antineoplastic therapy. It is prudent—some would say imperative—to ascertain well in advance of the emergency the goals of the patients and the wishes of patients and their families regarding intensive care unit support and full resuscitative measures.

C. Prevention. If possible, progressive steps to prevent or lessen the possibility of the development of respiratory failure should be undertaken. These include the following:

    1. Careful monitoring of granulocyte counts to be aware of patients at risk for bacterial infection.

    2. Routine lung auscultation of patients receiving agents with potential pulmonary toxicity followed by appropriate action in the event of pulmonary findings. This may include giving furosemide if indicated and discontinuing offending agents (such as bleomycin before the development of serious symptoms. Reasons for discontinuing bleomycin therapy include unexplained exertional dyspnea, fine bibasilar rales, fine bibasilar reticular shadows on chest radiograph, and significant fall in pulmonary function tests from pretreatment levels.

    3. Ensuring that patients are ambulatory or that antithrombotic precautions are taken for hospitalized patients who are bedridden.

    4. Consideration of underlying cardiopulmonary disease, prior chest irradiation, and so forth before patients are considered for systemic therapy is most important. Concurrent illnesses may proscribe the selection of or modify the dosing of cytotoxic agents (such as cisplatin, which requires substantial IV hydration) and biologic agents (such as IL-2, before which patients' cardiac and pulmonary function should be tested).

VI.   Tumor lysis syndrome. This syndrome may be seen with any tumor that is undergoing rapid cell turnover as a result of high growth fraction or high cell death due to therapy. In general, acute leukemia, high- and intermediate-grade lymphoma, and, less commonly, solid tumors such as small cell lung cancer and germ cell cancers undergoing therapy are the most commonly associated tumor types. Tumor lysis syndrome is characterized by the metabolic abnormalities of hyperuricemia, hyperkalemia, and hyperphosphatemia leading to hypocalcemia. Patients with underlying chronic renal insufficiency are more susceptible to developing tumor lysis syndrome because of their limited capacity to excrete the products of rapid tumor cell destruction. Severe clinical situations, including acute renal failure, and serious cardiac dysrhythmia, including ventricular tachycardia and ventricular fibrillation, may develop. It is therefore important for physicians to be aware of which patients might be at risk for this syndrome, attempt to prevent its onset, monitor patients' blood chemistry values carefully, and initiate treatment promptly.

    A. Prevention. It is useful to start all patients who have tumor types or therapy that predispose to this complication on allopurinol 600 to 1,200 mg/day PO in divided doses for

1 or 2 days at least 24 hours before initiating chemotherapy, and continuing with 300 mg PO b.i.d. for 2 to 3 days after the start of therapy. Thereafter, patients may receive allopurinol 300 mg/day PO.

For patients who must be treated immediately, allopurinol is started at the same dose just described, urine should be alkalinized (pH 7), and IV fluid hydration with a "brisk diuresis" of approximately 100 to 150 mL/hour of urine maintained. This can be achieved through the use of IV crystalloid, with 1 ampule (44.6 mEq) of sodium bicarbonate in each liter of IV solution. If the desired urine output is not reached after adequate hydration, furosemide 20 mg IV may be given to facilitate diuresis. If routine monitoring of urine shows pH less than 7.0, an additional ampule of sodium bicarbonate may be added to each liter of infused fluid. Acetazolamide 250 mg PO q.i.d. may also be added to keep the urine alkaline.

Recombinant urate oxidase, rasburicase, is a safe and effective alternative to allopurinol. The recommended dose of rasburicase is 0.15 to 0.2 mg/kg/day for 5 days, but excellent control of hyperuricemia may be achieved with a lower dose of 3 mg/day.

B. Monitoring. During the course of chemotherapy for patients at risk of tumor lysis syndrome, serum electrolytes, phosphate, calcium, uric acid, and creatinine levels should be checked before therapy and at least daily thereafter. Patients at high risk (e.g., high-grade lymphoma with large bulk) should have these parameters checked every 6 hours for the first 24 to 48 hours. In addition, patients who show any initial or subsequent abnormality in any of these parameters should have appropriate therapy initiated and have measurements of abnormal parameters repeated every 6 to 12 hours until completion of chemotherapy and normalization of laboratory values.

C. Treatment. Patients who have evidence of tumor lysis syndrome must have adequate hydration with half-normal saline solution. Oral aluminum hydroxide can be used to treat hyperphosphatemia.

Hyperkalemia may be treated in multiple ways. However, the clinician must differentiate between methods that reduce serum potassium by driving this ion intracellularly (as is done with dextrose and insulin or sodium bicarbonate) and methods that lead to actual potassium loss out of the body (as with furosemide through the urine and with sodium polystyrene sulfonate resin [Kayexalate] through the gut). If hyperkalemia or hypocalcemia occurs, an electrocardiogram should be obtained, with continuous monitoring of the cardiac rhythm until these abnormalities are corrected. In addition, because of the potential cardiac arrhythmias secondary to hyperkalemia with hypocalcemia, cardioprotection could be achieved through the use of IV calcium.

We recommend the following:

  1. For patients with mild elevation of potassium (serum potassium no higher than 5.5 mEq/L), increasing IV hydration using normal saline solution with a single dose (20 mg) of IV furosemide is often sufficient. An alternative to normal saline is the use of 2 ampules of sodium bicarbonate (89 mEq) in 1 L of 5% dextrose/water, although alkalinization per se is probably not beneficial.

2. For patients with serum potassium levels between 5.5 and 6.0 mEq/L, increased IV fluids, furosemide, and oral sodium polystyrene sulfonate resin 30 g with sorbitol may be used.

3. For patients with serum potassium levels of more than 6.0 mEq/L or evidence of cardiac arrhythmia, several options may be combined. IV calcium gluconate, 10 mL of a 10% solution or 1 ampule, is given first, followed by increased IV fluids, furosemide, plus 1 ampule of 50% dextrose and 10 U of regular insulin IV. Albuterol may be used to augment the effect of the insulin. Oral sodium polystyrene sulfonate resin with sorbitol also may be used except in patients with a history of congestive heart failure or reduced left ventricular function. Dialysis may be necessary for refractory hyperkalemia.

VII. Hypercalcemia

A. Causes of tumor hypercalcemia

1. Associated tumors. Hypercalcemia is relatively common in patients with malignancy. In one study, it was shown that the most common cause of hypercalcemia in hospitalized patients is malignancy. Hypercalcemia of malignancy can be associated with bone metastasis, or it may occur in the absence of any direct bone involvement by the tumor. On the basis of the findings of a study on 433 patients with hypercalcemia of cancer, 86% of the patients had identifiable bone metastasis. More than one-half (n = 225) of the cases were accounted for by patients with breast carcinoma, and cancer of the lung and kidneys accounted for a smaller proportion. Patients with hematologic malignancies accounted for approximately 15% of the cases. These patients usually had hypercalcemia in the presence of diffuse tumor involvement of bone, although in a small percentage there was no evidence of bone involvement.

2. Humoral mediators. In approximately 10% of the cases with malignancy, hypercalcemia develops in the absence of radiographic or scintigraphic evidence of bone involvement. In this group of patients, the pathogenesis of hypercalcemia appears to be secondary to humoral mediators, dominant of which is parathyroid hormone (PTH)–related protein (PTHrP), as well as other osteoclast-activating factors (OAFs). A number of other cytokines, with potential bone-resorbing activities, including IL-6 and tumor necrosis factor α (TNF-α), have been identified. These cytokines may account for the previously designated OAF. There is evidence indicating that prostaglandins (PGs) play a role in the hypercalcemia of malignancy. PGs are potent stimulators of bone resorption. There may also be the coexistence of tumor with primary hyperparathyroidism or other cause of hypercalcemia (e.g., vitamin D intoxication, sarcoidosis).

B. Symptoms, signs, and laboratory findings. Hypercalcemia often produces symptoms in patients with cancer and, in fact, may be the patients' major problem. Polyuria and nocturia, resulting from the impaired ability of the kidneys to concentrate the urine, occur early. Anorexia, nausea, constipation, muscle weakness, and fatigue are common. As the hypercalcemia progresses, severe dehydration, azotemia, mental obtundation, coma, and cardiovascular collapse may appear. In addition to hypercalcemia, the laboratory studies may reveal hypokalemia and increased blood urea nitrogen (BUN) and creatinine levels. Patients with hypercalcemia of malignancy frequently have hypochloremic metabolic alkalosis, whereas with primary hyperparathyroidism, metabolic acidosis is more common. The concentration of serum phosphorus is variable. PTH levels may be normal, low, or high, but marked elevations are rarely seen. Bone involvement is best evaluated by a bone scan, which is often positive in the absence of radiographic evidence of bone involvement.

C. Treatment. The management of hypercalcemia of malignancy has two objectives: reducing elevated levels of serum calcium and treating the underlying cause. When hypercalcemia is mild to moderate (corrected [for albumin concentration] serum calcium <12 to 13 mg/dL) and the patient is not symptomatic, adequate hydration and measures directed against the tumor (e.g., surgery, chemotherapy, or radiation therapy) may suffice. Severe hypercalcemia, on the other hand, is a life-threatening condition requiring emergency treatment. Therefore, for more severe degrees of hypercalcemia, other measures must be taken, including enhancement of calcium excretion by the kidney in patients with adequate renal function and the use of agents that decrease bone resorption.

The agents used for treatment of hypercalcemia have differences in the time of onset and duration of action as well as in their potency. Therefore, effective treatment of severe hypercalcemia requires the use of more than one modality of therapy.

A suggested approach to the treatment of severe hypercalcemia is as follows:

- Rehydration with 0.9% sodium chloride
- Bisphosphonate therapy—either pamidronate or zoledronic acid
- Continuing saline diuresis (0.9% sodium chloride + furosemide)

    1. Rehydration. Rehydration and restoration of intravascular volume comprise the most important initial step in the therapy of hypercalcemia. Rehydration should be accomplished using 0.9% sodium chloride (normal saline) and often requires the administration of 4 to 6 L over the first 24 hours. Rehydration alone causes only a mild decrease of the serum calcium levels (about 10%). However, rehydration improves renal function, facilitating urinary calcium excretion.

    2. Saline diuresis. After adequate restoration of intravascular volume, forced saline diuresis may be used. Sodium competitively inhibits the tubular resorption of calcium. Therefore, the IV infusion of saline causes a significant increase in calcium clearance. Because of the large amounts of saline that may be required to correct hypercalcemia, it is advisable to monitor the central venous pressure continuously. The infusion of normal saline (0.9% sodium chloride) at a rate of 250 to 500 mL/hour, accompanied by the IV administration of 20 to 80 mg of furosemide every 2 to 4 hours, results in significant calcium diuresis and mild lowering of the serum calcium in most patients. This type of therapy requires strict monitoring of cardiopulmonary status to avoid fluid overload. Also, it requires ready access to the laboratory to prevent electrolyte imbalance, because the urinary losses of sodium, potassium, magnesium, and water must be replaced to maintain metabolic balance. In some cases, the infusion of saline at rates of 125 to 150 mL/hour plus the addition of furosemide 40 to 80 mg IV once or twice a day may reduce the serum calcium until other measures aimed at inhibiting bone resorption take effect.

3. **Bisphosphonates**

   a. Mechanism of action. The bisphosphonates are potent inhibitors of normal and abnormal osteoclastic bone resorption. They bind to the surface of calcium phosphate crystals and inhibit crystal growth and dissolution. In addition, they may directly inhibit osteoclast resorptive activity.

   b. Pamidronate and zoledronic acid. Pamidronate and zoledronic acid are very potent inhibitors of bone resorption and highly effective agents for the treatment of hypercalcemia of malignancy. Pamidronate was the treatment of choice for hypercalcemia of malignancy for several years, but zoledronic acid, is at least as effective in the treatment of hypercalcemia and can be given over a shorter period of time.

   (1) Dosage and administration. For symptomatic, moderate hypercalcemia (corrected serum calcium 12 to 13.5 mg/dL), the recommended dose of pamidronate is 60 to 90 mg given IV as a single dose over 4 to 24 hours. The maximum recommended dose of zoledronic acid in hypercalcemia of malignancy is 4 mg, given as a single dose IV infusion over **no less than 15 minutes.** Doses may be repeated in 3 to 4 days if inadequate response has been seen.

   (2) Side effects. Pamidronate and zoledronic acid are usually well tolerated, and no serious acute side effects have been reported. Mild fever with temperature elevations of 1°C have been noted occasionally in patients after drug administration. The transient fever is presumed to be due to release of cytokines from osteoclasts. Pain, redness, swelling, and induration at the site of infusion occur in approximately 20% of patients. Hypocalcemia, hypophosphatemia, or hypomagnesemia may be seen in 15% of the patients. Both should be used with caution in patients with decreased renal function. Osteonecrosis of the jaw in association with dental procedures and conditions can be a debilitating side effect of the bisphosphonates and requires the skill of an experienced dentist or oral surgeon.

4. **Glucocorticoids.** Large initial doses of hydrocortisone 250 to 500 mg IV q8 hour (or its equivalent) can be effective

in the treatment of hypercalcemia associated with lympho-proliferative diseases such as non–Hodgkin's lymphoma and multiple myeloma and in patients with breast cancer metastatic to bone. However, it may take several days for glucocorticoids to lower the serum calcium level. Maintenance therapy should be started with prednisone 10 to 30 mg/day PO. The mechanisms by which glucocorticoids lower the serum calcium are multiple and involved.

5. Oral phosphate supplements (Neutra-Phos or Fleet Phospho-soda). Oral phosphate therapy is an adjunct for the chronic treatment of hypercalcemia of malignancy. Oral phosphate decreases the intestinal absorption of calcium and enhances the deposition of insoluble calcium salts in bone and tissue. Oral phosphate supplements at dosages of 1.5 to 3.0 g/day of elemental phosphorus can result in mild lowering of the serum calcium levels as well as a reduction in urinary calcium excretion. Diarrhea usually limits the amount of phosphate that can be given. Phosphate supplements should never be given to patients with renal failure or when hyperphosphatemia is present, as soft tissue calcification may occur. Monitoring of the level of calcium and phosphorus as well as the calcium times phosphorus ion product is important to prevent metastatic calcifications.

6. Other agents. Mithramycin is no longer used or recommended for hypercalcemia of malignancy. Salmon calcitonin use is uncommon, because of the requirement for frequent administration and the rapid development of therapeutic refractoriness. However, it does have a rapid duration of action and may be administered to patients with congestive heart failure and hypercalcemia. Calcitonin Salmon is given at 4 IU/kg every 12 hours SC or IM. The dose may be increased to 8 IU/kg every 12 hours after 24 to 48 hours if response is unsatisfactory.

VIII. Bone metastasis. Metastases to bone occur frequently from many types of tumors and have great potential for morbidity. Bone involvement can be a source of constant pain, limiting a patient's activity and quality of life. The consequences of spinal involvement have been discussed already. The occurrence of a pathologic fracture in a weight-bearing bone has catastrophic implications: patients who are consequently immobilized or bedridden are predisposed to a variety of complications including deep venous thrombi, pulmonary emboli, aspiration pneumonia, and decubitus ulcers as well as psychosocial consequences, including depression.

A. Clinical findings. Bone involvement with metastatic disease manifests as a spectrum of clinical presentations. This can vary from constant aching pain through nocturnal exacerbations of pain to sharp pains brought on by pressure, weight bearing, other use, or range of motion of the affected site. Tenderness of an affected bone area may or may not be present. Tenderness or sharp pain with weight bearing often implies a greater degree of disruption of the bony architecture and therefore a greater potential for fracture, particularly in a weight-bearing area.

B. Radiologic findings. These often depend on the type of malignancy involved as well as the extent of the metastases.

Multiple myeloma is a prime example of a malignancy that leads to pure osteolytic lesions. Consequently, radionuclide bone scans are rarely useful in the evaluation of patients with this disease. Rather, a metastatic skeletal survey (plain radiographs) is preferable. In contrast, prostate cancer most commonly has purely osteoblastic lesions. Therefore, a radionuclide bone scan would be the diagnostic test of choice. In general, most tumor types have the potential to yield either type of bone lesion or both. A radionuclide bone scan may be done to permit a "global view" in these patients. Although [^{18}F]fluorodeoxyglucose (FDG) positron emission tomography (FDG-PET) can also pick up bone metastasis, unless there is a reason to look at nonbony areas for other sites of disease it is not necessary to use it, and it is considerably more expensive.

The presence of "hot spots" in the spine, in weight-bearing bones such as the femur, or in other major long bones such as the humerus should lead the clinician to assess the patient further with plain radiographs of these bones. Patients who display significant cortical thinning of long bones or large lytic bone metastases are at high risk of developing pathologic fractures with great morbidity. These patients should be evaluated both by orthopedic surgery for consideration of prophylactic surgery to stabilize the affected bone and by radiation oncology for treatment of the tumor to permit regeneration of normal bone.

C. Treatment

1. **Surgery.** Because rapid return of the patient to as normal a life as possible is an overriding concern when treating patients with metastatic disease, surgical stabilization is most often the initial step in treating pathologic fractures of long bones. If the fracture is the initial manifestation of tumor relapse, biopsy confirmation can also be obtained. Whereas fractures at sites of significant residual bony architecture can be satisfactorily stabilized with an intramedullary rod or pin, marked lytic destruction may necessitate additional structural support such as methylmethacrylate cement to fill the intramedullary canal and cortical defects. Pathologic fractures of non–weight-bearing bones can be managed by splinting (ribs) or sling immobilization (humerus or clavicle) while delivering radiotherapy to promote healing. Fixation may also be used in the upper extremities to speed recovery of function, particularly of the humerus. Surgical stabilization of the spine may also be used in selected circumstances (provided the patient has an anticipated survival time of more than 3 months) with open or minimally invasive procedures such as kyphoplasty and vertebroplasty, and can result in significant pain relief and reduction in risk of cord and nerve root compression.

2. **External-beam therapy.** Radiation doses of 15 to 20 Gy in three to five fractions lead to complete relief of pain in approximately 50% of patients, with an additional 30% of patients having some decrease in pain, whereas 80% to 90% show significant improvement with 30 to 40 Gy. The alleviation of symptoms can be expected within 2 to 3 weeks. For patients who may be expected to have more

prolonged survival, higher doses over a larger number of fractions may be used. Most patients receive optimal results from courses of 30 Gy in 10 fractions (2 weeks) or 40 Gy in 15 fractions (3 weeks).

Radiotherapy fields should include the area of evident bone involvement, as shown on radiograph and bone scan, with a sufficient extension to prevent relapse at the portal margin. It is seldom necessary to treat an entire long bone unless the entire bone is involved because encroachment on marrow reserve may compromise any systemic chemotherapy that might also be indicated.

3. Strontium 89 (^{89}Sr) therapy. A different approach to the therapy of symptomatic bone metastases is through the use of radioisotopes, such as ^{89}Sr, which is given by IV injection. This isotope is highly selective for bone, is an emitter of β- radiation, and has low penetration into surrounding tissue. Strontium's affinity to metastatic bone disease is reported to be 2 to 25 times greater than its affinity to normal bone. This therapy is especially useful in patients with breast or prostate cancer who have many metastatic bone sites or who have received maximal external-beam irradiation to a specific site. Palliative effects may be seen in other types of tumors as well. Pain relief may occur as early as 1 to 2 weeks after the first injection. Multiple studies indicate that 10% to 20% of patients experience complete pain relief, whereas another 50% to 60% have at least a moderate reduction in symptoms. Responses last for 3 to 6 months. Patients who experience some relief of symptoms may receive multiple doses at 3-month intervals if there has been adequate hematologic recovery.

The toxicity of ^{89}Sr is primarily hematologic, involving both leukocytes and platelets. Approximately 10% of patients may experience a transient "flare" of their bone pain, similar to what is seen with tamoxifen therapy in breast cancer. This flare reaction often foreshadows a response to treatment. Other radioisotopes for the palliation of painful bone metastases include samarium 153 and rhenium 186.

4. Biphosphonates. Pamidronate and zoledronic acid are specific inhibitors of osteoclastic activity. They are not only effective for the treatment of hypercalcemia associated with malignancy but can reduce bone pain and reduce fractures, especially in multiple myeloma, breast cancer, and prostate cancer. Zoledronic acid appears to be more effective than pamidronate in reducing the risk of skeletal system–related events. Some improvement in survival may be seen in multiple myeloma.

SUGGESTED READINGS

Allon M, Shanklin N. Effect of bicarbonate administration on plasma potassium in dialysis patients: interactions with insulin and albuterol. *Am J Kidney Dis* 1996;28:508–514.

Arrambide K, Toto RD. Tumor lysis syndrome. *Semin Nephrol* 1993; 13:273–280.

Brown JE, Neville-Webbe H, Coleman RE. The role of bisphosphonates in breast and prostate cancers. *Endocr Relat Cancer* 2004; 11:207–224.

Ciesielski-Carlucci C, Leong P, Jacobs C. Case report of anaphylaxis from cisplatin/paclitaxel and a review of their hypersensitivity reaction profiles. *Am J Clin Oncol* 1997;20:373–375.

Cooper PR, Errico TJ, Martin R, et al. A systematic approach to spinal reconstruction after anterior decompression for neoplastic disease of the thoracic and lumbar spine. *Neurosurgery* 1993;32:1–8.

Courtheoux P, Alkofer B, Al Refai M, et al. Stent placement in superior vena cava syndrome. *Ann Thorac Surg* 2003;75:158–161.

Escalante CP. Causes and management of superior vena cava syndrome. *Oncology* 1993;7:61.

Garmatis CJ, Chu FC. The effectiveness of radiation therapy in the treatment of bone metastases from breast cancer. *Radiology* 1978;126:235.

Gray BH, Olin JW, Graor RA, et al. Safety and efficacy of thrombolytic therapy for superior vena cava syndrome. *Chest* 1991;99:54–59.

Greenberg A. Hyperkalemia: treatment options. *Semin Nephrol* 1998; 18:46–57.

Hauser MJ, Tabak J, Baier H. Survival of patients with cancer in a medical critical care unit. *Arch Intern Med* 1982;142:527.

Kademani D, Koka S, Lacy MQ, et al. Primary surgical therapy for osteonecrosis of the jaw secondary to bisphosphonate therapy. *Mayo Clin Proc* 2006;81:1100–1103.

Kanis JA, McCloskey EV, Taube T, et al. Rationale for the use of bisphosphonates in bone metastases. *Bone* 1991;12(Suppl 1): S13–S18.

Major P, Lortholary A, Hon J, et al. Zoledronic acid is superior to pamidronate in the treatment of hypercalcemia of malignancy: a pooled analysis of two randomized, controlled clinical trials. *J Clin Oncol* 2001;19:558–567.

Man Z, Otero AB, Rendo P, et al. Use of pamidronate for multiple myeloma osteolytic lesions. *Lancet* 1990;335:663.

Noel G, Bollet MA, Noel S, et al. Linac stereotactic radiosurgery: an effective and safe treatment for elderly patients with brain metastases. *Int J Radiat Oncol Biol Phys* 2005;63:1555–1561.

Porter AT, Davis LP. Systemic radionuclide therapy of bone metastases with strontium-89. *Oncology* 1994;8:93.

Rades D, Fehlauer F, Schulte R, et al. Prognostic factors for local control and survival after radiotherapy of metastatic spinal cord compression. *J Clin Oncol* 2006;24:3388–3393.

Rades D, Stalpers LJ, Schulte R, et al. Defining the appropriate radiotherapy regimen for metastatic spinal cord compression in non-small cell lung cancer patients. *Eur J Cancer* 2006;42:1052–1056.

Med Lett Drugs Ther. Samarium-153 lexidronam for painful bone metastases. 1997;39:83–84.

Seifert V, Zimmerman M, Stolke D, et al. Spondylectomy, microsurgical decompression and osteosynthesis in the treatment of complex disorders of the cervical spine. *Acta Neurochir (Wien)* 1993; 124:104–113.

Stafinski T, Jhangri GS, Yan E, et al. Effectiveness of stereotactic radiosurgery alone or in combination with whole brain radiotherapy compared to conventional surgery and/or whole brain radiotherapy for the treatment of one or more brain metastases: a systematic review and meta-analysis. *Cancer Treat Rev* 2006;32:203–213.

Thiebaud D, Leyvraz S, von Fliedner V, et al. Treatment of bone metastases from breast cancer and myeloma with pamidronate. *Eur J Cancer* 1991;27:37–41.

Weissman DE. Steroid treatment of CNS metastases. *J Clin Oncol* 1988;6:543–551.

Witham TF, Khavkin YA, Gallia GL, et al. Surgery insight: current management of epidural spinal cord compression from metastatic spine disease. *Nat Clin Pract Neurol* 2006;2:87–94.

CHAPTER 31

Malignant Pleural, Peritoneal, and Pericardial Effusions and Meningeal Infiltrates

Rekha T. Chaudhary

Malignant pleural, peritoneal, and pericardial effusions and malignant meningeal infiltrates are uncommon early in the course of the malignancy. They occur more frequently with disseminated disease and often herald a poor prognosis. Although pleural and peritoneal effusions may initially have little adverse effect on quality of life, when progressive, they (as well as pericardial effusions and meningeal infiltrates) can result in incapacitating disability and death. It is therefore necessary for the clinician to have a high index of suspicion for these problems and to be prepared to take appropriate action and deliver palliative treatment promptly.

I. **Pleural effusions**
   A. **Causes.** Malignant pleural effusions arise in association with malignant cells lining the pleura, exuded into the pleural space, or blocking veins or lymphatics. The most common malignancy associated with pleural effusions in women is carcinoma of the breast, whereas in men, it is carcinoma of the lung. Other causes of malignant pleural effusions include lymphoma, mesothelioma, and carcinomas of the ovary, gastrointestinal tract, urinary tract, and uterus. Malignancy is not the only cause of effusions, even in patients with known neoplastic disease; therefore, it is important to attempt to exclude other possible causes such as congestive heart failure, infection, and pulmonary infarction.
   B. **Diagnosis**
      1. **Clinical diagnosis.** Effusions may be asymptomatic or may be suspected because of respiratory symptoms such as shortness of breath with exertion or at rest, orthopnea, paroxysmal nocturnal dyspnea, or occasionally chest pressure or cough. The patient may feel more comfortable when lying on one side when the effusion is unilateral. On physical examination, dullness to percussion, decreased tactile fremitus, diminished breath sounds, and egophony are typical signs over the area of the effusion.
      2. **A chest radiograph** should be obtained to confirm the clinical impression. If fluid appears to be present, a lateral decubitus film must be obtained to help estimate the volume of the effusion and how free it is within the pleural space.
      3. **Diagnostic thoracentesis** should be performed. Ultrasonographic guidance is helpful if loculation is present. Fluid should be obtained for bacterial, acid-fast, and fungal cultures, for cytologic examination, and for determining

protein concentration (>3 g/dL in most exudates), lactate dehydrogenase (LDH) level, specific gravity, and cell count. The cytologic examination is important, because if the results are positive, as in 50% to 70% of patients with malignant effusion, the diagnosis is established. Other parameters of the pleural fluid that may be helpful in establishing that the fluid is an exudate and not a transudate include a specific gravity of more than 1.015, protein concentration that is more than 0.5 times the serum protein concentration, LDH level more than 0.6 times the serum LDH level, and low glucose level. A cytologic examination of fluid from a newly discovered pleural effusion is wise, regardless of whether the patient is known to have malignancy, because for nearly 50% of all malignant effusions, this finding is the first sign of malignancy. Analyzing pleural fluid for carcinoembryonic antigen (CEA) may be helpful in some patients. Levels higher than 20 ng/mL are suggestive of adenocarcinoma, although they do not substitute for a tissue diagnosis in patients who have no history of malignancy. CEA elevations may be seen in adenocarcinomas from various primary sites including the breast, lung, and gastrointestinal tract. Elevated levels between 10 and 20 ng/mL may reflect malignancy or benign disorders such as pulmonary infection. The role of assessing other tumor markers on a routine basis has not been established. Likewise, the utility of monoclonal antibodies and gene rearrangement studies in patients with lymphomas to distinguish reactive mesothelial or lymphocytic cells from malignant cells has yet to be determined. The routine use of a "panel of tumor markers" is costly and time consuming and is not recommended.

4. Pleural biopsy may be helpful in establishing the diagnosis in up to 20% of patients for whom the pleural fluid cytology results are negative.

5. Thoracotomy or pleuroscopy with direct biopsy may be done in patients who have negative cytology and pleural biopsy results but in whom there is still high suspicion of malignancy.

C. Treatment. As malignant pleural effusions are generally a sign of systemic rather than localized disease, the best therapy is treatment that effectively treats the malignancy systemically. Unfortunately, effective systemic treatment is often not possible, particularly when the malignancy is commonly refractory to systemic treatment (e.g., in non–small cell carcinoma of the lung) or in patients who have previously been heavily treated and in whom systemic therapy is no longer effective. In these circumstances, locoregional therapy is required for palliation of the patient's symptoms.

1. Drainage. Many malignant pleural effusions recur within 1 to 3 days after simple thoracentesis; approximately 97% recur within 1 month. Chest tube drainage (closed tube thoracotomy) allows the pleural surfaces to oppose each other and, if maintained for several days, may result in obliteration of the space and improvement in the effusion for several weeks to months. It does not appear to be as effective when used alone as when a cytotoxic or sclerosing agent is added, and therefore, one of these agents is commonly instilled into the space while the chest tube is in place.

2. **Cytotoxic and sclerosing agents.** The most widely used agents for intrapleural administration are bleomycin, doxycycline, and talc. Other agents including fluorouracil, interferon α, and methylprednisolone acetate have been less commonly used. Recent randomized studies have suggested that bleomycin may be more effective than doxycycline (in part because doxycycline sometimes requires multiple dose administrations) and that talc is either equal to or slightly better than bleomycin in terms of recurrence. The agents vary in toxicity, ease of administration, and cost. Additionally, institutional experience often determines the agent utilized. Nevertheless, for optimal effectiveness, drainage of pleural fluid as completely as possible is required before instillation.

   a. **Method of administration.** The drug to be used is diluted in 50 to 100 mL of saline and instilled through the thoracostomy tube into the chest cavity after the effusion has been drained for at least 24 hours and the rate of collection is less than 100 mL/24 hours. Throughout the procedure, care must be taken to avoid any air leak. The thoracostomy tube is clamped, and the patient is successively repositioned on his or her front, back, and sides for 15-minute periods during the next 2 to 6 hours. The tube is then reconnected to gravity drainage or suction for at least 18 hours to ensure that the pleural surfaces remain opposed and to prevent the rapid accumulation of any fluid in reaction to the instillation. Some clinicians repeat the instillation daily for a total of 2 to 3 days. For most of the agents, this has no proven benefit. Exceptions include methylprednisolone acetate and doxycycline, which appear to be more effective with additional doses. If the drainage is less than 40 to 50 mL over the previous 12 hours, the tube may be removed and a chest radiograph obtained to be certain that pneumothorax has not occurred during removal of the tube. If the thoracostomy tube continues to drain more than 100 mL/24 hours after the last instillation, it may be necessary to leave it in place for an additional 48 to 72 hours to ensure that a maximum amount of adhesion between the pleural surfaces has taken place. Because the use of sclerotic agents can be painful, it is prudent for the clinician to consider the use of scheduled narcotic analgesia, particularly during the initial 24 hours.

   b. **Recommended agents.** Efficacy, side effects, cost, and institutional (operator) experience must be considered when choosing a sclerosing agent. Bleomycin, in one prospective study, was shown to be more effective than tetracycline. It is also more expensive per dose than the other agents. Talc is the least expensive, but this must be balanced against the costs of related procedures, including thoracoscopy and anesthesia. Talc is probably superior to bleomycin in terms of recurrence rate of effusions at 90 days and later.

(1) Bleomycin 1 mg/kg or 40 mg/m^2 has relatively little myelosuppressive effect and is highly effective.

(2) Talc 5 g is given typically as a powder (poudrage). It is highly effective but requires thoracoscopy and general anesthesia. Rarely, adult respiratory distress syndrome has been reported, primarily with doses greater than 10 g.

(3) Doxycycline 500 mg may cause pleuritic chest pain. An injection of 10 mL of 1% lidocaine (100 mg) through the chest tube may reduce this symptom.

c. **Alternative agents**

(1) Fluorouracil 2 to 3 g (total dose) may have a theoretical advantage in sensitive carcinomas, but whether that advantage has practical significance is not established. Pain is generally minimal. Occasional patients may experience a depressed white blood cell count, especially at the higher dose.

(2) Interferon α 50×10^6 U typically causes influenza-like symptoms. Lower doses appear to be ineffective. Patients should be premedicated with acetaminophen 650 mg before and again 6 hours after interferon administration. Meperidine 25 mg IV by slow push may be given for rigors from interferon.

(3) Methylprednisolone acetate 80 to 160 mg appears to be well tolerated.

d. **Responses.** Chest tube drainage, together with instillation of one of the agents discussed in Section I.C.2.b or I.C.2.c, controls pleural effusions more than 75% of the time. The durations of response are often short with a median between 3 and 6 months unless the patient's systemic disease comes under adequate control. In that circumstance, the effusion may not recur for years or at least until the systemic disease once more emerges.

e. **Side effects** common to most agents include chest pain, fever, and occasional hypotension. These effects are usually not severe and may be controlled by standard symptomatic management. Fever after pleurodesis is usually not due to infection.

3. **Pleural catheter placement** is another option for patients who have recurrent pleural effusions. It involves placement of indwelling catheter in the pleural space. Patients must be willing to care for the catheter on an outpatient basis but in contrast to pleurodesis, it allows the patient to remain as outpatient. It has similar efficacy to pleurodesis, but carries an added risk of infection owing to the indwelling catheter.

4. **Thoracotomy and pleural stripping** may be tried subsequently for effusions refractory to other medical treatment.

II. **Peritoneal effusions**

A. **Causes.** Malignant peritoneal effusions usually occur in association with diffuse seeding of the peritoneal surface with small malignant deposits. The impairment of subphrenic lymphatic or portal venous flow may result in peritoneal effusions. Alternatively, it has been postulated that a "capillary leak" phenomenon mediated by tumor cells or immune effector cells could be a contributing factor. Carcinoma of the ovary is the most commonly associated malignancy in women, whereas in men, gastrointestinal carcinomas are most common. Other neoplasms that may cause peritoneal effusions include carcinoma of unknown primary, lymphoma, mesothelioma, and carcinomas of the uterus and breast. Liver metastasis by itself, unless it is far advanced, is not usually associated with symptomatic peritoneal effusions.

B. Diagnosis

1. **Symptoms and signs.** Patients may be completely symptom-free or have so much fluid that they have severe abdominal distention, abdominal pain, and respiratory distress. In the presence of peritoneal metastases, there may be abnormal bowel motility that at times resembles a paralytic ileus and may result in loss of appetite, early satiety, nausea, and vomiting. On examination, the lower abdomen and flanks bulge when the patient is supine. Confirmatory signs include shifting dullness, a fluid wave, diminished bowel sounds, or the "puddle sign" (periumbilical dullness when the patient rests on knees and elbows).

2. **Radiographic studies.** Ascites may be suggested on a recumbent film of the abdomen, although radiographs are less sensitive than computed tomography (CT) or ultrasound in detecting fluid. CT is also helpful in defining whether there are enlarged retroperitoneal nodes, tumor masses in the abdomen or pelvis, or liver metastases in association with the ascites.

3. **Paracentesis** is used to distinguish malignancy from other causes of peritoneal effusions, including congestive heart failure, hepatic cirrhosis, and peritonitis. Malignant cells are found in approximately 50% of patients in whom the effusion is due to malignancy. Other tests are less reliable, and treatment decisions must often be based on incomplete data. Elevated LDH and protein levels, along with a negative Gram stain and cultures, are supportive but nonspecific for malignancy. The use of monoclonal antibodies to identify tumor cells is still experimental.

C. Therapy. As with malignant pleural effusions, malignant peritoneal effusions as a rule are optimally treated with effective systemic therapy. (The possible exception to this is peritoneal effusions from carcinoma of the ovary. In this circumstance, there may be advantage to intraperitoneal therapy, at least as one component of therapy, because most systemic disease is on the peritoneal surface.) If the patient is resistant to all further systemic treatment, regional treatment should be tried, but the likelihood of success is less and the complications greater with peritoneal effusions than with pleural effusions. Success probably is less because of the greater likelihood of loculations to areas inaccessible to therapy and the impossibility of obliterating the peritoneal space in the same way that the pleural space can be obliterated. Complications are greater because of the increase in adhesions caused by instillation therapy and the resultant increase in obstructive bowel problems.

1. **Paracentesis** may be helpful in acutely relieving intraabdominal pressure. If the ascites has caused impairment

of respiration, paracentesis may give temporary relief. Rapid withdrawal of large volumes of fluid (more than 1 L) can result in hypotension and shock, however, and if frequent paracenteses are performed, severe hypoalbuminemia and electrolyte imbalance may result. Repeated procedures could also subject the patient to increased risk of peritonitis or bowel injury. This procedure thereby results in only temporary benefit.

2. Bed rest and dietary salt restriction, although helpful in the treatment of various nonmalignant causes of ascites, are of less benefit in malignant ascites.

3. Diuretics may be helpful in reducing ascites, but care must be taken not to be too vigorous in attempts at diuresis because of the possibility of dehydration and hypotension. A reasonable choice of diuretic is a combination of either furosemide 40 mg or hydrochlorothiazide 50 to 100 mg/day and spironolactone 50 to 100 mg/day.

4. Intracavitary therapy. Radioisotopes, cytotoxic drugs, and sclerosing agents have been used with some benefit for treating malignant ascites, but overall probably fewer than half the number of patients have a satisfactory response. The utility of these agents has less to do with direct tumor cytotoxicity and more with the induction of a local inflammatory response with subsequent sclerosis. The radioactive isotopes gold 198 and phosphorus 32 should be used only by those with experience and appropriate certification. Cytotoxic agents such as fluorouracil are associated with less risk to the person administering the therapy.

a. Method. The peritoneal fluid should be drained slowly through a Tenckhoff catheter over a 24- to 36-hour period. The potential distribution of the therapeutic agent can be determined by instilling ^{99m}Tc-glucoheptonate macroaggregated albumin in 50 mL of saline and obtaining an abdominal scintigram. Two liters of warmed 1.5% peritoneal dialysate solution is instilled, allowed to remain for 2 hours, and then drained. The chemotherapeutic agent is next mixed with 2 L of fresh 1.5% dialysate solution containing 1,000 U of heparin/L. After warming, this solution is instilled through the Tenckhoff catheter. For some agents, draining after 4 hours is recommended.

b. Agents

    (1) Cisplatin 50 to 100 mg/m^2 (especially for carcinoma of the ovary). Drainage is optional. Saline diuresis is recommended. Dosages higher than 100 mg/m^2 should not be used without protection by IV sodium thiosulfate. Cisplatin is repeated every 3 weeks.

    (2) Fluorouracil 1,000 mg (total dose) in normal saline with 25 mEq of sodium bicarbonate/L. Drainage is optional. Treatment is given on days 1 to 4 monthly.

    (3) Mitoxantrone 10 mg/m^2. Drainage is optional. This dose has been administered on a weekly basis, although white blood cell counts must be monitored.

(4) **Interferon** α 50 × 10⁶ U (for ovarian cancer). Drainage is optional. This dose has been administered weekly for 4 weeks or longer. Patients should be premedicated with acetaminophen before and every 4 hours thereafter on the day of therapy.

(5) **Floxuridine** (FUDR) 3 g in 1.5 to 2 L of normal saline given daily for 3 days every 3 to 4 weeks has been used in colon, gastric, and ovarian cancer.

(6) **Other agents** that have been used IP include carboplatin, paclitaxel, methotrexate, cytosine arabinoside, etoposide, bleomycin, thiotepa, and doxorubicin. High-dose interleukin-2 (IL-2) with lymphokine-activated killer cells has shown activity in ovarian and colorectal cancer but at the cost of significant toxicity, including peritoneal fibrosis, which in general has prevented the administration of more than one or two cycles. Lower-dose IL-2, 6 × 10⁶ IU, on days 1 and 7 has been used successfully.

5. **Peritoneal–venous shunts** (Denver shunt, LeVeen shunt) may offer palliative relief for refractory ascites because recurrent paracentesis leads to infection and leakage of peritoneal fluid through the paracentesis sites. Potential disadvantages are shunt occlusion, the systemic dissemination of cancer, and disseminated intravascular coagulation.

III. **Pericardial effusions.** Although 5% to 10% of patients dying with disseminated malignancy have cardiac or pericardial metastases, far fewer have symptomatic pericardial effusion. However, although malignant pericardial effusions are not particularly common, they are of great importance because of their potential to cause acute cardiac tamponade and death.

A. **Causes.** The most common neoplasms causing pericardial effusions are carcinomas of the lung and breast, lymphomas, and melanoma.

B. **Diagnosis**

1. **Clinical diagnosis.** Patients with developing cardiac tamponade may exhibit a variety of grave symptoms including extreme anxiety, dyspnea, orthopnea, precordial chest pain, cough, and hoarseness. On examination, they are likely to have engorged neck veins, generalized edema, tachycardia, distant heart tones, lateral displacement of the cardiac apex, a low systolic blood pressure and low pulse pressure, and a paradoxical pulse. They may also have tachypnea and a pericardial friction rub.

2. **Electrocardiogram** (ECG) may show nonspecific low-voltage, T-wave abnormalities, elevation of ST segments, and ventricular alternans or the more specific total electrical alternans. Premature beats and atrial fibrillation also occur.

3. **Chest radiograph** typically shows an enlarged cardiac silhouette, often with a bulging appearance suggestive of an effusion ("water-bottle heart"). There is frequently an associated pleural effusion.

4. **Echocardiography** can confirm the diagnosis and provide important information on the location of the effusion within the pericardium.

5. Pericardiocentesis reveals neoplastic cells on cytologic examination in more than 75% of patients.

C. Treatment

1. Volume expansion and vasopressor support are applied (if necessary) to maintain blood pressure. Adequate oxygenation must be maintained. Diuretics are contraindicated.

2. Pericardiocentesis under ECG and blood pressure monitoring should be done in emergent circumstances. If the patient can be stabilized or in cases of pericardial effusion without tamponade, pericardiocentesis under two-dimensional ECG is preferable because it significantly reduces the incidence of cardiac laceration, arrhythmia, and tension pneumothorax as a complication of the procedure.

3. Instillation of chemotherapeutic or sclerosing agents. Because pain may be associated with the intrapericardial therapy, lidocaine (Xylocaine) 100 mg may be administered intrapericardially as a local anesthetic. (Check with the cardiologist on the safety for each patient.) After the cytotoxic or sclerosing agent is instilled, the pericardial catheter is clamped for 1 to 2 hours and then allowed to drain. One of the following agents may be used:

a. Fluorouracil 500 to 1,000 mg in aqueous solution as supplied commercially. This dose is generally not repeated.

b. Thiotepa 25 mg/m^2 in 10 mL of normal saline may be preferred in tumor deemed sensitive to alkylating agents. Myelosuppression may occur. The dose is usually not repeated.

Complications of intrapericardial therapy include arrhythmias, pain, and fever.

4. Radiotherapy with radioisotopes or 2,000 to 4,000 cGy of external-beam therapy may help control effusions.

5. Systemic chemotherapy (with standard regimens) after pericardiocentesis is a possible alternative for newly diagnosed, potentially responsive malignancies such as lymphomas. Chemotherapy, intrapericardial or systemic, or radiotherapy controls the effusion for at least 30 days in 60% to 70% of patients.

6. Surgery to create a pericardial window may be necessary and can be effective for several months. It is not recommended, however, unless simpler measures fail.

IV. Malignant subarachnoid infiltrates

A. Causes. Leptomeningeal involvement with non–central nervous system cancer is an uncommon complication of most neoplasms, although in children with acute lymphocytic leukemia who have not received prophylactic treatment, the incidence approaches 50%. Of the nonleukemic diseases, breast carcinoma and lymphomas (primarily Burkitt's and T-cell lymphoblastic) account for approximately 30% each in cases of malignant subarachnoid infiltrates. Carcinoma of the lung and melanoma account for 10% to 12% each.

B. Diagnosis

1. Clinical diagnosis. Patients commonly present with headache, change in mental status, cranial nerve dysfunction, or spinal root–derived pain, paresthesia, or weakness.

Any onset of change in neurologic status, particularly of cerebral, cranial nerve, or spinal root origin, should alert the clinician to the possibility of subarachnoid infiltrates.

2. Diagnostic studies

a. CT or magnetic resonance imaging (MRI) of the head should be done to look for any intracranial mass. If none is present, a lumbar puncture should be done.

b. A lumbar puncture is done, and the following are evaluated or performed:

- Opening pressure
- Cytology of centrifugal specimen for malignant cells
- Total cell count and differential
- Cerebrospinal fluid (CSF) chemistry, including glucose and protein
- Microbiologic studies: India ink or cryptococcal antigen determination, Gram stain, cultures (routine, acid-fast, fungi), serum toxoplasma titer, CSF Epstein-Barr virus (EBV) polymerase chain reaction and other special studies as indicated by the clinical situation.

c. Magnetic resonance imaging (MRI) (or less commonly, myelography with CT follow-up) is performed if signs or symptoms of cord compression are present.

C. Treatment. Malignant subarachnoid infiltrates may be treated with radiotherapy, intrathecal chemotherapy, or a combination of the two.

1. Radiotherapy. The radiation field is usually limited to the most involved field (frequently the brain), and intrathecal chemotherapy is used to control the infiltrates elsewhere. This technique is used even though the entire neuraxis is usually involved because total craniospinal irradiation causes severe myelosuppression, which limits the patient's tolerance to concurrent or subsequent cytotoxic chemotherapy.

2. Chemotherapy may be administered by lumbar puncture or preferably into a surgically implanted (Ommaya) reservoir that communicates with the lateral ventricle. The latter has the advantages of being easily accessible in patients who require repeated treatments and of giving a better distribution of drug than can be obtained through lumbar puncture. When the Ommaya reservoir is used, a volume of CSF equal to that to be injected (6 to 10 mL) should be removed through the reservoir with a small-caliber needle. The chemotherapy should then be given as a slow injection. When the chemotherapy is given through lumbar puncture, the volume of injection (usually 7 to 10 mL) should be greater than that of the CSF withdrawn, so as to have a higher closing than opening pressure. This method facilitates distribution of the drug and minimizes post–lumbar puncture headache. The most commonly used drugs for intrathecal therapy are the following:

a. Methotrexate 12 mg/m^2 (maximum 15 mg) twice weekly until the CSF clears of malignant cells, then monthly.

b. Cytarabine 30 mg/m^2 (maximum 50 mg) twice weekly until the CSF clears of malignant cells, then monthly.

c. Liposomal cytarabine 50 mg (total dose) is given every 14 days for 2 doses. If the CSF clears, give 50 mg every 14 days for two additional doses. Then give 50 mg every 4 weeks for two additional doses (total of six doses).

d. Thiotepa 2 to 10 mg/m^2 twice weekly until the CSF clears of malignant cells, then monthly.

Each of the agents is given in preservative-free saline or, if available, buffered preservative-free diluent similar to Elliot's B solution. Any subsequent flush solution should be of similar composition. **Other drugs used to treat effusions (e.g., fluorouracil, mechlorethamine, or radioisotopes) must *not* be used to treat meningeal disease.**

D. Response to treatment. Most patients with meningeal leukemia or lymphoma respond to a combination of radiotherapy and intrathecal chemotherapy. Carcinomas are less likely to improve, but mild to moderate improvement may be seen in up to 50% of patients.

E. Complications. Aseptic meningitis or arachnoiditis, seizures, acute encephalopathy, myelopathy, leukoencephalopathy, and radicular neuropathy may result from intrathecal chemotherapy with or without radiotherapy. Bone marrow suppression is not usually severe unless the patient undergoes spinal irradiation or systemic chemotherapy as well. Oral leucovorin can be given after the intrathecal methotrexate (10 mg leucovorin PO every 6 hours for six to eight doses, starting either at the same time or 24 hours after the methotrexate) to prevent marrow toxicity. Serious complications are infrequent, however, and in patients with advanced metastatic disease, they are usually not a major problem.

SUGGESTED READINGS
Pleural Effusions

Andrews CO, Gora W. Pleural effusions: pathophysiology and management. *Ann Pharmacother* 1994;28:894–903.

de Campos JR, Vargas FS, de Campos Werebe E, et al. Thoracoscopy talc poudrage: a 15-year experience. *Chest* 2001;119:801–806.

Chernow B, Sahn SA. Carcinomatous involvement of the pleura: an analysis of 96 patients. *Am J Med* 1977;63:695.

Diacon AH, Wyser C, Bollinger CT, et al. Prospective randomized comparison of thoracoscopic talc poudrage under local anesthesia versus bleomycin instillation for pleurodesis in malignant pleural effusions. *Am J Respir Crit Care Med* 2000;162:1445–1449.

Fuller DK. Bleomycin versus doxycyclines: a patient-oriented, approach to pleurodesis. *Ann Pharmacother* 1993;27:794.

Goldman CA, Skinnider LF, Maksymiuk AW. Interferon instillation for malignant pleural effusions. *Ann Oncol* 1993;4:141–145.

Hamed H, Fentiman IS, Chaudary MA, et al. Comparison of intracavitary bleomycin and talc for control of pleural effusions secondary to carcinoma of the breast. *Br J Surg* 1989;76:1266–1267.

Herrington JD. Chemical pleurodesis, with doxycycline 1 g. *Pharmacotherapy* 1996;16:290–295.

Johnson WW. The malignant pleural effusion: a review of cytopathologic diagnoses of 584 specimens from 472 consecutive patients. *Cancer* 1985;56:905.

Kessinger A, Wigton RS. Intracavitary bleomycin and tetracycline in the management of malignant pleural effusions: a randomized study. *J Surg Oncol* 1997;36:81–83.

Patz EF Jr, McAdams HP, Erasmus JJ, et al. Sclerotherapy for malignant pleural effusions: a prospective randomized trial of bleomycin vs. doxycycline with small-bore catheter drainage. *Chest* 1998;113:1305–1311.

Putnam JB Jr, Light RW, Rodriguez RM, et al. A randomized comparison of indwelling pleural catheter and doxycycline pleurodesis in the management of malignant pleural effusions. *Cancer* 1999;86(10):1992–1999.

Van Hoff DD, LiVolsi V. Diagnostic reliability of needle biopsy of the parietal pleura: a review of 272 biopsies. *Am J Clin Pathol* 1975;64:200.

Walker-Renard PB, Vaughan LM, Sahn SA. Chemical pleurodesis for malignant pleural effusions. *Ann Intern Med* 1994;120:56–64.

Weissberg D. Bleomycin and talc for control of pleural effusions. *Br J Surg* 1990;77:955.

Peritoneal Effusions

Berek JS, Hacker NF, Lichtenstein A, et al. Intraperitoneal recombinant alpha-interferon for "salvage" immunotherapy in stage III epithelial ovarian cancer. A Gynecologic Oncology Group study. *Semin Oncol* 1986;13(Suppl 2):61.

Lacy JH, Wieman TJ, Shivley EH. Management of malignant ascites. *Surg Gynecol Obstet* 1984;159:397.

Lissoni P, Mandala M, Curigliano G, et al. Progress report on the palliative therapy of 100 patients with neoplastic effusions by intracavitary low-dose interleukin-2. *Oncology* 2001;60:308–312.

Muggia FM, Jeffers S, Muderspach L, et al. Phase I/II study of intraperitoneal floxuridine and platinums (cisplatin and/or carboplatin). *Gynecol Oncol* 1997;66:290–294.

Muggia FM, Liu PY, Alberts DS, et al. Intraperitoneal mitoxantrone or floxuridine: effects on time-to-failure and survival in patients with minimal residual ovarian cancer after second-look laparotomy: a randomized phase II study by the Southwest Oncology Group. *Gynecol Oncol* 1996;61:395–402.

Nicoletto MO, Fiorentino MW, Viante O, et al. Experience with intraperitoneal alpha2a interferon. *Oncology* 1992;49:467–473.

Speyer JL, Beller U, Colombo N, et al. Intraperitoneal carboplatin: favorable results in women with minimal residual ovarian cancer after cisplatin therapy. *J Clin Oncol* 1990;8:1335–1341.

Sugarbaker PH, Gianola FJ, Speyer JC, et al. Prospective, randomized trial of intravenous versus intraperitoneal 5-fluorouracil in patients with advanced primary colon or rectal cancer. *Surgery* 1985;95:414.

Pericardial Effusions

Buzaid AC, Garewal HS, Greenberg BR. Managing malignant pericardial effusion. *West J Med* 1989;150:174–179.

Callahan JA, Seward JB, Nishimura RA, et al. Two-dimensional echocardiographically guided pericardiocentesis: experience in 117 consecutive patients. *Am J Cardiol* 1985;55:476–479.

Helms SR, Carlson MD. Cardiovascular emergencies. *Semin Oncol* 1989;16:463.

Liu G, Crump M, Gross PE, et al. Prospective comparison of the sclerosing agents doxycycline and bleomycin for the primary management of malignant pericardial effusion and cardiac tamponade. *J Clin Oncol* 1996;14:3141–3147.

Maher ER, Buckman R. Intrapericardial installation of bleomycin in malignant pericardial effusion. *Am Heart J* 1986;111:613–614.

Shepherd FA, Ginsberg JS, Evans WK, et al. Tetracycline sclerosis in the management of pericardial effusion. *J Clin Oncol* 1985;3:1678–1682.

Malignant Subarachnoid Infiltrates

Glantz MJ, Jaeckle KA, Chamberlain MC, et al. A randomized controlled trial comparing intrathecal sustained-release cytarabine (Depocyt) to intrathecal methotrexate in patients with neoplastic meningitis from solid tumors. *Clin Cancer Res* 1999;5:3394–3402.

Gutin PH, Levi JA, Wiernik PH, et al. Treatment of malignant meningeal disease with intrathecal thiotepa: a phase II study. *Cancer Treat Rep* 1977;61:885–887.

Jaeckle KA, Phuphanich S, van den Bent MJ, et al. Intrathecal treatment of neoplastic meningitis due to breast cancer with a slow-release formulation of cytarabine. *Br J Cancer* 2001;84:157–163.

Olson ME, Chernik NL, Posner JB. Infiltration of the leptomeninges by systemic cancer. *Arch Neurol* 1974;30:122–137.

CHAPTER 32

Cancer Pain

Michael J. Fisch and Charles S. Cleeland

Eighty-five percent of patients with cancer could be free of significant pain with the techniques we have available today. Most pain from cancer can be adequately controlled with analgesics given by mouth. When this is not possible, various more sophisticated pain management techniques can provide good pain control. Unfortunately, poorly controlled pain and/or analgesic side effects have significant effects on the quality of life of patients and their families. For example, symptoms such as depressed mood, fatigue, anorexia, and sleep disturbance are associated with poor pain control. Likewise, opioid side effects may cause chronic nausea, anorexia, constipation, dehydration, sedation, and confusion. Consequently, overall performance status and adherence to anticancer treatment regimens may deteriorate in the presence of poor pain management. Desperate patients and families may seek relief through unproven therapies or even from physician-assisted suicide. Improving the practice of anticipating, evaluating, and treating pain will benefit most patients.

I. **Prevalence, severity, and risk for pain.** Most cancer patients with terminal disease need expert pain management; between 60% and 80% of such patients have significant pain. Pain is also a problem for many patients much earlier in the course of their disease. Patients with months or years to live may be similarly compromised by poorly controlled pain. Sometimes chronic pain will be expressed by the patient in confusing terms (*stiffness, nagging*) or masquerade as other symptoms (fatigue, apathy, anxiety, anorexia). For this reason, the estimates of the prevalence and impact of chronic pain in this population are probably conservative. Nevertheless, in the United States, 60% of all outpatients with metastatic disease have cancer-related pain, and one-third of them report pain so severe that it significantly impairs their quality of life. Multicenter studies indicate that approximately 40% of outpatients with cancer pain do not receive analgesics potent enough to manage their pain. Minority patients, female patients, and older patients are at greatest risk for poorly controlled pain.

II. **Etiology of cancer pain**

A. **Direct tumor involvement** is the most common cause of pain, and is present in approximately two-thirds of those with pain from metastatic cancer. Tumor invasion of bone is the physical cause of pain in approximately 50% of these patients. The remaining 50% of patients experience tumor-related pain that is due to nerve compression, tumor infiltration, or involvement of the gastrointestinal tract or soft tissue.

B. **Persistent pain after treatment** from long-term effects of surgery, radiotherapy, and chemotherapy, accounts for an additional 20% of all who report pain with cancer, with a small

residual group experiencing pain from non–cancer-related conditions. Chronic pain is a common problem for cancer survivors.
C. Complex, chronic pain. Most patients with advanced cancer have **pain at multiple sites** caused by multiple mechanisms. Pain **production** occurs either by stimulation of peripheral pain receptors or by damage to afferent nerve fibers. Peripheral pain receptors can be stimulated by pressure, compression, and traction as well as by disease-related chemical changes. Pain due to stimulation of pain receptors is called *nociceptive pain*. Damage to visceral, somatic, or autonomic nerve trunks produces *neurogenic* or *neuropathic pain.* Neuropathic pain is thought to be caused by spontaneous activity in nerves damaged by disease or treatment. Patients with cancer often simultaneously experience nociceptive and neuropathic pain. In addition to evaluating the broad possible causes of pain production, the evaluating clinician should also consider the relevant mechanisms of pain **perception** and **expression** (Fig. 32.1). Pain perception refers to the transmission of the nociception to the central nervous system (CNS). Peripheral nerve fibers include myelinated Aδ fibers that are responsible for the transmission of sharp pain and unmyelinated C fibers that carry dull and burning pain. These primary sensory afferents have their cell bodies in the dorsal horn, where the pathways decussate and ascend along the spinothalamic tracts to the thalamus and cortex. Repetitive or continuous stimulation of the peripheral nerves can increase the excitability of the secondary neurons and spread the neurologic region of pain perception and transmission. The *N*-methyl-D-aspartate (NMDA) receptor is involved in the neurobiology of this "wind-up" phenomenon as well as in the development of tolerance to opioid analgesics. Understanding this biology of pain perception helps one account for the observation that some patients experience pain that endures even after the tumor or injury has resolved, and

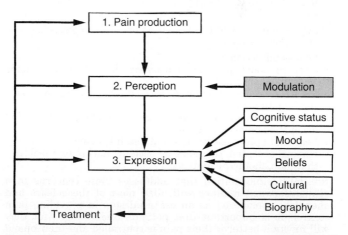

Figure 32.1.   Schema of the pain construct. (Courtesy of Dr. Eduardo Bruera.)

sometimes the pain is more severe than one might expect from the nerve or tissue insult itself. Of course, the clinician can directly observe only pain expression; the production and perception of the pain can be inferred only from indirect clues. Pain expression can be influenced by multiple factors (mood, cultural beliefs, etc.). For this reason, effective pain assessment and management necessitates a comprehensive understanding of the patient as a person.

III. Assessment of pain. Proper pain management requires a clear understanding of the characteristics of pain production, perception, and expression as described in the preceding text. The changing expression of cancer pain demands repeated assessment because new causes of pain can emerge rapidly and pain severity can increase quickly. In patients with advanced disease, pain from multiple causes is the rule and not the exception. A careful history includes asking questions concerning the location, severity, and quality of the pain as well as the aspects of the patient's daily routine that may be adversely affected by the pain experience.

A. Pain severity. Inadequate pain assessment and poor physician–patient communication about pain are major barriers to good pain care. Physicians and nurses tend to underestimate pain intensity, especially when it is severe. Patients whose physicians underestimate their pain are at high risk for poor pain management and compromised function. A small minority of patients with cancer may complain of pain in a dramatic manner, but **many more patients underreport the severity of their pain and the lack of adequate pain relief.**

Several studies have confirmed that there are multiple reasons for this hesitancy to report pain, including the following:

- Reluctance to acknowledge that the disease is progressing
- Reluctance to divert the physician's attention from treating the disease
- Reluctance to tell the physician that pain treatments are not working

Patients may not want to be put on opioid analgesics because of the following reasons:

- Fear of addiction
- Concern about possible neurotoxic side effects of opioids (sedation, confusion)
- Frustration over gastrointestinal side effects of opioids (nausea, constipation, anorexia)
- Fear that using opioids "too early" will endanger pain relief when they have more pain
- Fear that opioid use means that death is near
- Having accepted religious or societal norms or teachings that pain should be endured

Presenting information that addresses these concerns in a straightforward manner will allay most of these fears and should be considered as an essential step in providing pain control. It is important that patients understand that they will function better if their pain is controlled and their opioid side effects are prevented or managed effectively. Patient education materials available from state cancer pain initiatives and from the National Cancer Institute (www.cancer.gov), American Cancer Society (www.cancer.org), the NCCN (National Comprehensive Cancer Network) (www.nccn.org), and the American Society of Clinical Oncology (www.plwc.org) can be very useful for both patients and families and should be given to patients when they develop pain.

Communication about pain is greatly aided by having patients use a scale to rate the severity of their pain. A simple rating scale ranges from 0 to 10, with 0 being "no pain" and 10 being pain "as bad as you can imagine". Used properly, pain severity scales can be invaluable for titrating analgesics and monitoring increases in pain with progressive disease. Mild pain is often well tolerated with minimal impact on a patient's activities. However, there is a threshold beyond which pain is especially disruptive. This threshold has been reached when patients rate the severity of their pain at 5 or greater on a 0 to 10 scale. When pain is too great (7 or greater on this scale), it becomes the primary focus of attention and compromises most activities that are not directly related to pain. Although it may not be possible to eliminate pain totally, reducing its severity to 4 or less ought to be a minimum standard of pain therapy.

In some instances, patients may develop chronically high levels of pain expression that do not respond to appropriate initial analgesic dosing and coprescribing of medications to prevent nausea and constipation. The proper care of this subset of patients often requires a multidisciplinary approach and includes regular administration of pain medication plus counseling and sometimes use of antidepressants or anxiolytic agents. Skillful switching of opioid medications (often called *opioid rotation* or *opioid switching*) can produce a more favorable ratio of analgesia to opioid side effects. Interventional pain procedures may be appropriate in selected cases as well. Such procedures may include nerve blocks (such as a celiac plexus block) or neuraxial delivery of opioids and other adjuvant medications (such as epidural or intrathecal therapies).

B. Diagnostic steps. Those who treat patients with cancer should be familiar with the common pain syndromes associated with the disease:

1. Having the patient show the area of pain on a drawing of a human figure aids identification of the syndrome. This can be particularly helpful in indicating areas of referred pain that commonly coincide with nerve compression.

2. Careful questioning concerning the characteristics of the pain is essential for physical diagnosis. For example, pain characterized as "burning" or "shooting" may indicate neuropathic pain.

3. In addition to severity, these characteristics include the temporal pattern of the pain (constant or episodic) and its quality. Episodic or "incident" pain (such as severe pain when standing) requires a different strategy for management than chronic pain.

4. Other important characteristics of pain are its relationship to physical activity and what seems to alleviate the pain.

5. Physical examination includes examination of the painful area as well as neurologic and orthopedic

assessment. A brief assessment of mood and cognition is also appropriate. Impaired cognition can confound symptom assessment dramatically.

6. Because bone metastases are a common cause of pain and pain can occur with changes in bone density that is not detectable on radiographs, bone scans can be helpful. Magnetic resonance imaging (MRI) is useful in the evaluation of retroperitoneal, paravertebral, and pelvic areas as well as the base of the skull.

C. The impact of pain on the patient. When pain is of moderate or greater severity, we can assume that it has a negative impact on the patient's quality of life. That impact, including problems with sleep and depression, must be evaluated and treated when appropriate. A reduced number of hours of sleep as compared with the last pain-free interval, difficulties with sleep onset, frequent interruptions of sleep, and early morning awakening suggest the need for appropriate pharmacologic intervention. Just as patients hesitate to report severe pain, they may hesitate to report depression. Family caregivers can often provide important clues regarding the presence or absence of a mood disturbance. Significant depression should be treated. Treatment approaches may include use of antidepressants, counseling, and/or referral to a behavioral health specialist. Sometimes a patient will accept only one of the suggested options, thereby requiring some degree of flexibility on the part of the clinician in order to achieve the best results.

It is important to make an attempt to differentiate between physical pain and psychological distress. Accurate pain assessment in patients who are cognitively impaired, particularly those with agitation, may be extremely difficult. A small number of patients in severe psychosocial distress express their concerns as a report of physical pain. These patients present with symptoms that may be attributable to either agitated delirium or pain. Although it is important to recognize severe somatization and to provide psychiatric referral or counseling to these patients, it is equally important to recognize true physical pain. Often, the treatment approach for this difficult situation includes concomitant provision of pain treatment(s) and management of the patient's underlying psychological distress.

D. Addiction/aberrant drug-taking behaviors. Some patients with alcohol or drug addiction may request analgesics for their psychological effects or may have aberrant drug-taking behaviors. Aberrant drug-taking behaviors may include requests for frequent, early renewals, unauthorized dose escalations, reports of lost or stolen prescriptions, adamant requests for specific medications, and acquisition of similar drugs from other medical sources. Patients who are recovered alcoholics or drug abusers may also be difficult to treat because of their fear of exposure to opioid analgesics and potential relapse of addiction problems. In any case, these behaviors or fears should be discussed openly and in nonjudgmental terms with the patient. Ultimately, an agreement should be reached about the use of opioids for the management of pain (as opposed to mood alterations) and some details about the expectations and responsibilities of both the physician and the patient should be delineated. With this group of patients, long-acting opioids or continuous infusion is often preferable to short-acting opioids or patient-controlled analgesia. Although their care is more complex, patients with drug or alcohol addiction should not be denied appropriate pain medications.

IV. Treatment

   A. General aspects. All health care professionals who see patients with cancer should be familiar with standard guidelines for management of cancer pain such as those published by the NCCN or the AHRQ (Agency for Healthcare Research and Quality). An example of a cancer pain practice guideline is shown in Table 32.1. This guideline incorporates basic principles of cancer pain assessment, initial treatment, and routine management of opioid side effects.

   The prompt relief of pain from cancer frequently involves the use of simultaneously rather than serially administered combinations of drug and other adjunctive therapies. Identification of a treatable neoplasm as a factor in pain production calls for appropriate radiotherapy (e.g., to bone metastases), chemotherapy, or, in some instances, surgical debulking. Until such treatment can be effective (this may take days to weeks), the patient's pain must be managed with analgesics with or without other specific interventional pain procedures. In some instances, analgesics are the only effective palliative treatment available because of the patient's condition, the physical basis of the pain, or limited treatment options. The principles of pharmacologic management of pain are evolving through studies of analgesic effectiveness and research on the use of combinations of palliative medications.

   There is a growing consensus concerning the types of drugs to use, their routes of administration, and how best to schedule them. The first step is the choice of analgesic drug to be used (nonopioid, opioid, or a combination of both). The second step is the choice of adjuvant drugs, which can increase analgesic effectiveness and can produce other palliative effects to counter the disruptive consequences of pain.

   B. Nonsteroidal anti-inflammatory drugs (NSAIDs)

   1. Mechanism of action and selection of agents. NSAIDs constitute most nonopioid analgesics. Their effect on the inflammatory process is a key to their analgesic property. Tumor growth produces inflammatory and mechanical effects in adjacent tissues that can trigger the release of prostaglandins, bradykinin, and serotonin, which in turn may precipitate or exacerbate pain in the surrounding tissues. Prostaglandin-mediated actions on peripheral receptors probably include both direct activation and sensitization to other analgesic substances. Prostaglandins are frequently associated with painful bone metastasis because of their involvement in bone reabsorption. The NSAIDs appear to exert their analgesic, antipyretic, and anti-inflammatory actions by blocking the synthesis of prostaglandins. Table 32.2 gives the usual starting doses and dose ranges for several commonly used NSAIDs. There is new public concern about NSAIDs due to reports of cardiac toxicity associated with celecoxib as well as other agents in this class. It is appropriate to discuss the cardiac

Table 32.1. An example of a pain practice guideline

A. Comprehensive pain assessment
1. Evaluation of pain. Determine level using 0–10 intensity scale, location, onset, duration, frequency, quality (somatic, visceral, neuropathic), history, etiology, associated symptoms, what modifies the pain, side effects associated with treatment of pain, and response to other pain medications. No pain (0) Mild (1–3) Moderate (4–6) Severe (7–10)
2. Evaluation of past medical history (oncologic or other significant medical illnesses) to include medication history
3. Physical examination
4. Evaluation of relevant laboratory and imaging studies
5. Evaluation of risk factors for undertreatment of pain, including underreporting, extremes of age, gender, cultural barriers, communication barriers, and a history of substance abuse
6. Evaluation of psychosocial issues (patient distress, family support, psychiatric history, special issues relating to pain [meaning of pain for patient/family, patient/family knowledge of and beliefs surrounding pain])

B. Overall management plans
1. If pain = 0, reassess at each subsequent visit or interaction
2. Manage pain related to oncologic emergencies, if any
   a. Such pain requires assessment and treatment (e.g., surgery, steroids, radiotherapy, antibiotics) along with an emergent consultation
   b. Oncologic emergencies include
      - Bowel obstruction/perforation
      - Brain metastasis
      - Leptomeningeal metastasis
      - Fracture or impending fracture of weight-bearing bone
      - Epidural metastasis/spinal cord compression
      - Pain related to infection
3. Manage non–emergency-related pain

C. Management of non–emergency-related pain
1. If pain = 1–3
   - Nonsteroidal anti-inflammatory drugs (including COX-2 agents) and acetaminophen. If ineffective, opioids (hydrocodone scheduled or as needed)
   - Overall reassessment at each subsequent visit or interaction
2. If pain = 4–6
   - Oral opioids
   - Morphine 10 mg orally every 4 h as needed or scheduled
   - Oxycodone 5 mg orally every 4 h as needed or scheduled
   - Hydromorphone 2 mg orally every 4 h as needed or scheduled
   - Adjuvants: nonsteroidal anti-inflammatory drugs, antidepressants, antiepileptics, etc.
   - Overall reassessment in 24–48 h
3. If pain = 7–10 (possible pain crisis)
   - Oral opioids: morphine 20 mg orally every 4 h as needed (opioid naive)
   - 30% increase in current opioid regimen (sustained- and immediate-release [rescue] opioids)
   - Morphine, hydromorphone, or oxycodone for rescue dosing
   - Consider IV opioid titration (patient controlled analgesia [PCA] pump may be used to titrate)
   - Reassess frequently, based on clinical situation

D. Additional steps for pain that was rated 4–10
1. Re-evaluate opioid titration
2. Re-evaluate pain diagnosis
3. Consider consults from specialty services[a]
4. All patients receiving opioids should begin
   - Bowel regimen (such as oral senna 1 tablet twice daily)
   - Antiemetics as needed (such as metoclopramide 10 mg 30 min before meals and at bedtime)
   - Educational activities regarding pain management
   - Psychosocial support as needed

Table 32.1. (*Continued*)

E. At the time of re-evaluation for patients whose pain was 4–10
1. If pain now = 1–3
   - Consider conversion to a sustained-release agent with rescue medications
   - Continue adjuvants or add them as needed
   - Reassess and modify side effects of pain treatment
   - Provide psychosocial support
   - Provide educational activities
   - Reassess pain every week until comfortable, then every visit
2. If pain now = 4–6
   - Continue opioid titration
   - Consider specific pain problems
   - Consider consults from specialty services[a]
   - Continue psychosocial support
   - Continue educational activities
3. If pain now = 7–10[b] (possible pain crisis)
   - Continue opioid titration
   - Re-evaluate working diagnosis
   - Consider specific pain problems
   - Obtain consults from specialty services[a]
   - Continue psychosocial support

[a]Postoperative Pain Service, Cancer Pain Section, Department of Symptom Control and Palliative Care, or other specialties as needed (i.e., radiotherapy).
[b]Some patients with chronic pain syndromes will report high pain scores on an ongoing basis. Generally, this situation is not a crisis.
This practice guideline was created by the National Comprehensive Cancer Network (NCCN) and modified by the University of Texas M.D. Anderson Cancer Center under the supervision of Allen Burton, M.D., and Charles Cleeland, Ph.D.

toxicity of these agents in the context of the risk/benefit ratio relative to the condition(s) for which they are being prescribed.

By virtue of their different mechanisms of action and toxicity profiles, NSAIDs and opioids are often administered together. Enteric-coated aspirin is one of the first-choice drugs for mild to moderate cancer pain. Other NSAIDs

Table 32.2. **Starting doses and dose ranges of some nonsteroidal analgesic agents**

Drug	Starting Dose (mg)	Frequency	Dose Range
Aspirin	650	q4–6 h	Up to 1,300 mg q6 h
Choline magnesium trisalicylate	500	q6 h	Up to 1,000 mg q6 h
Diflunisal	500	q8–12 h	Up to 1,500 mg daily
Ibuprofen	400	q4–6 h	Up to 2,400 mg daily
Naproxen	250	q8–12 h	Up to 1,250 mg daily
Piroxicam	10	q12–24 h	Up to 20 mg daily
Tolmetin	400	q8 h	Up to 1,800 mg daily
Celecoxib	100	q24 h	Up to 400 mg daily

such as ibuprofen, diflunisal, naproxen, and choline magnesium trisalicylate (Trilisate) have established value in the management of clinical pain. These drugs are better tolerated than aspirin but are usually significantly more expensive. Individual differences in analgesic response to the various NSAIDs clearly occur but are not yet well understood.

Cyclooxygenase-2 (COX-2) NSAIDs are inhibitors of COX-2, the enzyme expressed in inflamed tissues, and have minimal or no effects on COX-1 (the enzyme expressed normally in the stomach and kidney). These NSAID drugs were widely used because of their once- or twice-daily dosing schedule and the roughly 50% relative reduction in significant gastrointestinal adverse events as compared with those induced by other NSAIDs. Rofecoxib was voluntarily withdrawn from the U.S. market in 2004 because of safety concerns of an increased risk for cardiovascular events, including heart attack and stroke. Celecoxib remains on the market as an analgesic. Acetaminophen is a peripherally acting analgesic that does not inhibit peripheral prostaglandin synthesis. Therefore, it does not have anti-inflammatory effects or the side effects associated with the use of NSAIDs. Acetaminophen may be safely combined with opioids and there is evidence that adding acetaminophen produces meaningful improvement in analgesic efficacy. Commercial preparations containing codeine or oxycodone and acetaminophen or aspirin are among the most widely prescribed scheduled analgesics and are frequently administered to patients with cancer.

2. Side effects. NSAIDs have a number of potentially serious side effects, including gastritis and gastrointestinal hemorrhage, bleeding due to platelet inhibition, renal failure, and cardiac toxicity. Most of these side effects are related to the prostaglandin-inhibitory effect of NSAIDs and are therefore common to all of these drugs. Renal failure due to the inhibition of renal medullary prostaglandins can be of particular concern for patients who are also receiving opioids. Decreased renal elimination of active opioid metabolites can result in somnolence, confusion, hallucinations, or generalized myoclonus. Therefore, kidney function should be monitored in patients receiving a combination of NSAIDs and opioids.

Gastrointestinal complications include gastric pain, nausea, vomiting, hemorrhage, and, in extreme cases, perforation. Gastrointestinal damage is mediated by prostaglandin inhibition. The most common form of nephrotoxicity associated with NSAIDs is renal failure, related to prostaglandin inhibition and consequent vasodilation. Hepatic injury has been reported with the use of aspirin, benoxaprofen, and phenylbutazone and, less commonly, with diclofenac, ibuprofen, indomethacin, naproxen, pirprofen, and sulindac. Sulindac, however, appears to be associated with a higher incidence of cholestasis.

NSAID use is also associated with various hypersensitivity reactions involving the skin (rash, eruption, itching), blood vessels (angioneurotic edema, vasomotor disorders), and respiratory system (rhinitis, asthma). In particular, aspirin may cause anaphylactic crisis, a syndrome characterized by dyspnea, sudden weakness, sweating, and collapse. Undesirable hematologic effects of NSAIDs include platelet dysfunction, aplastic anemia, and agranulocytosis. Factors often considered in the empiric selection of an NSAID for a given patient include its relative toxicity, cost, and dosage schedule and the patient's prior experience. The use of certain aspirin analogs (choline magnesium trisalicylate) has been associated with a low incidence of gastropathy and platelet dysfunction. The effects of NSAIDs used as single agents in the management of cancer pain are characterized by a ceiling effect, beyond which further increases in dose do not enhance analgesia.

C. **Opioid analgesics**

1. **When to start therapy.** The choice of using an opioid analgesic as opposed to a nonopioid analgesic follows from an assessment of the severity of pain. The decision is relatively easy when pain is mild (choose nonopioid) or severe (choose opioid, usually in combination with a nonopioid). The choice is more difficult when the patient reports moderate pain, especially when there is reason to suspect that the patient may be underreporting pain severity. Several studies have documented that many patients with cancer are inadequately managed because of the physician's reluctance to use opioids in dosages and with schedules known to be sufficient to relieve moderate pain.

Opioid analgesics should be prescribed promptly as soon as there is evidence that pain is not well controlled with nonopioid analgesics. When pain is moderate to severe, it is also appropriate to use a strong opioid as a first-line treatment for cancer pain.

2. **Schedule of treatment and selection of dose.** Except for a minority of patients whose pain is clearly episodic (often called *incidental pain*), analgesics should be given on an around-the-clock basis, with the time interval based on the duration of effectiveness of the drug and the patient's report of the duration of effectiveness. There is evidence that the total opioid requirement is lower when opioids are given on a scheduled basis, thereby preventing peaks of pain. Putting patients in the position of having to ask for medication or continually making a judgment about whether their pain is severe enough to take analgesics focuses their attention on pain, reminds them of their need for drugs, and allows pain to reach a severity not readily controlled by the same doses that would be effective with scheduled administration. Nevertheless, there may be large individual differences in the required dose of opioid, depending on such factors as the patient's opioid use history, activity level, and metabolism. The patient's report of pain severity and pain relief is the best guideline for opioid titration.

3. **The so-called "weak" opioids,** including codeine and hydrocodone, usually formulated in combination with acetaminophen or aspirin, can provide patients with good pain relief for long periods of time. As disease advances, oral

administration of the more potent opioids provides most patients with pain relief. There is considerable agreement that propoxyphene is not ideal for chronic use because of its low efficacy at commercially available doses and the presence of a toxic metabolite at higher doses that is a CNS stimulant, because it has a long serum half-life, and has no analgesic properties. Oral administration is preferred, but the physician must remain flexible to changes that are dictated by the patient's ability to use orally administered drugs. This may include the use of opioid and nonopioid suppositories and other alternative routes of administration (transdermal, sublingual, rectal, subcutaneous).

4. Oral morphine, either in an immediate- or sustained-release preparation, is the analgesic of choice for moderate to severe cancer pain. Long-acting formulations of morphine and other strong opioids may be convenient for both the patient and the health care staff, but they are usually most expensive. Immediate-release morphine is much cheaper, however, and is as effective for chronic pain relief when administered on a regular schedule. A typical starting dose for immediate-release oral morphine is 10 to 30 mg every 4 hours in patients who are not currently receiving opioids. When a patient is switching from another opioid (usually codeine or oxycodone) to morphine, it is important to calculate the equianalgesic morphine dose as a basis for determining the morphine-equivalent doses that are the threshold for pain control (Table 32.3). The starting dose may not be sufficient, and relatively rapid upward titration may be needed, especially if pain is severe.

Table 32.3.   Dose equivalence of selected opioids

Drug	Approximate Equianalgesic Dose	
	Oral	Parenteral
Morphine	30 mg q3–4 h[a]	10 mg q3–4 h
Hydromorphone	4–8 mg q3–4 h	1.5 mg q3–4 h
Levorphanol	4 mg q6–8 h	2 mg q6–8 h
Codeine[b]	130 mg q3–4 h	
Hydrocodone[b]	30 mg q3–4 h	
Oxycodone[b]	20 mg q3–4 h	
Transdermal fentanyl	25-μg/h patch = 8–22 mg/24 h IV or IM morphine sulfate = roughly 50 mg/day of oral morphine sulfate; 50-μg/h patch = roughly 60 mg MS-Contin q12 h	

[a]Slow-release formulations of oral morphine that are available have 8- to 12-h duration of analgesic action.
[b]Codeine, hydrocodone, and oxycodone are often given as combination products with aspirin, acetaminophen, or both.
Adapted from Weissman DE. *Handbook of Cancer Pain Management.* 4th ed. Madison: Wisconsin Cancer Pain Initiative, 1993.

The upward titration of morphine and other oral opioid analgesics can be done by giving a supplemental "boost" using 50% of the scheduled dose 2 hours after the scheduled dose if there is still significant pain and the patient is not overly sedated or lethargic. The scheduled dose is then set at 150% of the initial scheduled dose. Because of the time it takes to achieve a steady state, there may need to be some readjustment downward if the patient is unduly sleepy or is lethargic at the time of the scheduled dose. The supplemental dose may be given after any scheduled dose (even if there was an increase in the scheduled dose) as long as a sufficient time has passed for the drug to be absorbed from the stomach. An alternative way to titrate is simply to add 50% to the next scheduled dose, but staying with the previously determined schedule (usually every 4 hours). When the doses of opioid are higher (e.g., morphine 100 mg every 4 hours), some clinicians use less, for example, 20% to 30% (20 to 30 mg) as the boost, but incrementally add to the dose with each scheduled treatment until adequate pain relief has been achieved. Depending on the understanding of the patient and family, it is often best to have the patient check in with a physician or nurse 1 to 3 days after a significant dose or medication adjustment to be sure the treatment plan is understood, safe, and effective.

5. Long-acting preparations. When an effective dose of short-acting morphine has been established, the required 24-hour dose for a long-acting preparation can be calculated. An additional supply of short-acting morphine, given when necessary, will help the patient manage "breakthrough" pain. Consistent need for this additional short-acting morphine (e.g., three or four doses daily) dictates an upward adjustment of the dose of sustained-release drug. Orders for immediate-release morphine should allow for some upward titration of dose by the patient or by the nurse. Each dose of short-acting morphine for breakthrough pain is usually 5% to 15% of the 24-hour dose of long-acting morphine. If more than this is required, it is usually an indication for increasing the dose of the long-acting preparation or considering some other adjuvant or interventional approaches.

6. Although the **opioid agonist–antagonist analgesics** have established effectiveness in the control of acute (especially procedurally related) pain, their use in chronic cancer pain is limited by the possibility of precipitous withdrawal in the patient who has been taking morphine-type drugs, by their analgesic ceiling effect (when the drug does not provide more pain relief), and by the lack of an oral form of administration.

7. Methadone is an agonist opioid analgesic that has the advantages of extremely low cost (often 10- to 30-fold less expensive than other strong opioids), efficacy in neuropathic pain, slow development of tolerance, and lack of known active metabolites. Because of its long and unpredictable half-life and relatively unknown equianalgesic dose compared with other opioids, methadone has generally been used primarily by pain specialists with experience in

Table 32.4.   Suggested dosing of oral methadone based on Morphine-Equivalent Daily Dose (MEDD)

Oral MEDD (mg/day)	Initial Dose Ratio (oral morphine/oral methadone)
<30	2:1
30–99	4:1
100–180	6:1
181–249	8:1
250–300	10:1

Adapted from Fisch MJ, Appendix D: dosing strategies for oral methadone. In: Fisch MJ, Burton AW, eds. *Cancer pain management.* New York: McGraw-Hill, 2007:308.

its use. More recently, however, the utility of this agent in cancer pain has become more widely appreciated and it is being used in hospital and hospice settings. The methadone preparation widely utilized in the United States is a racemic mix of the D-isomer and L-isomer of methadone. The D-isomer has antagonist activity at the NMDA receptor, and this produces clinically relevant benefits in the control of neuropathic pain.

The relative potency of methadone increases with higher morphine-equivalent doses. Therefore, when converting from another opioid to methadone, the calculated equianalgesic dose of methadone should be decreased by 75% to 90%. A guideline for choosing an appropriate initial dose of methadone on the basis of the oral morphine-equivalent daily dose of the previous opioid is shown in Table 32.4. For example, a patient who has been using sustained-release morphine at 80 mg every 8 hours (240 mg/day) would be appropriately switched to methadone at a dose of 10 mg every 8 hours (30 mg/day, an 8:1 conversion ratio). In contrast, a patient who is taking sustained-release morphine at a total daily dose of 60 mg/day might be switched to an oral methadone dose of 5 mg every 8 hours (15 mg/day, a 4:1 conversion ratio).

Methadone is available as a pill, an elixir, and for parenteral use. The oral bioavailability of the drug is excellent (50% to 80%). Methadone administration through the IV or IM route is roughly twice as potent as the oral administration. Therefore, a patient with well-controlled pain on a stable oral methadone dose of 10 mg every 8 hours would be switched to IV methadone at 5 mg every 8 hours if necessary. SC use of methadone may cause skin irritation in some patients.

Methadone is metabolized primarily by the hepatic cytochrome P450 system isoenzyme CYP3A4, and to a lesser extent, by isoenzyme CYP2D6. Drugs that inhibit CYP3A4 cause the methadone levels to drift upward, and drugs that induce the metabolism of CYP3A4 will cause the methadone levels to drift downward. Important drugs to consider when prescribing methadone are summarized in Table 32.5.

Table 32.5.   Drugs affecting methadone serum levels

Drugs Causing Methadone Levels to Drift Upwards (higher effects)	Drugs Causing Methadone Levels to Drift Downwards (lower effects)
Ciprofloxacin	Rifampin
Ketoconazole, itraconazole, fluconazole	Phenytoin
Erythromycin, clarithromycin, doxycline	Corticosteroids
Grapefruit juice	Carbemazepine
HIV protease inhibitors Imatinib	St. John's wort
Nefazodone	

Methadone is one of a long list of medications that can cause prolongation of the Q-T interval and torsade de pointes ventricular tachycardia. This is caused by inhibition of the rapid component of the delayed rectifier potassium ion current. Other common drugs that share this attribute include haloperidol, chlorpromazine, clarithromycin, pentamidine, and others. The level of risk associated with these drugs is low, and depends on the dose and the population being treated. Oral methadone can be safely administered in the low doses (<100 mg/day) that are generally prescribed for the treatment of cancer pain, and routine electrocardiograms are not performed at our institution when prescribing oral methadone. Caution should be taken when prescribing methadone to certain patients who may be at higher risk of Q-T prolongation.

8. Alternative potent opioids include levorphanol, which has a longer half-life than morphine, and single-entity oxycodone and hydromorphone, which has a half-life similar to morphine. Equivalent starting doses can be selected from Table 32.3, but if the patient has been on high doses of morphine, care must be taken to reduce the dose to 50% to 75% of the calculated equianalgesic dose to account for incomplete cross-tolerance that may increase the relative potency of the newly prescribed agent.

9. Alternative routes. Approximately 70% of patients benefit from the use of an alternative route for opioid administration sometime before death. The duration for which patients need these routes varies between hours and months. Although intermittent injections can be effective for a brief period of time, this method is painful for the patient, time consuming for the nursing staff, and difficult to manage at home.

    a.   Intravenous (IV) infusion. Numerous studies have shown that IV infusions of opioids produce stable blood levels of drug and that they are safe and effective for treating both postoperative and cancer pain. IV infusion using a patient-controlled analgesia pump may be very effective in gaining rapid control over pain that has got out of hand. It may also be of value when the patient cannot take medications orally and does not wish to take suppositories. The main problem associated with continuous IV infusions is the prolonged maintenance of an IV line. Patients may need to be subjected to numerous venipunctures when peripheral IV lines are used. Totally implantable IV catheters represent a major improvement, permitting long-term IV access. However, these catheters are expensive and need to be surgically implanted, and their maintenance requires considerable nursing expertise and patient teaching. If such a catheter is already available in a patient with advanced cancer who has pain, it certainly could be used for the administration of opioids. Starting doses of morphine for severe pain are 2 to 3 mg/hour as a continuous infusion, with patient-controlled boosts of 1 mg every 6 to 15 minutes. At the end of 24 hours, 50% of the patient boosts can be added to the total 24-hour dose of the continuous infusion until the patient is requiring less than one boost hourly. At that time, a shift to oral analgesics can be started, if the patient is able to take oral medications. If the doses of IV morphine are high, shifting to appropriate oral doses may take several days. It is usually safe and effective to give a 24-hour dose of long-acting morphine orally that is equal in milligrams (not equianalgesic) to the 24-hour requirement IV and simultaneously to reduce the IV dose (continuous infusion rate) by half. Boosts can be given by mouth, but the patient should have the IV boost option as reassurance. The next day, the 24-hour IV dose required (continuous plus boosts) can be added orally to the previous day's oral dose (long-acting plus short-acting) and the infusion further reduced. The same process is repeated until the patient gets adequate pain relief with the oral morphine. The infusion can usually be stopped and needed boosts given orally by the third or fourth day.

b. Subcutaneous (SC) route. This route has been found to be safe and effective for the administration of morphine and hydromorphone. SC opioids can be administered as a continuous infusion using a pump (use as small a volume as possible, e.g., less than 5 mL/hour) or as an intermittent injection. A butterfly needle can be left under the skin for approximately 7 days, making both intermittent injections and continuous infusion painless. The needles are frequently inserted in the subclavicular region, anterior chest, or abdominal wall. This leaves the patients' limbs free.

c. Rectal route. Most of the experience reported in the literature is with the short-term use of rectal opioids for the management of acute pain. Both solid and liquid solutions have been used. Although there is considerable interindividual variation in the bioavailability of rectally administered morphine, there is general consensus that this drug is well absorbed after rectal administration. A number of authors have treated terminally ill cancer patients with rectal morphine, with good pain control until death. Advantages of the rectal route include the absence of the need for the insertion of needles and the use of portable pumps. However, rectal administration can be uncomfortable or psychologically distressing for some patients; absorption may be decreased by the presence of stool in the rectum, by diarrhea, or simply by normal bowel movements; and progressive titration may be difficult because of the limited availability of different commercial preparations.

d. Transdermal route. The recent development of a transdermal preparation of fentanyl citrate has revitalized an interest in this route. Pharmacokinetic data suggest that transdermal fentanyl is well absorbed, although there is considerable delay in reaching steady-state blood levels and a slowly declining plasma concentration after removal of the patch. The 72-hour dosing of the patch makes it convenient to use, and treatment appears to be well tolerated. The transdermal route is generally worth avoiding if the enteral route is readily available. Transdermal preparations are usually more expensive and more difficult to titrate compared with oral opioids. However, this route is quite useful for patients with chronic malignant bowel obstruction or similar chronic problems with the oral route.

e. Transmucosal route. Fentanyl citrate can also be formulated in a candied matrix to allow it to be administered orally as a lozenge on a stick. Oral transmucosal fentanyl citrate (OTFC) appears to be rapidly effective for breakthrough pain or for procedures. Dose-equivalency studies have suggested that OTFC is approximately 10 times more potent than parenteral morphine. Starting doses are usually 200 μg, with dosing intervals of 4 to 6 hours. Drug dose requires titrating up, as with other agents with single doses of up to 1,600 μg. This transmucosal route has been used sparingly because the lozenges are expensive and patients often try to use them economically, thus limiting their effectiveness.

f. Neuraxial route. Some patients suffering from localized pain syndromes might benefit from epidural or intrathecal administration of opioids. The advantage of the neuraxial route is the potential to spare side effects of opioids since a relatively small dose may be effective for the pain problem. The disadvantage is the need for the insertion of catheters into the epidural or intrathecal space, the need for expensive infusion pumps, and, in some patients, the rapid development of tolerance to the analgesic effect of different opioids. To overcome this rapid development of tolerance, some clinicians have used a combined infusion of opioids and local anesthetic. Another issue that has become recognized is catheter tip granuloma formation. This may present as gradual loss of pain control or new back pain, sometimes associated with neurologic deficits. This complication can be diagnosed by MRI and is most common with high concentrations of intrathecal opioids (such as morphine >25 mg/mL). Because of the complexity associated with this route, it should only be considered for selected patients and after an adequate trial of systemic opioids and adjuvant drugs. The insertion of the catheter and the maintenance of the spinal analgesic regimen should be under the control of a pain specialist.

10. Adverse effects of opioids. Fear of the inability to manage side effects is one of the main reasons cited by oncologists for limiting the use of opioids. Yet, most of the agents used in chemotherapy are associated with more potent side effects than opioids. The analgesic and side effects of opioid agonists are not identical for all patients. Some patients may require a higher equivalent dose of a certain opioid agonist to achieve adequate analgesia. This higher equivalent dose may result in a higher incidence of side effects such as nausea or sedation. Therefore, when significant toxicity occurs in a patient treated with a certain opioid agonist such as morphine, it may be appropriate to change to another opioid. In addition, after prolonged treatment, high dosages, or renal failure, patients may experience the accumulation of active metabolites of opioid agonists. Active metabolites have been identified for morphine, hydromorphone, oxycodone, and fentanyl. This accumulation results in CNS side effects such as sedation, generalized myoclonus, confusion, and, in some patients, agitated delirium or grand mal seizures. In these patients, it is also useful to change from one opioid to another.

This so-called opioid rotation (or "opioid switching") can produce improved analgesia and fewer adverse effects. Most often, such a switch occurs from morphine to a more potent opioid such as methadone, hydromorphone, fentanyl, or oxycodone. The dose guidelines for switching to methadone are shown in Table 32.4. When switching from morphine to hydromorphone or oxycodone, the initial dose should be 50% to 75% of the calculated equianalgesic dose. When switching from morphine to transdermal fentanyl, dose reduction is not needed because the dosing guidelines already incorporated the safety factor necessary for opioid rotation.

It is important to understand the side effect spectrum of these analgesics and be prepared to deal with side effects prophylactically or promptly when they do occur. *Most patients develop tolerance for side effects much more rapidly than they develop tolerance for the analgesic effects of the opioids.*

a. Sedation. This occurs in most patients during the beginning of opioid treatment or after a major increase in dose. Most patients develop rapid tolerance to this side effect, and while the sedation disappears within 3 to 5 days, the analgesic effect persists. When sedation occurs in patients with cancer receiving a stable dose of opioid, one should suspect the potential accumulation of active opioid metabolites such as morphine-6-glucuronide. This occurs most frequently in patients who are receiving high doses of opioids or who present with renal failure. It is also important to consider non–opioid-related causes such as hypercalcemia, because these patients are frequently very ill and metabolic problems or comorbidity may contribute to sedation. Opioid-induced sedation can be managed by opioid rotation (some opioids have a higher ratio of analgesic effects to sedation than others) or by the addition of psychostimulants such as methylphenidate or modafinil.

b. Nausea and vomiting. Most patients present with these symptoms after initial administration or a major increase in dose. Some authors propose the use of prophylactic antiemetics on a regular basis during the first days of treatment because in most patients, nausea disappears after that period. These side effects can be well managed with prokinetic agents such as metoclopramide (10 mg PO q.i.d.). Dexamethasone 2 to 4 mg PO q.i.d. is also a useful antiemetic that potentiates metoclopramide in these patients but it is prudent to taper this corticosteroid within 1 or 2 weeks. As with sedation, nausea is a syndrome with multiple possible etiologies in patients with cancer who are receiving opioids; severe constipation, cancer-induced autonomic dysfunction, gastritis, increased intracranial pressure, and opioid metabolite accumulation are all possible causes of nausea.

c. Constipation. This is probably the most common adverse effect of opioids, and it is necessary to anticipate constipation when opioid therapy is started. Opioids act at multiple sites in the gastrointestinal tract and spinal cord. The result is decreased intestinal secretions and peristalsis. Although tolerance to both sedation and nausea develops quickly, it develops very slowly as compared to the smooth muscle effects of opioids, so that constipation persists when these drugs are used for chronic pain. At the same time that the use of opioid analgesics is initiated, provision for a regular bowel regimen, including stimulants and stool softeners, should be instituted to diminish this adverse effect (see Chapter 27). Methylnaltrexone is an investigational peripheral opioid receptor antagonist, a quaternary derivative of naltrexone that does not cross the blood–brain barrier. Methylnaltrexone is being explored as a potential agent to block or reverse constipation without affecting analgesia or precipitating the opioid withdrawal symptoms.

d. Respiratory depression. This is the most serious adverse effect of opioid analgesics. Opioids can cause increasing respiratory depression to the point of apnea. In humans, death due to overdose of opioids is nearly always due to respiratory arrest. At equianalgesic doses, the morphine-like agonists produce an equivalent degree of respiratory depression. When respiratory depression occurs, it is usually in opioid-naive patients after acute administration of an opioid and is associated with other signs of CNS depression including sedation and mental clouding. Tolerance quickly develops to this effect with repeated drug administration, allowing the opioid analgesics to be used in the management of chronic cancer pain without significant risk of respiratory depression. If respiratory depression occurs, it can be reversed by the administration of the specific opioid antagonist naloxone. In patients chronically receiving opioids who develop respiratory depression, naloxone in a 1:10 dilution should be titrated carefully to prevent the precipitation of severe withdrawal syndromes while reversing the respiratory depression. Long-acting drugs such as methadone, fentanyl patches, or slow-release morphine or hydromorphone carry a greater risk of respiratory depression as compared to short-acting opioids. The simultaneous use of other depressants such as benzodiazepines or alcohol are also risk factors for respiratory depression. Although this is the most feared side effect of opioid analgesics, it seldom occurs in patients receiving chronic opioid therapy for the treatment of cancer pain.

e. Allergic reactions. These occur infrequently with opioids. However, patients are commonly described as being "allergic" to a number of opioid analgesics. This descriptor generally results from a misinterpretation by the patient or clinician of some of the common side effects of opioids, such as nausea, sedation, vomiting, diaphoresis, or pruritis. In most instances, a simple discussion with the patient is enough to clarify this issue.

f. Urinary retention. The increase in the tone of smooth muscle of the bladder induced by opioids results in increased sphincter tone, leading to urinary retention. This is most common in elderly patients. Attention should be directed to this potential transient side effect, and catheterization may be necessary, transiently, for management. Patients do accommodate to this side effect and it is seldom a barrier to effective pain management.

g. "Newer" side effects. During recent years, as a result of increased education in the assessment and management of cancer pain, patients have been receiving higher doses of opioids for longer periods of time than ever before. This more aggressive use of opioids is associated with additional side effects, usually seen only in patients with late-stage disease receiving high doses of opioids.

(1) Cognitive failure. Patients can experience a transient decrease in concentration and psychomotor coordination after starting opioids or after a sudden increase in the opioid dose. In some patients, opioid-induced cognitive failure can be permanent. Some of the cognitive effects can be reversed by the administration of amphetamine derivatives such as methylphenidate. Cognitive screening tools (such as the Mini-Mental State Examination and other similar bedside assessments) are useful in patients receiving high doses of opioids.

(2) Other central effects. Organic hallucinations, myoclonus, grand mal seizures, and even hyperalgesia have been observed in patients receiving high doses of opioids for long periods. These effects are likely due to the accumulation of active opioid metabolites. Sometimes, the development of these problems in a previously stable patient heralds the onset of renal insufficiency or renal failure. Improvement is frequently seen after renal function improves and/or there is an opioid rotation. Hallucinations may be treated symptomatically with low doses of haloperidol 0.5 to 2 mg b.i.d. while the underlying problem is being addressed. Myoclonus can be treated with clonazepam 0.5 mg PO b.i.d. initially, with titration every 3 days up to a maximum daily dose of 20 mg.

(3) Severe sedation and coma. When coma occurs in patients receiving a stable dose of opioids for a long period of time, it should be suspected that accumulation of active opioid metabolites has occurred. These patients usually improve quickly after discontinuation of opioids.

(4) Pulmonary edema. Although noncardiogenic pulmonary edema is a well-recognized complication of opioid overdose in addicts, it had not been recognized until recently as a potential complication of cancer pain treatment. Pulmonary edema usually occurs when patients have undergone rapid increases in dose, usually as a result of severe neuropathic pain. Even though the mortality of the syndrome is very low among patients presenting with acute opioid overdoses, because of the conservative nature of the treatment of terminally ill cancer patients, the mortality of pulmonary edema is much higher within this population.

V. Adjuvant drugs. Opioid analgesics are the most important drugs for the treatment of cancer pain. Although these drugs can, in most patients, control severe pain even when they are used appropriately, they may produce new symptoms or exacerbate preexisting symptoms, most notably nausea and somnolence. This aspect of treatment with opioid compounds is particularly problematic in patients with advanced cancer. The combination of severe pain, anorexia, chronic nausea, asthenia, and somnolence is a frequent finding in patients with advanced cancer. The term *adjuvant drug* has been used in a variety of ways, even in the context of cancer pain management. For the purposes of the following paragraphs, an adjuvant drug meets one or more of the following criteria:

- Increases the analgesic effect of opioids (adjuvant analgesia)
- Decreases the toxicity of opioids
- Improves other symptoms associated with terminal cancer

Most symptomatic patients with cancer receive more than one or two adjuvant drugs. Unfortunately, there is still limited consensus on the type and dose of the most appropriate adjuvant drugs.

Claims have been made for the adjuvant analgesic effect of many drugs, but unfortunately, most of the evidence for these effects is anecdotal. Controlled clinical trials are needed to define more clearly the indications and risk-to-benefit ratios. These agents, some of which have the potential to produce significant toxicity, can aggravate the toxicity of opioids.

A. Antidepressants. Tricyclic antidepressants have been found to be useful for various neuropathic pain syndromes, especially when pain has a prominent dysesthetic or burning character. Both amitriptyline and desipramine have been found to be effective in the management of postherpetic neuralgia, diabetic neuropathy, and other neurologic conditions. Amitriptyline or imipramine (25 mg at bedtime) may be started at low doses; if the drug is not overly sedating and the patient does not experience bothersome anticholinergic side effects, the dose may be increased every 3 days to a total daily dose of 150 mg. The toxic effects of these drugs are mainly autonomic (dry mouth, postural hypotension) and centrally mediated (somnolence, confusion). Cardiovascular side effects are also possible at therapeutic dosing levels, including increased heart rate, prolonged PR interval, intraventricular conduction delays, increased corrected Q-T interval (QTc), and flattened T waves. Because their use may contribute to symptoms already present in debilitated patients, they should be administered cautiously in those who are very ill.

Duloxetine is a serotonin/norepinephrine reuptake inhibitor indicated for the treatment of diabetic neuropathy. The appropriate dose for this indication is 60 mg once daily. Adults treated with any antidepressant medication should be watched closely for worsening of depression and/or suicidal behavior or suicidal ideation. Monitoring should be particularly vigilant during initiation of therapy and during any change in dosage. Overall, clinical experience and expert consensus suggest that tricyclic antidepressants or duloxetine may be tried for the management of pain that is of central, deafferentation, or neuropathic origin.

B. Anticonvulsants. Carbamazepine, phenytoin, valproic acid, lamotrigine, gabapentin, pregabelin, and clonazepam, alone or in combination with the tricyclic antidepressants, have been used successfully to treat neuropathic pain. On the basis of the well-documented efficacy for the treatment of trigeminal neuralgia, considerable experience and expert consensus suggest that these agents may be useful adjuvants for neuropathic cancer pain syndromes, including neural invasion by tumor, radiation fibrosis or surgical scarring, herpes zoster, and deafferentation. Some clinical improvement can be expected in one-half to two-thirds the number of patients whose predominant complaint is pain of a shooting, lancinating, burning, or hyperesthetic nature. Effective doses in the treatment of neuropathic pain in patients with cancer are not well established, and there is no clear-cut standard of care for use of these agents to guide the choice of agent or sequence of agents used in therapeutic trials.

C. Corticosteroids. Controlled studies suggest that the administration of corticosteroids to selected patients with advanced cancer results in decreased pain and improved appetite and activity. Unfortunately, the duration of the effects is probably short lasting. The mechanism by which corticosteroids appear to produce beneficial effects in patients with terminal cancer is unclear but may involve their euphoric effects or the inhibition of prostaglandin metabolism. The optimal drug and dosing regimens have not been established. For the treatment of painful conditions, prednisone or dexamethasone is often administered in doses totaling 30 to 60 mg PO daily and 8 to 16 mg PO daily, respectively. As soon as symptomatic relief is obtained, attempts should be made to decrease the dose progressively to the minimally effective dose. Although long-term side effects are not an important consideration in many patients with advanced cancer, treatment may produce limiting side effects in these patients, particularly immunosuppression (candidiasis occurs in most patients), proximal myopathy, and psychiatric symptoms. The incidence of psychologic disturbances ranges from 3% to 50%, with severe symptoms occurring in approximately 5% of patients. The spectrum of disturbances ranges from mild to severe affective disorders, psychotic reactions, and global cognitive impairment.

D. Clonidine. Clonidine, an α_2-adrenergic agonist developed for treatment of hypertension, can be administered orally or as part of an epidural regimen for control of cancer-related pain, especially neuropathic pain.

E. Approaches to metastatic bone pain

    1. Radioisotope therapy. Strontium 89 and samarium 153 are isotopes that have been found to be useful in providing systemic radiotherapy for palliation of pain in patients with bony metastases. These agents can be useful in patients with adequate bone marrow reserve who have multiple pain locations that limit the feasibility of external-beam radiation therapy. The main limitations of radioisotope therapy are its high cost and the potential for hematologic toxicity (mainly thrombocytopenia).

    2. Bisphosphonates. These agents have been found to be significantly better than placebo in patients with bone pain due to a variety of primary tumors. Pamidronate, clodronate, and zoledronate are the agents that have been most frequently studied. Because of their poor oral bioavailability, these drugs are most useful when given IV. In addition to pain control, these drugs can significantly reduce a number of other complications of osteolysis, such as hypercalcemia, fractures, and need for radiation therapy.

    3. External-beam radiotherapy. Radiation therapy can effectively control bone pain in approximately 70% of patients within 2 to 4 weeks. This treatment is most useful in patients with a single or small number of painful areas. A single administration may be as effective as multiple smaller fractions, reducing the cost and discomfort of transportation back and forth associated with multiple doses.

VI. Other procedures. Evaluation of the physical basis of the pain may indicate that a neuroablative procedure, in which the pain pathway is destroyed, would be of benefit for pain control. As aggressive opioid analgesia becomes more accepted, most patients with cancer do not require these neuroablative interventions. Destruction of the pain pathway can be accomplished surgically or through destructive nerve blocks using an agent such as phenol. The major barrier to the more widespread application of these techniques is the limited number of practitioners with expertise in their use. The most frequently used neurosurgical procedure is the anterolateral or spinothalamic cordotomy. This is often performed as closed percutaneous cordotomy by stereotactically placing a radiofrequency needle in the anterolateral quadrant of the cervical spinal cord. Unilateral interventions for pain control can unmask significant pain on the contralateral side of the body. Most often, performance of such interventional pain procedures does not eliminate the need to administer and monitor the effectiveness of systemic analgesics. Because of afferent regeneration, destructive procedures have had their greatest application in patients whose expected life span is only a few months.

Destructive anesthetic block of the celiac plexus has been used for several decades in the management of pain in the abdominal region. This block, which can be preceded by reversible diagnostic block, is a boon to many patients suffering from the severe pain accompanying cancer of the pancreas and may also be helpful for pain from cancers of the liver, gallbladder, or stomach. If success is achieved with the diagnostic block, lasting disruption of the pain pathway can be achieved using alcohol or phenol. Pain from rib metastases or tumors of the chest wall can be relieved with intercostal nerve blocks. Patients with bone metastases sometimes develop pathologic vertebral compression fractures. Percutaneous vertebroplasty is a surgical procedure that involves use of polymethylmethacrylate as bone cement that is injected at high pressure through a needle into the collapsed vertebral body in order to stabilize it and relieve pain. Another interventional technique with similar goals is called *kyphoplasty*. This procedure involves percutaneous insertion of a needle with an inflatable balloon placed into the fractured vertebra using fluoroscopic guidance. The balloon is inflated so that the vertebral end plates are elevated and bone height is restored. The resulting bone cavity is then filled with acrylic bone cement.

Finally, patients with painful metastatic lesions involving bone that have failed conventional treatments such as external-beam radiation therapy and chemotherapy may benefit from percutaneous radiofrequency ablation as a salvage procedure. This is an image-guided procedure, and a single ablation procedure is effective in most patients and well tolerated.

VII. Coping or behavioral skill techniques. Teaching specific skills to manage pain can be helpful to many patients, especially those who face pain for months to years. Evaluation and prescription of the specific skills most beneficial to the individual can often be obtained through consultation with a behavioral psychologist, psychiatrist, or nurse pain specialist. Such techniques should never be used as a substitute for appropriate analgesia. The skills include relaxation, self-hypnosis, and other distraction and cognitive control techniques. These measures can affect the sensation of pain by reducing muscle tension on pain-generating lesions as well as by maximizing the patient's ability to cope with the pain and remain as active as the disease permits. All patients need education about the nature of their pain, the methods that can be used to relieve it, and how they can cooperate with their health care providers to achieve good pain control.

SUGGESTED READINGS

Bennett G, Serafini M, Burchiel K, et al. Evidence-based review of the literature on intrathecal delivery of pain medication. *J Pain Symptom Manage* 2000;20:S12–S36.

Bruera E, Kim HN. Cancer pain. *J Am Med Assoc* 2003;290:2476–2479.

Bruera E, Palmer JL, Bosnjak S, et al. Methadone versus morphine as a first-line strong opioid for cancer pain: a randomized, double-blind study. *J Clin Oncol* 2004;22:185–192.

Carr DB, Goudas LC, Balk EM, et al. Evidence report on the treatment of pain in cancer patients. *J Natl Cancer Inst Monogr* 2004;32:23–31.

Cherney N, Ripamonti C, Pereira J, et al. Strategies to manage the adverse effects of oral morphine: an evidence-based report. *J Clin Oncol* 2001;19:2542–2554.

Cleeland CS, Gonin R, Hatfield AK, et al. Pain and its treatment in outpatients with metastatic cancer. *N Engl J Med* 1994;330:592–596.

Corbo M, Balmaceda C. Peripheral neuropathy in cancer patients. *Cancer Invest* 2001;19:369–382.

Davis MP, Weissman DE, Arnold RM. Opioid dose titration for severe cancer pain: a systematic, evidence-based review. *J Palliat Med* 2004;7:462–468.

Foley KM. Treatment of cancer-related pain. *J Natl Cancer Inst Monogr* 2004;32:103–104.

Fourney DR, Schomer DF, Nader R, et al. Percutaneous vertebroplasty and kyphoplasty for painful vertebral body fractures in cancer patients. *J Neurosurg (Spine 1)* 2003;98:21–30.

Goetz MP, Callstrom MR, Charboneau JW, et al. Percutaneous, image-guided radiofrequency ablation of painful metastases involving bone: a multicenter study. *J Clin Oncol* 2004;22(2):300–306.

Lawlor PG. The panorama of opioid-related cognitive dysfunction in patients with cancer. *Cancer* 2002;94:1836–1853.

de Leon-Casasola OA. Interventional procedures for cancer pain management: when are they indicated? *Cancer Invest* 2004;22:630–642.

Manfredi PL, Houde RW. Prescribing methadone, a unique analgesic. *J Support Oncol* 2003;1:216–220.

Mercadante S, Bruera E. Opioid switching: a systematic and critical review. *Cancer Treat Rev* 2006;32:304–315.

Morrison RS, Meier DE. Clinical practice. Palliative care. *N Engl J Med* 2004;350:2582–2590.

Pereira J, Lawlor P, Vigano A, et al. Equianalgesic dose ratios for opioids: a critical review and proposals for long-term dosing. *J Pain Symptom Manage* 2001;22:672–677.

Quigley C. Opioid switching to improve pain relief and drug tolerability. *Cochrane Database Syst Rev* 2004;25:169–178.

Stockler M, Vardy J, Pillai A, et al. Acetaminophen improves pain and well-being in people with advanced cancer already receiving a strong opioid regimen: a randomized, double-blind, placebo-controlled cross-over trial. *J Clin Oncol* 2004;22(16):3389–3394.

CHAPTER 33

Emotional and Psychiatric Problems in Patients with Cancer

Kathleen S. N. Franco-Bronson, and Kristi S. Williams

I. General principles. Clinical psychiatric disorders occur in up to 50% of patients with cancer at some point during their treatment. Delirium, depression, and anxiety are those most frequently seen and may coexist in the same patient. Vigilant monitoring for early symptoms of psychiatric distress is important to the care of these patients. The clinician should inquire regularly about symptoms in the affective and cognitive domains. Symptom clusters help differentiate anxiety, depression, and acute confusional states from other psychiatric disorders. Once an accurate diagnosis is made, safety, tolerability, efficacy, and price influence choice of medication. More than one psychiatric diagnosis may be present, requiring a hierarchical approach. For example, if both delirium and depression are present, the cause of the delirium should be determined and treated before starting antidepressant therapy (which could worsen the delirium). Once the delirium has improved, treatment for the depression can be considered. When major depression and an anxiety disorder coexist, treatment for the depression is started first and may adequately manage both disorders.

II. Acute confusional states. Approximately 15% of hospitalized patients with cancer experience delirium, but this can increase to 80% to 85% in those receiving palliative care.

A. Precepts. Attempting to treat delirium with psychotropic drugs, but without understanding the cause of the patient's confusion can have serious consequences. Delirium is characterized by fluctuating levels of alertness and consciousness, shortened attention and concentration, rapidly changing moods, irregular sleep–wake cycles, garbled or slurred speech, hypervigilance, and behavior not consistent with good judgment. The delirious patient may also have delusional ideas or hallucinations or appear depressed. Visual, auditory, tactile, and occasionally olfactory hallucinations can be present. The more sensory modalities that are involved in the hallucinations, the greater the likelihood that the patient is experiencing a medically induced confusional state.

B. Etiologies

1. Medications remain the most common reason for acute confusional states. The most frequently identified medications to cause delirium are sedatives, narcotic analgesics, anxiolytics, anticholinergic drugs, and corticosteroids. Antineoplastic and immunotherapeutic agents can cause delirium: cytarabine, methotrexate, asparaginase, fluorouracil, interferon, interleukins. Even histamine blockage from agents such as diphenhydramine or famotidine can lead to delirium.

2. Metabolic causes are often seen in patients with cancer and include hypernatremia and hyponatremia, hyperthyroidism and hypothyroidism, poorly controlled diabetes mellitus, vitamin deficiencies (B_{12}, folate, thiamine), and hypercalcemia.

3. Infections of the respiratory, urinary, central nervous, and other systems are common, especially in immunosuppressed patients.

4. Chemical withdrawal from benzodiazepines, alcohol, and other drugs can induce delirium.

5. Medical illness such as tumors, particularly in the brain, and brain metastases, cardiac arrhythmias, congestive heart failure, liver disease, trauma, strokes, and renal failure. Hyperviscosity syndrome with lymphoma, myeloma, and Waldenström's macroglobulinemia are unusual causes. After radiation to the brain, confusional states can occur, especially if the patient received very little steroid. An acute confusional state can occur secondary to a paraneoplastic syndrome frequently associated with lymphoma. In addition to the original illness, postoperative head and neck surgery, often for malignancy, carries a higher risk than many other surgical procedures for delirium.

C. Therapeutic approach. Once an acute confusional state is identified, the primary therapeutic approach is to treat the cause. The key is to determine when symptoms of delirium first occurred and to look for preceding changes in medications, vital signs, laboratory studies, or imagery/radiology. This helps determine how best to proceed with treatment, for example, withdrawing a medication or treating a urinary tract infection found on a urinalysis. When hypoactive delirium occurs, inclining the head to 30% reduces the risk for aspiration. Moving the patient frequently may prevent bed sores. Hyperactive patients with delirium are at high risk for falls and subsequent fractures. Research has demonstrated that a combined protocol of physical mobilization, cognitive exercise through conversation and reorientation, appropriate hydration, use of glasses or hearing aids from home, and minimizing sedatives at night can reduce the number, severity, and cost of delirium episodes. Antipsychotic medications may be helpful in managing symptoms such as hallucinations, delusions, and extreme agitation, but they do not treat the cause of the delirium.

1. Orientation (frequent reconnection) of the patient aids in reduction of confusion.

a. It is helpful to orient the patients frequently to the place and time, and why they are at the hospital and to give current explanations of procedures. This routine should be done once or more frequently per shift when the delirious patients are awake. Because patients' attention, concentration, and recent memory are frequently impaired, they often do not recall instructions given to them earlier. Leaving large, legibly written note cards with the patients' names, date, hospital name, and other data is beneficial in some instances.

b. A large calendar, a clock, and family pictures or mementos can assist the patients in feeling less estranged from their environment. It can be very reassuring to a patient if a family member can stay with them overnight.

c. Some patients are reassured by a small night light in their room, which cuts down on illusions or misinterpretations. Patients with compromised vision or hearing are particularly distraught when they are even less able to discern what is happening around them, and they should be provided with their regular hearing aids and glasses.

2. Medication helps control hallucinations, delusions, and psychotic agitation. The lowest dose to control symptoms is usually preferable.

a. Haloperidol (Haldol; Table 33.1) is a butyrophenone, an antipsychotic agent with potent dopamine-blocking action. It is less likely to produce cardiovascular, respiratory, gastrointestinal, and general anticholinergic side effects than many of the other antipsychotic medications. However, moderate doses may cause extrapyramidal symptoms. The starting dose in a patient with an acute confusional state is 0.25 to 2 mg PO or IM, on an as-needed or regular dosing schedule every 4 to 6 hours. A marked advantage of haloperidol is that sedation is minimized while controlling agitation. There are exceptions to the usually preferred low doses of antipsychotic medications. For example, if patients tolerate higher doses with few side effects, they may benefit by having improved pain control. IV haloperidol has not been approved by the U.S. Food and Drug Administration, although it is commonly used in the seriously agitated patient. There are much less extrapyramidal symptoms with IV haloperidol, but the half-life in this form is much shorter requiring more frequent administration. Avoid very high doses in patients with alcoholic cardiomyopathy, those prone to torsades de pointes or similar arrhythmias, and those with an excessively long QTc interval.

b. Risperidone (Risperdal) is less likely to produce extrapyramidal side effects, but is available only in oral form for short-acting (non-depot) use. **Olanzapine** (Zyprexa, Zydis) is sedating and can be given as a tablet that dissolves on the tongue or in an intramuscular form. **Ziprasidone** (Geodon) too can be given in a rapid onset IM preparation. **Quetiapine** (Seroquel) is only available orally, as is **aripiprazole** (Abilify). The latter acts slowly and would not help reduce symptoms quickly.

c. A delirious patient with vision or hearing impairment is likely to hallucinate during periods of excessive sedation especially if there is pulmonary compromise or a tendency toward hypoxia.

d. If the patient demonstrates a **predictable period of confusion,** such as during the early evening ("sundowning") when there is less environmental activity, a small once-a-day dose at that time may be adequate.

Table 33.1. Antipsychotic medications: prominent characteristics and dosage for patients with cancer

Agent	Starting Dose (mg)[a]	Characteristics
Phenothiazines		
Chlorpromazine (Thorazine)	10–25	Significant hypotension risk; lowers seizure threshold; highly sedating; anticholinergic
Thioridazine (Mellaril)	10–25	Similar to chlorpromazine but more likely to alter electrocardiogram; not available IM
Perphenazine (Trilafon)	4	Moderate sedation and hypotension
Trifluoperazine (Stelazine)	2	High frequency of extrapyramidal side effects
Others		
Haloperidol (Haldol)	0.5–2.0	Good for acute delirium; high frequency of extrapyramidal side effects; available IV, IM, or PO short acting; IV haloperidol has a very short half-life and must be given frequently, but there is much less extrapyramidal side effect; IM depot (2–4 weeks) form
Risperidone (Risperdal)	0.5–1.0	Some α-adrenergic effects; mild extrapyramidal side effects as dose increases; PO form for daily use; IM depot (2 weeks) form
Olanzapine (Zyprexa)	5	More sedation, weight gain, less extrapyramidal side effects; PO form regular capsule, liquid and tablet that dissolve on tongue; IM for acute use up to two times per day
Quetiapine (Seroquel)	25–50	More sedation; less extrapyramidal effects
Ziprasidone (Geodon)	20	Less weight gain; less extrapyramidal effects; IM for acute use up to two times per day
Aripiprazole (Abilify)	5–20	Less weight gain and extrapyramidal effects; can elevate mood, occasionally to hypomania

[a]Dose can generally be repeated every 4–6 h (other than risperidone, olanzapine, quetiapine, ziprasidone), on either an as-needed or a regular schedule (e.g., b.i.d.).

e. When increasing the dose of antipsychotic drugs, muscle spasms, restlessness, or pseudoparkinsonian symptoms may occur with older first-generation antipsychotics and some second generation agents such as risperidone or ziprasidone. Adding a small amount of trihexyphenidyl (Artane) 1 to 2 mg b.i.d., benztropine (Cogentin) 1 mg b.i.d., or diphenhydramine (Benadryl) 25 mg b.i.d. can often reduce the side effects. However, increasing the level of anticholinergic activity with these choices may cause an atropinic-like psychosis. Constipation, urinary retention, dry mouth, tachycardia, and increasing confusion are warnings of this potential problem, especially when multiple anticholinergic medications (e.g., antiemetics, analgesics) are being prescribed. Therefore, antiparkinsonian drugs are not prescribed prophylactically but only if clearly indicated. Ondansetron (Zofran), granisetron (Kytril), or dolasetron (Anzemet) may be substituted for other antiemetics, reducing extrapyramidal symptoms and avoiding the need for an antiparkinsonian medication. Some antiemetics (e.g., droperidol) are also antipsychotics, but these, like metoclopramide, can lead to extrapyramidal symptoms such as akathisia or dystonias.

f. Benzodiazepines such as **lorazepam** (Ativan) can be given 0.5 to 2.0 mg every 8 hours. They can be administered in small doses to a patient who needs some sedation without added anticholinergic activity or those whose cardiac status is at risk (i.e., heart block) if some antipsychotic medications were increased. Using both benzodiazepines and antipsychotics is sometimes helpful.

g. Increasing delirium. Too much medication may have been given if the patient's agitation increases with higher doses. Secondary hypoxia and akathisia should be excluded. High blood levels of longer-acting medications can accumulate, particularly if serum albumin and protein are low and hepatic and renal functioning are compromised.

h. Hypotension. Avoid adding a second antipsychotic, for example, chlorpromazine (Thorazine), as it may predispose to hypotension and shock. If the blood pressure does drop significantly, norepinephrine bitartrate (Levophed) or a similar choice may be necessary as antipsychotic medications such as haloperidol also block some peripheral action of dopamine.

III. Depression is roughly four times more common in patients with cancer than in age-matched controls. Oropharyngeal, pancreatic, lung, and breast cancer are associated with the highest rates of depression. Earlier studies indicated that patients with both cancer and depression had a higher risk of death, but larger meta-analysis did not find this to be true. However, patients who are depressed report poorer pain control, poorer compliance and more often choose to discontinue treatment.

Patients with cancer have various emotional responses to their diagnoses. The mourning period for some is brief, does not inhibit their ability to interact with family and friends, and does not hinder participation in their own treatment. Support from others, acceptance of their feelings, and time may be all that is necessary for them to continue the emotional work ahead. However, approximately one-fourth of patients with cancer develop longer, more severe depression. The greatest risk of depression is at the time of first relapse. There are many variables that influence this process, including emotional conflicts with loved ones, disproportionate guilt, previous losses that were never resolved, long-standing debilitating illness, individual personality characteristics such as dependency, and inadequate support systems. Any of these factors, along with a family history of depression, are warnings for the physician to heed.

Besides emotional response to the stress of having cancer and undergoing treatment, other causes of depression should be considered. Folate or vitamin B_{12} deficiencies, thyroid or parathyroid disorders, adrenal insufficiency, leptomeningeal disease, and brain metastases can induce depression. Interferon can sometimes precipitate sadness to suicidal proportions in patients who have never previously experienced depression. Some recommend that an antidepressant be started 2 weeks before starting interferon if a patient has a prior history of major depression.

Passive suicidal thoughts with depression are common. Patients who actually do commit suicide are more likely to be men, and have advanced disease, a history of psychiatric illness, substance abuse, and earlier attempts. Good pain control and efforts to reduce isolation can lessen suicidal thoughts and behavior.

A. Therapeutic approach
  1. Emotional support at frequent intervals from the physician is generally needed. Some patients explore old emotional conflicts, whereas others just need a safe person to whom they can express their feelings. It is important for patients to be able to hold on to hope. A degree of denial is acceptable, normal, and upheld. Only when this denial makes it impossible for a patient to make informed treatment decisions is it necessary to probe into the denial.

  Psychotherapy of a supportive nature is often provided by the primary care physician, oncologist, psychiatrist, clergy, nurse, family, or friend individually or in any combination. For patients who wish to explore ambivalence, a professional psychotherapist trained in psychodynamic or interpersonal therapy is a good option. Cognitive therapy is helpful in letting go of detrimental interpretations while increasing one's ability to deal with emotional pain.

  2. Psychiatric care may be particularly instrumental when the patient's preexisting personality style interferes with treatment. Anniversary responses to previous losses, important family events, or past hospitalizations may have a great impact on the presentation of the depression and deserve exploration by a psychotherapist if a pattern is found. If there is a designated psychiatric consultant, this individual must work closely with the rest of the oncology team, communicating in a helpful way to the patient, family, and staff.

  If a patient has felt depressed, distressed, or irritable for some time or describes a loss of pleasure from formerly enjoyable relationships or activities, inquiry about the following symptoms is necessary: insomnia or hypersomnia; alteration in appetite with unexpected weight change; reduced interest in family, sexuality, work, or hobbies; increased guilt; low energy level; poor concentration; thoughts of death or suicide; frequent crying episodes; and psychomotor hypoactivity or hyperactivity. When the diagnosis of depression in the medically ill patient is being made, the emphasis is placed on psychological features as opposed to physical ones. These include rumination or repetitive negative thoughts, increased tearfulness, hopeless–helpless feelings, withdrawal from family or friends, and anhedonia. These symptoms are characteristic of a major depressive disorder for which antidepressant medications, in addition to psychotherapy, are recommended. In some studies, group therapy for patients with breast cancer has improved quality of life and may prolong survival.

3. Medications. In the past, patients with cancer were often undertreated for major depression that was mistaken as an "understandable" consequence of their illness or as simple grief. Now, evidence exists that psychosocial adjustment and improved life adaptation, in general, occur when patients with cancer and major depression are treated with antidepressant medications.

  a. Selection of agents and their side effects. In addition to efficacy, an antidepressant medication should be selected on the basis of its safety and tolerability, including any tendency to sedate or activate, cause orthostatic changes, or produce anticholinergic effects. Medication selection should also be tailored to the patient's symptom cluster such as the need for sedation or weight gain versus the need for activation (Tables 33.2

Table 33.2. Characteristics of commonly used heterocyclic antidepressants

Antidepressant	Sedation[a]	Anticholinergic Actions[b]	Other Characteristics
Amitriptyline (Elavil, Endep)	+4 to +5[c]	+4 to +5	Also available IM; orthostasis; quinidine-like prolongation of conduction; good for neuropathic pain
Doxepin (Sinequan, Adapin)	+4	+3 to +4	Highest appetite increase; orthostasis; good for neuropathic pain
Nortriptyline (Pamelor, Aventyl)	+3	+3	Less likely than other tricyclic antidepressants to cause orthostasis

Note: Do not use tricyclic if QTc >450. Tricyclics can also suppress respiratory drive and reduce seizure threshold.
[a] Associated with histaminergic blockade; appetite increase follows somewhat similar trends.
[b] Constipation, dry mouth, and urinary retention.
[c] Scale of 1–5, where 1 is the least and 5 is the most.

Table 33.3. Characteristics of commonly used nonheterocyclic antidepressants

Antidepressant	Sedation[a]	Anticholinergic Actions[b]	Other Characteristics
Bupropion (Wellbutrin)	+1[c]	+1	Associated with increased seizure risk especially if organic brain pathology or eating disorder is present; more activating, less weight gain
Fluoxetine (Prozac)	+1	+1	May cause restlessness and gastrointestinal upset; more activating, less weight gain; safe in patients with renal disease but may accumulate in those with liver disease; self-tapers when discontinued
Sertraline (Zoloft)	+1	+1	Similar to fluoxetine; more diarrhea; few drug interactions; short half-life; should be tapered if discontinued
Paroxetine (Paxil)	+1	+2	Similar to fluoxetine; more anticholinergic than other SSRIs; should be tapered if discontinued
Citalopram (Celexa)	+1	+1	Similar to sertraline; few drug interactions
Escitalopram (Lexapro)	+1–2	+1	Similar to sertraline; few drug interactions
Venlafaxine (Effexor)	+1–2	+1	Both serotonin and norepinephrine reuptake inhibitor; increases blood pressure at higher doses; augments pain relief
Duloxetine (Cymbalta)	+1–2	+1	Similar to venlafaxine
Mirtazapine (Remeron)	+4	+2	Weight gain; potential increase in cholesterol; sedation; available as tablet that dissolves on tongue
Nefazodone	+3	+2	Some sedation; fewer sexual side effects; mild orthostasis; possible liver toxicity in some

SSRI, selective serotonin reuptake inhibitor.

[a] Associated with histaminergic blockade; appetite increase follows somewhat similar trends.

[b] Constipation, dry mouth, and urinary retention.

[c] Scale of 1–5, where 1 is the least and 5 is the most.

and 33.3). Route of metabolism and elimination, as well as an increased risk for seizures, should affect the choice. Agents such as venlafaxine and duloxetine can reduce depression in patients with or without anxiety and improve pain control. Starting with lower doses and titrating up can lessen the risk of added nausea.

There is increasing evidence that selective serotonin reuptake inhibitors (SSRI) inhibit platelet aggregation and prolong bleeding. Although this might be helpful to patients who also have cardiovascular disease, these agents should be discontinued when there is observed evidence of acute bleeding as indicated by rapid falls in hemoglobin and hematocrit.

Highly anticholinergic medications frequently produce dry mouth, blurred vision, tachycardia, and constipation. They can also produce urinary retention, ileus, and acute confusion. Antihistaminergic drugs can increase sedation and appetite and worsen hypotension. Both H_1- and H_2-blocking agents can cause delirium, whereas a proton pump inhibitor will not. Medications that produce α-adrenergic receptor blockade are associated with increased orthostatic hypotension, dizziness, and reflex tachycardia.

b. Dosages (Table 33.4). Weak, debilitated, or elderly patients need protection from side effects of psychotropic agents. Starting out with small doses and gradually increasing the dose is prudent. Splitting doses may also be helpful for minimizing side effects and maximizing pain relief from antidepressant medications.

If a patient has a personal history, family history, or previous response to medication (e.g., steroids) that reflects manic or hypomanic symptoms, proceed carefully,

Table 33.4. Dosages for antidepressant therapy

Drug	Starting Daily Dose (mg)	Average Daily Dose for Patient with Cancer (mg)
Amitriptyline	10–25	75–150
Bupropion	75–150	300
Citalopram	10–20	20–40
Doxepin	25	75–150
Duloxetine	20 b.i.d.	20–30 b.i.d.
Escitalopram	10	20
Fluoxetine	10–20	20
Mirtazapine	7.5–15	30+
Nefazodone	50	300
Nortriptyline	10–25	50–100
Paroxetine	10–20	20
Sertraline	25–50	100
Venlafaxine	25 or 37.5 (XR form)	75 (37.5 b.i.d.)

Table 33.5. Other medications used to treat affective disorders

Drug	Starting Dose	Average Dose for Cancer Patients	Disorders	Pretreatment Work-up	Follow-up Studies	Comment
Stimulants[a] to increase level of alertness						
Methylphenidate (Ritalin)	2.5–5 mg every morning	5–20 mg every morning and noon	Medically ill patient with depression and lethargy	CBC, vital signs	CBC	Watch for increases in blood pressure, heart rate, and respiratory rate with all stimulants
Long-acting methylphenidate (Concerta)	8 mg every morning	36–54 mg	Medically ill patient with depression and lethargy	CBC, vital signs	CBC	Same as above
Pemoline (Cylert)	18.75 mg every morning	37.5–56.25 mg every morning	Medically ill patient with depression and lethargy	Liver function tests, vital signs	Liver function tests	Can bite tablet and absorb sublingually
Modafinil (Provigil)	100–200 mg every morning	200–400 mg every morning	Medically ill patient with depression and lethargy	ECG, liver function tests	—	Reduce dose with hepatic impairment; do not use with cardiac disease

(continued)

Table 33.5. *(Continued)*

Drug	Starting Dose	Average Dose for Cancer Patients	Disorders	Pretreatment Work-up	Follow-up Studies	Comment
Mood stabilizers						
Lithium carbonate (Eskalith, Eskalith CR, Lithobid)	300 mg qhs	300 mg t.i.d.	Mania[b] (may need to add clonazepam or antipsychotic); depression[b] (may need to add antidepressant)	ECG, electrolytes, UA, BUN/Cr, thyroid (T$_4$ TSH), CBC (especially WBC and platelets)	Lithium level initially 2 times/week; gradually lengthen to q3 months; thyroid studies q6 months or earlier if indicated; UA/BUN/Cr, CBC if infection	Monitor blood level 12 h after evening dose and before morning dose; 0.8–1.0 mEq/L is most effective; watch for hypothyroidism, diabetes insipidus, nephropathy, dehydration
Carbamazepine[c] (Tegretol)	100 mg b.i.d.	200 mg t.i.d.	Mania or depression	CBC, reticulocytes, serum iron, liver function tests, UA, BUN, ECG	CBC, thyroid studies, blood level	Watch for leukopenia, thrombocytopenia, hepatotoxicity, decreased effect of warfarin (Coumadin)
Gabapentin (Neurontin)	100–300 mg t.i.d. or q.i.d.	300–800 mg t.i.d.	Insomnia, pain, panic disorder or other anxiety disorder, augmentation for other mood stabilizers	Cr clearance	Cr clearance	Can give larger dose (300–1,200 mg) at bedtime; can induce oversedation, occasional tremor or ataxia; useful for neuropathic pain

Drug	Starting dose	Therapeutic dose	Indication	Baseline labs	Follow-up labs	Comments
Lamotrigine (Lamictal)	25–50 mg q.d. (decrease starting dose if on valproate)	150–250 mg b.i.d.	Mania, depression	Liver function tests, Cr clearance	Liver function tests, Cr clearance	Increase dose every other week; high risk of Stevens–Johnson rash; used *only* if physician is familiar with this medication
Valproic acid (Depakene, Depakote)	15 mg/kg/d	500–750 mg/d (divided into t.i.d. doses)	Mania, depression	Liver function tests, CBC	Liver function tests, CBC, blood level	Watch for hepatotoxicity, especially in young children
Benzodiazepines						
Clonazepam (Klonopin)	0.5 mg qhs	≥2 mg/day	Mania, anxiety	CBC, liver function tests	CBC, liver function tests	Accumulates if impaired hepatic function and may cause respiratory distress; requires extremely cautious use; do not withdraw rapidly
Alprazolam (Xanax)	0.5 mg qhs	≥1 mg t.i.d.	Anxiety, minor depression	Liver function tests	—	Do not withdraw rapidly (reduce daily dose by 0.25 mg weekly); use cautiously if there is respiratory impairment

CBC, complete blood cell count; ECG, electrocardiogram; UA, urinalysis; BUN, blood urea nitrogen; Cr, creatinine; TSH, thyroid-stimulating hormone; WBC, white blood cells.

[a] Check on weight, pulse, and blood pressure. Tolerance may develop, and doses may require adjustment.
[b] Natural or corticosteroid induced.
[c] Caution required because of multiple drug interactions.

perhaps utilizing a mood stabilizer such as lithium or an anticonvulsant, and/or consult psychiatry (Table 33.5).

c. Monoamine oxidase inhibitors (MAOIs) may be used to treat major depression or panic disorders but are somewhat inconvenient owing to tyramine dietary restrictions and medication interactions requiring much attention. They are sometimes tried when other choices have failed. There is now a transdermal form of selegiline (Emsam) available that does not require dietary modification at the lowest dose of 6 mg/24 hours.

IV. Anxiety

A. Approach to the problem. As grieving is described as normal, so is anxiety in patients with cancer. However, anxiety varies in its cause, severity, and treatment. A detailed history of the onset, characteristics, and length of distress is important. Knowledge of the patient's previous symptoms, current and past physical illness, substance abuse, and medication usage is essential to the evaluation process. Like depression, anxiety also amplifies pain. Antianxiety agents may be helpful for alleviating patients' distress and helping them cope with other problems associated with their cancer (Table 33.6).

B. Problems that present as anxiety. The duration of the symptoms is one of the first factors to assess in the anxious patient.

1. Suspect an adjustment disorder when maladaptive anxious symptoms have persisted for less than 6 months and apparently represent an adjustment to learning the diagnosis or reactions to the treatment. This kind of anxiety may benefit from supportive therapy, relaxation therapy, or benzodiazepines.

2. Generalized anxiety. If the anxiety has been present for more than 6 months, is continuing no matter what environmental alterations occur, and is accompanied by signs of physical tension or poor attention to conversation or other daily activities, the patient is likely to have generalized anxiety. Supportive therapy, relaxation tapes, biofeedback, buspirone, gabapentin, and benzodiazepines are useful.

3. Brief, isolated episodes of anxiety that come and go lead the examiner to consider other diagnoses.

a. Panic attacks. If the patient has repeated "attacks" that have a rapid onset and last 20 minutes to a few hours and if they are accompanied by tachycardia, palpitations, shortness of breath, hyperventilation, choking, sweating, dizziness, and the wish to flee, without a physical or chemical explanation, they are most likely panic attacks. They may be treated with benzodiazepines such as clonazepam and alprazolam; however, antidepressants such as tricyclics, SSRIs, MAOIs, or mirtazapine are also effective. Antidepressants must be started at a very low dose (e.g., sertraline 12.5 mg, paroxetine 5.0 mg, or imipramine 10 mg) and increased slowly every 1 to 2 days to avoid increased anxiety. While the dose is brought up to that typically used in depression, benzodiazepines may be added if needed. Benzodiazepines

Table 33.6.   Antianxiety agents and nighttime sedatives

Agent	Half-life (h)	Onset	Starting Dose (mg)[a]
Benzodiazepines			
Triazolam (Halcion)	1.5–3.5	Rapid	0.125 (qhs)
Oxazepam (Serax)[b]	8–20	Moderate	10 (t.i.d.)
Lorazepam (Ativan)[b]	10–20	Rapid	0.5 (t.i.d.)
Temazepam (Restoril)[b]	12–24	Rapid	15 (qhs)
Alprazolam (Xanax)	12–24	Moderate	0.25 (t.i.d.)
Chlordiazepoxide (Librium)	12–48	Moderate	10 (b.i.d.)
Clonazepam (Klonopin)	20–30	Rapid	0.5 (b.i.d.)
Diazepam (Valium)	20–90	Rapid	2–5 (b.i.d.)
Clorazepate (Tranxene)	20–100	Rapid	7.5 (b.i.d.)
Flurazepam (Dalmane)	20–100	Rapid	15 (qhs)
Nonbenzodiazepine hypnotics			
Zolpidem (Ambien)[b]	1.5–4.5	Rapid	5 (qhs)
Zaleplon (Sonata)[b]	1.0	Rapid	5 (qhs)
Eszopiclone (Lunesta)	6	Rapid	1–2 (qhs)
Ramelteon(Rozerem)	1–2.5	Rapid	8 (qhs)

Antidepressants (for panic disorder)

Start at lower doses than for depression, i.e., an imipramine, starting dose of 10 mg t.i.d. Some antidepressants, like bupropion, have no efficacy for panic disorder

β-**Blockers** (for autonomic symptom control)

Propranolol (Inderal)	10–20 mg t.i.d.
Atenolol (Tenormin)	25–50 mg daily

Antipsychotics (for anxiety associated with delirium)

Antihistamines

May be safer in some cases when respiratory impairment is a complication; also used for insomnia

Diphenhydramine (Benadryl) 25 mg; starting doses b.i.d. or t.i.d.

Hydroxyzine (Vistaril) 50 mg; starting doses t.i.d. or q.i.d.

Note: Elderly or extremely debilitated patients should be given lower doses. Caution should be taken when prescribing long-acting sedating medications because they have been associated with a high incidence of falls and hip fracture.
[a]If chronic alcohol or benzodiazepine use exists, it is probable that the dose needed is at least double the starting doses listed.
[b]Preferred in the elderly.

with a short half-life, such as alprazolam, can induce breakthrough panic if tolerance develops, so those with longer half-lives, like clonazepam, may be preferred if tolerated. β-Blockers to block autonomic symptoms may be tried if performance anxiety around specific activities is identified, but they are less effective for panic disorder, as is buspirone.

b. Organic causes are often responsible for the anxiety

(1) Hypoxia. Repeating episodes of anxiety accompanied by alterations in intellectual functioning, poor orientation, reduced judgment, shortened attention, a rapidly fluctuating mood, and difficulty with memory suggest hypoxia. When anxiety is induced by hypoxia, it is wise to reduce central nervous system (CNS) depressant medications and give small doses of an antipsychotic drug if anxiety is accompanied by delirium. However, older antipsychotic and antiemetic medications as well as metoclopramide often produce akathisia, an extrapyramidal restlessness that mimics anxiety. Alternating the antipsychotic drug with small doses of a short–half-life benzodiazepine is one option for organically induced anxiety—if respiratory status or arterial blood gas measurements do not worsen. Newer antipsychotic agents are less likely to produce extrapyramidal akathisia but when used with benziazepines, still should be monitored with pulse oximetry measurements.

(2) Liver disease and other physical disorders. If anxiety is associated with liver disease, start by reducing CNS-depressant medications. When needed, small, infrequent doses of a short-acting benzodiazepine that requires conjugation but not oxidation in the liver are prescribed. These include lorazepam, oxazepam, and temazepam. Many other physical disorders can also produce anxious symptoms, including various brain tumors, pheochromocytoma, carcinoid, hyperthyroidism, cardiac arrhythmias, drug or alcohol withdrawal, and hyperparathyroidism. Gabapentin, which is renally cleared, may help with anxiety, sleep, and pain. It can also help augment other medications for mood stabilization and panic disorder.

(3) Medications such as theophylline, corticosteroids, antidepressants, and antipsychotic drugs can produce anxiety. Anxiety is frequently one of multiple symptoms associated with benzodiazepine or narcotic analgesic withdrawal. Akathisia mimics anxiety and often occurs with prochlorperazine, promethazine, perphenazine, and metoclopramide. It is generally wise to stop these medications to avoid prolonging this very uncomfortable, involuntary condition and find a suitable alternative.

c. Precipitating events can be identified in patients with cancer that initiate the previously discussed adjustment disorder lasting generally no longer than 6 months. Posttraumatic stress disorder (PTSD), less often seen in patients with cancer, follows a distressing event beyond what would be expected. Younger women with breast cancer are at higher risk for PTSD, especially if they have less education and lower income. More advanced disease, medical sequelae of treatments, and longer hospital admissions also contribute. More frequently observed, however, are patients who describe intense fears of needles, radiotherapy rooms, or confined-space scanning devices. Often, the history unfolds to describe previously existing phobias. These patients, like those with anticipatory anxiety about procedures or chemotherapy, may be assisted with relaxation or desensitization techniques, imagery, antianxiety medications, and assurance. If patients begin to experience procedures, treatments, or interpersonal situations as being particularly stressful, anticipatory anxiety intensifies the require-ment for larger doses of as-needed medication to attain some relief. Therefore, regular scheduling of antianxiety medication similar to that of pain medication is in order.

V. Insomnia

A. Principles. Difficulty falling asleep may be associated with anxiety, whereas awakening in the middle of the night is gen-erally more closely related to depression. In addition, there are a variety of physical disorders that cause sleep irregularities. The sleep–wake cycle is almost always disturbed in a delirious patient, no matter what the cause is. Pain often awakens a patient with cancer. Medications can awaken some patients directly (e.g., fluoxetine) or indirectly (e.g., diuretics). Aside from sorting out these influences, the physician must take into account the environment. Is the patient too hot or cold? Is the ward too brightly lit or too noisy? Do the patients awaken each time they are checked by the night staff? When any or several of these concerns are corrected, sleeping medication may not be necessary, although the need for sedatives remains in some patients.

B. Benzodiazepines (see Table 33.6). This class of drugs is most often prescribed if a patient needs nighttime seda-tion. The shorter–half-life benzodiazepines (i.e., lorazepam or temazepam) with a rapid onset produce less daytime grog-giness than those with a longer half-life. Short-acting agents tend to accumulate less and are safer for patients with liver dis-ease. On the other hand, longer–half-life drugs (i.e., diazepam or flurazepam) with a rapid onset produce less unwanted awakening very early morning.

C. Nonbenzodiazepine hypnotics (see Table 33.6). The four medications in this class help patients fall asleep quickly and do not leave the patient groggy in the morning. Clinical experience shows that tolerance can also develop to zolpidem, zaleplon and eszopiclone. Ramelteon, a melatonin receptor ag-onist, is a relatively new agent. It is contraindicated in patients taking fluvoxamine.

D. Antihistamines (see Table 33.6). These medications may be chosen if physicians are hesitant to prescribe benzodi-azepines, such as for patients with severe respiratory disease. A disadvantage may be the higher anticholinergic potential of these drugs, as compared with the benzodiazepine family, which can increase the risk of delirium.

E. Others. Chloral hydrate 500 to 1,000 mg, an old standby hypnotic, is occasionally used as long as patients are free of gastrointestinal or liver disease. Barbiturates such as amo-barbital sodium are occasionally used to treat some refractory sleep disturbances for a short time but are not routinely used because they induce respiratory depression and have addictive potential. Gabapentin, which is renally cleared and has few drug interactions, has become increasingly popular. Doses may vary from 300 to 1,200 mg at bedtime. It is always better to start with a lower dose.

SUGGESTED READINGS

Bezchlibnyk-Butler KZ, Jeffries JJ, eds. *Clinical handbook of psychotropic drugs*, 11th ed. Seattle: Hogrefe & Huber, 2001.

Breitbart W. Identifying patients at risk for and treatment of major psychiatric complications of cancer. *Support Care Cancer* 1995; 3:45.

Compton MT, Nemeroff CB. Depression and bipolar disorder. In: D Dale, D Federman, K Antman, et al. eds. *ACP medicine*, New York: WebMD Professional Publishing, 2006:2608–2619.

Davidson JR, Waisberg JL, Brundage MD, et al. Nonpharmacologic group treatment of insomnia: a preliminary study with cancer survivors. *Psychooncology* 2001;10:389–397.

Fromer MT. *Surviving childhood cancer*. Washington, DC: American Psychiatric Press, 1995.

Holland JC. *Psycho-oncology*. New York: Oxford University Press, 1998.

Homsi J, Walsh D, Nelson KA. Psychostimulants in supportive care. *Support Care Cancer* 2000;8:385–397.

Jacobson SA, Pies RW, Greenblatt DJ *Handbook of geriatric psychopharmacology*. Washington, DC: American Psychiatric Press, 2002.

Kane FJ, Remmel R, Moody S. Recognizing and treating delirium in patients admitted to general hospitals. *South Med J* 1993;86:985.

Koenig HG, McCullough ME, Larson DB *Handbook of religion and health*. New York: Oxford University Press, 2001:292–317.

Lieberman JA, Stroup TS, McEvoy JP, et al. Effectiveness of antipsychotic drugs in patients with chronic schizophrenia. *N Engl J Med* 2005;353:1209–1223.

Luebbert K, Dahme B, Hasenbring M. The effectiveness of relaxation training in reducing treatment-related symptoms and improving emotional adjustment in acute non-surgical cancer treatment: a meta-analytical review. *Psychooncology* 2001;10:490–502.

Marmelstein H, Lesko L, Holland JC. Depression in the cancer patient. *J Psychooncol* 1992;1:199.

Massie MJ, Greenberg DB. Oncology. In: Levinson J, ed. *Textbook of psychosomatic medicine*. Washington, DC: American Psychiatry Press, 2005:517–530.

McDaniel JS, Musselman DL, Nemeroff CB. Cancer and depression: theory and treatment. *Psychiatr Ann* 1997;27:360.

McDaniel JS, Musselman DL, Porter MR, et al. Depression in patients with cancer: diagnosis, biology and treatment. *Arch Gen Psychiatry* 1995;52:89.

Nasrallah H. CATIE'S surprises: in antipsychotics square-off, were there winners or losers? *Curr Psychiatry* 2006;5(2):49–65.

Olin J, Massand P. Psychostimulants for depression in hospitalized cancer patients. *Psychosomatics* 1996;37:57.

Patenaude AF, Last B. Cancer and children: where are we coming from? Where are we going? *Psychooncology* 2001;10:281–283.

Posner J. Neoplastic disorders. In: Dale D, Federman D, Antman K, et al. eds. *ACP medicine*. New York: WebMD Professional Publishing, 2006:2306–2321.

Potter EZ, Hollister LE. Antipsychotics and lithium. In: Katzung B, ed. *Basic and clinical pharmacology*, New York: McGraw Hill, 9th ed. 2005:462–474.

Potter WZ, Hollister LE. Antidepressants. In: Katzung B, ed. *Basic and clinical pharmacology*, 9th ed. 2005:484–494.

Roth AJ, Holland JH. Psychiatric complications in cancer patients. In: Brain MC, Carbone PP, eds. *Current therapy in hematology–oncology*, 5th ed. St. Louis: Mosby, 1995:609.

Roth AJ, McClear KZ, Massie MJ. Oncology. In: Stoudemire A, Fogel BS, Greenberg DB, eds. *Psychiatric care of the medically ill patient*. Oxford: Oxford University Press, 2000:733–756.

Shear MK. Anxiety disorders. In: Edit D, Dale D, Federman K, et al. eds. *ACP medicine*. New York: WebMD Professional Publishing, 2006:2651–2659.

Spiegel D, Bloom JR, Kraemer HC, et al. Effect of psychosocial treatment of patients with metastatic breast cancer. *Lancet* 1989;2:888–891.

APPENDIX A

Nomogram for Determining Body Surface Area of Adults from Height and Mass[a]

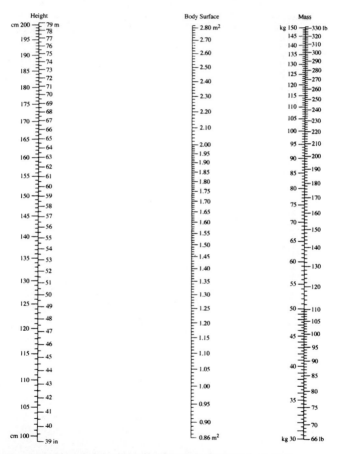

Height (cm / in), Body Surface (m^2), Mass (kg / lb)

[a] From the formula of Du Bois and Du Bois (*Arch Intern Med* 1916;17:863): $S = M^{0.425} \times H^{0.725} \times 71.84$, or $S = \log M \times 0.425 + \log H \times 0.725 + 1.8564$, where S is body surface (cm^2), M is mass (kg), and H is height (cm). (From Lenter C, ed. *Geigy scientific tables*, Vol 1, 8th ed. Basel: Ciba-Geigy, 1981:227.)

Nomogram for Determining Body Surface Area of Children from Height and Mass[a]

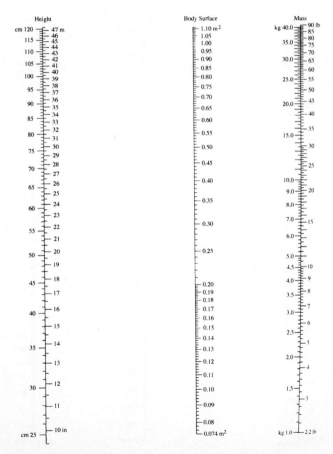

Height   Body Surface   Mass

[a] From the formula of Du Bois and Du Bois (*Arch Intern Med* 1916;17:863): $S = M^{0.425} \times H^{0.725} \times 71.84$, or $S = \log M \times 0.425 + \log H + 0.725 + 1.8564$, where S is body surface (cm²), M is mass (kg), and H is height (cm). (From Lenter C, ed. *Geigy scientific tables*, Vol 1, 8th ed. Basel: Ciba-Geigy, 1981:226.)

Cancer Screening Recommendations for Average-Risk Asymptomatic People by the American Cancer Society

Table C.1. Cancer screening recommendations for average-risk, asymptomatic people by the American Cancer Society

| Test or Procedure | Population | | Frequency |
	Sex	Age	
Fecal occult blood testing (FOBT) or fecal immunochemical test (FIT) and flexible sigmoidoscopy[a]	Men and women	50 and above	Annual FOBT or FIT, flexible sigmoidoscopy every 5 years
Or			
Flexible sigmoidoscopy			Every 5 years
Or			
FOBT or FIT			Annually
Or			
Colonoscopy			Every 10 years
Or			
Double-contrast barium enema (DCBE)			Every 5 years

Digital rectal examination (DRE) and prostate-specific antigen test (PSA)	Men	50 and over if life expectancy of at least 10 y. Higher risk men should start at 45.	Annually[b]
Pap test and pelvic examination	Women	18 and older	Annually until three or more consecutive satisfactory normal exams, then less frequently (every 2–3 years) at the discretion of physician
Breast self-examination	Women	20 and older	Monthly
Clinical breast examination	Women	20–39	Every 3 years
		40 and older	Annually
Mammography	Women	40 and older	Annually
Cancer-related check-up[c]	Men and women	20–39	At the discretion of patient and physician
		40 and older	

[a]Preferred over either alone.

[b]Information should be provided to men about the benefits and limitations of testing.

[c]Includes examination for thyroid, testicles, ovaries, lymph nodes, oral cavity, and skin; health counseling about tobacco, sun exposure, diet and nutrition, risk factors, sexual practices, and environmental and occupational exposures.
www.cancer.org—Cancer Detection Guidelines

Selected Oncology Web Sites

1. American Society of Hematology
   http://www.hematology.org/index.cfm
2. American Cancer Society (ACS statistics, other information, links to states)
   http://www.cancer.org/
3. American Society of Clinical Oncology (ASCO; physician site)
   http://www.asco.org
4. ASCO—People living with cancer (patient site)
   http://www.plwc.org
5. Agency for Health Care Research and Quality
   http://www.ahrq.gov
6. PubMed, National Library of Medicine (search medline and get abstracts)
   http://www.ncbi.nlm.nih.gov/entrez/query
7. Harvard Center for Cancer Prevention
   http://www.hsph.harvard.edu/cancer/
8. Health Services/Technology Assessment Text (a helpful collection of HSTAT guidelines, surgeon general reports, technology assessments, and reviews)
   http://hstat.nlm.nih.gov/
9. American Pain Society
   http://www.ampainsoc.org/
10. American Academy of Hospice and Palliative Medicine
    http://www.aahpm.org/
11. National Cancer Institute's Cancer Information home page (NCI information, including PDQ, clinical trials information, statistics)
    http://www.cancer.gov/
12. Cancer Therapy Evaluation Program (CTEP) home page (includes common toxicity criteria)
    http://ctep.cancer.gov/
13. Cancer Trials
    http://www.cancer.gov/clinicaltrials
    http://www.cancertrialshelp.org
14. Centers for Disease Control and Prevention (CDC)
    http://www.cdc.gov/
15. National Guideline Clearinghouse (guidelines for over 800 diseases and conditions, including many for cancer)
    http://www.guideline.gov/
16. National Comprehensive Cancer Network (NCCN) Complete Library of Clinical Practice Guidelines in Oncology, for health professionals (free registration required) and patients.
    http://www.nccn.org
17. Association of Community Cancer Centers (includes the Compendia-Based Drug Bulletin)
    http://www.accc-cancer.org/

18. Rxlist—Internet Drug Index (primarily for patients; includes alternative medicines)
    http://www.rxlist.com

19. FDA Oncology Tools web site (contains information about approved cancer therapies, product labels, approval summaries, what drugs are approved for what diseases, and considerations for making decisions about therapies, including advice on when to contemplate using unapproved drugs and how to obtain access to unapproved drugs)
    http://www.fda.gov/cder/cancer/

20. Drugs@FDA—A catalog of FDA Approved Drugs—Drug approval letters, labels, and review packages.
    http://www.accessdata.fda.gov/scripts/cder/drugsatfda/

Index

Note: Page numbers followed by *f* indicate figures; those followed by *t* indicate tables.